Amyotrophic Lateral Sclerosis: Diagnosis and Management

Amyotrophic Lateral Sclerosis: Diagnosis and Management

Editor: Antonio Chavez

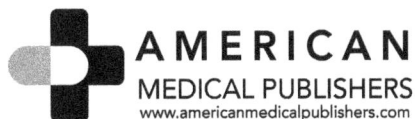

AMERICAN
MEDICAL PUBLISHERS
www.americanmedicalpublishers.com

AMERICAN
MEDICAL PUBLISHERS
www.americanmedicalpublishers.com

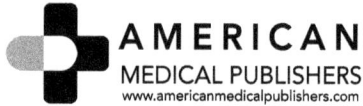

Cataloging-in-Publication Data

Amyotrophic lateral sclerosis : diagnosis and management / edited by Antonio Chavez.
    p. cm.
Includes bibliographical references and index.
ISBN 978-1-63927-280-8
1. Amyotrophic lateral sclerosis. 2. Amyotrophic lateral sclerosis--Diagnosis. 3. Amyotrophic lateral sclerosis--Treatment.
4. Motor neurons--Diseases. 5. Neuromuscular diseases. I. Chavez, Antonio.
RC406.A24 A49 2022

616.839--dc23

American Medical Publishers,
41 Flatbush Avenue,
1st Floor, New York,
NY 11217, USA

ISBN 978-1-63927-280-8 (Hardback)

Contents

Preface

A condition that causes the death of neurons which control the voluntary muscles of the body is known as amyotrophic lateral sclerosis (ALS). It is also referred to as Lou Gehrig's disease or motor neurone disease. Patients with ALS exhibit signs of muscle stiffness, muscle twitching and muscle wasting. The person may experience progressive difficulty in speaking or swallowing, and weakness in the arms or legs. The diagnosis of ALS is based on a study of the clinical signs and symptoms, full medical history and neurologic examinations. Blood tests and MRIs can rule out the likelihood of other diseases. ALS has no medical cure. Its management is focused on providing supportive care, treating symptoms and improving quality of life. Medicines like riluzole prolong survival by 2-3 months, while edaravone slows functional decline to some extent but at the cost of quality of life. Respiratory failure is managed with non-invasive ventilation. For patients with advanced ALS, invasive ventilation is an option that can prolong survival even as the disease continues to progress and body functions decline. The various studies that are constantly contributing towards advancing diagnosis and treatment of amyotrophic lateral sclerosis are examined in detail in this book. It presents researches and studies performed by experts across the globe. This book will prove to be immensely beneficial to students and researchers in the field of neuroscience.

The information contained in this book is the result of intensive hard work done by researchers in this field. All due efforts have been made to make this book serve as a complete guiding source for students and researchers. The topics in this book have been comprehensively explained to help readers understand the growing trends in the field.

I would like to thank the entire group of writers who made sincere efforts in this book and my family who supported me in my efforts of working on this book. I take this opportunity to thank all those who have been a guiding force throughout my life.

Editor

Directly converted patient-specific induced neurons mirror the neuropathology of FUS with disrupted nuclear localization in amyotrophic lateral sclerosis

Su Min Lim[1,2†], Won Jun Choi[3†], Ki-Wook Oh[2,4], Yuanchao Xue[5], Ji Young Choi[2], Sung Hoon Kim[2], Minyeop Nahm[2], Young-Eun Kim[6], Jinhyuk Lee[7,8], Min-Young Noh[2], Seungbok Lee[9], Sejin Hwang[10], Chang-Seok Ki[6*], Xiang-Dong Fu[11] and Seung Hyun Kim[1,2,4*]

Abstract

Background: Mutations in the fused in sarcoma (FUS) gene have been linked to amyotrophic lateral sclerosis (ALS). ALS patients with FUS mutations exhibit neuronal cytoplasmic mislocalization of the mutant FUS protein. ALS patients' fibroblasts or induced pluripotent stem cell (iPSC)-derived neurons have been developed as models for understanding ALS-associated FUS (ALS-FUS) pathology; however, pathological neuronal signatures are not sufficiently present in the fibroblasts of patients, whereas the generation of iPSC-derived neurons from ALS patients requires relatively intricate procedures.

Results: Here, we report the generation of disease-specific induced neurons (iNeurons) from the fibroblasts of patients who carry three different FUS mutations that were recently identified by direct sequencing and multi-gene panel analysis. The mutations are located at the C-terminal nuclear localization signal (NLS) region of the protein (p.G504Wfs*12, p.R495*, p.Q519E): two de novo mutations in sporadic ALS and one in familial ALS case. Aberrant cytoplasmic mislocalization with nuclear clearance was detected in all patient-derived iNeurons, and oxidative stress further induced the accumulation of cytoplasmic FUS in cytoplasmic granules, thereby recapitulating neuronal pathological features identified in mutant FUS (p.G504Wfs*12)-autopsied ALS patient. Importantly, such FUS pathological hallmarks of the patient with the p.Q519E mutation were only detected in patient-derived iNeurons, which contrasts to predominant FUS (p.Q519E) in the nucleus of both the transfected cells and patient-derived fibroblasts.

Conclusions: Thus, iNeurons may provide a more reliable model for investigating FUS mutations with disrupted NLS for understanding FUS-associated proteinopathies in ALS.

Keywords: Amyotrophic lateral sclerosis, Fused in sarcoma, Human cell models, Induced neuron, Nuclear localization signal, Stress granules, Neuronal cytoplasmic inclusion

* Correspondence: changski@skku.edu; kimsh1@hanyang.ac.kr
†Equal contributors
[6]Department of Laboratory Medicine and Genetics, Samsung Medical Center, Sungkyunkwan University School of Medicine, Seoul 135-710, Republic of Korea
[1]Department of Translational Medicine, Graduate School of Biomedical Science and Engineering, Hanyang University, Seoul 133-792, Republic of Korea
Full list of author information is available at the end of the article

Background

Fused in sarcoma (FUS) is a multifunctional DNA/RNA-binding protein involved in various aspects of cellular RNA metabolism and executes its main functions predominantly in the cell nucleus. Initially discovered as a fusion onco-gene, mutations in the *FUS* gene resulting in FUS protei-nopathies were recently linked to amyotrophic lateral sclerosis (ALS), responsible for ~4 % of familial and ~1 % of sporadic ALS cases [1–3]. *FUS* mutations cluster either in the glycine-rich region of the protein or in the RGG-rich C-terminal domain, where they disrupt the nuclear localization signal (NLS) and result in altered subcellular localization of the FUS protein. ALS-associated *FUS* (ALS-FUS) mutations have been reported to cause cytoplasmic mislocalization of the protein in the brain and spinal cord of ALS patients [4, 5]. Moreover, cytoplasmic FUS tends to aggregate to form inclusions in degenerating motor neurons of ALS patients [6–8]. As a consequence, both toxic gain-of-function in the cytoplasm and loss-of-function in the nucleus are proposed to be causative events in ALS development [9, 10].

Key pathological features have been documented based on immunocytochemical studies on cultured fibroblasts from ALS patients or immunohistological analysis on autopsy samples [11, 12]. These studies revealed abnormal cytoplasmic mislocalization of the FUS protein in ALS patients with *FUS* mutations in its NLS. When modeled on fibroblasts, however, mutant FUS proteins were predominantly detected in the nucleus, with minimal association with pathological signatures detected with those mutations in vivo [11, 13, 14]. Patient-derived induced pluripotent stem cells (iPSC) with the ability to differentiate into neural cells were found to be suitable for studying ALS-FUS pathology [15], but neuronal induction and differentiation processes using iPSC require tedious and labor-intensive procedures. Hence, it would be advantageous to develop rapid and simple FUS-associated ALS patient-derived cell models to study ALS-related neuronal pathology.

To overcome the limitations associated with the current cell modeling systems, we examined FUS pathology in a more disease-relevant cell model. We used our previously described method of repressing a polypyrimidine-tract-binding (PTB) protein to directly convert patient fibroblasts carrying *FUS* mutations and those from age-matched healthy controls into functional neurons (iNeuron) [16]. We have recently identified *FUS* mutations (p.G504Wfs*12, p.R495*, and p.Q519E) by direct sequencing and multi-gene panel testing [17–19]. In this study, we examined the pathophysiological and biochemical properties of the three different *FUS* mutations at NLS region. Analysis of brain and spinal cord autopsy samples from FUS (p.G504Wfs*12) patient demonstrated the expected pathologic features including nuclear clearance and cytoplasmic accumulation of FUS in neurons. To generate a cell model that recapitulates

key pathological features found in autopsy, we compared cellular localization and aggregation-prone properties of the endogenous FUS in fibroblasts, HEK-293 cells and rat primary cortical neurons and directly converted iNeurons in the presence or absence of stress. Directly converted iNeurons from patient fibroblasts was the only model that recapitulated the mutant FUS-associated neurological pathology that is observed in autopsied brain and spinal cord. Moreover, we showed that the FUS neuropathology of the familial ALS patient with p.Q519E mutation could be demonstrated in directly converted iNeurons but not in transfected cells or patient-derived fibroblasts. These findings suggest that directly converted iNeurons have a potential to become reliable disease-relevant models for dissecting pathophysiologies of FUS-related proteinopathies in ALS.

Results and discussion

Clinical and genetic characteristics of three ALS patients harboring *FUS* mutations in the NLS region

Among ten diverse, recently identified FUS mutants or variants [17, 19], two *de novo* FUS mutants (p.G504Wfs*12, p.R495*) confirmed by trio study in sporadic ALS [18] and one FUS variant (p.Q519E) in familial ALS [19] were included in this study. The residues of the three mutants are located in the C-terminal region containing the nuclear localization signal (NLS). As diagrammed in Fig. 1, the Q519E mutation is a missense mutation in the C-terminal NLS region; the mutation (p.G504Wfs*12) causes a frame shift in exon 15, leading to a truncated FUS; and the mutation (p.R495*) creates a premature codon to eliminate the NLS. The mutation (p.R495*) is associated with an aggressive clinical phenotype of ALS [20–22], and the mutation (p.G504Wfs*12) is a pathogenic truncation mutant associated with sporadic ALS [18, 23]. In order to investigate whether FUS (p.Q519E) variant has the significance in disease pathogenesis, we established structural analysis of the mutation with Transportin-1 (Protein Data Bank, PDB (ID: 4FDD)) (Additional file 1: Figure S1). FUS is a nuclear protein that its nuclear import is mediated by interaction between Transportin-1 and the C-terminal NLS region of FUS [24, 25]. Hence, we analyzed the hydrogen bonding pattern of FUS-Transportin-1 complexes and observed that one hydrogen bond is relevant to the FUS Q519 residue. The distance between acceptor atom (oxygen; atom type: OE1) of E509 from Transportin-1 and donor atom (nitrogen; atom type: NE2) of Q519 from FUS was measured as 3.21 Å. Since the experimental structure has no hydrogen atoms, the angle of hydrogen bond was measured between acceptor (OE1 of E509 from Transportin-1), donor (NE2 of Q519 from FUS), and the prior atom connected on donor (CD of Q519 from FUS), which comes to 134.7°. This is a possible hydrogen bonding between FUS-Transportin-1 complexes. If the Q519 on FUS is mutated to E519, the length of side chain is decreased by one

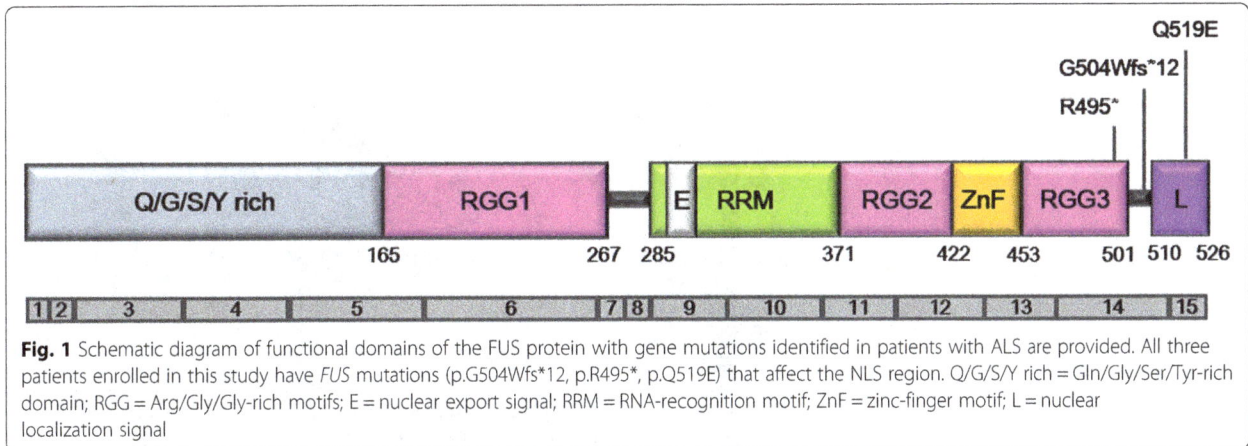

Fig. 1 Schematic diagram of functional domains of the FUS protein with gene mutations identified in patients with ALS are provided. All three patients enrolled in this study have *FUS* mutations (p.G504Wfs*12, p.R495*, p.Q519E) that affect the NLS region. Q/G/S/Y rich = Gln/Gly/Ser/Tyr-rich domain; RGG = Arg/Gly/Gly-rich motifs; E = nuclear export signal; RRM = RNA-recognition motif; ZnF = zinc-finger motif; L = nuclear localization signal

carbon chain (from 4 to 3) and the polar property changes to negative from neutral. In the end, the found Q519 (FUS)-E509 (Transportin-1) hydrogen bond in wild-type will disappear in the Q519E mutant. In addition, the negative-negative repulsion (E519-E509) in Q519E mutant may result in the deactivation on FUS-Transportin-1 binding, thus providing a significance of the FUS (p.Q519E) variant in disease pathogenesis.

Detailed clinical and epidemiological characteristics of three ALS patients with different *FUS* mutations, one sporadic ALS patient, and four healthy controls enrolled in this study are summarized in Table 1.

FUS pathology in ALS-FUS patient brain and spinal motor neurons

Human autopsy samples were used to reveal the distribution of FUS in the brain and spinal cord of FUS (G504Wfs*12) patient compared to a normal control (CTL 4) and a sporadic ALS patient without any known mutation. Immunohistochemical profiles demonstrated that wild-type FUS was confined predominantly to the

nucleus in the majority of neurons in the control brain. A similar distribution of FUS immunoreactivity was also seen in a sporadic ALS patient. In contrast, prominent cytoplasmic or decreased nuclear staining of FUS with ring-like perinuclear inclusions was observed in the FUS (G504Wfs*12) case (Fig. 2a). To confirm cytoplasmic accumulation of FUS in neuronal cells from the FUS (G504Wfs*12) patient, we performed double-label immunohistochemistry for NeuN (neuronal nuclei marker) and FUS. This demonstrated co-labeling of NeuN in the nucleus and the mutant FUS in the cytoplasmic of the same neurons from the ALS-FUS patient, in contrast to the localization of the FUS protein in the nucleus of neurons from healthy control and a sporadic ALS patient (Fig. 2b, Additional file 2: Figure S2).

We also determined the pathogenic features of the mutant FUS in spinal cord motor neurons. Consistent with findings in the precentral motor cortex, immunohistochemistry for FUS in NeuN-positive cells revealed the same pathological feature in the ventral horn of spinal cords (Fig. 2c, d). The sections of spinal cords from both

Table 1 Patients and controls whose skin fibroblasts were studied

Characteristic	ID	MND	Sex	Exon	FUS genotype	Age at biopsy, yr	Age of onset, yr	Familial history	Site of onset	ALSFRS-R	delta-FS	Survival, mo	Autopsy
ALS-FUS	HS374	777	M	15	Q519E[a]	34	34	Yes	Limb	46	0.10	>61 [c]	N/A
	HS131	402	F	14	G504Wfs*12[b]	34	31	No	Limb	36	0.92	46	Yes
	HS197	502	F	14	R495*[b]	31	27	No	Bulbar	23	1.92	54	N/A
Sporadic ALS	HS250	551	M	N/A	N/A	N/A	57	No	N/A	39	0.82	68	Yes
CTL 1	N/A	N/A	F	N/A	N/A	35	N/A	N/A	N/A	N/A	N/A	N/A	N/A
CTL 2	N/A	N/A	F	N/A	N/A	40	N/A	N/A	N/A	N/A	N/A	N/A	N/A
CTL 3	N/A	N/A	M	N/A	N/A	45	N/A	N/A	N/A	N/A	N/A	N/A	N/A
CTL 4	N/A	N/A	N/A	N/A	N/A	N/A	N/A	N/A	N/A	N/A	N/A	N/A	Purchased

FUS, fused in sarcoma, *ALSFRS-R* a revised ALS functional rating scale, *ALS* amyotrophic lateral sclerosis, *F* female, *N/A* not applicable, *M* male, *CTL* control
ALSFRS-R and delta FS were evaluated at the first visit
[a]Reported previously (Kim H-J et al., 2015). [b]Reported previously (Kwon MJ et al., 2012; Kim YE et al., 2014).
[c]>61 means that more than 61 months have passed since symptom onset and the patient is still alive on the last follow-up

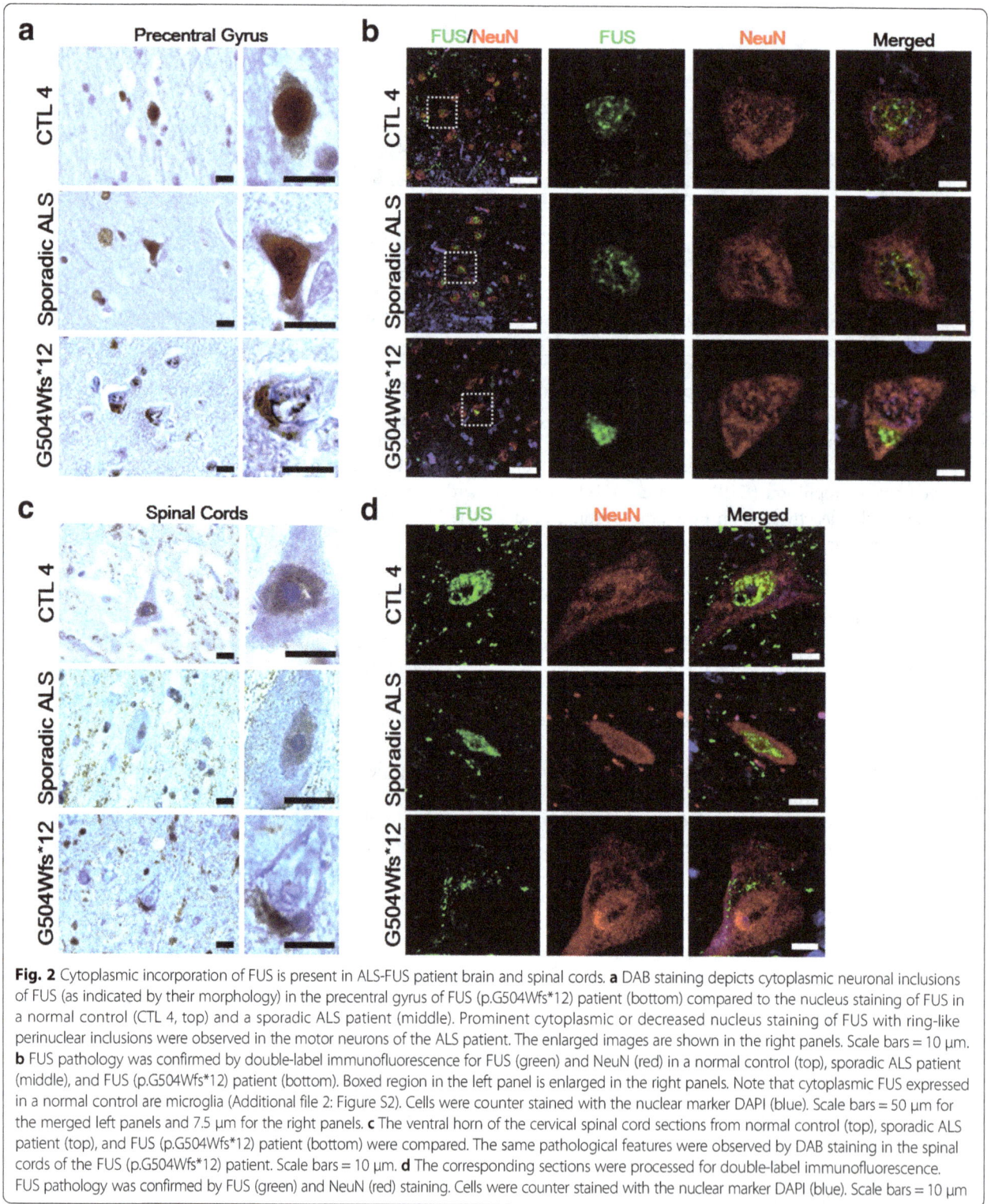

Fig. 2 Cytoplasmic incorporation of FUS is present in ALS-FUS patient brain and spinal cords. **a** DAB staining depicts cytoplasmic neuronal inclusions of FUS (as indicated by their morphology) in the precentral gyrus of FUS (p.G504Wfs*12) patient (bottom) compared to the nucleus staining of FUS in a normal control (CTL 4, top) and a sporadic ALS patient (middle). Prominent cytoplasmic or decreased nucleus staining of FUS with ring-like perinuclear inclusions were observed in the motor neurons of the ALS patient. The enlarged images are shown in the right panels. Scale bars = 10 μm. **b** FUS pathology was confirmed by double-label immunofluorescence for FUS (green) and NeuN (red) in a normal control (top), sporadic ALS patient (middle), and FUS (p.G504Wfs*12) patient (bottom). Boxed region in the left panel is enlarged in the right panels. Note that cytoplasmic FUS expressed in a normal control are microglia (Additional file 2: Figure S2). Cells were counter stained with the nuclear marker DAPI (blue). Scale bars = 50 μm for the merged left panels and 7.5 μm for the right panels. **c** The ventral horn of the cervical spinal cord sections from normal control (top), sporadic ALS patient (top), and FUS (p.G504Wfs*12) patient (bottom) were compared. The same pathological features were observed by DAB staining in the spinal cords of the FUS (p.G504Wfs*12) patient. Scale bars = 10 μm. **d** The corresponding sections were processed for double-label immunofluorescence. FUS pathology was confirmed by FUS (green) and NeuN (red) staining. Cells were counter stained with the nuclear marker DAPI (blue). Scale bars = 10 μm

the normal controls and the sporadic ALS patient demonstrated FUS in the nucleus of those neurons. By contrast, mutant FUS were excluded from the nucleus of ALS-FUS patient neurons.

Interestingly, FUS was predominantly nuclear in the postcentral gyrus and dorsal horn neurons of FUS (p.G504Wfs*12) patient indicating that FUS abnormalities are FUS abnormalities are observed in the motor system to a greater extent than that observed for the patient sensory neurons (Additional file 3: Figure S3). This is the first report on the case of FUS (p.G504Wfs*12) pathology on autopsy ALS samples.

Endogenous mutant FUS pathology in primary patient fibroblasts

The residues of the three mutants (p.G504Wfs*12, p.R495*, p.Q519E) are all located in the C-terminal NLS-containing domain of FUS. To examine the presence of ALS-FUS pathology in ALS patient fibroblasts, a punch skin biopsy were obtained from normal controls and ALS patients to isolate their fibroblasts. Primary fibroblasts from healthy individuals (CTL 1, 2, and 3) showed endogenous FUS entirely in the nucleus (Fig. 3a, left panels). Contrary to the report showing endogenous neuronal FUS harboring the G504Wfs*12 or R495* mutation in the cytoplasm with decreased staining in the nucleus [26], we observed more abundant nuclear immunoreactivity of FUS and somewhat diffuse cytoplasmic immunoreactivity on patient-derived fibroblasts that harbor either the G504Wfs*12 or R495* mutation. Surprisingly, FUS (p.Q519E) did not even show any cytosolic mislocalization. These results suggested that either FUS (p.Q519E) does not contribute to the pathogenic potential of ALS or that its mislocalization failed to be captured in the fibroblast model.

Stress agents are known to induce cytoplasmic granules, and various ALS-causing *FUS* mutations have previously been reported to be recruited to those stress granules under stress conditions [21]. Sodium arsenite (referred to as arsenite) is widely used to induce oxidative stress in cells. To determine whether the cytoplasmic FUS protein in the patient fibroblasts could be recruited into stress granules, we stressed cells with arsenite, and observed the shift of dispersed FUS G504Wfs*12 or R495* proteins to cytoplasmic stress granules, which is similar to the response of the eukaryotic translation initiation factor 4G (eIF4G) (Fig. 3a, right panels, and Fig. 3b, c). Again, the Q519E mutant remained in the nucleus under such stress conditions. In addition to oxidative stress induced by sodium arsenite, we tested hyperosmotic stress induced by 0.4 M sorbitol for 1 hr [7]. In response to sorbitol stress, the amount of FUS in the cytoplasm increased with corresponding decrease in the nucleus. Importantly, the accumulation of cytoplasmic FUS granules in mutant fibroblasts is clearly much greater than that in healthy controls (Additional file 4: Figure S4).

Subcellular fractionation of fibroblasts was performed to further investigate the localization of endogenous FUS. In agreement with the immunofluorescence results, the shorter G504Wfs*12 and R495* mutants could be distinguished from the longer wild-type FUS by Western blotting, showing that the mutants were more detectable in the cytosol and that the wild type was exclusively detected in the nucleus. In contrast, the Q519E mutant was detected in only the nucleus (Fig. 3d). These data suggest that patient-derived fibroblasts may not fully reflect the ALS pathology with disease-associated mutations in FUS.

Mutant FUS pathology in transfected HEK-293 cells and primary neurons

We aimed to examine whether the similar mutant FUS characteristics of patient fibroblasts, carrying the Q519E mutation, i.e., predominant nucleus FUS staining, was also observed in transfected cells. We overexpressed the cDNA encoding an N-terminal green fluorescence protein (GFP)-tagged wild-type or a mutant FUS in HEK-293 cells. The transiently transfected G504Wfs*12 and R495* mutants showed both nuclear and cytosolic distribution, whereas the Q519E mutant like the wild-type FUS resided predominantly in the nucleus (Fig. 3e, left panels). To determine whether the cytoplasmic mutant FUS could be incorporated into stress granules under oxidative stress conditions, we exposed the cells to arsenite. Both the G504Wfs*12 and R495* mutants showed the incorporation of their cytoplasmic FUS into eIF4G-containing granules, but the Q519E mutant still behaved like the wild-type FUS (Fig. 3e, right panels).

The neuropathology of ALS is characterized by degenerating neurons in the brain and spinal cord, which is coincident with neuronal cytoplasmic inclusions of ALS-associated FUS proteins [27]. To determine the distribution of wild-type or mutant FUS constructs in neurons, we cultured cortical neurons from rats on embryonic day 18 rats and transfected them with GFP-tagged FUS constructs. The neurons were first cultured for 21 days and then transfected for 48 hrs before fixation. As shown in HEK-293 cells, both G504Wfs*12 and R495* mutants resided largely in the cytosol, which is contrary to the patterns that were observed in patient fibroblasts (Fig. 3f, left panels). When rat cortical neurons were exposed to oxidative stress, the cytosolic FUS (p.G504Wfs*12 and p.R495*) was further incorporated in eIF4G-positive stress granules (Fig. 3f, right panels). Interestingly, both the Q519E mutant and the wild-type FUS continued to reside in the nucleus before and after stress induction. These findings suggest that neurons from murine models may fail to reflect certain neuronal pathologies in human ALS-FUS brain or spinal cord samples. Moreover, overexpressed FUS may also cause deleterious effects that may be unrelated to ALS pathologies in transfected cells [28].

Endogenous mutant FUS that recapitulates autopsied ALS pathology is iNeuron-specific

To develop more accurate disease models for ALS, we trans-differentiated ALS patient fibroblasts into induced neurons (iNeurons) by repressing a single RNA binding

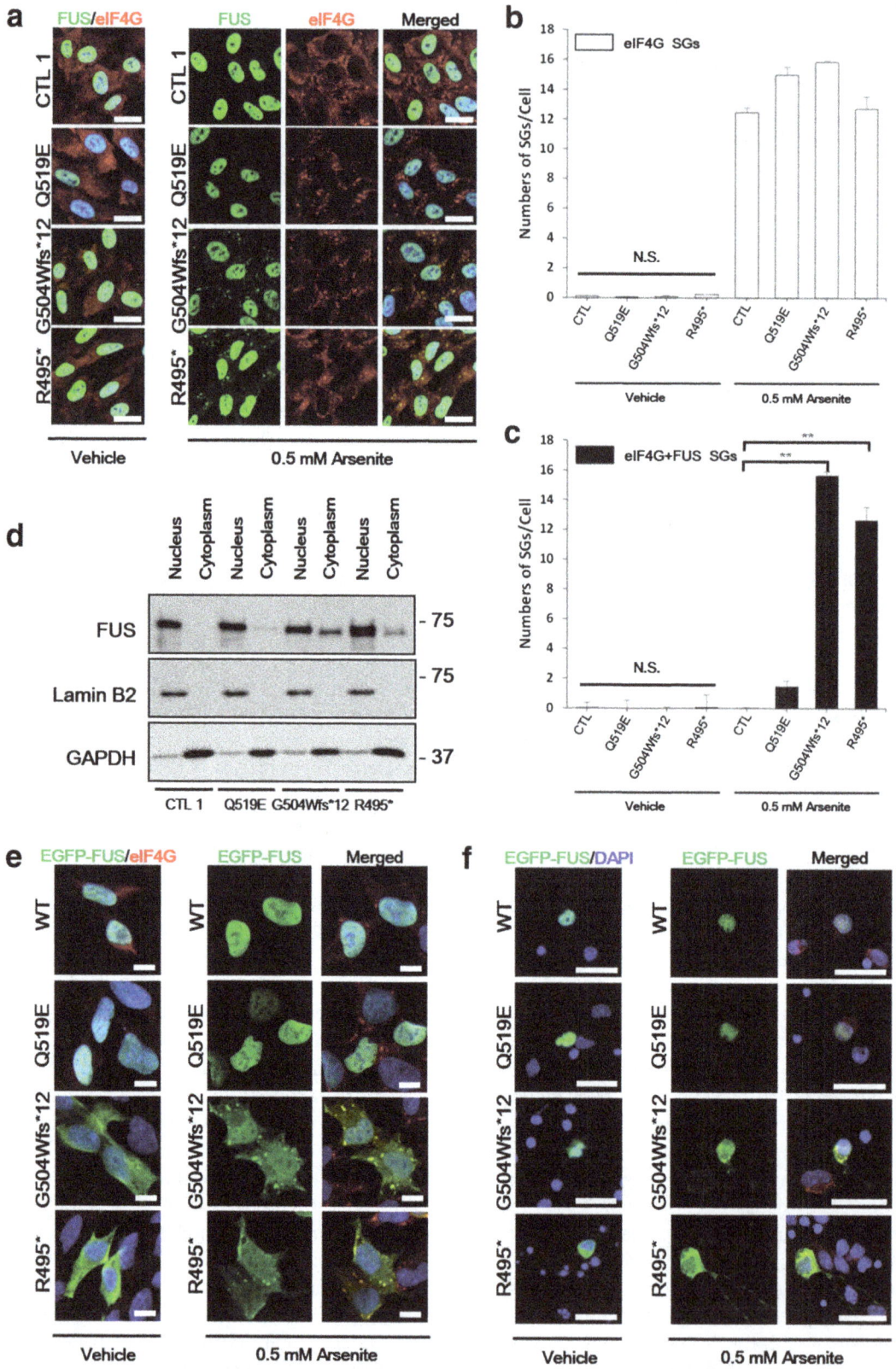

Fig. 3 (See legend on next page.)

(See figure on previous page.)

Fig. 3 Endogenous FUS is partially mislocalized in patient fibroblasts with G504Wfs*12 and R495* mutations. **a** Primary fibroblasts cultures examined by confocal microscopy. A representative control image shows intense staining for FUS (green) in the nuclei (DAPI) and the stress granule markers eIF4G (red) in the cytoplasm. Patients with the G504Wfs*12 and R495* mutations near the NLS region also show that a majority of FUS protein in the nuclei with a slight increase of cytoplasmic FUS. In response to oxidative stress conditions, cytoplasmic FUS-positive inclusion bodies of G504Wfs*12 and R495* mutation co-localized with eIF4G stress granules (red). Cells were counter stained with the nuclear marker DAPI (blue). Scale bars = 25 µm. Bar graphs represent **b** the numbers of stress granules and **c** the numbers of FUS-positive stress granules (SGs). Data are from three experiments (the mean ± SEM, n = 20). One-way ANOVA followed by Tukey multiple comparisons test; **$p < 0.001$; N.S., not significant. **d** Cell fractionation analysis of cultured fibroblasts from ALS patients and controls showing an increased cytoplasmic expression of FUS in G504Wfs*12 and R495* patients compared with a representative control and Q519E patient. The upper band of FUS in the nucleus fraction of FUS (p.R495*) patient fibroblasts presumably an allele without a mutation and the lower band indicates the allele with the truncated R495* fragment. Lamin B2 and GAPDH are loading controls for the nuclear and cytoplasmic fractions, respectively. **e** HEK-293 cells were transfected with green fluorescent protein (GFP) wild-type FUS or FUS containing the ALS-associated mutations and treated with vehicle or 0.5 mM arsenite for 30 min. The cells were then processed for immunofluorescence analysis. Localization of GFP-tagged FUS wild type or the indicated FUS mutations (green), eIF4G stress granules (red) are shown. Cytosolic eIF4G co-localizes with FUS aggregates after oxidative stress. GFP (green) and eIF4G (red) show an increased overlap between mutant FUS (p.G504Wfs*12, p.R495*) and eIF4G as compared to wild-type FUS (WT) and eIF4G. Nuclei are shown by DAPI staining. Scale bars = 10 µm. **f** Rat E18 primary cortical neurons were cultured for 21 days and were transfected with constructs expressing wild-type FUS or ALS-associated mutants of FUS (green). After stress, redistribution of mutant FUS aggregates (green) into eIF4G (red) under oxidative stress is demonstrated. Nuclei are shown by DAPI staining. Scale bars = 25 µm.

polypyrimidine-tract-binding (PTB) protein. To generate human iNeurons, we infected both patient and control fibroblasts with a lentivirus-repressing PTBP1, according to and modified from our recently published methods [16]. The subsequent culture conditions are provided in the schematic overview in Fig. 4a. In confocal cellular immunostaining assays, cells exhibited typical neuronal morphology, and nearly all cells were strongly positive for TUJ1 (the early neuronal marker βIII-tubulin). Within a day of neuronal induction, the cells were positive for TUJ1, and from 5–21 days, an increase in MAP2 (neuronal dendrites marker) immunostaining was observed (Fig. 4b). The maturated morphology of iNeurons with dendritic branching were confirmed with MAP2, NeuN (neuronal nuclei marker), and synapsin (neuronal synapsis marker) immunostaining at day 10 of neuronal induction (Fig. 4c). The percentage of neuronal tubulin marker TUJ1-positive iNeuron cells of the controls and three ALS patients with different types of *FUS* mutations were similar (Fig. 4d).

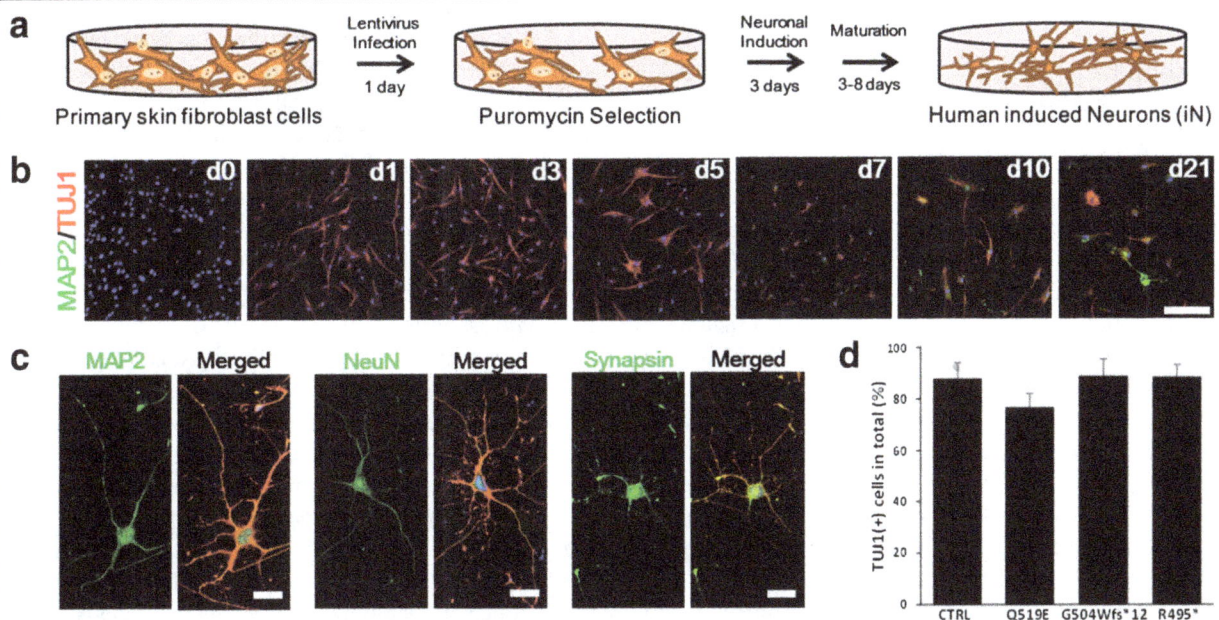

Fig. 4 Direct conversion. **a** Schematic of the experimental protocol. **b** Cells probed with a mature neuronal marker anti-MAP2 (green) and a tubulin marker anti-TUJ1 (red) revealed that mature iNeurons are detected from day 7. Cells were counter stained with the nuclear marker DAPI (blue). Scale bars = 250 µm. **c** Expression of mature neuronal markers in iNeurons. Green: MAP2, NeuN, Synapsin; red: TUJ1; blue: DAPI. Scale bars: 50 µm. **d** Quantification of iNeurons based on TUJ1-positive cells divided by the number of initial plating cells in response to PTBP1 shRNA. Cells untreated with shPTBP1 had no TUJ1-positive staining. Data are from three experiments (the mean ± SEM, $n = 30$–82).

In control iNeurons, endogenous FUS was predominantly nuclear (Fig. 5a and b left panels). In contrast, the patient iNeurons of G504Wfs*12 or R495* exhibited reduced endogenous FUS immunoreactivities in the nucleus along with increased cytoplasmic FUS. Considering that FUS was predominantly distributed in the nucleus of patient fibroblasts, FUS expression in iNeuron models seem to more closely mirror the FUS neuropathology found in ALS patients than those observed in patient fibroblasts. Intriguingly, the FUS (p.Q519E) patient also showed cytoplasmic localization of FUS with less nuclear distribution in the iNeuron model.

To determine whether the cytosolic FUS (p.Q519E) could be induced to stress granules in iNeurons, we treated iNeurons with arsenite, and in line with the results with the cytoplasmic FUS in G504Wfs*12 or R495* patient iNeurons, we observed co-localization of the FUS (p.Q519E) mutant with arsenite-induced stress granules, which was further validated by the detection of the colocalization of the Ras-GTPase-activating protein SH3 domain binding protein (G3BP), another known component of stress granules (Fig. 5b, right panels). Co-localization of the cytosolic FUS inclusions with eIF4G under oxidative stress was also confirmed and quantified (Additional file 5: Figure S5, and Fig. 5c, d). These findings suggest that unlike patient-derived fibroblasts and transfected cell models, only patient iNeurons are able to fully capture the neuropathology of *FUS* mutations with a disrupted NLS region.

Conclusions

Mutations in *FUS* have been strongly implicated as the genetic cause of ALS [2, 29]. In this study, we performed functional analysis of three different *FUS* mutations found in ALS patients, including the two *de novo* mutations (p.G504Wfs*12, p.R495*) we previously identified by trio study in sporadic ALS [30] and a novel variant (p.Q519E) by multi-gene panel testing in familial ALS (Table 1). All these mutations were located in the C-terminal region that contains the nuclear localization signal (NLS). FUS accumulation in neuronal cytoplasmic inclusions along with a degree of nuclear clearance are histopathological hallmarks of patients with FUS-mediated ALS, especially for the mutations located at the NLS region [2, 31]. Consistently, we show for the first time that FUS (p.G504Wfs*12) exhibited the accumulation of cytoplasmic FUS and the depletion of nuclear FUS in patient brain and spinal cord motor neurons. The autopsy results demonstrated typical ALS-FUS features of cytoplasmic aggregation and nuclear clearance of FUS in neurons, which have also been described in the autopsy of patients with other FUS mutations in the NLS region.

As of now, cultured patient fibroblasts have been used as cellular models for disease studies. Induced pluripotent stem cell (iPSC)-derived neurons from patients with a *FUS* mutation appear to provide a suitable model for understanding pathophysiological mechanisms of *FUS* mutations; however, one of the problems in skin fibroblast models is that some common FUS-associated pathological hallmarks found in autopsy cases are not consistently identified in patient fibroblasts [13]. Although iPSC-based models are useful in identifying the molecular and cellular defects in neuronal abnormality and instrumental for in vitro drug screening for therapeutic effects, the process of generating iPSC-derived neurons from human fibroblasts is intricate. To develop disease models more efficiently, we directly converted the fibroblasts from patients with *FUS* mutations into induced neuron (iNeuron) by repressing a polypyrimidine-tract-binding (PTB) protein. As PTB is naturally down-regulated during neuronal induction in development, PTB regulation enhanced the neurogenesis program in the fibroblasts [16]. As shown in the present data, iNeuron is a rapid and highly disease-relevant cell model. Compared to the majority of nuclear FUS distribution in patient fibroblasts carrying mutations in the NLS region, iNeurons demonstrated a clear increase in cytoplasmic distribution and a concurrent decrease in the nuclear distribution of mutant FUS. Moreover, cytosolic aggregates of FUS could be induced under oxidative stress conditions. The analysis on iNeurons from a FUS (p.G504Wfs*12) patient recapitulated all key features of FUS pathology found in the patient brain and spinal cord motor neurons, thus confirming that iNeurons as a more disease-relevant in vitro model that accurately mirrors disease pathology of the patient. Intriguingly, the FUS (p.Q519E) patient who had endogenous FUS distributed in only the nucleus in fibroblast models or transiently transfected cells demonstrated a cytosolic mislocalization and aggregation of FUS only in the iNeuron model. These findings further support this new model as a useful research tool for studying ALS-FUS pathogenesis.

FUS proteinopathies in ALS neuronal degeneration have been poorly understood due to the lack of clinically relevant cell models for the disease. The identification of disease-causing genes and the development of patient-specific and disease-relevant cell models for functional analysis are critical for advancing our understanding of the pathophysiology in ALS. Studies using patient iNeurons may reveal additional features of FUS pathology in the cytoplasm that may have escaped previous studies on patient fibroblasts [11]. Similarly, mutant FUS cDNA constructs of patients whose fibroblasts or each cDNA construct does not display typical FUS pathology may have distinct pathologic features, which can now be dissected in iNeurons.

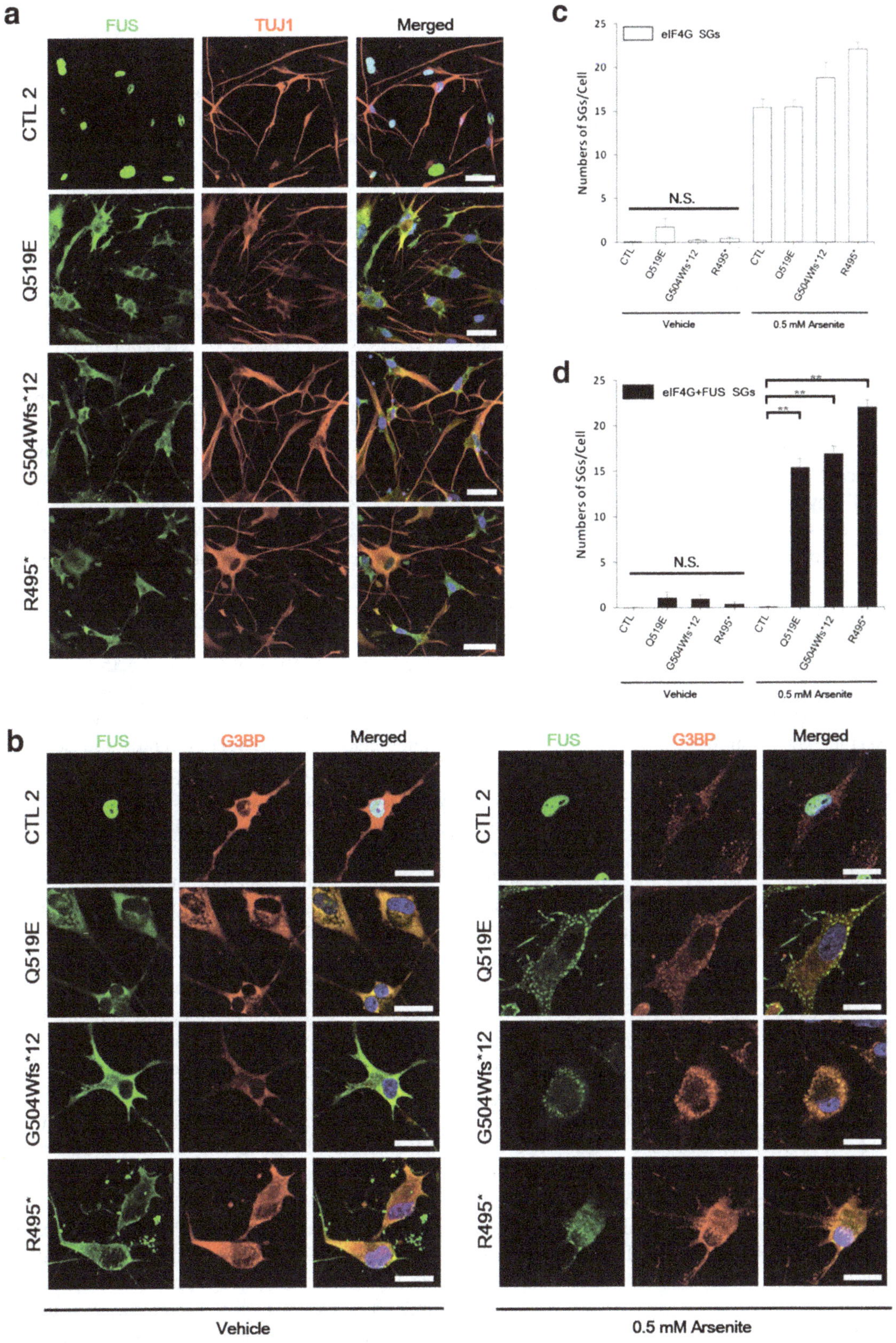

Fig. 5 (See legend on next page.)

(See figure on previous page.)

Fig. 5 Endogenous FUS is mislocalized to the cytoplasm and is incorporated into cytoplasmic stress granules in response to arsenite in patient iNeurons. **a** A representative control shows intense staining for FUS (green) in the nuclei (DAPI) in TUJ1-positive (red) iNeurons at day 10 of neuronal induction, whereas the patients show a majority of FUS protein in the cytoplasm. Cells were counter stained with the nuclear marker DAPI (blue). Scale bars = 50 μm. **b** Confocal images of vehicle treated iNeurons (left panel) as compared to cells treated with 0.5 mM arsenite for 30 min (right panel) at day 10 are shown. A representative control shows FUS protein predominantly localized to the nuclei. ALS-FUS patient with Q519E mutation recapitulated the FUS neuropathology only in iNeurons: iNeurons from the patient show a majority of FUS protein (green) in the cytoplasm. In response to oxidative stress conditions, cytoplasmic FUS-positive inclusion bodies (green) in iNeurons were co-localized with G3BP stress granules (red). Cells were fixed and probed by immunofluorescence for DAPI (blue). Scale bars = 25 μm. Bar graphs represent (**c**) the numbers of stress granules and (**d**) the numbers of FUS-positive stress granules (SGs). Data are from three experiments (the mean ± SEM, $n = 20$). One-way ANOVA followed by Tukey multiple comparisons test; **$p < 0.001$; N.S., not significant

ALS-FUS patient fibroblast models present endogenous cytoplasmic FUS incorporation into stress granules; however, FUS in patient fibroblasts are predominantly expressed in the nucleus. Murine neurons transiently transfected with mutant FUS constructs revealed both decreases in the nucleus and increases in the cytosol, and upon stress, cytosolic FUS could be induced into stress granules. Yet, murine neurons may be insufficient to capture all key mechanism in neuronal pathology in human brain or spinal cords.

Development of more disease-relevant experimental models from ALS patients that recapitulate the characteristics of neuronal dysfunction found in human post-mortem tissues will open new doors to both understanding pathophysiologic mechanisms in ALS-FUS and developing new therapeutic strategies. Therefore, simple, reliable, and reproducible iNeuron models are promising in that they may greatly accelerate ALS research.

Methods

Subjects

Three ALS patients with different types of *FUS* mutations were enrolled in this study. We have recently identified *FUS* mutations (p.G504Wfs*12, p.R495*, and p.Q519E) by direct sequencing and multi-gene panel testing [17, 19, 32]. These patients showed onset at age 27 to 34 with various disease progression. Skin fibroblasts were obtained from these ALS patients with disrupted NLS region and three healthy controls. Autopsy tissues were obtained from two patients: one ALS-FUS patient (p.G504Wfs*12) and one sporadic ALS patient without any known mutation in *FUS, C9orf72, SOD1, ALS2, SPG11, UBQLN2, DAO, GRN, SQSTM1, SETX, MAPT, TARDBP*, and *TAF15*. The clinical and genetic findings are summarized in Table 1. The study protocol was approved by the Institutional Review Board of Hanyang University Hospital, and written informed consents were obtained from all patients involved in the study (IRB# 2011-R-63).

Structural modelling

For a structural analysis, we sought for an applicable protein structure in PDB (ID: 4FDD), which contains Transportin-1 and FUS domains. Because the FUS domain includes the Q519 residue, the influence of Q519E mutation on the complex can be examined. The PDB complex consists of Transportin-1 (chain A: residue number from 371 to 890) and FUS (chain B: residue number from 498 to 526). The missing part (residue number from 321 to 370) and N-terminal region (from 1 to 320) in Transportin-1 was removed from the original PDB structure because they are not relevant to direct interactions with the FUS domain. The FUS missing residues from 498 to 506 were generated and minimized to find their local minima with keeping the rest atomic coordinates unchanged. To examine the effect of Q519E mutation on the FUS-Transportin-1 binding, a hydrogen bonding analysis was performed between FUS and Transportin-1 structures. Because the structure has no hydrogen atoms, we used an implicit hydrogen bonding analysis with the following loose criteria, the bond distance below 5 Å between acceptor and donor atom and the angle above 90°, among acceptor, donor, and the prior atom connected to the donor atom. The analysis was performed in CHARMM (Chemistry at Harvard Macromolecular Mechanics) [33], and the structure was visualized using Jmol (an open-source Java viewer for chemical structures in 3D. http://www.jmol.org/)

Immunohistochemistry and immunofluorescence

Autopsied samples of brain and spinal cord were obtained from one ALS-FUS patient (p.G504Wfs*12), one sporadic ALS patient, and one healthy control. Immunohistochemistry was performed on 5 μm thick paraffin sections. Tissues were deparaffinized, rehydrated in serial changes of xylene and ethanol gradients and autoclaved for 10 min in 10 mM citric acid, pH 8.0. Sections were then blocked with 10 % normal goat serum (vol/vol) in PBS. For immunostaining, rabbit polyclonal antibodies reactive to FUS (Abnova) were applied on the precentral motor cortex and postcentral gyrus, and mouse antibodies against FUS (Proteintech) were used on spinal cord tissue. The sections were colorimetrically developed using the 3,3'-diaminobenzidine DAB substrate kit (Vector Labs) for 1 min and counter stained with haematoxylin (Sigma-Aldrich), dehydrated, and coverslipped in Permount medium. Images were acquired with a Leica DM5000B microscope.

For double labeling immunofluorescence, paraffin-embedded sections were blocked with 10 % normal goat serum (vol/vol). The primary antibodies used were mouse antibodies against FUS (Proteintech) and rabbit polyclonal antibodies against NeuN (Millipore), GFAP (Dako), and Iba-1 (Wako). The secondary antibodies included Alexa Fluor 488-conjugated mouse and tetramethylrhodamine B isothiocyanate (TRITC)-conjugated rabbit antibodies. Images were acquired using a Leica TCS SP5 confocal microscope.

Plasmids and site-directed mutagenesis
N-terminally GFP-tagged wild-type human FUS cDNA was cloned into the pReceiver vector (Genecopoeia). To make the mutant DNA (p.Q519E, p.G504Wfs*12, p.R495*), in vitro mutagenesis of the GFP-tagged FUS cDNA was conducted using the EZchange™ site-directed mutagenesis kit (Enzynomics) according to the manufacturer's protocol.

Cell culture and reagents
HEK-293 cells were cultured in Dulbecco's modified Eagle's medium (DMEM) supplemented with 10 % fetal bovine serum (Gibco), sodium bicarbonate, sodium pyruvate (Sigma-Aldrich), and antibiotics. Primary rat neurons were maintained in Neurobasal medium supplemented with 2 % (vol/vol) B27, 1 % (vol/vol) GlutaMAX, 100X insulin-transferrin-selenium (ITS) (all from Invitrogen), and antibiotics.

HEK-293 and primary rat neurons were transiently transfected with GFP-tagged wild-type or mutant human FUS cDNA using Lipofectamine 2000 (Invitrogen) according to the manufacturer's instructions. After 48 hrs, the cells were fixed in the presence or absence of stress for immunofluorescence staining as described below.

For oxidative stress induction, vehicle (water) or 1 M stock solution of sodium arsenite (Sigma-Aldrich) dissolved in water was added to the media at a final concentration of 0.5 mM for up to 30 min. For hyperosmotic stress induction, vehicle (growth media) or 0.4 M sorbitol (Sigma-Aldrich) dissolved directly into the growth media for up to 1 hr.

Conversion of human skin fibroblasts to iNeurons
Fibroblasts were obtained from forearm skin with a punch biopsy (Table 1). Fibroblasts were cultured and maintained in DMEM supplemented with 20 % FBS, non-essential amino acids (all from Gibco), sodium bicarbonate (Sigma-Aldrich), and 1 % (vol/vol) Penicillin/Streptomycin/Fungizone (Cellgro). In all experiments, passage-matched fibroblasts (passages 3–5) were used. Fibroblast were seeded at a density of 1×10^4 cells/cm^2

and used for experiments after cell synchronization by serum starvation at matched time points.

For direct conversion, human fibroblasts were seeded onto matrigel (BD Biosciences)-coated 24-well tissue culture dishes or cell culture flasks (Nunc). Induced neurons (iNeurons) were generated from patient-derived fibroblasts using lentiviral transduction of the shRNAs against human PTBP1 (Sigma-Aldrich MISSION) according to our previously described protocol [16, 34]. Thirty hours after the shRNA treatment, the cells were selected with 1 μg/ml puromycin for another 30 hrs. Selected cells were replaced for 3 days in N3 media (DMEM/F12 (Gibco) supplemented with 25 μg/ml Insulin, 50 μg/ml apo-transferrin, 20 nM progesterone, 100 nM putrescine, and 30 nM sodium selenite (all Sigma-Aldrich)), 10 ng/ml bFGF (Gibco), supplemented with BDNF, CNTF, GDNF, and NT3 (all PeproTech) as previously described [16]. From day 4 to the day of analysis, the cells were maintained in N3 media supplemented with 2 % FBS.

Immunocytochemistry and confocal microscopy
Fibroblasts, HEK-293, primary rat neurons, and iNeurons were washed with 1 × PBS, fixed with 4 % paraformaldehyde (PFA) for 15 min at room temperature and then washed three more times with PBS. Cells were permeabilized by incubation in 0.3 % Triton X-100 for 10 min at room temperature, washed with PBS, and then blocked for 1 hr in 5 % normal goat serum (Vector Labs). Cells were incubated with primary antibodies for 2 hrs at room temperature, washed three times with 1 × PBS, and incubated with secondary antibodies for 1 hr at room temperature. After three additional washings with 1 × PBS, nuclei were stained with DAPI. Coverslips were mounted on glass slides with Fluoromount-G (Southern-Biotech). The primary antibodies used included mouse monoclonal antibodies against C-terminus FUS (Santa Cruz Biotechnology), FUS (Proteintech), G3BP (BD Transduction Laboratories), and rabbit polyclonal antibodies against eIF4G (Santa Cruz Biotechnology), FUS (Abnova). For neuronal cell markers, mouse monoclonal antibody reactive to β-tubulin III (TUJ1; Covance) and rabbit polyclonal antibody to MAP2 (Cell Signaling Technology), NeuN (Millipore), and Synapsin I (Chemicon) were used. Secondary antibodies were Alexa Fluor 488-conjugated and/or TRITC-conjugated mouse or rabbit antibodies (Gibco). Images were acquired with a Leica TCS SP5 confocal microscope. The stress granules were counted manually. Twenty cells from each patient fibroblasts or iNeurons were chosen based on DAPI staining of nuclei ($n = 3$). Significance between stress granule formations was calculated using one-way ANOVA followed by Tukey multiple comparisons test.

Nuclear-cytoplasmic fractionation and immunoblot analysis

Cell fractionation was performed using the NE-PER Nuclear and Cytoplasmic Extraction Reagents kit (Thermo Fisher Scientific) according to the manufacturer's protocol. Nuclear and cytoplasmic extracts from fibroblasts were analyzed by Western blotting. Equal amounts of protein from each sample were separated by 10 % sodium dodecyl sulfate polyacrylamide gel electrophoresis (SDS-PAGE) and transferred to a PVDF membrane (GE Healthcare). Membranes were blocked with 5 % skim milk. The primary antibodies used were mouse monoclonal antibodies against Lamin B2 (AbCam) and rabbit polyclonal antibodies against FUS (Abnova) and GAPDH (Santa Cruz Biotechnology). The membranes were probed with horseradish peroxidase-conjugated secondary antibodies (Santa Cruz Biotechnology) and developed using West-Q Chemiluminescent Substrate Plus Kits (GenDEPOT).

Additional files

Additional file 1: Figure S1. Structures of FUS-Transportin-1 complexes. (a) Overall structure of FUS-Transportin-1 complexes are presented in blue sphere and white surface, respectively. The position of FUS (p.Q519) is marked by red sphere models. (b) The focused view around the mutation (p.Q519). The structure of FUS and Transportin-1 complexes are consisted of a ball-and-stick representation. Stick models are colored by atom (N: blue, O: red, C: gray, respectively). The important position of the mutation (p.Q519) is depicted in a red ball-and-stick representation. A possible hydrogen bonding between Q519 of FUS and E509 of Transportin-1 is shown in the red circle with the acceptor-donor distance (3.21 Å).

Additional file 2: Figure S2. FUS is distributed in the cytoplasm in microglia but is absent in astrocytes. FUS (green) is (a) apparently not expressed in GFAP-positive astrocytes, (red) and is (b) cytoplasmic in Iba-1-positive microglia (red, arrows) in the precentral gyrus of a normal control (CTL 4, top), sporadic ALS patient (middle), and FUS (p.G504Wfs*12) patient (bottom). Boxed region in the left panel is enlarged in the right panels. Cells were counter stained with the nuclear marker DAPI (blue). Scale bars = (a) 50 μm for the merged left panels and 10 μm for the right panels, and (b) 25 μm. Cells were counter stained with the nuclear marker DAPI (blue).

Additional file 3: Figure S3. FUS is distributed in the nucleus in ALS-FUS patient postcentral gyrus and dorsal horn. (a) DAB staining depicts predominant nucleus localization of FUS (as indicated by their morphology) in the postcentral gyrus of a normal control (CTL 4, top), sporadic ALS patient (middle), and FUS (p.G504Wfs*12) patient (bottom). The enlarged images are shown in the right panels. Scale bars = 10 μm. (b) The dorsal horn of the spinal cord sections from normal control (top), sporadic ALS patient (top), and FUS (p.G504Wfs*12) patient (bottom) were compared. The same predominant nucleus staining of FUS were observed by DAB staining in the dorsal horn neurons (as indicated by their morphology) of a normal control (top), sporadic ALS patient (middle), and FUS (p.G504Wfs*12) patient (bottom). Scale bars = 10 μm.

Additional file 4: Figure S4. Endogenous FUS is partially redistributed to the cytoplasm in response to sorbitol. Primary fibroblasts of a representative control and the patient with the Q519E mutation shows intense staining for FUS (green) in the nuclei (DAPI) and the stress granule markers eIF4G (red) in the cytoplasm. Patients with the G504Wfs*12 and R495* mutations also show that a majority of FUS protein in the nuclei with a slight increase of cytoplasmic FUS (left panel). Cells treated with 0.4 M sorbitol for 1 hr are shown on the right panel. In response to sorbitol stress, slight decrease of nucleus FUS and increase of cytoplasmic FUS-positive inclusion bodies co-localized with eIF4G stress granules were observed.

The accumulation of cytoplasmic FUS granules in mutant fibroblasts were much greater than that in healthy controls. Cells were counter stained with the nuclear marker DAPI (blue). Scale bars = 10 μm.

Additional file 5: Figure S5. Endogenous FUS cytoplasmic incorporation into stress granule marker eIF4G in response to arsenite in patient iNeurons. Immunocytochemistry performed on vehicle treated iNeurons (left panel) as compared to cells treated with 0.5 mM arsenite for 30 min (right panel) at day 10 are shown. A representative control shows FUS protein predominantly localized to the nuclei. All three ALS-FUS patients show a majority of FUS protein (green) in the cytoplasm of iNeurons. Cytoplasmic FUS-positive inclusion bodies (green) were detectable in eIF4G-positive stress granules (red) in patients. Cells were fixed and probed by immunofluorescence for DAPI (blue). Scale bars = 25 μm.

Abbreviations
ALS: Amyotrophic lateral sclerosis; ALS-FUS: ALS-associated FUS; eIF4G: Eukaryotic translation initiation factor 4G; FUS: Fused in sarcoma; G3BP: Ras-GTPase-activating protein SH3 domain binding protein; iNeurons: Induced neurons; iPSC: Induced pluripotent stem cell; NLS: Nuclear localization signal; PTB: Polypyrimidine-tract-binding.

Competing interests
The authors declare that they have no competing interests.

Authors' contributions
SML, WJC, C-SK, and SeHK participated in the design of the research. SML and YX performed the neuronal conversion experiments. SML, SuHK, MN, and SH performed and analyzed immunohistochemical experiments. SML, JYC, and M-YN performed immunocytochemical and biochemical experiments. JL performed protein structural modeling experiments. SML, WJC, K-WO, MN, Y-EK, JL, SL, C-SK, X-DF, and SeHK participated in the preparation of the manuscript. All authors read and approved the final manuscript.

Acknowledgements
This work is supported in part by grants from the Korean Health Technology R&D Project, Ministry for Health, Welfare & Family Affairs, Republic of Korea (HI12C0135), supported in part by the US National Human Genome Research Institute grant (HG004659) to X-D.F, and supported in part by grants from the KOBIC Research Support Program to JL.

Author details
¹Department of Translational Medicine, Graduate School of Biomedical Science and Engineering, Hanyang University, Seoul 133-792, Republic of Korea. ²Cell Therapy Center, Hanyang University Hospital, Seoul 133-792, Republic of Korea. ³Department of Neurology, Sheikh Khalifa Specialty Hospital, Ras Al Khaimah, United Arab Emirates. ⁴Department of Neurology, College of Medicine, Hanyang University, Seoul 133-792, Republic of Korea. ⁵Key Laboratory of RNA Biology, Institute of Biophysics, Chinese Academy of Sciences, Beijing 100101, China. ⁶Department of Laboratory Medicine and Genetics, Samsung Medical Center, Sungkyunkwan University School of Medicine, Seoul 135-710, Republic of Korea. ⁷Korean Bioinformation Center, Korea Research Institute of Bioscience and Biotechnology, Daejeon 305-806, Republic of Korea. ⁸Department of Bioinformatics, University of Sciences and Technology, Daejeon 305-806, Republic of Korea. ⁹Department of Brain and Cognitive Sciences, College of Natural Sciences, Seoul National University, Seoul 110-744, Republic of Korea. ¹⁰Department of Anatomy and Cell Biology, College of Medicine, Hanyang University, Seoul 133-792, Republic of Korea. ¹¹Department of Cellular Molecular Medicine, University of California, La Jolla, San Diego, CA 92093, USA.

References
1. Renton AE, Chio A, Traynor BJ. State of play in amyotrophic lateral sclerosis genetics. Nat Neurosci. 2014;17(1):17–23. doi:10.1038/nn.3584.
2. Kwiatkowski Jr TJ, Bosco DA, Leclerc AL, Tamrazian E, Vanderburg CR, Russ C, et al. Mutations in the FUS/TLS gene on chromosome 16 cause familial amyotrophic lateral sclerosis. Science. 2009;323(5918):1205–8. doi:10.1126/science.1166066.

3. Lagier-Tourenne C, Polymenidou M, Cleveland DW. TDP-43 and FUS/TLS: emerging roles in RNA processing and neurodegeneration. Hum Mol Genet. 2010;19(R1):R46–64. doi:10.1093/hmg/ddq137.

4. Neumann M, Bentmann E, Dormann D, Jawaid A, DeJesus-Hernandez M, Ansorge O, et al. FET proteins TAF15 and EWS are selective markers that distinguish FTLD with FUS pathology from amyotrophic lateral sclerosis with FUS mutations. Brain. 2011;134(Pt 9):2595–609. doi:10.1093/brain/awr201.

5. Lashley T, Rohrer JD, Bandopadhyay R, Fry C, Ahmed Z, Isaacs AM, et al. A comparative clinical, pathological, biochemical and genetic study of fused in sarcoma proteinopathies. Brain. 2011;134(Pt 9):2548–64. doi:10.1093/brain/awr160.

6. Dormann D, Rodde R, Edbauer D, Bentmann E, Fischer I, Hruscha A, et al. ALS-associated fused in sarcoma (FUS) mutations disrupt Transportin-mediated nuclear import. EMBO J. 2010;29(16):2841–57. doi:10.1038/emboj.2010.143.

7. Sama RR, Ward CL, Kaushansky LJ, Lemay N, Ishigaki S, Urano F, et al. FUS/TLS assembles into stress granules and is a prosurvival factor during hyperosmolar stress. J Cell Physiol. 2013;228(11):2222–31. doi:10.1002/jcp.24395.

8. Mackenzie IRA, Rademakers R, Neumann M. TDP-43 and FUS in amyotrophic lateral sclerosis and frontotemporal dementia. Lancet Neurol. 2010;9(10):995–1007. doi:10.1016/s1474-4422(10)70195-2.

9. Armstrong GA, Drapeau P. Loss and gain of FUS function impair neuromuscular synaptic transmission in a genetic model of ALS. Hum Mol Genet. 2013;22(21):4282–92. doi:10.1093/hmg/ddt278.

10. Sun S, Ling SC, Qiu J, Albuquerque CP, Zhou Y, Tokunaga S, et al. ALS-causative mutations in FUS/TLS confer gain and loss of function by altered association with SMN and U1-snRNP. Nat Commun. 2015;6:6171. doi:10.1038/ncomms7171.

11. Schwartz JC, Podell ER, Han SS, Berry JD, Eggan KC, Cech TR. FUS is sequestered in nuclear aggregates in ALS patient fibroblasts. Mol Biol Cell. 2014;25(17):2571–8. doi:10.1091/mbc.E14-05-1007.

12. Shelkovnikova TA, Robinson HK, Troakes C, Ninkina N, Buchman VL. Compromised paraspeckle formation as a pathogenic factor in FUSopathies. Hum Mol Genet. 2014;23(9):2298–312. doi:10.1093/hmg/ddt622.

13. Vance C, Scotter EL, Nishimura AL, Troakes C, Mitchell JC, Kathe C, et al. ALS mutant FUS disrupts nuclear localization and sequesters wild-type FUS within cytoplasmic stress granules. Hum Mol Genet. 2013;22(13):2676–88. doi:10.1093/hmg/ddt117.

14. Sabatelli M, Moncada A, Conte A, Lattante S, Marangi G, Luigetti M, et al. Mutations in the 3' untranslated region of FUS causing FUS overexpression are associated with amyotrophic lateral sclerosis. Hum Mol Genet. 2013;22(23):4748–55. doi:10.1093/hmg/ddt328.

15. Lenzi J, De Santis R, de Turris V, Morlando M, Laneve P, Calvo A et al. ALS mutant FUS proteins are recruited into stress granules in induced Pluripotent Stem Cells (iPSCs) derived motoneurons. Dis Model Mech. 2015. doi:10.1242/dmm.020099

16. Xue Y, Ouyang K, Huang J, Zhou Y, Ouyang H, Li H, et al. Direct conversion of fibroblasts to neurons by reprogramming PTB-regulated microRNA circuits. Cell. 2013;152(1–2):82–96. doi:10.1016/j.cell.2012.11.045.

17. Kwon MJ, Baek W, Ki CS, Kim HY, Koh SH, Kim JW et al. Screening of the SOD1, FUS, TARDBP, ANG, and OPTN mutations in Korean patients with familial and sporadic ALS. Neurobiol Aging. 2012;33(5):1017 e17-23. doi:10.1016/j.neurobiolaging.2011.12.003.

18. Kim YE, Oh KW, Kwon MJ, Choi WJ, Oh SI, Ki CS et al. De novo FUS mutations in 2 Korean patients with sporadic amyotrophic lateral sclerosis. Neurobiol Aging. 2015;36(3):1604 e17-9. doi:10.1016/j.neurobiolaging.2014.10.002.

19. Kim H-J, Oh K-W, Kwon M-J, Oh S-i, Park J-s, Kim Y-E et al. Identification of mutations in Korean patients with amyotrophic lateral sclerosis using multigene panel testing. Neurobiology of Aging. 2015. doi:10.1016/j.neurobiolaging.2015.09.012

20. Waibel S, Neumann M, Rabe M, Meyer T, Ludolph AC. Novel missense and truncating mutations in FUS/TLS in familial ALS. Neurology. 2010;75(9):815–7. doi:10.1212/WNL.0b013e3181f07e26.

21. Bosco DA, Lemay N, Ko HK, Zhou H, Burke C, Kwiatkowski Jr TJ, et al. Mutant FUS proteins that cause amyotrophic lateral sclerosis incorporate into stress granules. Hum Mol Genet. 2010;19(21):4160–75. doi:10.1093/hmg/ddq335.

22. King A, Troakes C, Smith B, Nolan M, Curran O, Vance C, et al. ALS-FUS pathology revisited: singleton FUS mutations and an unusual case with both a FUS and TARDBP mutation. Acta Neuropathol Commun. 2015;3:62. doi:10.1186/s40478-015-0235-x.

23. Zou ZY, Cui LY, Sun Q, Li XG, Liu MS, Xu Y et al. De novo FUS gene mutations are associated with juvenile-onset sporadic amyotrophic lateral sclerosis in China. Neurobiol Aging. 2013;34(4):1312 e1-8. doi:10.1016/j.neurobiolaging.2012.09.005.

24. Dormann D, Madl T, Valori CF, Bentmann E, Tahirovic S, Abou-Ajram C, et al. Arginine methylation next to the PY-NLS modulates Transportin binding and nuclear import of FUS. EMBO J. 2012;31(22):4258–75. doi:10.1038/emboj.2012.261.

25. Neumann M, Valori CF, Ansorge O, Kretzschmar HA, Munoz DG, Kusaka H, et al. Transportin 1 accumulates specifically with FET proteins but no other transportin cargos in FTLD-FUS and is absent in FUS inclusions in ALS with FUS mutations. Acta Neuropathol. 2012;124(5):705–16. doi:10.1007/s00401-012-1020-6.

26. Al-Chalabi A, Jones A, Troakes C, King A, Al-Sarraj S, van den Berg LH. The genetics and neuropathology of amyotrophic lateral sclerosis. Acta Neuropathol. 2012;124(3):339–52. doi:10.1007/s00401-012-1022-4.

27. Mackenzie IR, Ansorge O, Strong M, Bilbao J, Zinman L, Ang LC, et al. Pathological heterogeneity in amyotrophic lateral sclerosis with FUS mutations: two distinct patterns correlating with disease severity and mutation. Acta Neuropathol. 2011;122(1):87–98. doi:10.1007/s00401-011-0838-7.

28. McGoldrick P, Joyce PI, Fisher EM, Greensmith L. Rodent models of amyotrophic lateral sclerosis. Biochim Biophys Acta. 2013;1832(9):1421–36. doi:10.1016/j.bbadis.2013.03.012.

29. Vance C, Rogelj B, Hortobagyi T, De Vos KJ, Nishimura AL, Sreedharan J, et al. Mutations in FUS, an RNA processing protein, cause familial amyotrophic lateral sclerosis type 6. Science. 2009;323(5918):1208–11. doi:10.1126/science.1165942.

30. Hubers A, Just W, Rosenbohm A, Muller K, Marroquin N, Goebel I et al. De novo FUS mutations are the most frequent genetic cause in early-onset German ALS patients. Neurobiol Aging. 2015;36(11):3117 e1-6. doi:10.1016/j.neurobiolaging.2015.08.005.

31. Zhou Y, Liu S, Liu G, Ozturk A, Hicks GG. ALS-associated FUS mutations result in compromised FUS alternative splicing and autoregulation. PLoS Genet. 2013;9(10):e1003895. doi:10.1371/journal.pgen.1003895.

32. Kim YE, Oh KW, Kwon MJ, Choi WJ, Oh SI, Ki CS et al. De novoFUS mutations in 2 Korean patients with sporadic amyotrophic lateral sclerosis. Neurobiology of aging. 2014. doi:10.1016/j.neurobiolaging.2014.10.002

33. Brooks BR, Brooks 3rd CL, Mackerell Jr AD, Nilsson L, Petrella RJ, Roux B, et al. CHARMM: the biomolecular simulation program. J Comput Chem. 2009;30(10):1545–614. doi:10.1002/jcc.21287.

34. Liu Y, Xue Y, Ridley S, Zhang D, Rezvani K, Fu XD, et al. Direct Reprogramming of Huntington's Disease Patient Fibroblasts into Neuron-Like Cells Leads to Abnormal Neurite Outgrowth, Increased Cell Death, and Aggregate Formation. PloS One. 2014;9(10):e109621. doi:10.1371/journal.pone.0109621.

2

ADAMTS-4 promotes neurodegeneration in a mouse model of amyotrophic lateral sclerosis

Sighild Lemarchant*, Yuriy Pomeshchik, Iurii Kidin, Virve Kärkkäinen, Piia Valonen, Sarka Lehtonen, Gundars Goldsteins, Tarja Malm, Katja Kanninen and Jari Koistinaho

Abstract

Background: A disintegrin and metalloproteinase with thrombospondin motifs (ADAMTS) proteoglycanases are specialized in the degradation of chondroitin sulfate proteoglycans and participate in mechanisms mediating neuroplasticity. Despite the beneficial effect of ADAMTS-4 on neurorepair after spinal cord injury, the functions of ADAMTS proteoglycanases in other CNS disease states have not been studied. Therefore, we investigated the expression, effects and associated mechanisms of ADAMTS-4 during amyotrophic lateral sclerosis (ALS) in the SOD1^{G93A} mouse model.

Results: ADAMTS-4 expression and activity were reduced in the spinal cord of SOD1^{G93A} mice at disease end-stage when compared to WT littermates. To counteract the loss of ADAMTS-4, SOD1^{G93A} and WT mice were treated with saline or a recombinant ADAMTS-4 before symptom onset. Administration of ADAMTS-4 worsened the prognosis of SOD1^{G93A} mice by accelerating clinical signs of neuromuscular dysfunctions. The worsened prognosis of ADAMTS-4-treated SOD1^{G93A} mice was accompanied by increased degradation of perineuronal nets enwrapping motoneurons and increased motoneuron degeneration in the lumbar spinal cord. Motoneurons of ADAMTS-4-treated SOD1^{G93A} mice were more vulnerable to degeneration most likely due to the loss of their extracellular matrix envelopes. The decrease of neurotrophic factor production induced by ADAMTS-4 in vitro and in vivo may also contribute to a hostile environment for motoneuron especially when devoid of a net.

Conclusions: This study suggests that the reduction of ADAMTS-4 activity during the progression of ALS pathology may be an adaptive change to mitigate its neurodegenerative impact in CNS tissues. Therapies compensating the compromised ADAMTS-4 activity are likely not promising approaches for treating ALS.

Keywords: A disintegrin and metalloproteinase with thrombospondin motifs, Amyotrophic lateral sclerosis, Extracellular matrix, Neurodegeneration, Perineuronal net, Chondroitin sulfate proteoglycan, Astrogliosis, Nerve growth factor, Brain-derived neurotrophic factor, Glial cell-derived neurotrophic factor

Background

A disintegrin and metalloproteinase with thrombospondin motifs type 4, ADAMTS-4, belongs to the subfamily of ADAMTS proteases capable of degrading proteoglycans. The subfamily is composed of ADAMTS-1, −4, −5, −8, −9, −15 and −20 [1, 2]. Increasing evidence suggests that some ADAMTS proteoglycanases, for instance ADAMTS-1 and −4, may play critical roles in the control of synaptic plasticity during CNS development and aging via both protease-dependent and independent mechanisms [2–4]. In addition, administration of ADAMTS-4 has been recently described as a promising therapeutic strategy to improve axonal regeneration/collateral sprouting after spinal cord injury in rats by degrading chondroitin sulfate proteoglycans [5, 6]. While deregulated expression of ADAMTS proteoglycanases has been previously reported during acute CNS injuries, such as stroke [7–9] and spinal cord injury [5, 6, 10], the

* Correspondence: sighild.lemarchant@uef.fi
Department of Neurobiology, A. I. Virtanen Institute for Molecular Sciences, Biocenter Kuopio, University of Eastern Finland, P.O. Box 1627, 70211 Kuopio, Finland

expression and function of ADAMTS proteoglycanases have not been studied in neurodegenerative diseases, such as amyotrophic lateral sclerosis (ALS).

ALS is a devastating neurodegenerative disease characterized by the selective death of upper and lower motoneurons. Muscle wasting and weakness are early signs of ALS, and finally, the patient's death occurs usually within 3–5 years after disease onset. In 90 % of ALS cases, no apparent familial linkage has been identified, but in the remaining 10 % of the patients, the disease is inherited [11]. Autosomal dominant mutations in the *Cu, Zn-superoxide dismutase (SOD1)* gene account for 20 % of the familial disease form [12, 13]. The two forms of ALS are clinically indistinguishable and share many pathogenic features including oxidative damage, mitochondrial dysfunction, endoplasmic reticulum stress, excitotoxicity and inflammation [14]. Riluzole is the only FDA-approved drug for the treatment of ALS but it unfortunately has a modest impact of prolonging the life span of patients by only 2–3 months [15]. Therefore, it is essential to further understand mechanisms underlying ALS development in order to find new approaches for diagnostics and therapy.

Considering the beneficial effect of ADAMTS-4 on neuroplasticity, we aimed at investigating the expression, effects and associated mechanisms of ADAMTS-4 in ALS. While the expressions of ADAMTS-1, −5 and −9 were increased in the lumbar spinal cord of SOD1^{G93A} mice compared to corresponding WT littermates, the expression and activity of the most expressed proteoglycanase, ADAMTS-4, were reduced at the end-stage of the disease. To counteract the loss of ADAMTS-4 expression in the spinal cord, recombinant ADAMTS-4 was administered to SOD1^{G93A} mice early prior to the onset of symptoms by intracerebroventricular injections. Surprisingly, ADAMTS-4 treatment promoted the degeneration of lumbar spinal motoneurons by degrading their perineuronal nets and led to a detrimental functional outcome in SOD1^{G93A} mice. Our results also show that ADAMTS-4 decreased the synthesis and release of neurotrophic factors by astrocytes and microglia in vitro and in vivo.

While ADAMTS-4 has a beneficial impact on neuroplasticity and the subsequent functional outcome of injured rats after spinal cord injury, it may represent a damageable target in the context of ALS by accelerating neurodegeneration and clinical signs of neuromuscular dysfunctions in the SOD1^{G93A} mouse model. The modulation of the synthesis and release of neurotrophic factors by endogenous or exogenous ADAMTS-4 shows that ADAMTS-4 functions are not limited solely to the degradation of the extracellular matrix.

Results

ADAMTS-4 is the most expressed ADAMTS proteoglycanase in the central nervous system

We first studied the differential expression of ADAMTS proteoglycanases (ADAMTS-1, −4, −5, −9) in the lumbar spinal cord and in the cortex of adult WT mice by RT-PCR. ADAMTS-4 was at least 8-fold more expressed than the other ADAMTS proteoglycanases in the spinal cord and in the cortex of WT mice (Fig. 1a: $P = 0.0209$ and $P = 0.0495$, respectively). Confocal imaging revealed that the expression of ADAMTS-4 was widespread within the spinal cord in the grey matter and also in the white matter. Its expression was particularly abundant in ventral horn neurons (Fig. 1b), astrocytes (Fig. 1c) and oligodendrocytes (Fig. 1d). Negative controls with only the secondary antibody used for ADAMTS-4 staining failed to reveal any fluorescence (Fig. 1e).

Decrease of ADAMTS-4 activity in the lumbar spinal cord of SOD1^{G93A} mice at disease end-stage

We next studied the time course of the expression of ADAMTS proteoglycanases (ADAMTS-1, −4, −5, −9) in the lumbar spinal cord of SOD1^{G93A} and age-matched WT mice by RT-PCR at key time points of ALS progression (*eg.* presymptomatic (PS), symptomatic (SS) and end (ES) stages). ADAMTS-4 mRNA levels were considerably decreased in SOD1^{G93A} male mice compared to WT at the symptomatic and end-stages of the disease (Fig. 2a: −53.7 % at SS, −85.7 % at ES compared to age-matched WT, $P = 0.0209$). Contrary to ADAMTS-4, ADAMTS-1 (Fig. 2b: +92.1 % at SS, +410.7 % at ES compared to age-matched WT, $P = 0.0433$, $P = 0.0209$, respectively), ADAMTS-5 (Fig. 2c: +148.9 % at ES compared to age-matched WT, $P = 0.0339$) and ADAMTS-9 (Fig. 2d: +149.6 % at ES compared to age-matched WT, $P = 0.0209$) mRNA levels were significantly increased in the lumbar spinal cord of SOD1^{G93A} male mice compared to WT at the symptomatic and/or end-stages of the disease. Similarly, ADAMTS-4 mRNA levels were considerably decreased in the lumbar spinal cord of SOD1^{G93A} female mice compared to WT at all the stages of the disease (Fig. 2e: −38.9 % at PS, −48.9 % at SS, −82.7 % at ES compared to age-matched WT, $P = 0.0339$, $P = 0.0209$, $P = 0.0339$, respectively). Conversely, ADAMTS-1 (Fig. 2f: +60.5 % at SS, +472 % at ES compared to age-matched WT, $P = 0.0209$, $P = 0.0339$, respectively), ADAMTS-5 (Fig. 2g: +33.6 % at SS, +171 % at ES compared to age-matched WT, $P = 0.0209$, $P = 0.0339$, respectively) and ADAMTS-9 (Fig. 2h: +35.8 % at SS, +114,9 % at ES compared to age-matched WT, $P = 0.0209$, $P = 0.0339$, respectively) mRNA levels were significantly increased in the lumbar spinal cord of SOD1^{G93A} female mice compared to WT at the symptomatic and end-stages of the disease.

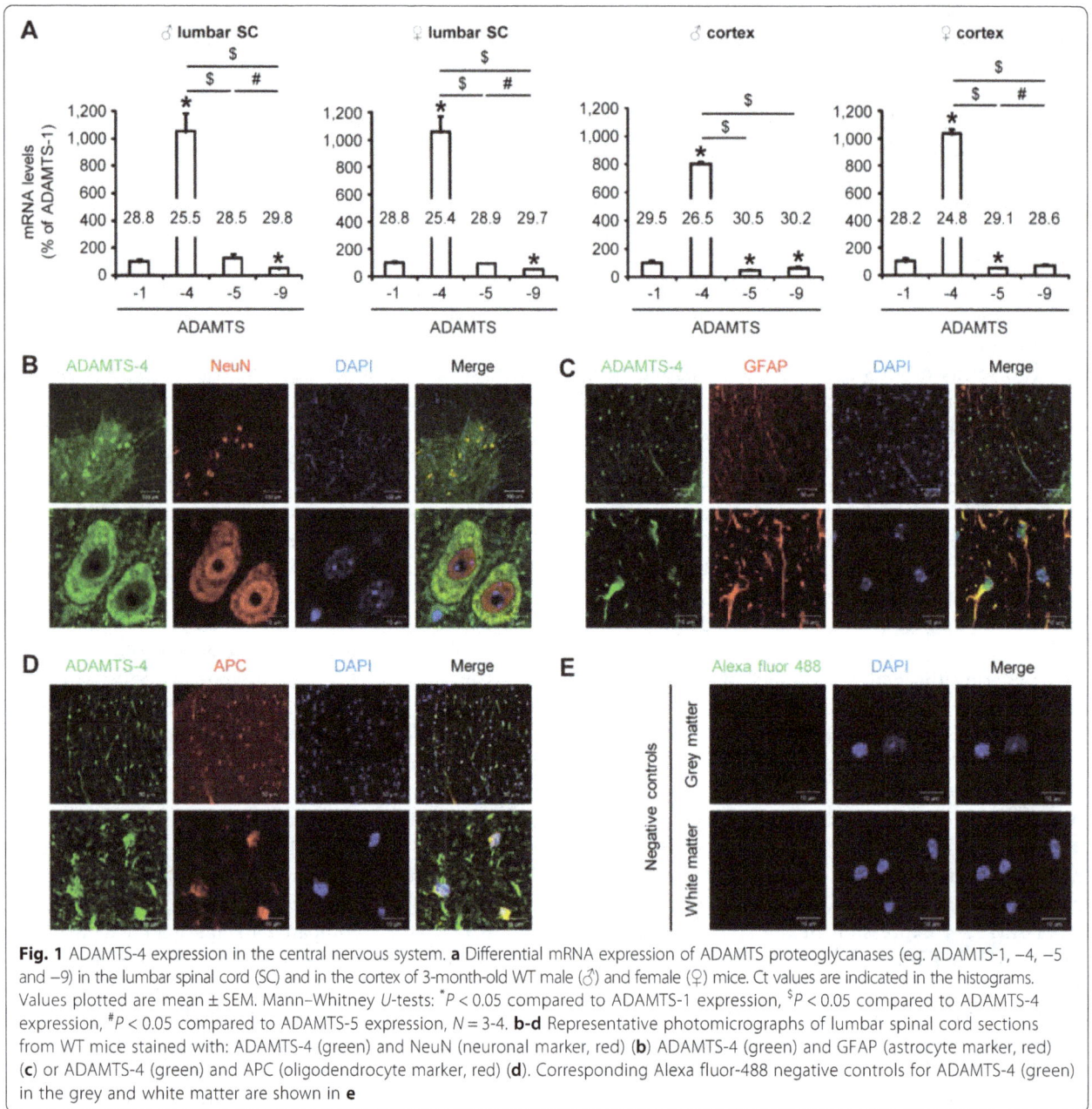

Fig. 1 ADAMTS-4 expression in the central nervous system. a Differential mRNA expression of ADAMTS proteoglycanases (eg. ADAMTS-1, −4, −5 and −9) in the lumbar spinal cord (SC) and in the cortex of 3-month-old WT male (♂) and female (♀) mice. Ct values are indicated in the histograms. Values plotted are mean ± SEM. Mann–Whitney U-tests: *$P < 0.05$ compared to ADAMTS-1 expression, $^$P < 0.05$ compared to ADAMTS-4 expression, #$P < 0.05$ compared to ADAMTS-5 expression, $N = 3$-4. b-d Representative photomicrographs of lumbar spinal cord sections from WT mice stained with: ADAMTS-4 (green) and NeuN (neuronal marker, red) (b) ADAMTS-4 (green) and GFAP (astrocyte marker, red) (c) or ADAMTS-4 (green) and APC (oligodendrocyte marker, red) (d). Corresponding Alexa fluor-488 negative controls for ADAMTS-4 (green) in the grey and white matter are shown in e

Confocal imaging revealed an abundant expression of ADAMTS-4 in ventral horn neurons of WT mice (Fig. 1b), and a loss/degeneration of motoneurons occurring at disease end-stage in SOD1^G93A mice (Fig. 2i).

No modifications of ADAMTS-4 protein levels were observed between WT and SOD1^G93A male mice at the presymptomatic and symptomatic stages (Fig. 2j-k: $P = 0.1482$ and $P = 0.5637$, respectively). However, at the end-stage of the disease, the decrease of ADAMTS-4 mRNA levels in the lumbar spinal cord of SOD1^G93A male mice was accompanied by a decrease of the protein levels of the mature form of ADAMTS-4 (p68) (Fig. 2l: −50.1 % at ES compared to age-matched WT, $P = 0.0209$) and an increase of its

truncated form (p53) (Fig. 2l: +898.5 % at ES compared to age-matched WT, $P = 0.0209$). As previously observed for SOD1^G93A male mice, no modifications of ADAMTS-4 protein levels were observed between WT and SOD1^G93A female mice at the presymptomatic and symptomatic stages (Fig. 2m-n: $P = 0.5637$ and $P = 0.2482$, respectively), but at the end-stage of the disease, the decrease of ADAMTS-4 mRNA levels in the lumbar spinal cord of SOD1^G93A female mice was accompanied by a decrease of the protein levels of the mature form of ADAMTS-4 (p68) (Fig. 2o: −52.4 % at ES compared to age-matched WT, $P = 0.0143$) and an increase of its truncated form (p53) (Fig. 2o: +218 % at ES compared to age-matched WT,

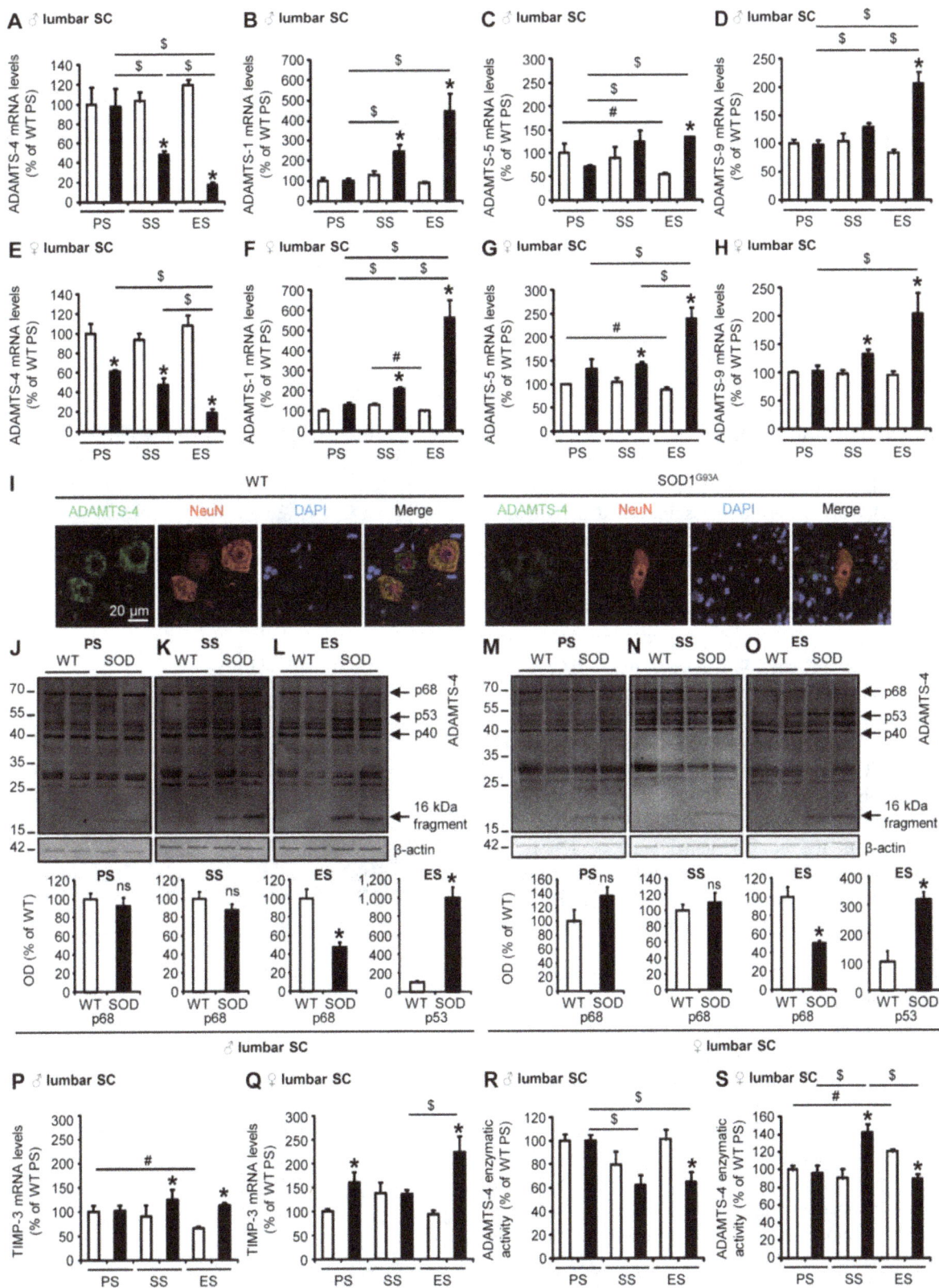

Fig. 2 (See legend on next page.)

(See figure on previous page.)
Fig. 2 Decrease of ADAMTS-4 activity in the lumbar spinal cord of SOD1^{G93A} mice at disease end-stage. **a-h** Quantitative RT-PCR for ADAMTS-4 (**a, e**) ADAMTS-1 (**b, f**) −5 (**c, g**) and −9 (**d, h**) expression in the lumbar spinal cord (SC) of WT (blank bar) and SOD1^{G93A} (black bar) male (♂; **a, b, c, d**) or female (♀; **e, f, g, h**) mice at presymptomatic (PS), symptomatic (SS) and end (ES) stages. Values plotted are mean ± SEM. Mann–Whitney U-tests: *$P < 0.05$ compared to corresponding WT mice, $^{S}P < 0.05$ compared to SOD1^{G93A} mice at other stages, #$P < 0.05$ compared to WT mice at other stages, N = 3-4. **i** Representative photomicrographs of ventral horns in lumbar spinal cord sections from WT and SOD1^{G93A} mice at end-stage stained with ADAMTS-4 (green) and NeuN (neuronal marker, red). Scale bar = 20 m. **j-o** Immunoblot for ADAMTS-4 in the lumbar spinal cord of WT and SOD1^{G93A} male (**j-l**) and female (**m-o**) mice at PS, SS and ES. The immunoblots revealed ADAMTS-4 mature form (p68), ADAMTS-4 truncated forms (p53, p40) and a 16 kDa fragment. Values plotted are mean ± SEM. Mann–Whitney U-tests: *$P < 0.05$ compared to corresponding WT mice, N = 4-5. **p-q** Quantitative RT-PCR for TIMP-3 in the lumbar spinal cord of WT and SOD1^{G93A} male (**p**) and female (**q**) mice at PS, SS and ES. Values plotted are mean ± SEM. Mann–Whitney U-tests: *$P < 0.05$ compared to corresponding WT mice, $^{S}P < 0.05$ compared to SOD1^{G93A} mice at other stages, #$P < 0.05$ compared to WT mice at other stages, N = 3-4. **r-s** ADAMTS-4 enzymatic activity assay in the lumbar spinal cord of WT and SOD1^{G93A} male (**r**) and female (**s**) mice at PS, SS and ES. Values plotted are mean ± SEM. Mann–Whitney U-tests: *$P < 0.05$ compared to corresponding WT mice, $^{S}P < 0.05$ compared to SOD1^{G93A} mice at other stages, #$P < 0.05$ compared to WT mice at other stages, N = 4

$P = 0.0209$). No significant modifications of ADAMTS-4 truncated form (p40) were observed (Figs. 2l, o: quantifications not shown).

Then, quantitative RT-PCR was performed for the mRNA expression of the most potent inhibitor of ADAMTS-4, TIMP-3 (type 3 tissue inhibitor of metalloproteinases) [16], in the lumbar spinal cord of WT and SOD1^{G93A} male and female mice at the different stages of the disease. TIMP-3 mRNA levels were found to be increased in the lumbar spinal cord of SOD1^{G93A} male mice compared to WT at the symptomatic and end-stages of the disease (Fig. 2p: +38.3 % at SS, +70.8 % at ES compared to age-matched WT, $P = 0.0339$, $P = 0.0209$, respectively). For female mice, TIMP-3 mRNA levels were also increased in the lumbar spinal cord of SOD1^{G93A} mice compared to WT at the presymptomatic and end-stages of the disease (Fig. 2q: +59.6 % at PS, +138.8 % at ES compared to age-matched WT, $P = 0.0339$).

Consequently, the enzymatic activity of ADAMTS-4 was reduced in the lumbar spinal cord of SOD1^{G93A} male (Fig. 2r: −35.8 % at ES compared to age-matched WT, $P = 0.0209$) and female (Fig. 2s: −25.9 % at ES compared to age-matched WT, $P = 0.0209$) mice at disease end-stage

To further examine whether the loss of ADAMTS-4 at disease end-stage was specific to the lumbar spinal cord, we studied the expression of ADAMTS-4 in the cervical and thoracic parts of the spinal cord, as well as in the cortex, of WT and SOD1^{G93A} mice by western blot. Interestingly, there was a decrease of ADAMTS-4 expression in the cervical and thoracic spinal cord of SOD1^{G93A} male mice compared to WT (Fig. 3a-b: −65.5 % in the cervical (A) and −38.2 % in the thoracic (B) spinal cord at ES compared to age-matched WT, $P = 0.0209$), but no significant modification of ADAMTS-4 expression in the cortex was observed (Fig. 3c: $P = 0.1489$). For females, no modification of ADAMTS-4 expression was observed in the cervical spinal cord of SOD1^{G93A} mice compared to WT (Fig. 3d: $P = 0.1489$), but we observed a significant decrease of ADAMTS-4 expression in the thoracic spinal

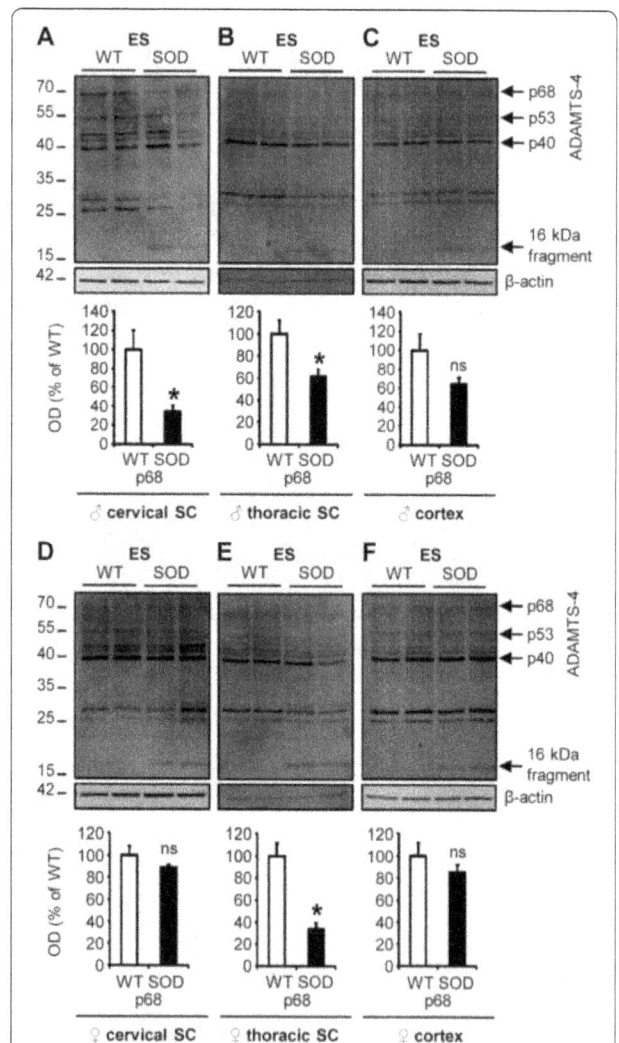

Fig. 3 Spinal cord-specific decrease of ADAMTS-4 expression in SOD1^{G93A} mice at disease end-stage. **a-f** Immunoblot for ADAMTS-4 in the cervical or thoracic spinal cord (SC) and in the cortex of WT (blank bar) and SOD1^{G93A} (black bar) male (♂; **a, b, c**) or female (♀; **d, e, f**) mice at disease end-stage (ES). Values plotted are mean ± SEM. Mann–Whitney U-tests: *$P < 0.05$ compared to corresponding WT mice, N = 4

cord of SOD1^{G93A} mice compared to WT (Fig. 3e: –66.3 % in the thoracic spinal cord at ES compared to age-matched WT, $P = 0.0209$). Again, no modification of ADAMTS-4 expression was observed in the cortex (Fig. 3f: $P = 0.2207$). No significant modifications of ADAMTS-4 truncated forms (p53 and p40) were observed (Figs. 3a-f; quantifications not shown). We also observed the appearance of a 16 kDa fragment in protein extracts of both spinal cords and cortices of SOD1^{G93A} mice at all the stages of the disease, even when the mature form of ADAMTS-4 (p68) was unchanged when compared to corresponding WT mice (Fig. 2j-o, Fig. 3a-f).

Then, we studied the expression of ADAMTS-5 in the lumbar spinal cord of WT and SOD1^{G93A} mice by western blot. Surprisingly, while the mRNA levels of ADAMTS-5 were increased in the lumbar spinal cord at the end-stage in SOD1^{G93A} male mice and at the symptomatic and end-stages in SOD1^{G93A} female mice, no modifications were found at the protein levels between

WT and SOD1^{G93A} mice at any stage of the disease (Fig. 4a-c: $P = 0.0833$, $P = 0.3865$, $P = 0.2482$ at PS, SS and ES respectively compared to age-matched male WT; Fig. 4d-f: $P = 0.5637$, $P = 0.2482$, $P = 0.5637$ at PS, SS and ES respectively compared to age-matched female WT).

To summarize, the expression and the synthesis of ADAMTS-4 and its inhibitor TIMP-3, as well as ADAMTS-4 proteolytic cleavage profile, were considerably altered in the spinal cord of SOD1^{G93A} mice at the end-stage of the disease, representing a series of events leading to the decrease of ADAMTS-4 enzymatic activity.

Presymptomatic treatment with recombinant ADAMTS-4 worsens the prognosis of SOD1^{G93A} mice

To prevent the loss of ADAMTS-4 activity at disease end-stage, a human recombinant ADAMTS-4 previously shown to be biologically active and to support neuroplasticity [5] was administered to SOD1^{G93A} mice early before the onset of symptoms by intracerebroventricular

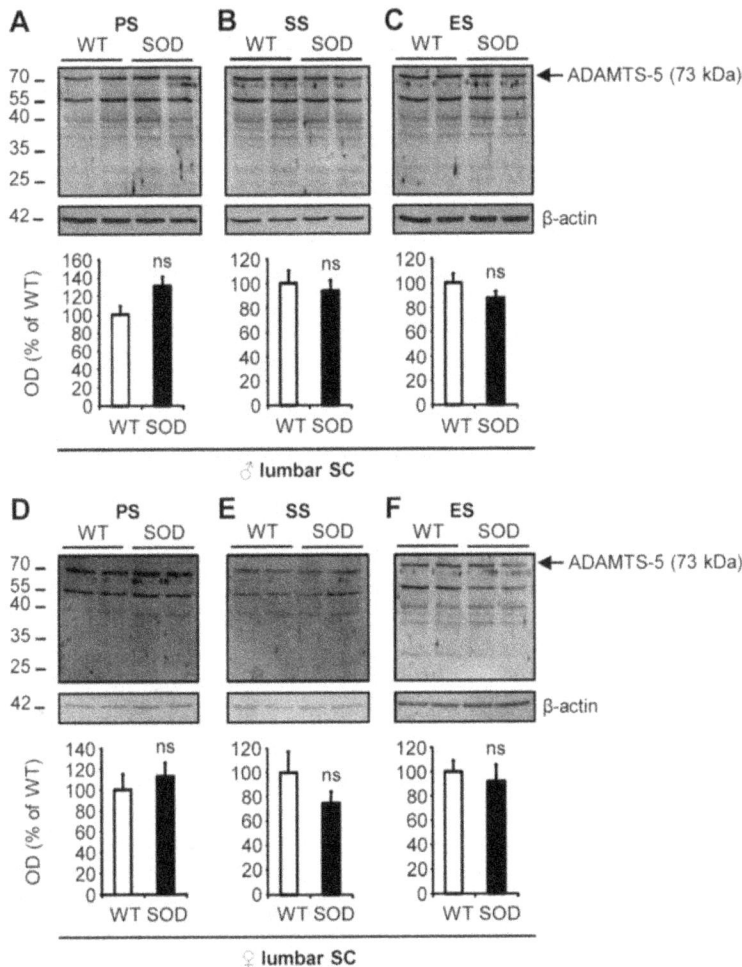

Fig. 4 No modification of ADAMTS-5 expression in the lumbar spinal cord of SOD1^{G93A} mice at any stage of the disease. **a-f** Immunoblot for ADAMTS-5 (73 kDa) in the lumbar spinal cord of WT and SOD1^{G93A} male (**a-c**) and female (**d-f**) mice at PS, SS and ES. Values plotted are mean ± SEM. Mann–Whitney U-tests: $P > 0.05$ compared to corresponding WT mice, $N = 4$

injections. Control SOD1^{G93A} mice were injected with saline in the same conditions. Age-matched WT mice were also treated with saline or ADAMTS-4. The onset of symptoms was determined by the appearance of clinical signs of neuromuscular dysfunction, measured by the loss of ability for SOD1^{G93A} mice to hold onto an inverted lid. ADAMTS-4 treatment was detrimental in SOD1^{G93A} male mice by bringing forward the probability of onset of symptoms compared to saline-treated SOD1^{G93A} male mice (Fig. 5a: median asymptomatic survival: 189 d for control and 174 d for ADAMTS-4 SOD1^{G93A}, $P = 0.0488$). Accordingly, there was a significant decrease of the age at symptom onset in ADAMTS-4-treated SOD1^{G93A} male mice (Fig. 5b: average age of onset: 197.8 ± 8.5 d for control and 176.2 ± 3.9 d for ADAMTS-4 SOD1^{G93A}, $P = 0.0423$). No change in the latency to fall was observed during the first week following the symptom onset between ADAMTS-4-treated and saline-treated SOD1^{G93A} male mice (Fig. 5c: time latency to fall: 156.7 ± 14.0 s for control and 160.4 ± 5.2 s for ADAMTS-4 SOD1^{G93A}, $P = 0.7573$). Surprisingly, ADAMTS-4 treatment did not affect the probability of symptom onset (Fig. 5d: median asymptomatic survival: 241 d for control and 240.5 d for ADAMTS-4 SOD1^{G93A}, $P = 0.4787$) or the age at symptom onset in ADAMTS-4-treated SOD1^{G93A} female mice compared to untreated mice (Fig. 5e: average age of onset: 236.0 ± 5.0 d for control and 240.3 ± 6.2 d for ADAMTS-4 SOD1^{G93A}, $P = 0.3798$). However, the latency to fall during the first week following the symptom onset was significantly reduced in ADAMTS-4-treated SOD1^{G93A} female mice compared to untreated mice (Fig. 5f: time latency to fall: 157.6 ± 5.3 s for control and 107.8 ± 18.5 s for ADAMTS-4 SOD1^{G93A}, $P = 0.0455$). Failure to gain body weight is another indicator of disease onset and progression in SOD1^{G93A} mice, therefore the weight of WT and SOD1^{G93A} mice was recorded from 150 to 190 days for males (Fig. 5g) and from 200 to 240 days for females (Fig. 5h). While no genotype effect was evident in male mice at any time point, there was a genotype effect in female mice. Contrary to WT female mice, the SOD1^{G93A} female mice failed to gain weight over time. We did not observe any change in the weight of ADAMTS-4-treated WT mice (Figs. 5g-h: $P > 0.05$). Overall, our data show that preventing the loss of endogenous ADAMTS-4 activity by exogenous provision of an active human recombinant protein is detrimental for functional outcome in the context of ALS.

ADAMTS-4 treatment accelerates neurodegeneration in the ventral horn of the lumbar spinal cord in SOD1^{G93A} mice

Motoneuron survival in the ventral horn of lumbar spinal cord of WT and SOD1^{G93A} mice was quantified

to determine whether the decline of motor function in ADAMTS-4-treated SOD1^{G93A} mice was a result of accelerated spinal cord pathology. In SOD1^{G93A} mice, there was an approximately 50 % loss of motoneurons compared to age-matched WT mice (Fig. 6: $P < 0.001$). ADAMTS-4 did not affect the severity of motoneuron loss in SOD1^{G93A} male mice (Fig. 6a, b: $P = 0.8297$). However, the size of the remaining motoneurons was significantly smaller in ADAMTS-4-treated SOD1^{G93A}-mice (Fig. 6a, c: -13.8 % for ADAMTS-4-treated SOD1^{G93A} mice compared to untreated SOD1^{G93A} mice, $P = 0.0496$). On the contrary, the number of motoneurons was decreased by approximately 2-fold in ADAMTS-4-treated SOD1^{G93A} female mice compared to untreated SOD1^{G93A} female mice (Fig. 6d, e: -55.7 % for ADAMTS-4-treated SOD1^{G93A} mice compared to untreated SOD1^{G93A} mice, $P = 0.0347$). However, the size of the remaining motoneurons was not different from those of untreated SOD1^{G93A} female mice (Fig. 6d, f: $P = 0.6961$). ADAMTS-4 treatment had no effect on motoneurons in WT mice. Overall, the results demonstrate that ADAMTS-4 promotes neurodegeneration in ALS pathology.

ADAMTS-4 treatment reduces perineuronal nets enwrapping motoneurons in the ventral horn of the lumbar spinal cord in SOD1^{G93A} mice

To further understand how ADAMTS-4 promotes degeneration/cell death of motoneurons, we then quantified perineuronal nets (PNNs) enwrapping motoneurons, which are protective extracellular matrix (ECM)-envelopes containing chondroitin sulfate proteoglycans (CSPGs), well-known substrates for ADAMTS-4 [17]. For this purpose, lumbar spinal cord sections of SOD1^{G93A} and age-matched WT mice treated or not with ADAMTS-4 were stained with Wisteria Floribunda Agglutin (WFA), a common marker for PNNs [18, 19]. In SOD1^{G93A} mice, there was an approximately 70 % loss of PNNs compared to age-matched WT mice at symptomatic stage (Fig. 7: $P < 0.001$). The amount of the remaining PNNs was even smaller in ADAMTS-4-treated SOD1^{G93A} male (Fig. 7a-b: -69.4 % for ADAMTS-4-treated SOD1^{G93A} mice compared to untreated SOD1^{G93A} mice, $P = 0.0040$) and female (Fig. 7c-d: -74 % for ADAMTS-4-treated SOD1^{G93A} mice compared to untreated SOD1^{G93A} mice, $P = 0.0210$) mice. Additionally, the amount of PNNs was positively correlated with the number of motoneurons in the ventral horn of the spinal cords (Fig. 7e: $P = 0.0002$, $R = 0.5474$). Again, ADAMTS-4 treatment had no effect on PNNs of WT mice. To determine why the PNNs of SOD1^{G93A} mice were sensitive to ADAMTS-4 treatment while PNNs of WT mice were not, RT-qPCR were carried out for the expression of several PNN components in the lumbar spinal cord of WT and SOD1^{G93A} mice: aggrecan (a CSPG present exclusively

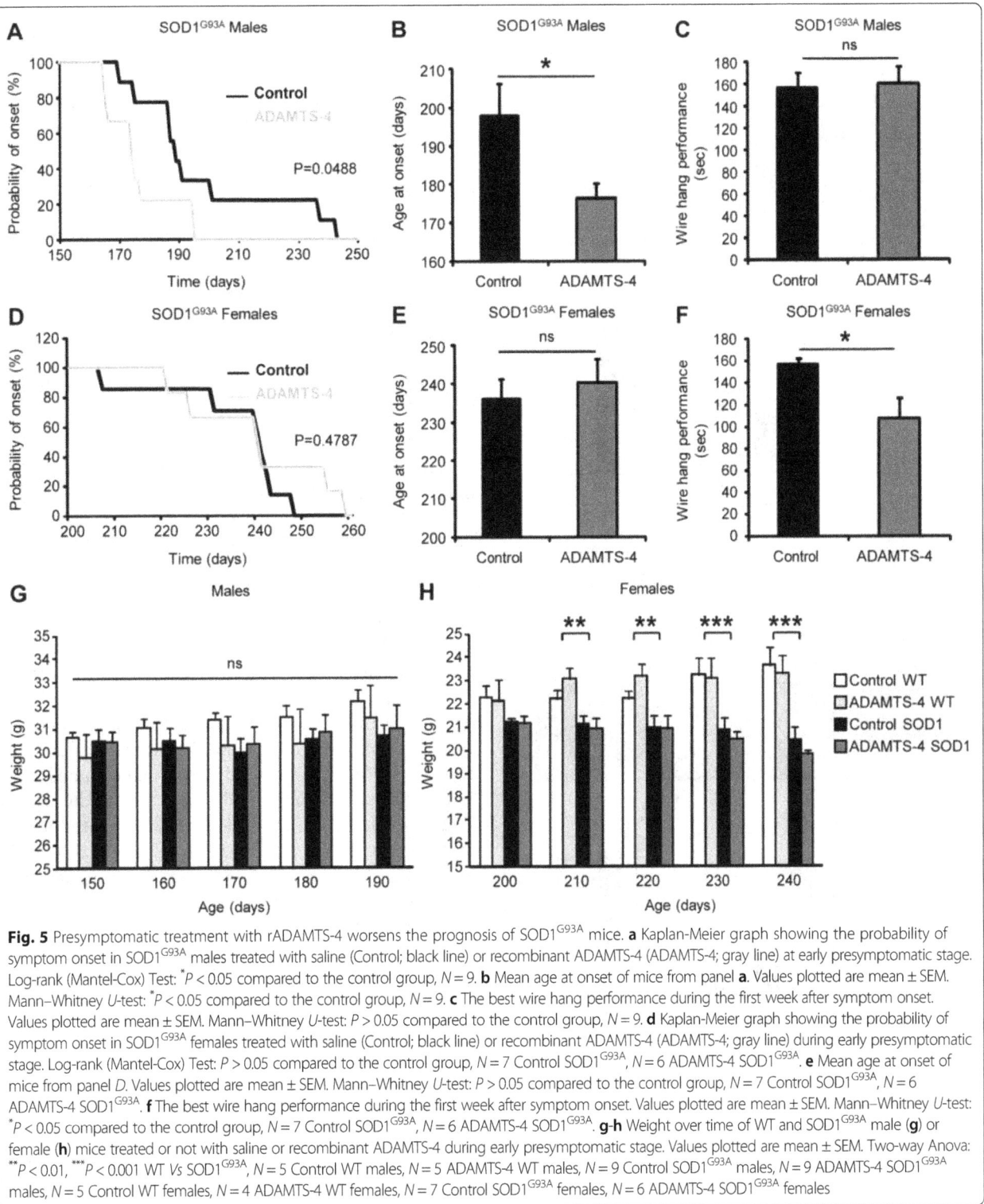

Fig. 5 Presymptomatic treatment with rADAMTS-4 worsens the prognosis of SOD1^{G93A} mice. **a** Kaplan-Meier graph showing the probability of symptom onset in SOD1^{G93A} males treated with saline (Control; black line) or recombinant ADAMTS-4 (ADAMTS-4; gray line) at early presymptomatic stage. Log-rank (Mantel-Cox) Test: *$P < 0.05$ compared to the control group, $N = 9$. **b** Mean age at onset of mice from panel **a**. Values plotted are mean ± SEM. Mann–Whitney U-test: *$P < 0.05$ compared to the control group, $N = 9$. **c** The best wire hang performance during the first week after symptom onset. Values plotted are mean ± SEM. Mann–Whitney U-test: $P > 0.05$ compared to the control group, $N = 9$. **d** Kaplan-Meier graph showing the probability of symptom onset in SOD1^{G93A} females treated with saline (Control; black line) or recombinant ADAMTS-4 (ADAMTS-4; gray line) during early presymptomatic stage. Log-rank (Mantel-Cox) Test: $P > 0.05$ compared to the control group, $N = 7$ Control SOD1^{G93A}, $N = 6$ ADAMTS-4 SOD1^{G93A}. **e** Mean age at onset of mice from panel D. Values plotted are mean ± SEM. Mann–Whitney U-test: $P > 0.05$ compared to the control group, $N = 7$ Control SOD1^{G93A}, $N = 6$ ADAMTS-4 SOD1^{G93A}. **f** The best wire hang performance during the first week after symptom onset. Values plotted are mean ± SEM. Mann–Whitney U-test: *$P < 0.05$ compared to the control group, $N = 7$ Control SOD1^{G93A}, $N = 6$ ADAMTS-4 SOD1^{G93A}. **g-h** Weight over time of WT and SOD1^{G93A} male (**g**) or female (**h**) mice treated or not with saline or recombinant ADAMTS-4 during early presymptomatic stage. Values plotted are mean ± SEM. Two-way Anova: **$P < 0.01$, ***$P < 0.001$ WT Vs SOD1^{G93A}, $N = 5$ Control WT males, $N = 5$ ADAMTS-4 WT males, $N = 9$ Control SOD1^{G93A} males, $N = 9$ ADAMTS-4 SOD1^{G93A} males, $N = 5$ Control WT females, $N = 4$ ADAMTS-4 WT females, $N = 7$ Control SOD1^{G93A} females, $N = 6$ ADAMTS-4 SOD1^{G93A} females

in PNNs), HPLAN1 (hyaluronan and proteoglycan link protein 1; involved in the interaction between hyaluronan and CSPGs) and tenascin R (involved in the interaction between the cell surface and CSPGs). Importantly, we observed a decrease of aggrecan expression in the lumbar spinal cord of SOD1^{G93A} male mice compared to WT at the presymptomatic and end-stages of the disease (Fig. 7f: −20.5 % at PS, −30 % at ES compared to age-matched WT, $P = 0.0339$). For female mice, aggrecan mRNA levels were also decreased in the lumbar spinal cord

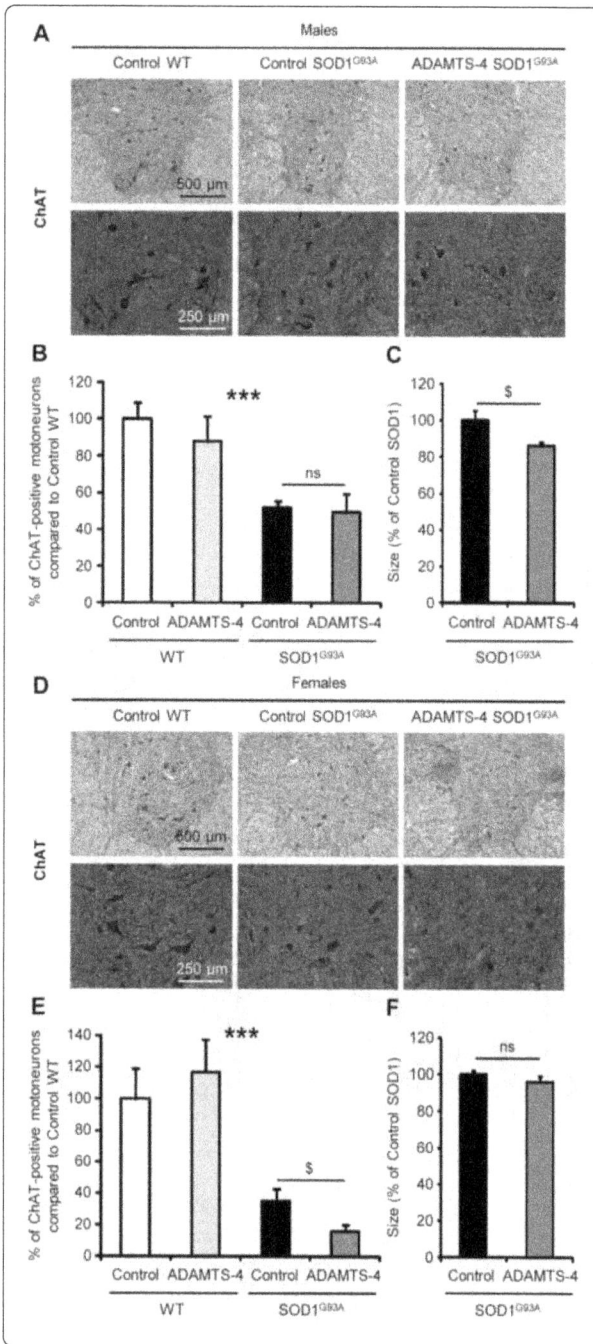

Fig. 6 rADAMTS-4 accelerates neurodegeneration in the lumbar spinal cord of SOD1^{G93A} mice. **a** Representative photomicrographs of ventral horns in lumbar spinal cord sections from WT and control or ADAMTS-4-treated SOD1^{G93A} male mice stained with ChAT. Scale bar: 500 or 250 m. **b-c** Quantification of average spinal motoneuron number (**b**) and size (**c**) in male mice from (**a**). Values plotted are mean ± SEM. Two-way ANOVA: $^{***}P < 0.001$ WT Vs SOD1^{G93A}. Unpaired two-tailed t-Test: $P > 0.05$ (Number) or $^{\$}P < 0.05$ (Size) Control Vs ADAMTS-4 SOD1^{G93A}, $N = 3$ Control WT, $N = 5$ ADAMTS-4 WT, $N = 8$ Control SOD1^{G93A}, $N = 7$ ADAMTS-4 SOD1^{G93A}. **d** Representative photomicrographs of ventral horns in lumbar spinal cord sections from WT and control or ADAMTS-4-treated SOD1^{G93A} female mice stained with ChAT. Scale bar: 500 or 250 m. **e-f** Quantification of average spinal motoneuron number (**e**) and size (**f**) in female mice from (**d**). Values plotted are mean ± SEM. Two-way ANOVA: $^{***}P < 0.001$ WT Vs SOD1^{G93A}. Unpaired two-tailed t-Test: $^{\$}P < 0.05$ (Number) or $P > 0.05$ (Size) Control Vs ADAMTS-4 SOD1^{G93A}, $N = 5$ Control WT, $N = 3$ ADAMTS-4 WT, $N = 5$ Control SOD1^{G93A}, $N = 6$ ADAMTS-4 SOD1^{G93A}

of SOD1^{G93A} mice compared to WT at the end-stage of the disease (Fig. 7g: –34 % at ES compared to age-matched WT, $P = 0.0339$). Then, we observed a decrease of HAPLN1 expression in the lumbar spinal cord of SOD1^{G93A} male mice compared to WT at the presymptomatic and end-stages of the disease (Fig. 7h: –30.7 % at PS, –42.7 % at ES compared to age-matched WT, $P = 0.0339$). For female mice, HAPLN1 mRNA levels were also decreased in the lumbar spinal cord of SOD1^{G93A} mice compared to WT at the end-stage of the disease (Fig. 7i: –48.1 % at ES compared to age-matched WT, $P = 0.0339$). Finally, we observed an increase of tenascin R expression in the lumbar spinal cord of SOD1^{G93A} male and female mice compared to WT at the symptomatic and end-stages of the disease (Fig. 7j: +33.6 % at SS, +74.3 % at ES compared to age-matched male WT, $P = 0.0339$; Fig. 7k: +25.3 % at SS, +47.7 % at ES compared to age-matched female WT, $P = 0.0433$ and 0.0339 respectively). To determine whether the degradation of CSPG core protein present in PNNs was specific of ADAMTS-4 recombinant protein, we exposed or not lumbar spinal cord protein extracts from SOD1^{G93A} male mice at symptomatic stage to human recombinant ADAMTS-1, ADAMTS-4 or ADAMTS-5 *ex vivo* for 24 h at 37 °C. Interestingly, we evidenced that only ADAMTS-4 recombinant protein was successful to degrade CSPG core proteins *ex vivo* (Fig. 7l: –53 % of CSPG core proteins in ADAMTS-4-incubated protein extracts compared to the control condition, $P = 0.0209$; $P > 0.05$ between ADAMTS-1 or ADAMTS-5-incubated protein extracts and the control condition).

ADAMTS-4 treatment increases astrogliosis in the ventral horn of the lumbar spinal cord of female SOD1^{G93A} mice
Astrogliosis and microgliosis are classical hallmarks of ALS pathology and strongly contribute to neurodegeneration.

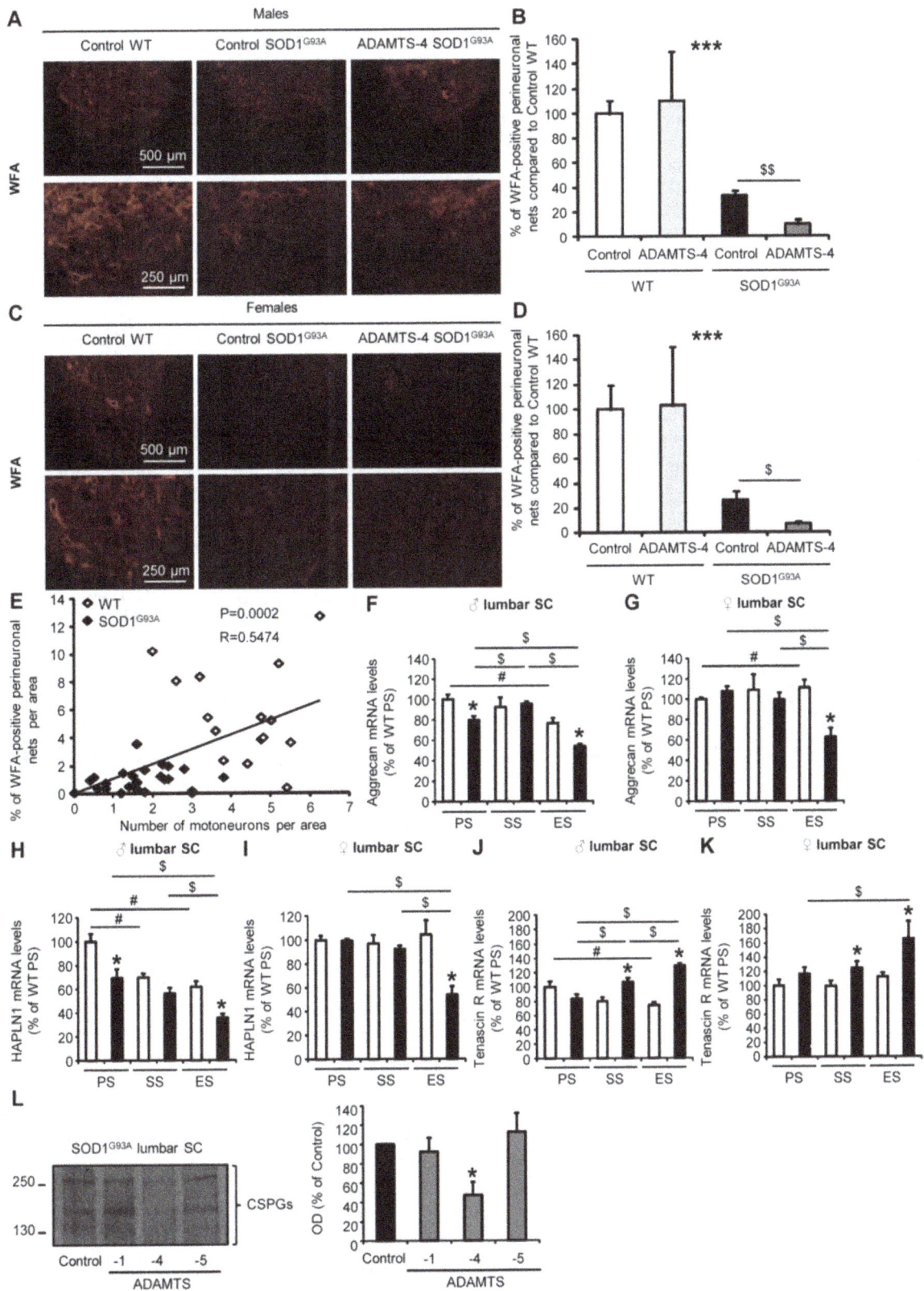

Fig. 7 (See legend on next page.)

(See figure on previous page.)

Fig. 7 rADAMTS-4 reduces perineuronal nets enwrapping motoneurons in the lumbar spinal cord of SOD1^{G93A} mice. **a** Representative photomicrographs of ventral horns in lumbar spinal cord sections from WT and control or ADAMTS-4-treated SOD1^{G93A} male mice stained with WFA, a marker of perineuronal nets. Scale bar: 500 or 250 m. **b** Quantification of WFA immunoreactivity per area from male mice (**a**). Values plotted are mean ± SEM. Two-way ANOVA: $^{***}P < 0.001$ WT Vs SOD1^{G93A}. Unpaired two-tailed t-Test: $^{\$\$}P < 0.01$ Control Vs ADAMTS-4 SOD1^{G93A}, N = 3 Control WT, N = 5 ADAMTS-4 WT, N = 8 Control SOD1^{G93A}, N = 7 ADAMTS-4 SOD1^{G93A}. **c** Representative photomicrographs of ventral horns in lumbar spinal cord sections from WT and control or ADAMTS-4-treated SOD1^{G93A} female mice stained with WFA. Scale bar: 500 or 250 m. **d** Quantification of WFA immunoreactivity per area from female mice (**c**). Values plotted are mean ± SEM. Two-way ANOVA: $^{***}P < 0.001$ WT Vs SOD1^{G93A}. Unpaired two-tailed t-Test: $^{\$}P < 0.05$ Control Vs ADAMTS-4 SOD1^{G93A}, N = 5 Control WT, N = 3 ADAMTS-4 WT, N = 5 Control SOD1^{G93A}, N = 6 ADAMTS-4 SOD1^{G93A}. **e** Positive correlation between the percentage of WFA-positive perineuronal nets per area and the number of motoneurons in male and female WT (N = 15; blank diamond) and SOD1^{G93A} (N = 24; black diamond) symptomatic mice from figs. 4-5. Spearman's rank correlation: $^{***}P < 0.001$. R represents the coefficient of correlation. **f-k** Quantitative RT-PCR for aggrecan (**f-g**) HAPLN1 (**h-i**) and tenascin R (**j-k**) in the lumbar spinal cord of WT and SOD1^{G93A} male (**f, h, j**) and female (**g, i, k**) mice at PS, SS and ES. Values plotted are mean ± SEM. Mann–Whitney U-tests: $^{*}P < 0.05$ compared to corresponding WT mice, $^{\$}P < 0.05$ compared to SOD1^{G93A} mice at other stages, $^{\#}P < 0.05$ compared to WT mice at other stages, N = 3-4. **l** Immunoblot for CSPG (chondroitin sulfate proteoglycans) core proteins in lumbar spinal cord protein extracts of SOD1^{G93A} mice exposed to human recombinant ADAMTS-1, ADAMTS-4 or ADAMTS-5 ex vivo for 24 h at 37 °C. Quantification of total CSPG core proteins. Values plotted are mean ± SEM. Mann–Whitney U-tests: $^{*}P < 0.05$ between control and ADAMTS-4 conditions, N = 4

Therefore, we next investigated whether ADAMTS-4 increases gliosis in the ventral horn of the lumbar spinal cord of SOD1^{G93A} compared to untreated SOD1^{G93A} mice. In SOD1^{G93A} mice, there was a remarkable increase of the astrocyte marker, GFAP (glial fibrillary acidic protein), compared to age-matched WT mice (Fig. 8a-c: $P < 0.001$). While no modification of GFAP expression was observed in ADAMTS-4-treated SOD1^{G93A} male mice compared to untreated SOD1^{G93A} male mice (Fig. 8b: $P = 0.8514$), ADAMTS-4 significantly increased GFAP immunoreactivity in SOD1^{G93A} female mice (Fig. 8c: +126.7 % for ADAMTS-4-treated SOD1^{G93A} mice compared to untreated SOD1^{G93A} mice, $P = 0.0414$). In SOD1^{G93A} mice, there was an approximately 10-fold increase of the microglial marker, Iba1 (ionized calcium-binding adapter molecule-1), compared to age-matched WT mice (Fig. 8d-f: $P < 0.001$). No change in Iba1 expression was observed in ADAMTS-4-treated SOD1^{G93A} mice compared to untreated SOD1^{G93A} mice (Fig. 8e-f: $P = 0.1146$ for males and $P = 0.5893$ for females). GFAP and Iba1 immunoreactivities in WT mice were not altered by ADAMTS-4 treatment.

ADAMTS-4 treatment does not directly affect neuronal survival in vitro

Glutamate-induced excitotoxicity represents a key pathophysiological process in ALS contributing to neurodegeneration through activation of Ca^{2+}-dependent enzymatic pathways [14]. We therefore aimed at determining whether ADAMTS-4 directly influenced neuronal death in vitro using cortical neurons exposed or not to glutamate for 24 h. Exogenous ADAMTS-4 was not toxic to neurons in control conditions (Fig. 9a: $P = 0.4158$). When neurons were exposed to glutamate, the amount of viable cells was decreased by about 40 % (Fig. 9b, d: $P < 0.0001$). However, ADAMTS-4 did not promote glutamate-induced toxicity (Fig. 9b: $P = 0.3559$, $P = 0.1962$, $P = 0.2505$, $P = 0.2423$ for cell viability when neurons were

exposed to glutamate compared to glutamate in presence of ADAMTS-4 at 20, 100, 200, 500 ng/ml respectively). Similarly, we did not observe any influence of exogenous ADAMTS-1 on neuronal viability in control conditions (Fig. 9c: $P = 0.5896$) or after glutamate exposure (Fig. 9d: $P > 0.9999$, $P = 0.7782$, $P = 0.8880$, $P = 0.5732$ for cell viability when neurons were exposed to glutamate compared to glutamate in presence of ADAMTS-1 at 20, 100, 200, 500 ng/ml respectively).

Exogenous and endogenous ADAMTS-4 modulate the expression and release of neurotrophic factors by glial cells in vitro

Since ADAMTS-4 did not influence directly neuronal survival in vitro (Fig. 9), we aimed at investigating secondary pathways through which ADAMTS-4 may confer the neurodegeneration/death observed in vivo (Fig. 6). For that purpose, we investigated whether ADAMTS-4 may modulate the expression and/or release of neurotrophic factors such as NGF (nerve growth factor), GDNF (glial cell-derived neurotrophic factor) and BDNF (brain-derived neurotrophic factor), in astrocyte and microglia cultures. ADAMTS-4 was found to decrease the mRNA levels of NGF (Fig. 10a: −30.2 % or −28.1 % for astrocytes treated with ADAMTS-4 at 20 or 100 ng/ml compared to control astrocytes, $P = 0.0209$), GDNF (Fig. 10b: −11.9 % for astrocytes treated with ADAMTS-4 at 200 ng/ml compared to control astrocytes, $P = 0.0209$) and BDNF (Fig. 10c: −25.2 %, −25.6 % or −14.9 % for astrocytes treated with ADAMTS-4 at 20, 100 or 200 ng/ml compared to control astrocytes, $P = 0.0209$) in astrocytes. The reduction of NGF mRNA levels by ADAMTS-4 (Fig. 10a) was accompanied by a decrease of NGF present in the culture media (Fig. 10d: −15.9 % or −23.1 % for astrocytes treated with ADAMTS-4 at 20 or 100 ng/ml compared to control astrocytes, $P = 0.0495$). This effect was specific to ADAMTS-4, since a human recombinant ADAMTS-1 did not change the levels of NGF present in

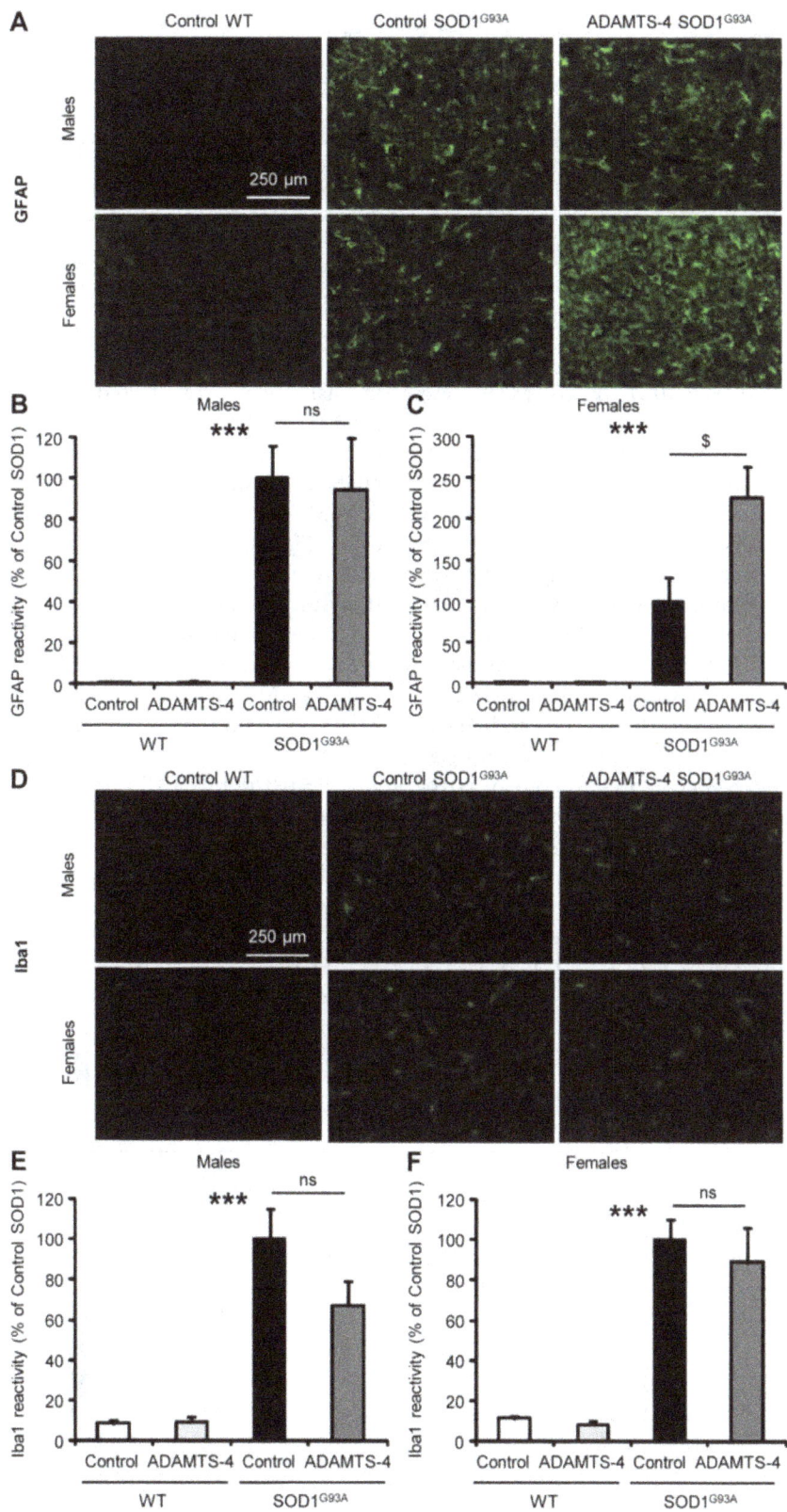

Fig. 8 (See legend on next page.)

(See figure on previous page.)
Fig. 8 rADAMTS-4 increases astrogliosis in the lumbar spinal cord of female SOD1^{G93A} mice. **a** Representative photomicrographs of ventral horns in lumbar spinal cord sections from WT and control or ADAMTS-4-treated SOD1^{G93A} mice stained with GFAP. Scale bar: 250 m. **b** Quantification of GFAP immunoreactivity per area from male mice (**a**). Values plotted are mean ± SEM. Two-way ANOVA: $^{***}P < 0.001$ WT Vs SOD1^{G93A}. Unpaired two-tailed t-Test: $P > 0.05$ Control Vs ADAMTS-4 SOD1^{G93A}, $N = 3$ Control WT, $N = 5$ ADAMTS-4 WT, $N = 8$ Control SOD1^{G93A}, $N = 7$ ADAMTS-4 SOD1^{G93A}. **c** Quantification of GFAP immunoreactivity per area from female mice (**a**). Values plotted are mean ± SEM. Two-way ANOVA: $^{***}P < 0.001$ WT Vs SOD1^{G93A}. Unpaired two-tailed t-Test: $^{$}P < 0.05$ Control Vs ADAMTS-4 SOD1^{G93A}, $N = 5$ Control WT, $N = 3$ ADAMTS-4 WT, $N = 5$ Control SOD1^{G93A}, $N = 6$ ADAMTS-4 SOD1^{G93A}. **d** Representative photomicrographs of ventral horns in lumbar spinal cord sections from WT and control or ADAMTS-4-treated SOD1^{G93A} mice stained with Iba1. Scale bar: 250 m. **e** Quantification of Iba1 immunoreactivity per area from male mice (**d**). Values plotted are mean ± SEM. Two-way ANOVA: $^{***}P < 0.001$ WT Vs SOD1^{G93A}. Unpaired two-tailed t-Test: $P > 0.05$ Control Vs ADAMTS-4 SOD1^{G93A}, $N = 3$ Control WT, $N = 5$ ADAMTS-4 WT, $N = 8$ Control SOD1^{G93A}, $N = 7$ ADAMTS-4 SOD1^{G93A}. **f** Quantification of Iba1 immunoreactivity per area from female mice (**d**). Values plotted are mean ± SEM. Two-way ANOVA: $^{***}P < 0.001$ WT Vs SOD1^{G93A}. Unpaired two-tailed t-Test: $P > 0.05$ Control Vs ADAMTS-4 SOD1^{G93A}, $N = 5$ Control WT, $N = 3$ ADAMTS-4 WT, $N = 5$ Control SOD1^{G93A}, $N = 6$ ADAMTS-4 SOD1^{G93A}

the culture media (Fig. 10e: $P = 0.5127$). ADAMTS-4 was not toxic to cultured astrocytes.

To confirm these results, we transfected astrocytes for 2 h with silencing siRNAs targeting ADAMTS-4 or with an empty vector (mock) as a control. After 48 h, ADAMTS-4 gene expression was decreased by 69 % in astrocytes transfected with siRNAs silencing ADAMTS-4 expression compared to control astrocytes (Fig. 10f: $P = 0.0209$). Interestingly, we observed an increase of the mRNA levels of NGF (Fig. 10g: +46.1 % for astrocytes transfected with siRNAs targeting ADAMTS-4 compared to control astrocytes, $P = 0.0209$) and GDNF (Fig. 10h: +46.8 % for astrocytes transfected with siRNAs targeting ADAMTS-4 compared to control astrocytes, $P = 0.0209$), but not BDNF (Fig. 10i: $P = 0.2482$),

in astrocytes transfected with siRNAs silencing ADAMTS-4 expression compared to control astrocytes. In the culture media, we observed an increase of NGF in astrocytes transfected with siRNAs silencing ADAMTS-4 expression compared to control astrocytes (Fig. 10j: +16.9 % for astrocytes transfected with siRNAs targeting ADAMTS-4 compared to control astrocytes, $P = 0.0209$).

To determine whether this effect was astrocyte-specific, we repeated the same experiments in microglia cultures. ADAMTS-4 decreased the mRNA levels of NGF (Fig. 10k: –9.4 % for microglia treated with ADAMTS-4 at 100 ng/ml compared to control microglia, $P = 0.0209$), GDNF (Fig. 10l: –15.1 % for microglia treated with ADAMTS-4 at 100 ng/ml compared to

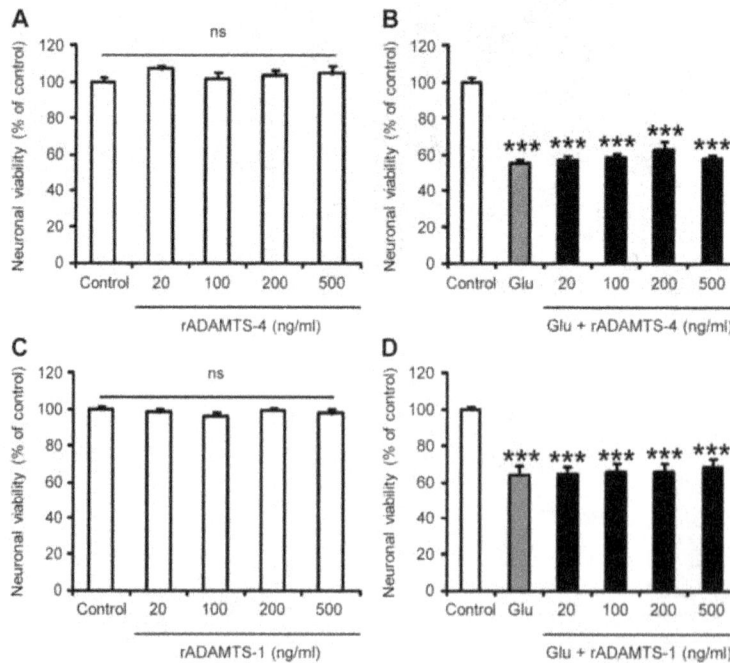

Fig. 9 rADAMTS-4 is not toxic to cortical neurons *in vitro*. Neuronal viability assessed by MTT assay in primary cortical neuron cultures treated or not with a human recombinant ADAMTS-4 (**a-b**) or ADAMTS-1 (**c-d**) at different doses (20, 100, 200, 500 ng/ml) 30 min before exposure (**b, d**) or not (**a, c**) to glutamate 400 M (Glu) during 24 h. Values plotted are mean ± SEM. Mann–Whitney U-tests: $P > 0.05$ control Vs ADAMTS, $^{***}P < 0.001$ control Vs glutamate, $P > 0.05$ glutamate Vs glutamate + ADAMTS, $N = 11$-12 from 3 independent experiments

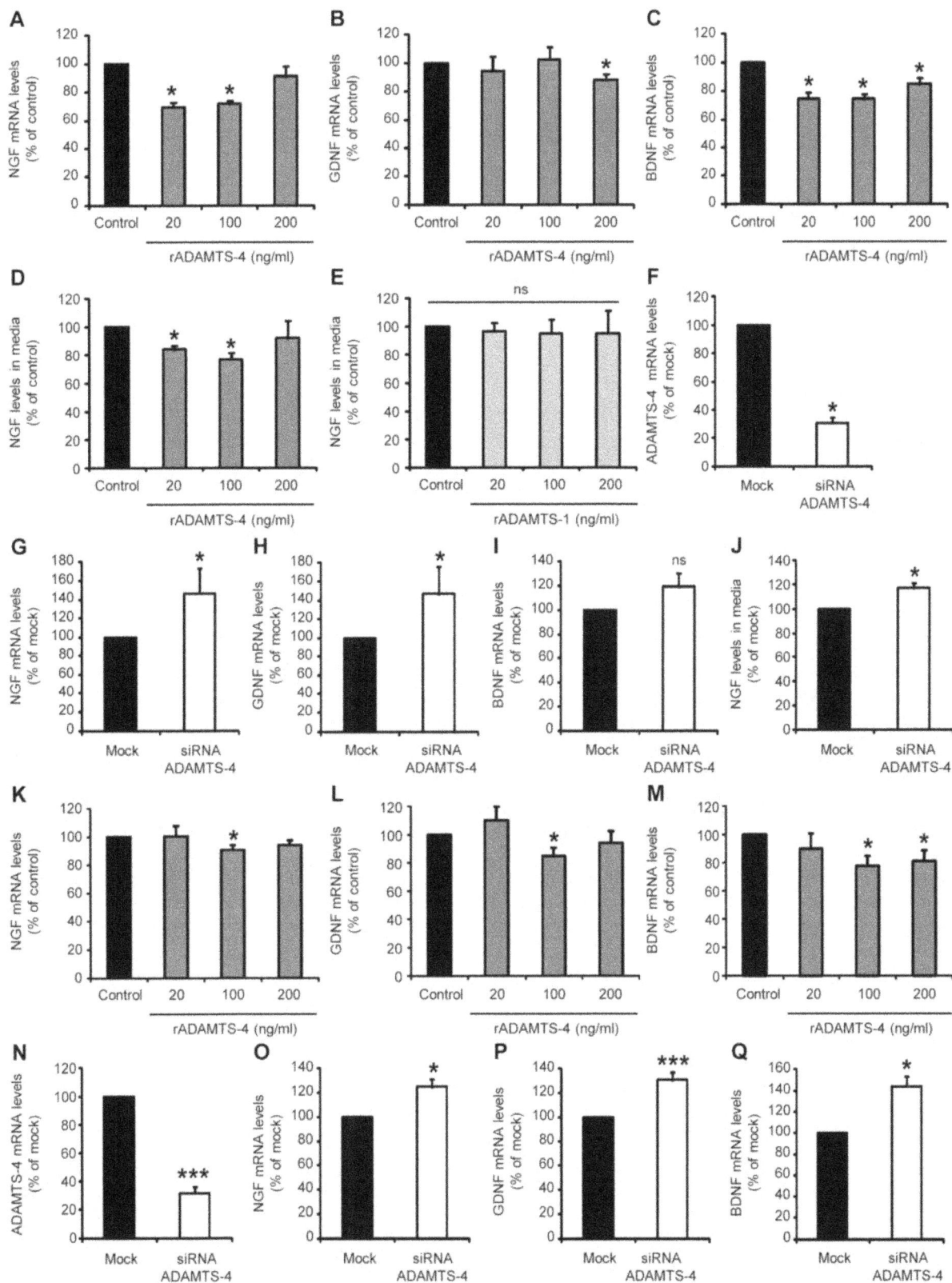

Fig. 10 (See legend on next page.)

(See figure on previous page.)
Fig. 10 ADAMTS-4 modulates the synthesis/release of neurotrophic factors by glial cells *in vitro*. **a-c** Quantitative RT-PCR for NGF (**a**) GDNF (**b**) and BDNF (**c**) expression in mouse adult cortical astrocyte cultures treated or not for 48 h with a human recombinant ADAMTS-4 (20, 100, 200 ng/ml). Values plotted are mean ± SEM. Mann–Whitney *U*-tests: $^*P < 0.05$ compared to control, $N = 4$. **d-e** ELISA-measurements of NGF released in the media of mouse adult cortical astrocyte cultures treated or not for 48 h with a human recombinant ADAMTS-4 (**d**) or ADAMTS-1 (**e**) at different doses (20, 100, 200 ng/ml). Values plotted are mean ± SEM. Mann–Whitney *U*-tests: $^*P < 0.05$ (ADAMTS-4) or $P > 0.05$ (ADAMTS-1) compared to control, $N = 3$. **f-i** Quantitative RT-PCR for ADAMTS-4 (**f**) NGF (**g**) GDNF (**h**) and BDNF (**i**) expression in mouse adult cortical astrocyte cultures transfected or not for 48 h with empty vector (mock) or silencing RNAs (siRNAs) targeting the expression of ADAMTS-4. Values plotted are mean ± SEM. Mann–Whitney *U*-tests: $^*P < 0.05$ (ADAMTS-4, NGF, GDNF) or $P > 0.05$ (BDNF) compared to mock, $N = 4$. **j** ELISA-measurements of NGF released in the media of mouse adult cortical astrocyte cultures transfected or not for 48 h with mock or siRNAs targeting the expression of ADAMTS-4. Values plotted are mean ± SEM. Mann–Whitney *U*-tests: $^*P < 0.05$ compared to control, $N = 4$. **k-m** Quantitative RT-PCR for NGF (**k**) GDNF (**l**) and BDNF (**m**) expression in mouse neonatal cerebral microglia cultures treated or not for 48 h with a human recombinant ADAMTS-4 (20, 100, 200 ng/ml). Values plotted are mean ± SEM. Mann–Whitney *U*-tests: $^*P < 0.05$ compared to control, $N = 4$. **n-q** Quantitative RT-PCR for ADAMTS-4 (**n**) NGF (**o**) GDNF (**p**) and BDNF (**q**) expression in mouse neonatal cerebral microglia cultures transfected or not for 48 h with mock or siRNAs targeting the expression of ADAMTS-4. Values plotted are mean ± SEM. Mann–Whitney *U*-tests: $^*P < 0.05$ (NGF, BDNF), $^{***}P < 0.001$ (ADAMTS-4, GDNF) compared to mock, $N = 8$

control microglia, $P = 0.0209$) and BDNF (Fig. 10m: −22.4 % or −18.9 % for microglia treated with ADAMTS-4 at 100 or 200 ng/ml compared to control microglia, $P = 0.0209$) in microglia cultures. ELISA failed to detect NGF in microglia culture media (data not shown). ADAMTS-4 was not toxic to cultured microglia.

To confirm these results, we transfected microglial cells for 2 h with silencing siRNAs targeting ADAMTS-4 or with an empty vector (mock) as a control. After 48 h, ADAMTS-4 gene expression was decreased by 68 % in microglial cells transfected with siRNAs silencing ADAMTS-4 expression compared to control microglia (Fig. 10n: $P = 0.0008$). Importantly, we observed an increase in the mRNA levels of NGF (Fig. 10o: +25.1 % for microglia transfected with siRNAs targeting ADAMTS-4 compared to control microglia, $P = 0.0117$), GDNF (Fig. 10p: +30.7 % for microglia transfected with siRNAs targeting ADAMTS-4 compared to control microglia, $P = 0.0008$) and BDNF (Fig. 10q: +44.2 % for microglia transfected with siRNAs targeting ADAMTS-4 compared to control microglia, $P = 0.0117$) in microglial cells transfected with siRNAs silencing ADAMTS-4 expression compared to control microglia.

ADAMTS-4 treatment decreases NGF expression in the ventral horn of the lumbar spinal cord of male SOD1^{G93A} mice

We next aimed to determine whether the regulation of neurotrophic factor expression and release by ADAMTS-4 evidenced in vitro (Fig. 10) may contribute at least partly to the deleterious effects of ADAMTS-4 observed in vivo in SOD1^{G93A} mice. For that purpose, we immunostained NGF in lumbar spinal cord sections of SOD1^{G93A} mice treated or not with ADAMTS-4. Interestingly, we observed a 2-fold decrease of NGF expression in the ventral horn of the lumbar spinal cords of SOD1^{G93A} male mice treated with ADAMTS-4 compared to untreated SOD1^{G93A} mice (Fig. 11a-b: −54.9 %

for ADAMTS-4-treated SOD1^{G93A} mice compared to untreated SOD1^{G93A} mice, $P = 0.0209$). However, no difference of NGF expression was found between SOD1^{G93A} female mice treated or not with ADAMTS-4 (Fig. 11c-d: $P = 0.9907$).

Discussion

ADAMTS-4 is a metalloproteinase specialized in the degradation of chondroitin sulfate proteoglycans (CSPGs) whose functions during neurodegenerative diseases, including ALS, have not been investigated. Here, we demonstrated that (i) ADAMTS-4 activity is decreased at disease end-stage in the spinal cord of SOD1^{G93A} mice, and that (ii) provision of exogenous ADAMTS-4 promoted the degradation of perineuronal nets (PNNs) and decreased glial production of neurotrophic factors, possibly thereby enhancing neurodegeneration and subsequent motor impairments in SOD1^{G93A} mice (Fig. 12a).

In contrast to other ADAMTS proteoglycanases, ADAMTS-4 is highly expressed in the CNS in all types of cells [1, 20–23]. However, ADAMTS proteoglycanases display different potency for CSPGs. For example, ADAMTS-5 is more potent than ADAMTS-4 for the proteolysis of aggrecan [24, 25], a CSPG found exclusively in PNNs. Nevertheless, ADAMTS functions extend beyond proteolysis by regulating synaptic protein expression (ADAMTS-1) [3] or neurotrophic factor expression/release (ADAMTS-4). Modifications of ADAMTS-4 expression/activity have been reported during spinal cord injury (SCI), experimental autoimmune encephalomyelitis and multiple sclerosis [1]. Here, we showed that ADAMTS-4 activity was decreased in the lumbar spinal cord of SOD1^{G93A} mice compared to WT mice at disease end-stage. This reduction could be related to a myriad of events, including a decrease of ADAMTS-4 gene/protein expression, an increase of the proteolytic cleavage of ADAMTS-4 mature form, and an increase of its inhibitor TIMP-3.

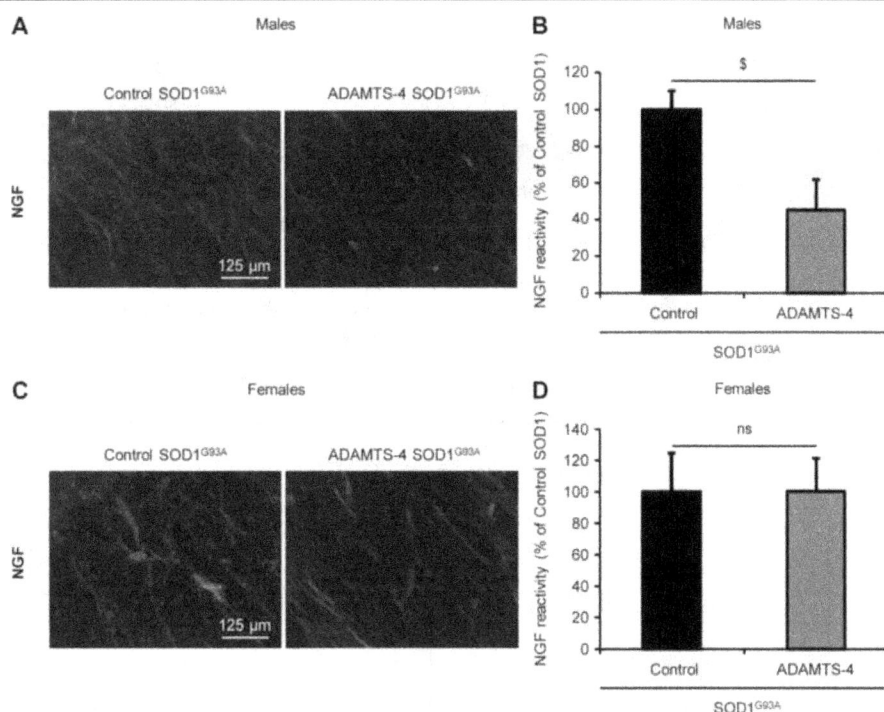

Fig. 11 rADAMTS-4 decreases NGF expression in the lumbar spinal cord of male SOD1^{G93A} mice. **a** Representative photomicrographs of ventral horns in lumbar spinal cord sections from control or ADAMTS-4-treated SOD1^{G93A} male mice stained with NGF. Scale bar: 125 m. **b** Quantification of NGF immunoreactivity per area from male mice (**a**). Values plotted are mean ± SEM. Unpaired two-tailed t-Test: $^{\$}P < 0.05$ Control Vs ADAMTS-4 SOD1^{G93A}, $N = 8$ Control SOD1^{G93A}, $N = 7$ ADAMTS-4 SOD1^{G93A}. **c** Representative photomicrographs of ventral horns in lumbar spinal cord sections from control or ADAMTS-4-treated SOD1^{G93A} female mice stained with NGF. Scale bar: 125 m. **d** Quantification of NGF immunoreactivity per area from female mice (**c**). Values plotted are mean ± SEM. Unpaired two-tailed t-Test: $P > 0.05$ Control Vs ADAMTS-4 SOD1^{G93A}, $N = 5$ Control SOD1^{G93A}, $N = 6$ ADAMTS-4 SOD1^{G93A}

TIMP-3 is also an inhibitor for ADAMTS-1 and –5, which may impair their activities although their expressions are increased in the lumbar spinal cord of SOD1^{G93A} mice.

We and others have previously shown that exogenous supply of ADAMTS-4 after SCI in rats promotes neuroplasticity by degrading CSPGs and subsequent functional recovery [5, 6]. One possible reason why ADAMTS-4 is beneficial after SCI while it is deleterious during ALS may rely on the impact of CSPGs/PNNs degradation in these two diseases. Indeed, while it is clear that CSPGs are highly induced after SCI and represent strong inhibitors for neuroregeneration in this context, their expression and role during neurodegenerative diseases including ALS are poorly understood [18, 26–28]. Nevertheless, increasing evidence shows that the neurons devoid of a net are less protected against neurodegeneration compared to PNNs-bearing neurons in Alzheimer disease (AD) or oxidative stress animal models [29–31]. Forostyak and colleagues have shown that the PNNs enwrapping spinal motoneurons of SOD1^{G93A} rats are considerably degraded at disease end-stage compared to WT rats. Additionally, they showed that PNNs are partly preserved in SOD1^{G93A}

rats after transplantation of bone marrow mesenchymal stromal cells and that this effect is associated with an increase of motoneuron survival and an increase of SOD1^{G93A} rats survival [18]. Similarly, we showed here a decrease of PNNs around motoneurons of the lumbar spinal cord of SOD1^{G93A} mice at the symptomatic stage. Disorganized SOD1^{G93A}-PNNs may facilitate local degradation of the remaining aggrecan by ADAMTS-4 since PNNs were even more damaged in ADAMTS-4-treated SOD1^{G93A} mice. This was associated with an increased neurodegeneration and a poor functional outcome. Our results suggest that digestion of PNNs by ADAMTS-4 may be harmful for motoneurons during ALS pathology. Because PNNs only contain 2 % of total CSPGs [32], we cannot exclude that ADAMTS-4 may have an effect on digestion of the 98 % remaining CSPGs.

Neurotrophic factors have been extensively described to protect dying motoneurons and represent a potential therapeutic strategy in ALS [33, 34]. Here we described for the first time that ADAMTS-4 decreased the expression of several neurotrophic factors in astrocytes and microglia. Accordingly, decreasing ADAMTS-4 expression by siRNA approach led to an increase of neurotrophic factor expression. This demonstrates that

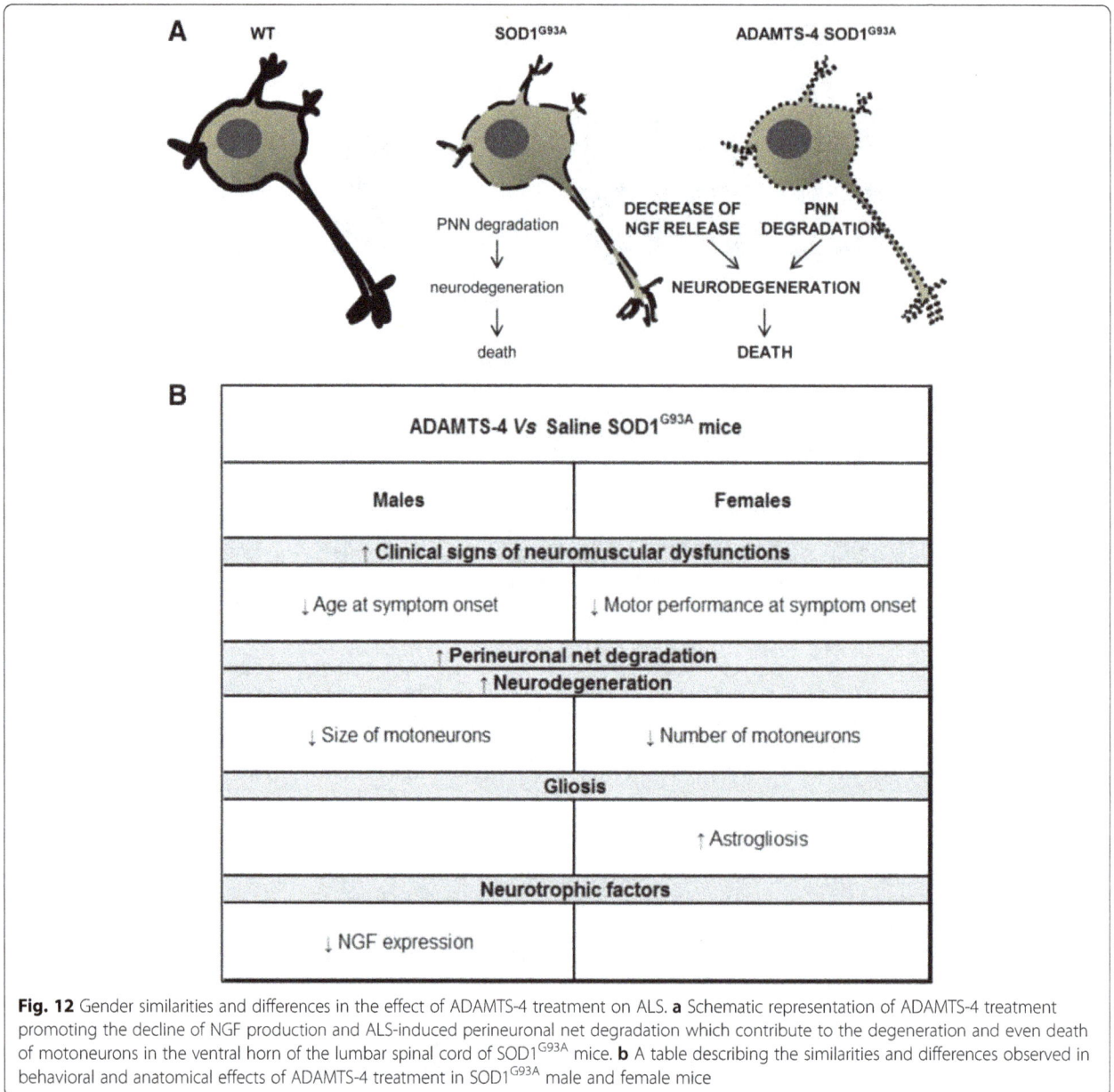

Fig. 12 Gender similarities and differences in the effect of ADAMTS-4 treatment on ALS. **a** Schematic representation of ADAMTS-4 treatment promoting the decline of NGF production and ALS-induced perineuronal net degradation which contribute to the degeneration and even death of motoneurons in the ventral horn of the lumbar spinal cord of SOD1^{G93A} mice. **b** A table describing the similarities and differences observed in behavioral and anatomical effects of ADAMTS-4 treatment in SOD1^{G93A} male and female mice

ADAMTS-4 functions are not limited only to CSPGs degradation. It would be interesting to determine whether ADAMTS-4 may induce mechanisms previously described to downregulate neurotrophic factor production, for instance, by modulating the nuclear translocation of transcription factors such as the histone deacetylase HDAC6 (negative regulator) [35], CREB (cAMP response element-binding protein) or NF-κB (nuclear factor kappa B) (positive regulators) [36–38], and/or by modulating micro-RNAs (miR) production such as miR-15a, miR-132, miR-134, miR-221 or Let-7 miR [39–41]. Because ADAMTS-4 did not increase glutamate-induced neuronal death in vitro, we hypothesize that ADAMTS-4-dependent decrease of neurotrophic factors released by glial cells around dying motoneurons during ALS may participate in the accelerated neurodegeneration induced by ADAMTS-4 in vivo. The neurotrophic factor production after ADAMTS-4 treatment has not been studied in SCI studies so far, but we could hypothesize that even if ADAMTS-4 also induced a decrease of neurotrophic factor production in the context of SCI, its impact may be negligible compared to the great benefit of the CSPGs/PNNs degradation-induced neuroregeneration [5, 6]. Among the neurotrophic factors modulated by ADAMTS-4, NGF is of particular interest as it exerts dual roles on neuronal survival/cell death depending on whether it activates the tyrosine kinase receptor TrkA or the tumor necrosis factor receptor p75^{NTR} [42], two receptors induced after injury and in ALS [43, 44]. Although astrocyte-derived NGF was described to promote motoneuron cell death through the activation of p75^{NTR} receptor during ALS [45, 46], it was also described that the surviving motoneurons expressed the TrkA receptor [43], suggesting that NGF-TrkA signaling also plays a critical role in the survival of motoneurons. Additionally, NGF-p75^{NTR} signaling reduces astrocyte proliferation in vitro and in vivo in an autocrine manner [47]. ADAMTS-4-mediated reduction in NGF release by astrocytes may contribute to neurodegeneration in ADAMTS-4-treated SOD1^{G93A} mice by preventing TrkA signaling in surviving motoneurons. The decrease of astrocytic NGF-p75^{NTR} signaling could also explain the increase in astrocyte activation/proliferation observed in ADAMTS-4-treated SOD1^{G93A} females. Contrary to ADAMTS-4-treated SOD1^{G93A} males, no modification of NGF expression was identified in the lumbar spinal cords of ADAMTS-4-treated SOD1^{G93A} females. Nevertheless, we cannot rule out that: i) the decrease of NGF in ADAMTS-4-treated SOD1^{G93A} females may have occurred earlier than the time point studied here. ii) the main source of NGF is provided by astrocytes, therefore the increased astrogliosis observed in the lumbar spinal cord of ADAMTS-4-treated SOD1^{G93A} females might mask the reducing effect of ADAMTS-4 on NGF astrocytic expression.

This study reveals intriguing gender-specific effects of ADAMTS-4 at the functional and anatomical levels (Fig. 12b). While ADAMTS-4-treated SOD1^{G93A} males presented clinical signs of neuromuscular dysfunctions 20 days earlier than untreated SOD1^{G93A} males, ADAMTS-4-treated SOD1^{G93A} females had symptoms of neuromuscular dysfunctions at the same age as untreated SOD1^{G93A} females. Even though we evidenced that the motor performance of ADAMTS-4-treated SOD1^{G93A} females was more impaired than untreated SOD1^{G93A} females at symptom onset, it is clear that ADAMTS-4 more severely impaired the functional outcome of SOD1^{G93A} males than females. Surprisingly, this does not reflect what happened at the anatomical level, since ADAMTS-4 caused motoneuron death in SOD1^{G93A} females and only mild motoneuron degeneration in SOD1^{G93A} males. It is difficult to explain such non-linear relationship between functional and anatomical outcomes in ADAMTS-4-treated SOD1^{G93A} males (severe functional impairment/mild neurodegeneration) or females (mild functional impairment/severe neurodegeneration). However, the fact that motoneuron degeneration obviously led to cell death in ADAMTS-4-treated SOD1^{G93A} females but not yet in males may be due to the increased astrogliosis induced by ADAMTS-4 in SOD1^{G93A} females, but not in males. Estrogens may

most likely play a role in some of the mechanisms mediated by ADAMTS-4. Gender-specific effects of another ADAMTS proteoglycanase, ADAMTS-1, have been previously observed in the CNS where a decline of synaptic proteins was evidenced in the frontal cortex of ADAMTS-1 knock-out female mice during development, but not in males [3].

Conclusions
To conclude, our results provide the first evidence that ADAMTS-4 promotes neurodegeneration in the context of ALS. It would be interesting to determine if: (i) endogenous ADAMTS-4 contributes to neurodegeneration in mice expressing high copy number of mutant SOD1 as well as in other model of ALS such as WT or mutant TDP43 (TAR DNA-binding protein 43) rodent models, or even in frontotemporal dementia or AD models; (ii) therapeutic approaches aimed at decreasing ADAMTS-4 expression/activity would represent potential targets to slow down neurodegeneration in chronic CNS diseases.

Methods
Ethics
Animal experiments were conducted according to the national regulation of the usage and welfare of laboratory animals, approved by the National Animal Experiment Board of Finland and followed the Council of Europe legislation and regulation for animal protection.

Animals
Transgenic male and female mice over-expressing the human superoxide dismutase SOD1^{G93A} mutation were also purchased from the Jackson laboratory (Bar Harbor, Maine, USA) and maintained on C57BL/6 J congenic background. Transgenic genotypes were identified by polymerase chain reaction (PCR) amplification of ear DNA a few days after birth and of liver DNA after death to confirm the results of the first genotyping. PCR revealed a low copy number of mutated SOD1 in the mice used in this study. The mice were housed under controlled temperature, humidity and light conditions (12 h light and dark cycles) with free access to food and water. Animals of the same sex were housed in groups of up to 5 in cages. WT and SOD1^{G93A} mice were used for the 2 studies described hereafter.

Study 1: ADAMTS-4 expression in the time course of ALS

- *Characterization of the disease stage in SOD1^{G93A} mice.* Male and female SOD1^{G93A} mice and WT littermates from generations 18–19 were sacrificed at key time points during the development of the ALS pathology: presymptomatic (m/f: ~13/14.5 weeks-old), symptomatic (m/f: ~20.5/22 weeks-old) and end-stages (m/f: ~27/28 weeks-old). The symptomatic stage was estimated based on the symptom onset of SOD1^{G93A} mice from the previous cohort, and confirmed when the mice developed abnormal hindlimb splay reflexes when suspended by their tails. The end-stage was defined as the age when the mice suffered from functional paralysis of the hindlimbs. At disease end-stage, SOD1^{G93A} mice were given macerated food for easier food uptake and hydration. Mice were sacrificed by terminal perfusion with heparinized saline, followed or not by paraformaldehyde (PFA) perfusion (as described in the immuno-histochemistry section) for respectively RNA ($N = 3$-4 in each group)/protein ($N = 4$ in each group) (cortices, cervical, thoracic and lumbar spinal cords) or staining ($N = 3$ in each group) (lumbar spinal cords) purposes.

Study 2: ADAMTS-4 treatment and functional outcome in ALS

– *Intracerebroventricular injection of recombinant ADAMTS-4.* Male and female WT and SOD1^{G93A} mice from generations 20–22 were randomized into treatment groups using GraphPad Quickcalcs (GraphPad Software Inc., La Jolla, CA, USA): $N = 5$ Control WT males, $N = 5$ ADAMTS-4 WT males, $N = 9$ Control SOD1^{G93A} males, $N = 9$ ADAMTS-4 SOD1^{G93A} males, $N = 5$ Control WT females, $N = 4$ ADAMTS-4 WT females, $N = 7$ Control SOD1^{G93A} females, $N = 6$ ADAMTS-4 SOD1^{G93A} females. The anesthesia of mice was induced by 5 % isoflurane in a 70 %/30 % mixture of NO_2/O_2 and maintained at 2 % isoflurane during the surgery. The temperature of the mice was controlled by a homeothermic control system connected to a heating blanket and rectal probe (Harvard apparatus, Pan Lab, Barcelona, Spain). A 4-µl volume containing saline or 40 ng of a human recombinant ADAMTS-4 (CC1028, Merck Millipore, Darmstadt, Germany) was injected bilaterally into lateral ventricles using a 5-µl Hamilton syringe (Hamilton company, Reno, Nevada, USA) at the age of 9 and 13 weeks (coordinates from Bregma: mediolateral = ± 1 mm, anteroposterior = – 0.5 mm, dorsoventral = – 3 mm).

– *Assessment of functional outcome.* Disease onset was determined by the wire hang test [48]. Each mouse was placed on a wire lid of a conventional cage which was turned upside down and the latency of the mouse to fall was recorded. Deficits in motor performance were defined by the inability to hang for more than 3 min. If the mouse fell, the test was repeated for the second time. The test was performed 3 times a week. In parallel, the weight of the transgenic mice was recorded 3 times a week

using a normal digital balance, while WT mice were only weighted once a week. The testing was performed blinded to the experimental groups. Mice were sacrificed during the symptomatic stage (m/f: ~29/35 weeks-old) by terminal perfusion with heparinized saline, followed by PFA perfusion (as described in the immunohistochemistry section) for staining (lumbar spinal cords) purposes.

Quantitative real-time PCR

Total RNAs were isolated by homogenizing spinal cords or cortex in TRIzol (Life technologies, Carlsbad, CA, USA) according to manufacturer's instructions utilizing 5-mm stainless steel beads and a Tissuelyzer II homogenizer (Qiagen, Leusden, NL, USA). Total RNAs from cells were isolated with the RNeasy Mini Kit (Qiagen). Synthesis of cDNA was performed by using 500 ng of total RNA, Maxima reverse transcriptase, dNTP and random hexamer primers (Life technologies). The final concentration of cDNA was 2.5 ng/µl. The relative expression levels of mRNAs encoding the selected genes were run in duplicates and measured according to the manufacturer's protocol by quantitative RT-PCR (StepOne Plus™ Real-Time PCR system; Life technologies) and using specific assays-on-demand target mixes (Life technologies) as follows: ADAMTS-1: Mm00477355_m1; ADAMTS4: Mm005 56068_m1; ADAMTS-5: Mm00478620_m1; ADAM TS-9: Mm00614433_m1; TIMP-3 (type 3 tissue inhibitor of metalloproteinases): Mm00441826_m1; Aggrecan: Mm00545794_m1; BDNF (brain-derived neurotrophic factor): Mm0133402_m1; NGF (nerve growth factor): Mm00443039_m1; GDNF (glial cell-derived neurotrophic factor): Mm00599849_m1; HAPLN1 (hyaluronan and proteoglycan link protein 1): Mm00488952_m1; Tenascin R: Mm00659075_m1; GAPDH (glyceraldehyde-3-phosphate dehydrogenase): 4352932E (Applied Biosystems, Warrington, UK). The expression levels were normalized to GAPDH. Relative mRNA transcription was expressed as a percentage of control conditions using the $2^{-\text{ }Ct}$ method where Ct is the threshold-cycle value. The relative expression of ADAMTS proteoglycanases was expressed as a percentage of ADAMTS-1 gene expression using the $2^{-\text{ }Ct}$ method: $2^{-((\text{ }Ct\text{ ADAMTS-1} - \text{ }Ct\text{ GAPDH}) - (\text{ }Ct\text{ ADAMTS-4, 5 or 9} - \text{ }Ct\text{ GAPDH}))}$.

Protein extraction

Cortices as well as cervical, thoracic or lumbar spinal cords were dissociated in ice-cold TNT buffer (50 mM Tris–HCl pH 7.4; 150 mM NaCl; 0.5 % Triton X-100) containing EDTA/EGTA (ethylene diamine/glycol tetraacetic acid, 1 mM), protease (Sigma-Aldrich, St Louis, MO, USA) and phosphatase (Roche Diagnostics, Mannheim, Germany) inhibitors. For the ADAMTS-4 fluorimetric assay, lumbar spinal cords were dissociated in TNT buffer without protease and phosphatase inhibitors. Debris were removed by centrifugation (12,000 g at 4 °C, 15 min). Supernatants were stored at −70 °C until further processing. Protein quantification was performed according to the BCA protein method (Pierce, Rockford, USA).

Western blot

Proteins (5 μg) were resolved on 12 % polyacrylamide gel under denaturing conditions and transferred onto a polyvinylidene difluoride membrane. Membranes were blocked with phosphate buffered saline (PBS) tween (0.2 % Tween-20; Sigma-Aldrich) and 5 % of milk. Blots were incubated overnight at 4 °C with the rabbit anti-ADAMTS-4 (1/5000; AbCam, Cambridge, UK) or the rabbit anti-ADAMTS-5 (1/1000; AbCam) primary antibodies diluted in PBS-tween containing 5 % of bovine albumin serum (BSA). After a 2-h incubation at room temperature (RT) with the peroxidase-conjugated anti-rabbit secondary antibody (1/2000; GE Healthcare life sciences, Uppsala, Sweden), proteins were revealed with an enhanced chemiluminescence ECL-Plus kit immunoblotting detection system (GE Healthcare life sciences) and visualized using Storm^{TM} FluorImager system. Mouse anti-β-actin (1/5000; Sigma-Aldrich) was used as a loading control and visualized by Alexa fluor 647-conjugated anti-mouse secondary antibody (1/1000; Jackson ImmunoResearch laboratories Inc., West Grove, PA, USA).

Ex vivo CSPG proteolysis by ADAMTS human recombinant proteins

Sixteen μg of lumbar spinal cord protein extracts from symptomatic SOD1^{G93A} male mice were exposed or not to 1 μg of human recombinant ADAMTS-1 (2197-AD-020), ADAMTS-4 (4307-AD-020) or ADAMTS-5 (2198-AD-020; all recombinant proteins were from R&D SYSTEMS, Minneapolis, MN, USA) in the aggrecanase buffer (50 mM TrisHCl, 125 mM NaCl, 5 mM CaCl$_2$, pH 7.5) within a final volume of 55 μl, for 24 h at 37 °C ($N = 4$ per condition). The reaction was stopped by heating the samples at 75 °C for 10 min. Twelve μl of each condition of the above preparations were resolved in a 6 % polyacrylamide gel, the membrane probed with the mouse anti-CSPG antibody (1/1000; Sigma-Aldrich), then with the peroxidase-conjugated anti-mouse secondary antibody (1/5000; GE Healthcare life sciences) and finally revealed by ECL detection, as previously described in the Western Blot section.

Fluorimetric assay for ADAMTS-4

A fluorogenic substrate (5-FAM/TAMRA; SensoLyte® 520 Aggrecanase-1 assay kit, Eurogentec, San Jose, CA) was incubated with protein extracts of lumbar spinal cords (25 μg in 50 μl) of WT and SOD1^{G93A} male and female mice at presymptomatic, symptomatic and end-stages ($N = 4$ in each group). Measurements were performed at 37 °C over 60 min using a multiplate reader. The slope of each absorbance curve was then determined between 10 and 20 min.

Immunohistochemistry

Anesthetized mice were perfused with cold heparinized saline and, thereafter, with a solution containing 4 % PFA in 0.1 M phosphate buffer (PB) pH 7.4. Lumbar spinal cords were removed and rinsed in a PB containing 20 % sucrose for cryoprotection for 24 h. The spinal cords were embedded and frozen in OCT (Optimal Cutting Temperature; Sakura Finetek, Tokyo, Japan). Five 12-μm-transverse sections 200 μm apart covering a 1-mm-length of each lumbar spinal cord were cut on a cryostat, collected on lysine glasses (Thermo Scientific, UK), and stored at −70 °C until analysis. After washing with PB, PBS and PBS-tween (0.05 % Tween-20), sections were treated as required with PBS-TritonX-100 (0.4 %, Sigma-Aldrich) and unspecific binding was blocked with 1 h incubation with 10 % normal goat or rabbit serum (NGS or NRS; Vector Laboratories Ltd, Burlingame, CA) or 0.5 % mouse on mouse reagent (MOM; Vector Laboratories Ltd). Incubation with primary antibodies was conducted overnight at RT with dilutions as follows: rabbit anti-ADAMTS-4 (1/500; AbCam), rabbit anti-GFAP (glial fibrillary acidic protein, 1/200; Dako, Glostrup, Denmark), mouse anti-GFAP (1/400; Merck Millipore), rabbit anti-Iba1 (ionized calcium-binding adapter molecule-1, 1/250; Wako Pure Chemical Industries, Ltd, Tokyo, Japan), mouse anti-NeuN (1/200; Chemicon, Billerica, MA, USA), rabbit anti-NGF (1/100; AbCam), mouse anti-APC (Adenomatous polyposis coli, 1/200; Merck Millipore) or lectin from Wisteria Floribunda (WFA, Wisteria Floribunda Agglutin, 1/1000; Sigma-Aldrich). After washing with PBS-tween, sections were incubated with corresponding fluorescent Alexa fluor −488 or −568-conjugated secondary antibodies (1/200; Life technologies) or with a fluorescent Alexa fluor-568 secondary antibody conjugated to streptavidin (for WFA staining, 1/500; Life technologies) for 2 h at RT, then washed again and finally mounted in Vectashield with DAPI (Vector Laboratories Ltd). For choline acetyltransferase (ChAT) staining, sections were incubated in 0.3 % H$_2$O$_2$ diluted in MeOH for 30 min to block endogenous peroxidase activity followed by heat-mediated antigen retrieval for 30 min in 0.05 M citrate buffer, pH 6.0. After blocking unspecific binding, sections were incubated in primary antibody (1/500; Chemicon), followed on the next day by 1-h incubation in biotinylated secondary antibody (1/200) and then incubation in avidin-biotin complex solution (Vectastain Elite kit, both from Vector Laboratories Inc., USA). The staining was visualized using nickel-enhanced diaminobenzidine (Sigma-Aldrich) with 0.075 % H_2O_2 as chromogen/substrate reagent solution. Negative controls for unspecific binding of the secondary antibodies were conducted in parallel sections following the same procedures described above except the incubation in primary antibodies.

For GFAP, Iba1, WFA, ChAT and NGF analyses, the ventral horn of the lumbar spinal cords were imaged using 10x (GFAP, Iba1, ChAT), 20x (WFA) or 40x (NGF) magnification on an AX70 microscope (Olympus corporation, Tokyo, Japan) coupled to a digital camera (Color View 12, soft Imaging System, Muenster, Germany) using Soft Imaging software: $N = 3$ Control WT males, $N = 5$ ADAMTS-4 WT males, $N = 8$ Control SOD1^{G93A} males, $N = 7$ ADAMTS-4 SOD1^{G93A} males, $N = 5$ Control WT females, $N = 3$ ADAMTS-4 WT females, $N = 5$ Control SOD1^{G93A} females, $N = 6$ ADAMTS-4 SOD1^{G93A} females. Immunoreactivity for GFAP, Iba1, WFA or NGF were quantified using Image-Pro Plus software (Media Cybernetics, Rockville, MO, USA) at a pre-defined range, measured as the relative immunoreactive area for GFAP, Iba1, WFA or NGF. The number and size of ChAT-positive motoneurons were measured by using Image-Pro Premier software (Media Cybernetics). Co-localization of NeuN, GFAP or APC with ADAMTS-4 were assessed by a Zeiss LSM 700 confocal microscope coupled to a digital camera using Zen 2009 Image Analysis Software (Zeiss Inc., Maple Grove, USA).

Primary neuron culture

Primary neuron cultures were prepared as described previously [49]. Cortices were isolated from 14 day-old mouse embryos in sterile Krebs solution containing 125 mM NaCl, 5 mM KCl, 1 mM NaH_2PO_4, 15 mM D-glucose, 25 mM HEPES, 0.05 mM BSA and 2 mM $MgSO_4$. Cortices were then incubated for 15 min at 37 °C in Krebs solution containing 0.1 mM trypsin (Sigma-Aldrich). Krebs solution containing 25 nM DNAse (Sigma-Aldrich) and 130 nM soy bean trypsin inhibitor (Sigma-Aldrich) was added to the suspension (1:1 dilution), and then centrifuged at 250 g for 3 min. The pellet was resuspended in new Krebs solution, and centrifuged again. The cells were finally resuspended in Neurobasal medium supplemented with 2 % B-27 supplement and 0.5 mM L-glutamine. Neurons were plated on 48 well-plates at a density of 125 000 cells/well previously coated with 5 µg/ml poly-D-lysine and were used for experiments 6 days after plating. After 5 days, half of the medium was changed to complete Neurobasal medium.

Treatment of neurons with recombinant proteins

Cultured neurons were treated with either a human recombinant ADAMTS-1 (2197-AD-020) or a human recombinant ADAMTS-4 (4307-AD-020; R&D SYSTEMS) at 20, 100, 200 or 500 ng/ml 30 min before exposure or not to 400 µM glutamate (Sigma-Aldrich) ($N = 11$-12 from 3 independent experiments).

MTT assay

After 24 h' exposure to glutamate, the neuron viability was assessed by measuring 3-(4,5-dimethylthiazol-2-yl)-2,5-diphenyltetrazolium bromide reduction (MTT; Sigma-Aldrich). For that purpose, cells were incubated with 120 µM MTT for 1 h before lysing in dimethyl sulfoxide (DMSO; J.T.Baker, Deventer, The Netherlands) and quantifying absorbance at 540 nm.

Adult astrocyte culture

Primary cortical astrocyte cultures were prepared as described previously [50] with some modifications. Briefly, cortices were isolated from 6–8 week-old C57Bl/6 J mice and the tissue was suspended in Hank's Balanced Salt Solution (HBSS, GIBCO, Life technologies) and centrifuged at 400 g for 5 min at RT. After the addition of 0.25 % trypsin-EDTA (GIBCO, Life technologies), the suspension was incubated at 37 °C for 30 min with occasional shaking. Fresh culture medium containing serum was added to neutralize the effect of trypsin and the suspension was centrifuged at 400 g for 5 min. The cells were treated with Percoll (Sigma-Aldrich) and centrifuged at 400 g for 10 min to separate the phases. The supernatant was discarded and the layer of glial cells was washed once with fresh culture media. The cells were plated onto poly-L-lysine coated flasks in Dulbecco's Modified Eagle Medium Nutrient Mixture F-12 (DMEM/F12, GIBCO, Life technologies) containing 10 % heat-inactivated fetal bovine serum (FBS, GIBCO, Life technologies), 2 mM L-Glutamine (GIBCO, Life technologies), 100 U/ml penicillin/streptomycin (P/S, GIBCO, Life technologies) and G5 supplement (Invitrogen, Life technologies). The astrocytic culture contains on average 99 % of GFAP-positive cells. The microglial cells were removed by shaking at 200 g for 2 h prior to the experiments. Astrocytes were plated on 12 well-plates at a density of 50 000 cells/well and used for experiments 3 days after plating.

Primary microglial culture

Primary microglial cultures were prepared as described previously [51, 52]. Brains were isolated from neonatal C57Bl/6 J mice (P1-2), washed in PBS containing 1 % glucose and mechanically and enzymatically dissociated using trypsin (TrypLE Express, GIBCO, Life technologies). The suspension was incubated at 37 °C for 20 min. Fresh culture medium containing FBS was added to neutralize the effect of trypsin. The suspension was plated in 15 cm-petradish in DMEM-F12 Glutamax

(GIBCO, Life technologies) containing 1 % P/S and 10 % FBS (complete media). After 3 weeks, cells were shaken at 200 g and then washed with PBS before addition of 0.08 % trypsin-EDTA for 45 min in order to peel off the astrocytes. After removal of astrocytes, microglial cells were washed with PBS and 0.25 % trypsin-EDTA was added for 5 min. After neutralizing trypsin with complete media, cells were dislodged and centrifuged at 400 g for 5 min. Cells were resuspended in complete media. Microglia were plated on 24-well plates at a density of 200 000 cells/well. After one day, cells were placed in serum-free media and used for experiments 2 or 3 days after plating.

Treatment of astrocytes and microglia with recombinant proteins

Cultured cortical astrocytes and neonatal microglia were treated with either a human recombinant ADAMTS-4 (4307-AD-020) or a human recombinant ADAMTS-1 (2197-AD-020; R&D SYSTEMS) at 20, 100 or 200 ng/ml for 48 h. The culture media were collected for ELISA assays ($N = 3$ in each group) and the RNAs ($N = 4$ in each group) were isolated from the corresponding cell layers for quantitative real-time PCR.

siRNA assays

Silencing small-interfering RNAs (siRNAs) targeting the expression of ADAMTS-4 (Sigma-Aldrich) were transiently transfected in cultured cerebral microglia or cortical astrocytes with the lipofectamine 2000 reagent (Invitrogen, Life technologies) using the protocol provided by the manufacturer. For each well of a 12 well-plate, 2 μg of siRNA and 4 μl of lipofectamine were added to astrocytes previously deprived of serum. For each well of a 24 well-plate, 1 μg of siRNA and 2 μl of lipofectamine were added to microglial cells in serum-free fresh media. After 2 h of transfection, astrocytes or microglia were rinsed and fresh culture medium containing FBS (astrocytes) or not (microglia) was added. After 48 h, cells were rinsed with PBS and RNA/culture media were collected as described above. ADAMTS-4 siRNA sequences used were: Mm01-00044319, 5 -CC CAUAUCCUUGUACGGCA-3 and 3 -UGCCGUACAA GGAUAUGGG-5 . As a control, empty vector (mock) was used (Mission siRNA Universal negative control #1, Sigma-Aldrich). ADAMTS-4 gene expression was significantly decreased by 69 % in astrocyte cultures ($N = 4$ in each group) and by 68 % in microglia cultures ($N = 8$ in each group) transfected with siRNA silencing ADAMTS-4 compared to mock.

NGF ELISA

The NGF protein concentrations were measured in astrocyte ($N = 3$ and 4 in each group for respectively recombinant and siRNA experiments) or microglia ($N = 4$ and 5 in each group for respectively recombinant and siRNA experiments) culture media using the *ChemiKine*™ NGF sandwich ELISA (Merck Millipore) following the manufacturer's instructions.

Statistical analyses

The data are expressed as mean ± SEM. An alpha level of $P < 0.05$ was used for determination of significance in all statistical tests. Molecular and cellular statistical analyses were performed with the Statview software package (v5.0). Kruskal-Wallis test was used for intergroup multiple comparisons. In significant cases, Mann–Whitney U-test was applied as post hoc test. Behavior and immunohistochemistry statistical analyses were performed using GraphPad Prism 5 (GraphPad Software Inc.). Kaplan-Meier survival analyses and log-rank test were used to compare the symptom onset of untreated SOD1^{G93A} and ADAMTS-4-treated SOD1^{G93A} mice. Two-way ANOVA was used to compare anatomical differences between genotypes. Unpaired two-tailed t-test was used for multiple comparisons.

Abbreviations

AD: Alzheimer disease; ADAMTS: a disintegrin and metalloproteinase with thrombospondin motifs; ALS: amyotrophic lateral sclerosis; APC: Adenomatous polyposis coli; BDNF: brain-derived neurotrophic factor; BSA: bovine albumin serum; ChAT: choline acetyltransferase; CNS: central nervous system; CREB: cAMP response element-binding protein; CSPG: chondroitin sulfate proteoglycan; DMEM: Dulbecco's Modified Eagle Medium; DMSO: dimethyl sulfoxide; ECM: extracellular matrix; EDTA: ethylene diamine tetraacetic acid; EGTA: ethylene glycol tetraacetic acid; ES: end stage; FBS: fetal bovine serum; FDA: Food and Drug Administration; GAPDH: glyceraldehyde-3-phosphate dehydrogenase; GDNF: glial cell-derived neurotrophic factor; GFAP: glial fibrillary acidic protein; HBSS: Hank's Balanced Salt Solution; HDAC6: histone deacetylase; HPLAN1: hyaluronan and proteoglycan link protein 1; Iba1: ionized calcium-binding adapter molecule-1; KO: knock-out; miR: Micro-RNA; MOM: mouse on mouse; MTT: 3-(4,5-dimethylthiazol-2-yl)-2,5-diphenyltetrazolium bromide reduction; NF-
 B: nuclear factor kappa b; NGF: nerve growth factor; NGS: normal goat serum; NMJ: neuromuscular junction; NRS: normal rabbit serum; OCT: Optimal Cutting Temperature; p75NTR: tumor necrosis factor receptor; PB: phosphate buffer; PBS: phosphate buffered saline; PFA: Paraformaldehyde; PNN: perineuronal net; PS: presymptomatic stage; RNA: ribonucleic acid; RT: room temperature; RT-PCR: real time polymerase chain reaction; SC: spinal cord; SCI: spinal cord injury; SEM: standard error of the mean; siRNA: small interference silencing RNA; SOD1: superoxide dismutase 1; SS: symptomatic stage; TDP43: TAR DNA-binding protein 43; TIMP-3: type 3 tissue inhibitor of metalloproteinases; TrkA: tyrosine kinase receptor A; WFA: Wisteria Floribunda Agglutin; WT: wild-type.

Competing interests
The authors declare that they have no competing interests.

Authors' contributions
SLem, JK, KK, TM, GG designed research, analyzed and/or interpreted the data. SLem, YP, IK, VK, PV, SLeh, KK performed experiments. SLem wrote the article and JK, KK and YP gave critical comments on the draft of the manuscript. All authors read and approved the final version of the manuscript.

Acknowledgements
We thank Mrs Laila Kaskela and Mrs Mirka Tikkanen for their technical assistance, and Mrs Sanna Loppi and Dr Eveliina Pollari for occasional help with behavioral testing. We also thank Dr Piia Vehviläinen for scientific discussions. This work was supported by the Academy of Finland.

References

1. Lemarchant S, Pruvost M, Montaner J, Emery E, Vivien D, Kanninen K, et al. ADAMTS proteoglycanases in the physiological and pathological central nervous system. J Neuroinflammation. 2013;10:133.
2. Hamel MG, Mayer J, Gottschall PE. Altered production and proteolytic processing of brevican by transforming growth factor beta in cultured astrocytes. J Neurochem. 2005;93:1533–41.
3. Howell MD, Torres-Collado AX, Iruela-Arispe ML, Gottschall PE. Selective decline of synaptic protein levels in the frontal cortex of female mice deficient in the extracellular metalloproteinase ADAMTS1. PLoS One. 2012;7:e47226.
4. Krstic D, Rodriguez M, Knuesel I. Regulated proteolytic processing of Reelin through interplay of tissue plasminogen activator (tPA), ADAMTS-4, ADAMTS-5, and their modulators. PLoS One. 2012;7:e47793.
5. Lemarchant S, Pruvost M, Hébert M, Gauberti M, Hommet Y, Briens A, et al. tPA promotes ADAMTS-4-induced CSPG degradation, thereby enhancing neuroplasticity following spinal cord injury. Neurobiol Dis. 2014;66:28–42.
6. Tauchi R, Imagama S, Natori T, Ohgomori T, Muramoto A, Shinjo R, et al. The endogenous proteoglycan-degrading enzyme ADAMTS-4 promotes functional recovery after spinal cord injury. J Neuroinflammation. 2012;9:53.
7. Zamanian JL, Xu L, Foo LC, Nouri N, Zhou L, Giffard RG, et al. Genomic analysis of reactive astrogliosis. J Neurosci. 2012;32:6391–410.
8. Reid MJ, Cross AK, Haddock G, Allan SM, Stock CJ, Woodroofe MN, et al. ADAMTS-9 expression is up-regulated following transient middle cerebral artery occlusion (tMCAo) in the rat. Neurosci Lett. 2009;452:252–7.
9. Cross AK, Haddock G, Surr J, Plumb J, Bunning RA, Buttle DJ, et al. Differential expression of ADAMTS-1, −4, −5 and TIMP-3 in rat spinal cord at different stages of acute experimental autoimmune encephalomyelitis. J Autoimmun. 2006;26:16–23.
10. Demircan K, Yonezawa T, Takigawa T, Topcu V, Erdogan S, Ucar F, et al. ADAMTS1, ADAMTS5, ADAMTS9 and aggrecanase-generated proteoglycan fragments are induced following spinal cord injury in mouse. Neurosci Lett. 2013;544:25–30.
11. Ajroud-Driss S, Siddique T. Sporadic and hereditary amyotrophic lateral sclerosis (ALS). Biochim Biophys Acta. 1852;2015:679–84.
12. Ticozzi N, Tiloca C, Morelli C, Colombrita C, Poletti B, Doretti A, et al. Genetics of familial Amyotrophic lateral sclerosis. Arch Ital Biol. 2011;149:65–82.
13. Rosen DR, Siddique T, Patterson D, Figlewicz DA, Sapp P, Hentati A, et al. Mutations in Cu/Zn superoxide dismutase gene are associated with familial amyotrophic lateral sclerosis. Nature. 1993;362:59–62.
14. Vucic S, Rothstein JD, Kiernan MC. Advances in treating amyotrophic lateral sclerosis: insights from pathophysiological studies. Trends Neurosci. 2014;37:433–42.
15. Miller RG, Mitchell JD, Moore DH. Riluzole for amyotrophic lateral sclerosis (ALS)/motor neuron disease (MND). Cochrane Database Syst Rev. 2012;3:CD001447.
16. Murphy G. Tissue inhibitors of metalloproteinases. Genome Biol. 2011;12:233.
17. Salter RC, Ashlin TG, Kwan AP, Ramji DP. ADAMTS proteases: key roles in atherosclerosis? J Mol Med (Berl). 2010;88:1203–11.
18. Forostyak S, Homola A, Turnovcova K, Svitil P, Jendelova P, Sykova E. Intrathecal delivery of mesenchymal stromal cells protects the structure of altered perineuronal nets in SOD1 rats and amends the course of ALS. Stem Cells. 2014;32:3163–72.
19. Wang D, Ichiyama RM, Zhao R, Andrews MR, Fawcett JW. Chondroitinase combined with rehabilitation promotes recovery of forelimb function in rats with chronic spinal cord injury. J Neurosci. 2011;31:9332–44.
20. Levy C, Brooks JM, Chen J, Su J, Fox MA. Cell-specific and developmental expression of lectican-cleaving proteases in mouse hippocampus and neocortex. J Comp Neurol. 2015;523:629–48.
21. Cross AK, Haddock G, Stock CJ, Allan S, Surr J, Bunning RA, et al. ADAMTS-1 and −4 are up-regulated following transient middle cerebral artery occlusion in the rat and their expression is modulated by TNF in cultured astrocytes. Brain Res. 2006;1088:19–30.
22. Haddock G, Cross AK, Plumb J, Surr J, Buttle DJ, Bunning RA, et al. Expression of ADAMTS-1, −4, −5 and TIMP-3 in normal and multiple sclerosis CNS white matter. Mult Scler. 2006;12:386–96.
23. Hamel MG, Ajmo JM, Leonardo CC, Zuo F, Sandy JD, Gottschall PE. Multimodal signaling by the ADAMTSs (a disintegrin and metalloproteinase with thrombospondin motifs) promotes neurite extension. Exp Neurol. 2008;210:428–40.
24. Glasson SS, Askew R, Sheppard B, Carito B, Blanchet T, Ma HL, et al. Deletion of active ADAMTS5 prevents cartilage degradation in a murine model of osteoarthritis. Nature. 2005;434:644–8.
25. Stanton H, Rogerson FM, East CJ, Golub SB, Lawlor KE, Meeker CT, et al. ADAMTS5 is the major aggrecanase in mouse cartilage in vivo and in vitro. Nature. 2005;434:648–52.
26. Mizuno H, Warita H, Aoki M, Itoyama Y. Accumulation of chondroitin sulfate proteoglycans in the microenvironment of spinal motor neurons in amyotrophic lateral sclerosis transgenic rats. J Neurosci Res. 2008;86:2512–23.
27. Gottschall PE, Howell MD. ADAMTS expression and function in central nervous system injury and disorders. Matrix Biol. 2015;44-46:70-6.
28. Burnside ER, Bradbury EJ. Manipulating the extracellular matrix and its role in brain and spinal cord plasticity and repair. Neuropathol Appl Neurobiol. 2014;40:26–59.
29. Suttkus A, Rohn S, Jäger C, Arendt T, Morawski M. Neuroprotection against iron-induced cell death by perineuronal nets - an in vivo analysis of oxidative stress. Am J Neurodegener Dis. 2012;1:122–9.
30. Morawski M, Brückner G, Jäger C, Seeger G, Arendt T. Neurons associated with aggrecan-based perineuronal nets are protected against tau pathology in subcortical regions in Alzheimer's disease. Neuroscience. 2010;169:1347–63.
31. Morawski M, Brückner MK, Riederer P, Brückner G, Arendt T. Perineuronal nets potentially protect against oxidative stress. Exp Neurol. 2004;188:309–15.
32. Deepa SS, Carulli D, Galtrey C, Rhodes K, Fukuda J, Mikami T, et al. Composition of perineuronal net extracellular matrix in rat brain: a different disaccharide composition for the net-associated proteoglycans. J Biol Chem. 2006;281:17789–800.
33. Tovar-Y-Romo LB, Ramírez-Jarquín UN, Lazo-Gómez R, Tapia R. Trophic factors as modulators of motor neuron physiology and survival: implications for ALS therapy. Front Cell Neurosci. 2014;8:61.
34. Schulte-Herbrüggen O, Braun A, Rochlitzer S, Jockers-Scherübl MC, Hellweg R. Neurotrophic factors–a tool for therapeutic strategies in neurological, neuropsychiatric and neuroimmunological diseases? Curr Med Chem. 2007;14:2318–29.
35. Sen A, Nelson TJ, Alkon DL. ApoE4 and Aβ Oligomers Reduce BDNF Expression via HDAC Nuclear Translocation. J Neurosci. 2015;35:7538–51.
36. Corbett GT, Roy A, Pahan K. Sodium phenylbutyrate enhances astrocytic neurotrophin synthesis via protein kinase C (PKC)-mediated activation of cAMP-response element-binding protein (CREB): implications for Alzheimer disease therapy. J Biol Chem. 2013;288:8299–312.
37. Zaheer A, Yorek MA, Lim R. Effects of glia maturation factor overexpression in primary astrocytes on MAP kinase activation, transcription factor activation, and neurotrophin secretion. Neurochem Res. 2001;26:1293–9.
38. Woodbury D, Schaar DG, Ramakrishnan L, Black IB. Novel structure of the human GDNF gene. Brain Res. 1998;803:95–104.
39. Shi J. Regulatory networks between neurotrophins and miRNAs in brain diseases and cancers. Acta Pharmacol Sin. 2015;36:149–57.
40. Gao Y, Su J, Guo W, Polich ED, Magyar DP, Xing Y, et al. Inhibition of miR-15a Promotes BDNF Expression and Rescues Dendritic Maturation Deficits in MeCP2-Deficient Neurons. Stem Cells. 2015;33:1618–29.
41. Huang W, Liu X, Cao J, Meng F, Li M, Chen B, et al. miR-134 regulates ischemia/reperfusion injury-induced neuronal cell death by regulating CREB signaling. J Mol Neurosci. 2015;55:821–9.
42. Skaper SD. The biology of neurotrophins, signalling pathways, and functional peptide mimetics of neurotrophins and their receptors. CNS Neurol Disord Drug Targets. 2008;7:46–62.
43. Nishio T, Sunohara N, Furukawa S. Neutrophin switching in spinal motoneurons of amyotrophic lateral sclerosis. Neuroreport. 1998;9:1661–5.
44. Seeburger JL, Tarras S, Natter H, Springer JE. Spinal cord motoneurons express p75NGFR and p145trkB mRNA in amyotrophic lateral sclerosis. Brain Res. 1993;621:111–5.
45. Pehar M, Cassina P, Vargas MR, Castellanos R, Viera L, Beckman JS, et al. Astrocytic production of nerve growth factor in motor neuron apoptosis: implications for amyotrophic lateral sclerosis. J Neurochem. 2004;89:464–73.

46. Turner BJ, Cheah IK, Macfarlane KJ, Lopes EC, Petratos S, Langford SJ, et al. Antisense peptide nucleic acid-mediated knockdown of the p75 neurotrophin receptor delays motor neuron disease in mutant SOD1 transgenic mice. J Neurochem. 2003;87:752–63.
47. Cragnolini AB, Huang Y, Gokina P, Friedman WJ. Nerve growth factor attenuates proliferation of astrocytes via the p75 neurotrophin receptor. Glia. 2009;57:1386–92.
48. Pollari E, Savchenko E, Jaronen M, Kanninen K, Malm T, Wojciechowski S, et al. Granulocyte colony stimulating factor attenuates inflammation in a mouse model of amyotrophic lateral sclerosis. J Neuroinflammation. 2011;8:74.
49. Moujalled D, James JL, Yang S, Zhang K, Duncan C, Moujalled DM, et al. Phosphorylation of hnRNP K by cyclin-dependent kinase 2 controls cytosolic accumulation of TDP-43. Hum Mol Genet. 2015;24:1655–69.
50. Pihlaja R, Koistinaho J, Kauppinen R, Sandholm J, Tanila H, Koistinaho M. Multiple cellular and molecular mechanisms are involved in human Aβ clearance by transplanted adult astrocytes. Glia. 2011;59:1643–57.
51. Malm T, Mariani M, Donovan LJ, Neilson L, Landreth GE. Activation of the nuclear receptor PPARζ is neuroprotective in a transgenic mouse model of Alzheimer's disease through inhibition of inflammation. J Neuroinflammation. 2015;12:7.
52. Rolova T, Puli L, Magga J, Dhungana H, Kanninen K, Wojciehowski S, et al. Complex regulation of acute and chronic neuroinflammatory responses in mouse models deficient for nuclear factor kappa B p50 subunit. Neurobiol Dis. 2014;64:16–29.

3

Stathmin 1/2-triggered microtubule loss mediates Golgi fragmentation in mutant SOD1 motor neurons

Sarah Bellouze[1†], Gilbert Baillat[1†], Dorothée Buttigieg[1], Pierre de la Grange[2], Catherine Rabouille[3] and Georg Haase[1*]

Abstract

Background: Pathological Golgi fragmentation represents a constant pre-clinical feature of many neurodegenerative diseases including amyotrophic lateral sclerosis (ALS) but its molecular mechanisms remain hitherto unclear.

Results: Here, we show that the severe Golgi fragmentation in transgenic mutant $SOD1^{G85R}$ and $SOD1^{G93A}$ mouse motor neurons is associated with defective polymerization of Golgi-derived microtubules, loss of the COPI coat subunit β-COP, cytoplasmic dispersion of the Golgi tether GM130, strong accumulation of the ER-Golgi v-SNAREs GS15 and GS28 as well as tubular/vesicular Golgi fragmentation. Data mining, transcriptomic and protein analyses demonstrate that both SOD1 mutants cause early presymptomatic and rapidly progressive up-regulation of the microtubule-destabilizing proteins Stathmins 1 and 2. Remarkably, mutant SOD1-triggered Golgi fragmentation and Golgi SNARE accumulation are recapitulated by Stathmin 1/2 overexpression but completely rescued by Stathmin 1/2 knockdown or the microtubule-stabilizing drug Taxol.

Conclusions: We conclude that Stathmin-triggered microtubule destabilization mediates Golgi fragmentation in mutant SOD1-linked ALS and potentially also in related motor neuron diseases.

Background

Structural alterations of the Golgi apparatus are among the earliest and most constant pathological features in neurodegenerative diseases and have been widely studied in the motor neuron disease amyotrophic lateral sclerosis (ALS) [16, 23, 57]. The Golgi alterations are detectable in degenerating ALS motor neurons of spinal cord and cerebral motor cortex [20, 36], are common to both sporadic [22] and familial forms of the disease [21, 24, 31, 36, 58], and manifest at presymptomatic stage [36, 65, 66].

The Golgi apparatus of normal motor neurons is made of stacked membrane-bound cisternae that are laterally connected to form the Golgi ribbon [5]. Earlier studies in particular by Gonatas and colleagues have characterized the structural Golgi alterations in ALS motor neurons as

fragmentation [22], i.e. transformation of the Golgi ribbon into disconnected stacks or into tubules and vesicles [5], and as atrophy [22, 36], i.e. loss or dispersion of Golgi membranes. In the most widely studied ALS mouse model, transgenic mutant $SOD1^{G93A}$ mice, Golgi fragmentation can affect up to 75 % of spinal cord motor neurons at symptomatic stage [36, 65].

The Golgi apparatus is a highly dynamic cellular organelle that ensures the processing and sorting of proteins form their site of synthesis in the endoplasmic reticulum (ER) en route to their final destination, which is reflected by its functional division into a cis(entry) side and a trans(exit) side. Intra-Golgi transport involves COPI-coated vesicles [2] which are formed through recruitment of coatomers α-ζ [43], tethered by Rabs and Golgins [37] and fused/docked to target membranes by Golgi SNAREs [29].

While the molecular mechanisms of Golgi fragmentation in ALS remain largely to be deciphered, at least two mechanisms can been proposed. The first mechanism involves an impairment in transport from endoplasmic reticulum (ER) to Golgi [4, 52] and from Golgi to plasma

---
* Correspondence: georg.haase@univ-amu.fr
†Equal contributors
[1]Institut de Neurosciences de la Timone, UMR 7289, Centre National de la Recherche Scientifique (CNRS) and Aix-Marseille Université, 27 bd Jean Moulin, 13005 Marseille, France
Full list of author information is available at the end of the article

membrane [54]. Both could in turn affect Golgi structure. The second mechanism involves potential microtubule alterations [36]. Microtubules are indeed closely associated with the Golgi [30, 50] and nucleated at its membrane [8, 14] in motor neurons [5]. Furthermore, pharmacological microtubule disruption with colchicine or nocodazole causes reversible Golgi fragmentation and dispersal [15, 47, 61]. Finally, we have recently demonstrated that defective polymerization of Golgi-derived microtubules causes Golgi fragmentation in motor neurons of *pmn* mice with progressive motor neuronopathy which are mutated in the tubulin-binding cofactor E (Tbce) gene [5].

The role of microtubules in mutant SOD1-linked Golgi fragmentation remained however unclear. Indeed, microtubules appeared normal in motor neuron cell bodies with a fragmented Golgi [53] despite their early alterations in axons [17, 70]. In addition, dys-regulation of a microtubule-severing protein (Stathmin-1) was seen only in a fraction of motor neurons with Golgi fragmentation and only at late disease stage [55], suggesting that it may represent a compensatory event.

To analyze the mechanisms of Golgi pathology in ALS, we here investigated two transgenic mouse lines with similar disease course due to either dismutase active (G93A) or inactive (G85R) human SOD1. Mutant SOD1^{G93A} mice (line G1del) develop limb weakness between day 165 to 240 and fatal paralysis about 40 days later [1]. Mutant SOD1^{G85R} mice (line 148) develop limb weakness between day 240 to 280 and die about 15 days later [6]. As controls, we used non-transgenic litter mice and mice expressing wild type human SOD1 (SOD1^{wt}, line 76) at a similar level as in the mutants. In addition, we used NSC-34 cells transfected with mutant or wildtype SOD1 as in vitro system. We show that the early Golgi pathology observed in mutant SOD1^{G85R} and SOD1^{G93A} motor neurons involves disruption of the Golgi-nucleated somatic microtubule network due to up-regulation of the two microtubule-severing proteins Stathmin 1 and 2. This in turn leads to Golgi fragmentation with early presymptomatic and rapidly progressive accumulation of the ER-Golgi v-SNAREs GS28 and GS15. These data, together with our findings in ALS-like *pmn* mice [5], lead us to propose that a disruption of Golgi-nucleated microtubules underlies Golgi fragmentation in human SOD1-linked ALS and related degenerative motor neuron diseases.

Results

To confirm the reported Golgi alterations in mutant SOD1 motor neurons [36, 65, 66], we first examined lumbar spinal cord cryosections from 240-day-old mice by confocal microscopy using GM130 antibodies. We demonstrate that Golgi membranes form a dense ribbon in the cell bodies of control and SOD1^{wt} motor neurons, but

appear fragmented or atrophied in motor neurons of mutant SOD1^{G85R} and SOD1^{G93A} mice (Fig. 1a). Golgi fragmentation was confirmed by GM130 membrane modeling demonstrating an ~4 fold increase in the number of individual Golgi profiles in SOD1^{G85R} and SOD1^{G93A} motor neurons when compared to control (Fig. 1a,b). Loss of Golgi area in SOD1^{G85R} and SOD1^{G93A} motor neurons was quantified by a reduction in its cross-sectional area to ~35 % of normal (Fig. 1a,c, Additional file 1: Figure S1A).

To confirm that Golgi fragmentation precedes disease onset in ALS [36, 65, 66], we analyzed mutant SOD1^{G93A} mice and SOD1^{G85R} mice, respectively one month before (age 130 days) and two months before (age 180 days) the onset of first clinical symptoms and before any reported loss of motor neurons. Up to 19 % of mutant SOD1 motor neurons displayed signs of Golgi fragmentation labelled by GM130, as compared to < 1 % of motor neurons in non-transgenic and SOD1^{wt} mice (Fig. 1d and Additional file 1: Figure S1B). This compares very well with published results at least in mutant SOD1^{G93A} mice, where Golgi fragmentation is scored in 25-30 % of motor neurons about 10 days later at 20 weeks of age [65].

To confirm and characterize the changes of the Golgi architecture, we analyzed presymptomatic mutant SOD1 mice aged 140 days at the ultrastructural level by electron microscopy. In control mice (Fig. 1e, upper left panel) and in transgenic SOD1^{wt} mice (not shown), the Golgi apparatus exhibits the typical morphology of stacked cisternae as described in [5]. Conversely, in motor neurons of mutant SOD1 mice, we observe a fragmentation of the Golgi ribbon into many disconnected Golgi stacks, small tubules and vesicles that appear uncoated as well as unlinked (Fig. 1e, arrows in lower left panels).

To analyze the molecular basis of the observed Golgi fragmentation in mutant SOD1 motor neurons, we investigated the status of Golgi vesicle coats, tethers and SNAREs using biochemical methods. We found that the level of the COPI vesicle subunit β-COP is lower in mutant SOD1^{G85R} and SOD1^{G93A} spinal cords than in control spinal cords, whereas the level of the COPII vesicle subunit Sec23 remains normal (Fig. 1f, upper panels).

The Golgi tethering protein GM130 is normally associated with the cytoplasmic face of cis-medial Golgi membranes and binds the Golgi tether p115 present on incoming vesicles [38]. We found that the total levels of GM130 and p115 are unchanged in mutant SOD1 spinal cords when compared to control (Fig. 1f, lower panels). Since the membrane association of GM130 and p115 is critical for their function [37], we investigated a potential subcellular redistribution of both Golgi tethers in mutant SOD1 mice by biochemical fractionation of spinal cords into membrane (P10), vesicle (P100) and cytosol (S100) fractions. We found that GM130 is significantly redistributed from its typical Golgi membrane localization in

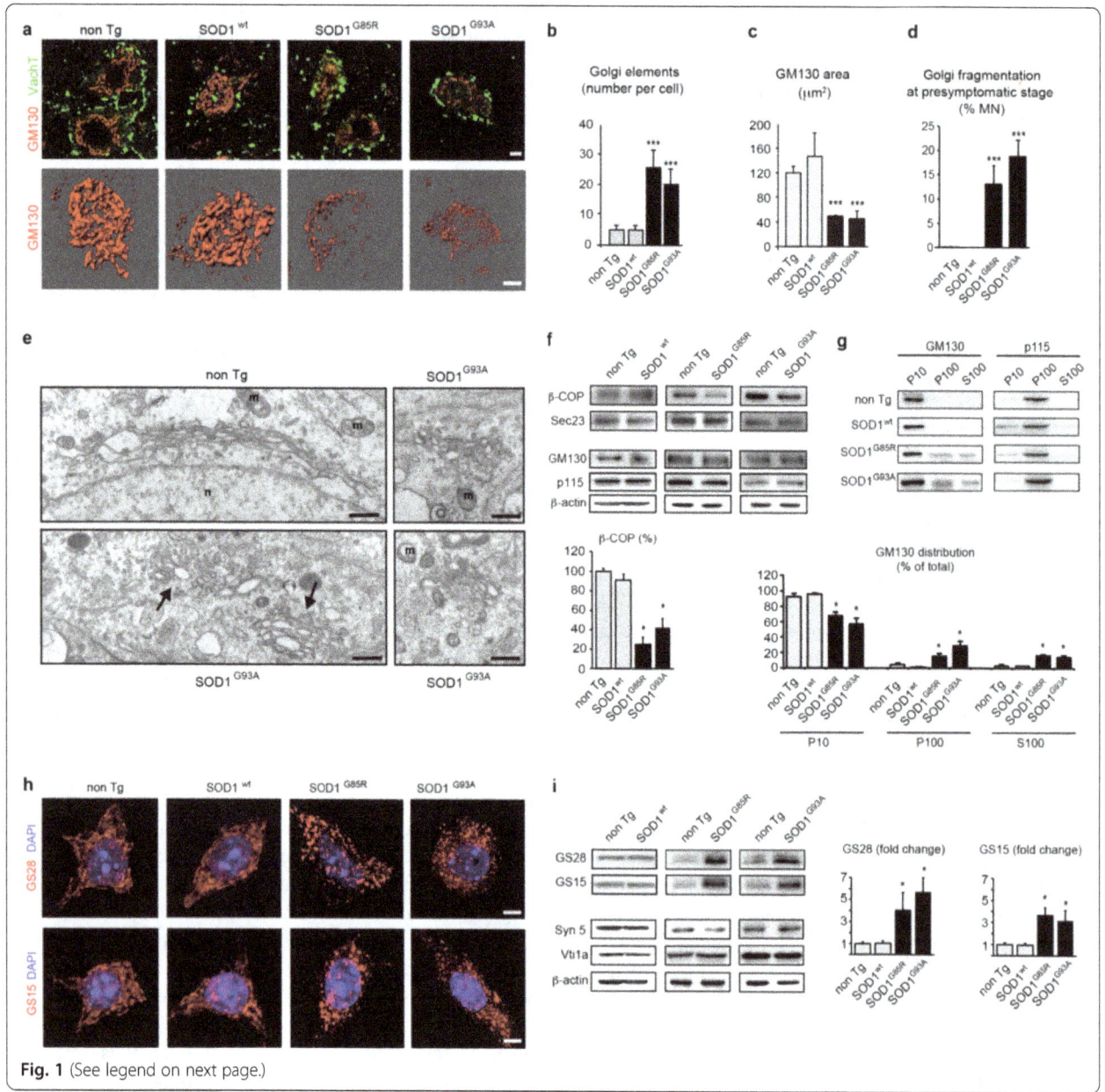

Fig. 1 (See legend on next page.)

(See figure on previous page.)

Fig. 1 Morphological and molecular Golgi alterations in motor neurons of mutant SOD1 mice. **a.** Confocal z-stacks (upper panels) show fragmentation of GM130-labeled Golgi membranes in lumbar motor neurons of 240-day-old mutant SOD1^{G85R} and SOD1^{G93A} mice as compared to non-transgenic mice and transgenic SOD1^{wt} mice. Motor neurons are identified by expression of VaChT (vesicular acetylcholine transporter). 3D-modeling (lower panels) of GM130-labelled Golgi membranes in entire motor neurons confirms Golgi fragmentation. Scale bars 10 μm. **b.** Increased number of GM130-stained Golgi elements in mutant SOD1^{G85R} and SOD1^{G93A} motor neurons determined by 3D modeling of Golgi membranes in entire cells (mean ± sd, n = 12 motor neurons from three mice per genotype, *** p < 0.0001 by student's t-test, unpaired. **c.** Decreased cross-sectional area of GM130-labeled Golgi area in mutant SOD1^{G85R} and SOD1^{G93A} motor neurons as compared to control motor neurons (mean ± sd, *** p < 0.001, n = 50 motor neurons from three mice per genotype, student's t test). See also Additional file 1: Figure S1. **d.** Percentage of motor neurons with GM130-labeled Golgi fragmentation at presymptomatic stage (mean ± sd, *** p < 0.001 by student's t-test, n > 250 motor neurons from four mice per genotype were analyzed at presymptomatic stage corresponding to age 130 days (SOD1^{G93A}, non Tg) or 180 days (SOD1^{G85R}, SOD1^{wt}). **e.** Electron microscopy of a lumbar motor neuron from a non-transgenic mouse aged 140 days showing a typical Golgi apparatus (upper panel) that is easily distinguished from unlinked, partially swollen and vesiculated Golgi profiles observed in mutant SOD1^{G93A} motor neurons (arrows in lower panel, magnifications on the right). n: nucleus, m: mitochondria. Scale bars 500 nm (left panels), 200 nm (right panels). **f.** Western blots showing decreased levels of β-COP in mutant SOD1 mice, and normal levels of Sec23, GM130 and p115. Loading control β-actin. Shown is one representative blot per genotype out of four. The diagram below shows that β-COP levels (normalized to β-actin) are reduced to 25 ± 7.7 % and 42.5 ± 9.6 % of non Tg (mean ± sd, n = 4 per genotype, * p < 0.01 by Mann Whitney test). **g.** Subcellular fractionation of spinal cords. Western blot analyses show redistribution of GM130 in mutant SOD1 mice, as indicated by shift from its normal membrane localization in control and SOD^{wt} mice into fragmented membranes and vesicles in SOD1^{G85R} and SOD1^{G93A} mice and cytosol. P115 is not redistributed. Each blot is representative of three independant experiments on mice of the indicated genotypes. The diagram below shows densitometric determination of protein distribution (mean ± sd, n = 3 per genotype, * p < 0.01 by Mann Whitney test). **h.** Confocal imaging reveals accumulation of Golgi v-SNARE protein GS28 (upper panels) and GS15 (lower panels) in small vesicle-like punctae of motor neurons in mutant SOD1 mice, as compared to controls. Scale bars 10 μm. **i.** Western blots (upper two panels) demonstrating massively increased levels of Golgi v-SNAREs GS28 and GS15 in mutant SOD1^{G85R} and SOD1^{G93A} lumbar spinal cords, as compared to non-transgenic and SOD1^{wt} spinal cords. Western blots (lower three panels) showing normal expression of the Golgi t-SNARE Syntaxin-5a and the endosomal v-SNARE Vti1a. β-actin indicates equal protein loading. Each blot is representative of three independant experiments on mice of the indicated genotypes. The diagrams show increased spinal cord protein levels of GS28 by 4 ± 1.6 (SOD1^{G85R}) and by 3.7 ± 1.3 (SOD1^{G93A}) fold and of GS15 by 3.7 ± 0.7 (SOD1^{G85R}) and by 3.2 ± 1 (SOD1^{G93A}) as compared to non Tg control (mean ± sd, * p < 0.001 by Mann Whitney test)

control mice to vesicles, membrane fragments and cytosol in SOD1^{G85R} and SOD1^{G93A} mice (Fig. 1g, blots and diagram). Interestingly, this subcellular redistribution is specific for GM130 since p115 remains associated with the vesicle fraction as in control mice (Fig. 1g). The purity of the P10, P100 and S100 fractions was confirmed by analysis of molecular markers L1, Vt1a and GAPDH (Additional file 1: Figure S2). These data suggest that mutant SOD1 expression leads to defective tethering of Golgi vesicles due to redistribution of GM130.

Last, Golgi SNAREs mediate vesicle fusion through interaction of v-SNAREs (present on vesicles) and t-SNAREs (present on target membranes) [26, 29]. Using immunofluorescence, we found that the ER-Golgi v-SNAREs GS28 [56] and GS15 [71] are present in small dispersed profiles in mutant SOD1^{G85R} and SOD1^{G93A} motor neurons when compared to control motor neurons (Fig. 1h). Furthermore, Western blots showed that the total spinal cord levels of GS28 and GS15 are increased by > 4 fold and >3 fold respectively in mutant SOD1^{G85R} mice and SOD1^{G93A} mice when compared to control mice (Fig. 1i, upper panels and diagrams). This is specific for GS15 and 28 because, by contrast, the levels of Syntaxin5a, the major Golgi t-SNARE cognate of GS28 and GS15, and of the endosomal v-SNARE Vti1a, are unchanged in mutant SOD1 mice (Fig. 1i, lower panels). Importantly in SOD1^{wt} spinal cords, the levels of all tested SNARE proteins are identical to those in non-transgenic mice (Fig. 1h, upper panels), indicating a

specific and significant increase of Golgi v-SNAREs GS28 and GS15 in mutant SOD1 spinal cords.

In order to set up a tractable in vitro model, we reproduced these Golgi alterations in cultured NSC-34 motor neurons [7] expressing mutant SOD1 (Fig. 2). Using MannII-GFP or GM130 as Golgi markers, the Golgi appears as a compact juxtanuclear structure in control cells transfected with empty or SOD1^{wt} plasmids but is fragmented in cells transfected with SOD1^{G85R} or SOD1^{G93A} plasmids (Fig. 2a,b and Additional file 1: Figure S1C). Expression of both SOD1 mutants also triggers dispersal of GS28, as shown by IF (Fig. 2a,c) and a >2 fold increase in protein levels of GS28 and GS15, as shown by Western blot (Fig. 2d).

Taken together, these results show that both in spinal motor neurons and in NSC-34 cells, expression of mutant SOD1^{G85R} and SOD1^{G93A} causes loss of β-COP, redistribution of GM130 and strong accumulation of Golgi SNAREs GS28 and GS15, in line with the observed Golgi fragmentation. Importantly, these alterations closely resemble those that we previously observed in *pmn* mice [5].

Mutant SOD1 proteins localize to the Golgi and impede the polymerization of Golgi-derived microtubules

Given that the molecular features observed in *pmn* mice are triggered by a point mutation in Golgi-localized TBCE that affects the Golgi microtubule network, we wondered whether mutant SOD1 also impairs Golgi-derived microtubules.

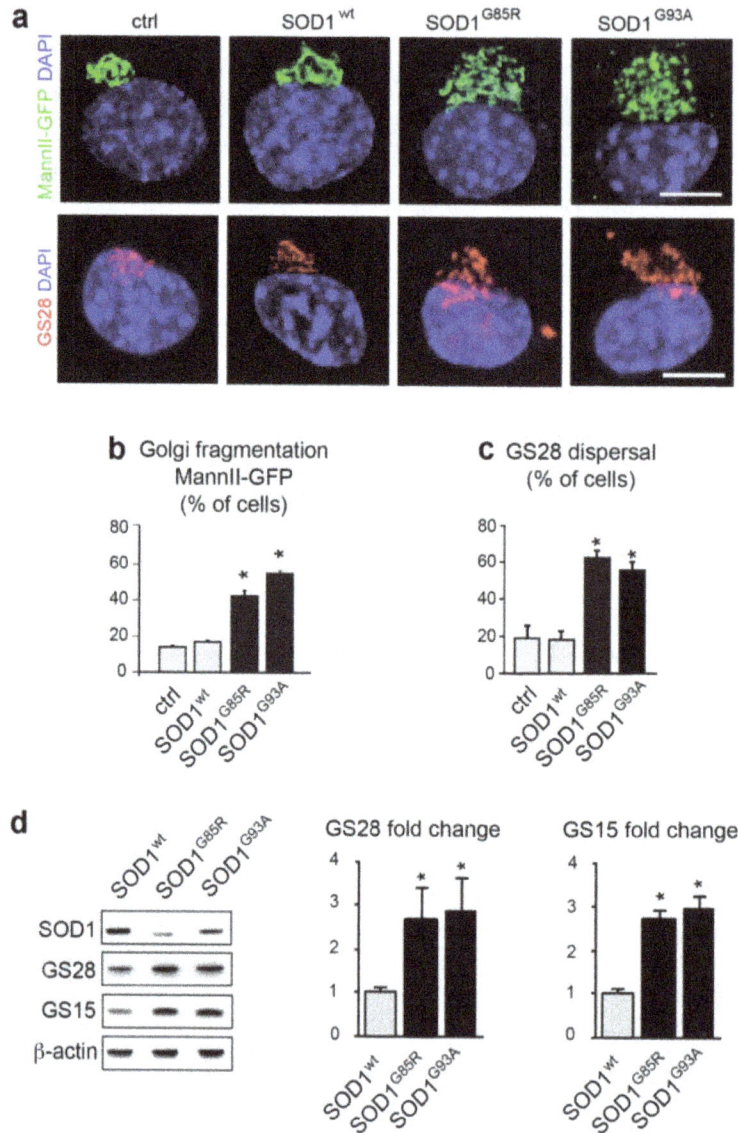

Fig. 2 Golgi alterations in mutant SOD1-transfected NSC-34 motor neurons. **a.** Confocal images (upper panels) showing Golgi fragmentation with the marker MannII-GFP in NSC-34 cells transfected for 4 DIV with mutant SOD1, as compared to the situation in control or wildtype SOD1-transfected cells. Confocal images (lower panels) showing GS28 dispersal after transfection with mutant SOD1, as compared to the situation in control or wildtype SOD1 cells. Scale bar 10 μm. **b.** Percentage of cells (mean ± sd) with Golgi fragmentation labeled for MannII-GFP. More than 300 cells per condition were analyzed on quadruplicate wells per condition. Statistical significance * p < 0.01 by Mann–Whitney test, as compared to mock and SOD^{wt}. Data represent one out of three experiments yielding similar results. **c.** Percentage of transfected cells with dispersal of GS28. More than 200 cells per condition were analyzed on quadruplicate wells per condition. Statistical significance * p < 0.01 by Mann–Whitney test, as compared to mock and SOD^{wt}. **d.** Western blot analysis of NSC-34 cells demonstrating that GS28 protein levels are increased to 2.7 ± 0.7 and 2.9 ± 0.8 by SOD1^{G85R} and SOD1^{G93A}, respectively, as compared to those in control SOD^{wt}. GS15 protein levels are increased to 2.7 ± 0.2 and 3.0 ± 0.3 fold, respectively. The diagrams show densitometric quantification of protein levels relative to SOD^{wt} (mean ± sd). Cellular extracts from three independently transfected cultures were blotted and analyzed each in duplicate. Statistical significance * p < 0.01 by Mann Whitney test

Previous studies in non-motor neuronal cells have localized a significant fraction of SOD1 to Golgi membranes [63, 64]. To confirm this, we transfected RFP-tagged forms of wildtype and mutant SOD1 together with MannII-GFP in NSC-34 cells. After extraction of soluble proteins, co-localization and Pearson correlation analysis showed that both RFP-tagged SOD1^{wt}, SOD1^{G85R} and SOD1^{G93A} indeed significantly co-localize with MannII-GFP-labeled Golgi membranes whereas RFP is mainly nuclear (Fig. 3a, upper three panels).

Since the Golgi membrane is a major site of microtubule polymerization and nucleation in motor neurons

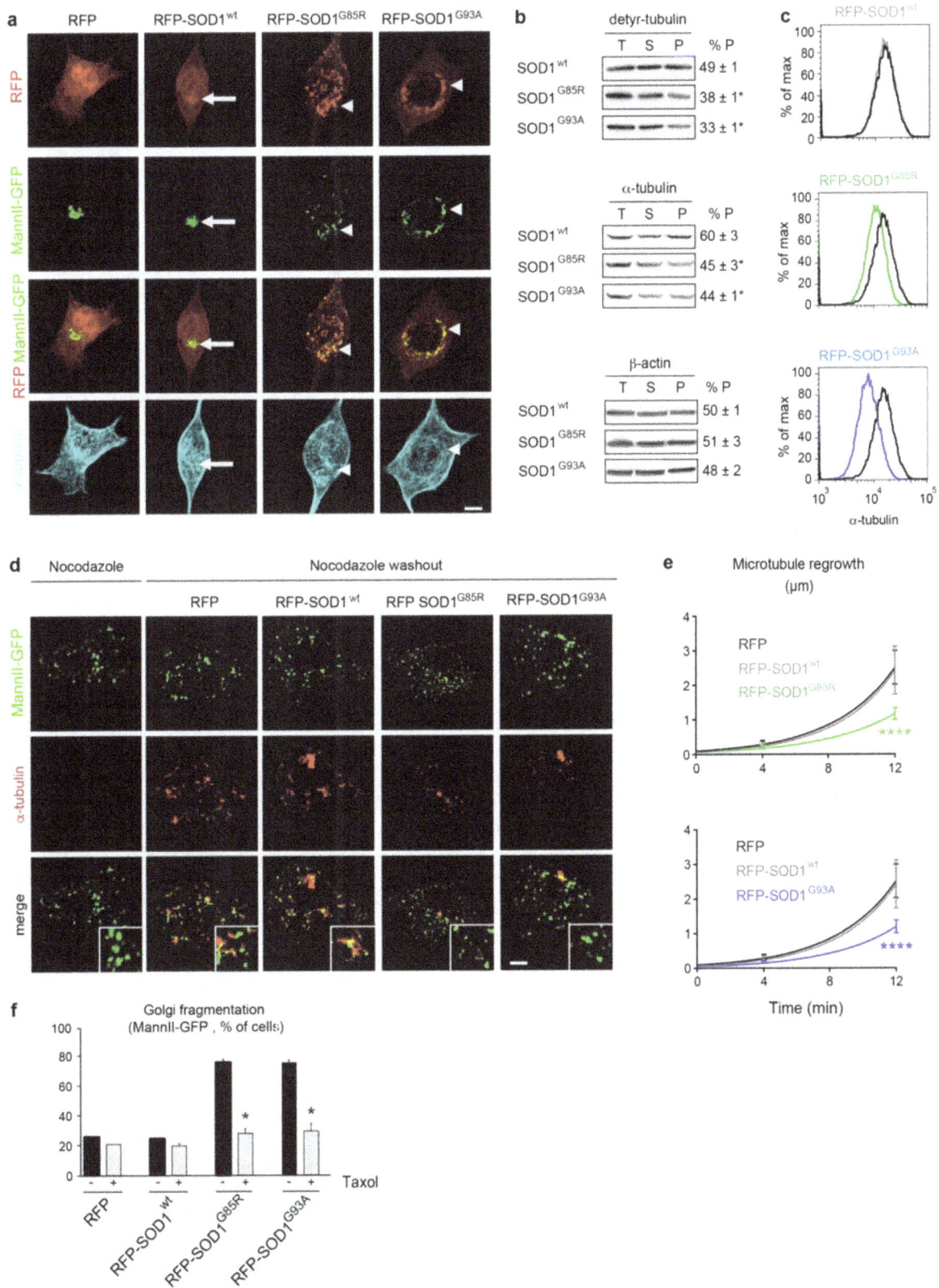

Fig. 3 (See legend on next page.)

(See figure on previous page.)

Fig. 3 SOD1 mutants impair polymerization of Golgi-derived microtubules. **a**. Images show NSC-34 cells expressing RFP or SOD1 variants tagged with RFP after extraction for soluble proteins and labeling with MannII-GFP (Golgi) and antibodies against α-tubulin (microtubules). Merged RFP/MannII-GFP images show that both wildtype SOD1 (arrow) and mutant SOD1 (arrowheads) localize to Golgi membranes. This is confirmed by Pearson's correlation analysis (RFP-SOD1^{wt} 0.74 ± 0.09, RFP-SOD1^{G85R} 0.72 ± 0.09, RFP-SOD1^{G93A} 0.77 ± 0.14, RFP 0.13 ± 0.14, statistical significance SOD1 variants vs RFP : p < 0.0006 by student's t-test). Mutant SOD1^{G85R} and SOD1^{G93A} specifically cause rarefaction of microtubules around fragmented Golgi profiles (arrowheads in lower panel). **b**. Biochemical fractionation of total (T), soluble (S) and polymerized (P) tubulins. Cells expressing SOD1^{G85R} or SOD1^{G93A} display a decreased ratio of polymerized detyrosinated (detyr-) tubulin. The ratio of polymerized α-tubulin is also decreased. Polymerization of β-actin is not affected by mutant SOD1. % P is equivalent to P/(P + S), * p < 0.01 by Mann–Whitney test, n = 3 experiments each. **c**. Flow cytometry of cellular microtubules in NSC-34 cells after extraction of soluble tubulins, microtubule stabilization and intracellular labeling with α-tubulin-FITC antibodies. Cells expressing SOD^{wt} (in grey, upper panel) display normal levels of α-tubulin-containing microtubules in comparison to cells expressing RFP (in black). Cells expressing mutant SOD1^{G85R} (in green, middle panel) or mutant SOD1^{G93A} (in blue, lower panel) show decreased levels of cellular microtubules. Median fluorescence signal per cell: 15.800 (RFP), 15.900 (SOD1wt), 11.600 (SOD1^{G85R}), 8.418 (SOD1^{G93A}). Statistical significance by chi square test, * T(x) > 200, ns T(x) = 0. **d**. Images showing transfected NSC-34 cells that were treated with Nocodazole (left column) and restored to drug-free medium for 12 min (right four columns). Cells were identified by RFP expression (not shown), Golgi profiles were identified by MannII-GFP and growing microtubules with antibodies against α-tubulin (pseudocolored in red). Mutant SOD1^{G85R} and SOD1^{G93A} impede regrowth of Golgi-derived microtubules (zoomed insets). Scale bar 5 μm. **e**. Diagrams showing reduced growth rate of Golgi-derived microtubules in cells expressing RFP- SOD1^{G85R} (upper panel) or RFP- SOD1^{G93A} (lower panel) as compared to cells expressing RFP- SOD1^{wt} or RFP. Microtubule length represents mean of mean of >12 cells per time point and condition and a total of 1495 microtubules analyzed. Statistical significance **** p < 0.0001 (RFP-SOD1^{G85R} vs RFP or vs SOD1^{wt}) and **** p < 0.0001 (RFP-SOD1^{G93A} vs RFP or vs SOD1^{wt}) by ANOVA test and Tukey's multiple comparison test. **f**. Diagrams showing Taxol-mediated rescue of MannII-GFP-labeled Golgi fragmentation in cells expressing mutant SOD1^{G85R} or SOD1^{G93A} each tagged to RFP. Statistical significance * p < 0.01 (Taxol vs mock) by Mann–Whitney test, n ≥ 50 cells per well and 4 replicate wells were analyzed per condition

[5, 8, 14], we then tested whether SOD1 mutants affect the polymerization of microtubules. By IF, microtubules appear disorganized and rarefied around MannII-GFP-labeled Golgi punctae in mutant SOD1 cells when compared to control cells (Fig. 3a, lower panel). To confirm this, we biochemically analyzed detyrosinated tubulins, which are markers of Golgi-associated microtubules [50, 60], by determining their total, soluble and polymerized fractions (Fig. 3b). The ratio of polymerized versus total detyrosinated tubulin is significantly lower in mutant SOD1^{G85R} cells and SOD1^{G93A} cells than in SOD1^{wt} cells (Fig. 3b, upper panels). The ratio of polymerized versus total α-tubulin in mutant SOD1 cells is also decreased, albeit to a lower extent (Fig. 3b, middle panels). These data indicate that both SOD1 mutants impede the polymerization of Golgi-derived microtubules.

To determine the microtubule content in individual cells, we extracted soluble tubulins, labeled polymerized microtubules with FITC-coupled antibodies against α-tubulin and performed flow cytometry. This method accurately measures cellular microtubules since the flow cytometry signals of cells are increased after treatment with the microtubule-stabilizing drug Taxol, decreased after treatement with the microtubule-disrupting drug Nocodazole and correlated with the amount of biochemically fractionated microtubules (Additional file 1: Figure S3A-B). Using this technique, we found significantly less polymerized microtubules in cells expressing RFP-tagged SOD1^{G85R} or SOD1^{G93A} than in cells expressing RFP-SOD1^{wt} or RFP (Fig. 3c), confirming the mutant SOD1-triggered loss of cellular microtubules.

To directly measure the polymerization rate of microtubules at the Golgi, we incubated control and mutant SOD1 NSC-34 cells with Nocodazole, restored the cells to drug-free medium and measured the regrowth of Golgi-derived microtubules over 12 min using α-tubulin/MannII-GFP labeling (Fig. 3d). In control cells expressing RFP or RFP-SOD1^{wt}, small microtubule asters form at Golgi profiles within few minutes after nocodazole washout. These microtubules then grow rapidly, confirming the capacity of Golgi membranes to nucleate microtubules [5, 8, 14]. In mutant SOD1 expressing cells, however, Golgi-derived microtubule asters are rare and grow slowly. Their mean growth rate is reduced by over 50 % in SOD1^{G85R} and SOD1^{G93A} cells in comparison to RFP expressing cells (Fig. 3e). Wildtype SOD1 does not impede growth of Golgi-derived microtubules (Fig. 3e). Taken together, these data indicate that SOD1 mutants decrease the growth rate and steady state levels of Golgi-derived microtubules.

Last, to test whether these microtubule defects are responsible for the observed Golgi alterations, we stabilized microtubules in mutant SOD1- and control-transfected cells by treating the cultures with Taxol (10 nM) from 0 to 4 DIV. We found that Taxol significantly reduces the percentage of mutant SOD1-transfected cells harboring MannII-GFP-labeled Golgi alterations (Fig. 3f), indicating that microtubule defects mediate the mutant SOD1-triggered Golgi alterations.

Mutant SOD1 causes up-regulation of Stathmin 1 and 2 gene expression

To identify the upstream triggers of microtubule loss and tubular/vesicular Golgi fragmentation in mutant SOD1 motor neurons, we performed data mining and bioinformatic analyses. We first analyzed five studies comparing the gene expression profiles of SOD1^{G93A} and control motor neurons isolated by laser capture microdissection from adult spinal cord [19, 28, 33, 40, 42]. Two studies showed that cytoskeleton-related genes annotated to the Gene Ontology (GO) terms "cytoskeletal part/ GO:0044430" and "cytoskeleton/GO:0005856" are significantly dys-regulated: 14 genes at presymptomatic stage [33]), 76 genes at early disease stage [33]) and 42 genes at end stage [42]). Among those, genes annotated to the microtubule cytoskeleton (GO:0015630) display significant dys-regulation [33].

To identify individual dys-regulated genes linked to microtubules, we then compared by bioinformatics analysis the publically available gene expression profiles from mutant SOD1 G93A and control motor neurons deposited in the Gene Omnibus database by Ferraiuolo et al. as GSE10953 [19] and by Nardo et al. as GSE46298

[40]. Given the similarities between *pmn* and SOD1, we first focused on tubulin binding co-factors but found that the six genes Tbca, Tbcb, Tbcc, Tbcd, Tbce and Tbcel (Tbce-like) are not significantly dys-regulated in mutant SOD1 motor neurons at any time point (fold change < 1.5, p > 0.05, Table 1).

By contrast, we found three Stathmin genes whose expression was significantly modulated in presymptomatic mutant SOD1^{G93A} motor neurons when compared to control. Stathmin 1 and Stathmin 2 were up-regulated by 1.87 and 1.63 fold respectively, whereas Stathmin 3 was down-regulated by 1.71 fold at P60 (p < 0.05, Table 2). Stathmin 1 up-regulation (by 1.68 fold) also tended to occur at end stage in an independent dataset of Perrin et al. [42], although not reaching statistical significance (p = 0.06, Table 2).

Table 1 Gene expression profiles of tubulin-binding cofactors in mutant SOD1 motor neurons

Ferraiuolo et al. 2007	Presymptomatic G93A vs. Ctrl (P60)			Symptomatic G93A vs. Ctrl (P90)			Endstage G93A vs. Ctrl (P120)		
Gene Symbol	Regulation	Fold-Change	P-Value	Regulation	Fold-Change	P-Value	Regulation	Fold-Change	P-Value
Tbca	up	1,74	1,61 E-01	up	1,13	6,11E-01	down	1,63	9,62E-02
Tbcb	up	1,03	9,24E-01	down	1,08	7,49E-01	down	1,33	6,17E-02
Tbcc	down	1,09	8,24E-01	down	1,25	4,57E-01	up	1,03	9,71E-01
Tbcd	down	1,14	8,10E-01	up	1,07	7,65E-01	down	1,03	9,32E-01
Tbce	up	1,29	6,22E-01	up	1,01	9,87E-01	down	1,07	9,18E-01
Tbcel	down	1,07	9,21 E-01	down	1,12	7,91 E-01	up	1,10	8,09E-01
Nardo et al. 2013	Presymptomatic C57 G93A vs. Ctrl			Onset C57 G93A vs. Ctrl			Symptomatic C57 G93A vs. Ctrl		
Gene	Regulation	Fold-Change	P-Value	Regulation	Fold-Change	P-Value	Regulation	Fold-Change	P-Value
Tbca	up	1,23	1,81 E-01	down	1,03	8,53E-01	up	1,04	3,83E-01
Tbcb	up	1,06	7,17E-01	down	1,15	5,21 E-01	down	1,04	8,46E-01
Tbcc	up	1,16	2,81 E-01	down	1,10	2,12E-01	up	1,07	6,83E-01
Tbcd	up	1,09	6,15E-01	up	1,01	9,47E-01	up	1,10	5,20E-01
Tbce	up	1,11	6,02E-01	up	1,17	2,70E-01	up	1,10	1,05E-02
Tbcel	up	1,06	6,01 E-01	up	1,10	4,47E-01	down	1,09	6,51E-01
Nardo et al. 2013	Presymptomatic 129sv G93A vs. Ctrl			Onset 129sv G93A vs. Ctrl			Symptomatic 129sv G93A vs. Ctrl		
Gene	Regulation	Fold-Change	P-Value	Regulation	Fold-Change	P-Value	Regulation	Fold-Change	P-Value
Tbca	up	1,11	5,19E-01	down	1,11	2,51 E-01	down	1,10	4,67E-01
Tbcb	up	1,22	2,89E-01	down	1,45	3,00E-03	down	1,45	1,61E-02
Tbcc	up	1,20	1,50E-01	down	1,23	4,28E-02	down	1,06	3,85E-01
Tbcd	up	1,28	1,37E-01	down	1,11	4,26E-01	down	1,06	5,97E-01
Tbce	up	1,17	2,44E-01	down	1,20	8,76E-03	down	1,05	5,69E-01
Tbcel	up	1,10	6,18E-01	up	1,01	9,11E-01	down	1,02	8,61E-01

Gene expression profiles from mutant SOD1 G93A and control motor neurons isolated by laser capture microdissection at different stage of disease [19, 40] respectively were downloaded from the Gene Omnibus database and analyzed with EASANA software based on FAST DB annotations [12, 13]. Gene dysregulation was considered significant at fold changes >1.5 and p-values < 5E-02
Genes encoding tubulin-binding cofactors Tbca to Tbcel are not significantly dys-regulated in mutant SOD1 motor neurons at any time point in the datasets GSE10953 [19] or GSE46298 [40]
Note that mutant SOD1 G93A mice with genetic backgrounds C57BL/6 and 129sv and corresponding control mice were analyzed in the study of Nardo and colleagues [40]. Here, onset of disease was defined when mice showed first signs of paw grip strength impairment and when body weight started to decline. Symptomatic disease was defined when mice displayed a decrease of 50 % in their latency on grip strength and when body weight declined by >5 %

Table 2 Gene expression profiles of Stathmins in mutant SOD1 motor neurons

Ferraiuolo et al. 2007	Presymptomatic G93A vs. Ctrl (P60)			Symptomatic G93A vs. Ctrl (P90)			Endstage G93A vs. Ctrl (P120)		
Gene	Regulation	Fold-Change	P-Value	Regulation	Fold-Change	P-Value	Regulation	Fold-Change	P-Value
Stmnl	**up**	**1,87**	**3,80E-02**	up	1,21	4,54E-01	down	1,40	3,32E-01
Stmn2	down	1,03	9,47E-01	down	1,39	2,65E-01	up	1,91	3,96E-01
Stmn3	**down**	**1,71**	**9,50E-03**	down	1,44	2,73E-01	down	1,21	2,92E-01
Stmn4	down	1,02	9,61 E-01	up	1,39	5,15E-01	up	1,09	8,50E-01

Nardo et al. 2013	Presymptomatic C57 G93A vs. Ctrl			Onset C57 G93A vs. Ctrl			Symptomatic C57 G93A vs. Ctrl		
Gene	Regulation	Fold-Change	P-Value	Regulation	Fold-Change	P-Value	Regulation	Fold-Change	P-Value
Stmnl	down	1,35	9,31 E-02	up	1,17	1,49E-01	up	1,16	3,48E-01
Stmn2	down	1,05	8.98E-01	down	1,52	2,38E-01	up	1,36	4,89E-01
Stmn3	up	1,07	7.28E-01	down	1,24	1,41 E-02	down	1,14	1,50E-02
Stmn4	down	1,06	6,69E-01	up	1,43	1,63E-01	up	1,36	3,15E-02

Nardo et al. 2013	Presymptomatic 129v G93A vs. Ctr			Onset 129sv G93A vs. Ctrl			Symptomatic 129sv G93A vs. Ctrl		
Gene	Regulation	Fold-Change	P-Value	Regulation	Fold-Change	P-Value	Regulation	Fold-Change	P-Value
Stmnl	up	1,05	5,50E-01	up	1,06	3,40E-01	down	1,04	7,57E-01
Stmn2	**up**	**1,63**	**1.98E-02**	down	1,46	1,76E-01	down	1,71	9,08E-02
Stmn3	up	1,08	6,24E-01	down	1,25	6,38E-03	down	1,30	1,18E-02
Stmn4	down	1,13	3,75E-01	up	1,15	3,11E-01	up	1,23	2,98E-03

Perrin et al. 2006	Presymptomatic G93A vs. Ctrl (P60)			Symptomatic G93A vs. Ctrl (P90)			Endstage G93A vs. Ctrl (P120)		
Gene	Regulation	Fold-Change	P-Value	Regulation	Fold-Change	P-Value	Regulation	Fold-Change	P-Value
Stmnl	down	1,38	nc	down	1,38	nc	up	1,68	6,00E-02
Stmn2	up	1,20	nc	up	1,30	1,36E-01	up	1,12	6,44E-01
Stmn3	down	1,03	nc	up	1,07	5,63E-01	down	1,02	8,36E-01
Stmn4	up	1,75	nc	up	1,30	6,49E-01	up	1,85	nc

Gene expression profiles from mutant SOD1 and control motor neurons were analyzed with EASANA software based on FAST DB® annotations, see Table 1. Gene dysregulation was considered significant at fold changes >1.5 and p-values < 5E-02. nc: non calculated
The Stmn1 and Stmn2 genes are significantly up-regulated at presymptomatic disease stage in datasets GSE10953 [19] and GSE46298/129sv [40] respectively, whereas the Stmn3 gene is significantly down-regulated in dataset GSE10953 [19]. Stathmin-1 also tended to be up-regulated in the dataset kindly provided by F. Perrin [42]

Stathmins represent a family of four proteins (Stathmins 1 to 4), which destabilize microtubules either by sequestering tubulin dimers or by increasing the frequency of microtubule catastrophes, i.e. their transition from steady growth to rapid depolymerization [3, 10]. All Stathmins are highly expressed in neurons, several of them localize to the Golgi [10] and Stathmin 1 protein levels were found increased in spinal cords of paralyzed (late stage) SOD1^{G93A} mice [55]. We therefore considered Stathmins as good candidates for mutant SOD1-linked microtubule alterations and Golgi fragmentation.

We analyzed whether one of the four Stathmins is dysregulated at the protein level in the spinal cord of mutant SOD1 mice. Using Western blot, we found that levels of Stathmin 1 (19 kD) and Stathmin 2 (also called SCG10, ~22 kD) are both increased by more than 3 fold in mutant SOD1^{G85R} and SOD1^{G93A} spinal cords at age 240 days (Fig. 4a) whereas they are not in SOD1^{wt} mice (not shown). Of note, this up-regulation is not observed for Stathmin 3

(RB3, ~26 kD) (not shown) and Stathmin 4 (RB3', ~24 kD) is undetectable. We therefore validate that expression of mutant SOD1 triggers up-regulation of Stathmins 1 and 2 in motor neurons and conclude that this could cause the observed microtubule defects and Golgi fragmentation.

Early and progressive co-accumulation of Stathmins and GS28 in mutant SOD1 motor neurons

We then set out to test whether Stathmin up-regulation could be causative of the Golgi fragmentation. As a first prerequisite to this, Stathmin up-regulation should have kinetics matching the early onset and progression of Golgi pathology in mutant SOD1 spinal cord [36, 65, 66]. To establish this, we monitored the kinetics of Stathmin 1 and Stathmin 2 protein levels from early pre-symptomatic stage (postnatal days P8 and P30) to disease endstage (P240) and compared it to GS28 increase as a molecular sign of Golgi pathology. The levels of Stathmin 1 and 2 in spinal cords of mutant SOD1^{G85R} and SOD1^{G93A} mice are already significantly

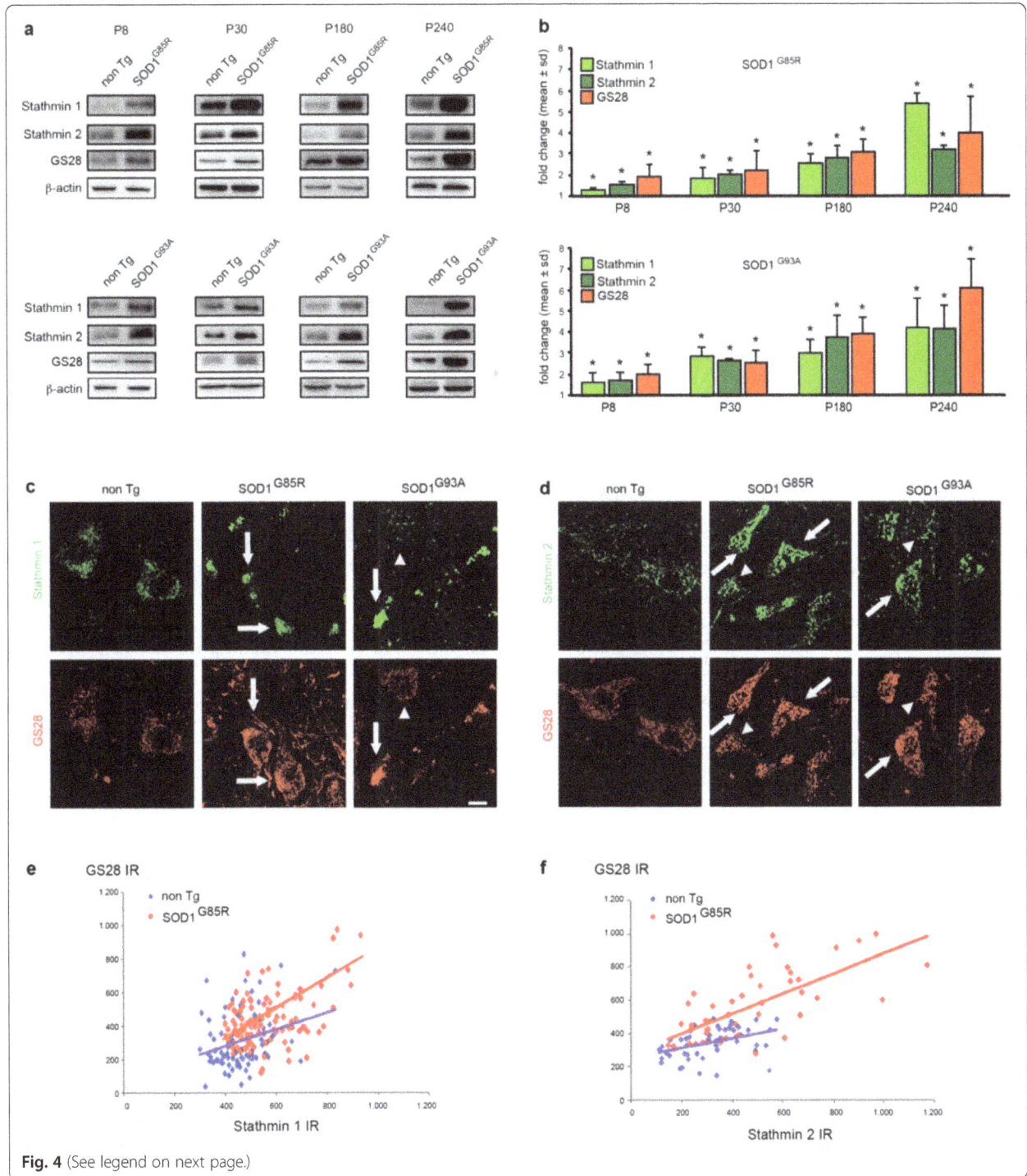

Fig. 4 (See legend on next page.)

(See figure on previous page.)
Fig. 4 Early and rapidly progressive co-accumulation of Stathmin 1, Stathmin 2 and GS28 in motor neurons of mutant SOD1 mice. **a**. Western blots show expression of Stathmin 1, Stathmin 2 and GS28 in lumbar spinal cords of SOD1^{G85R} mice (upper panels), SOD1^{G93A} mice (lower panels) and corresponding litter mates. Analyses were performed at ages P8, P30, P180 and P240. Loading control β-actin. Each blot was performed in duplicate and is representative of four animals per genotype. **b**. Diagrams showing kinetics of Stathmin 1, Stathmin 2 and GS28 protein levels in lumbar spinal cords of mutant SOD1^{G85R} mice and SOD1^{G93A} mice. Stathmin 1 and 2 levels are already significantly increased at P8. Fold changes (mean ± sd) are determined from four spinal cords per genotype and time point and expressed relative to the levels in non-transgenic littermate controls (set to 1). Differences between mutant SOD1 and control are statistically significant as measured by Mann Whitney test (*, p < 0.01). **c-d**. Confocal images of lumbar spinal cord cross sections from non-transgenic, SOD1^{G85R} and SOD1^{G93A} mice aged 240 days showing accumulation of Stathmin 1 (C, upper panels), Stathmin 2 (D, upper panels) and GS28 (C-D, lower panels) in motor neurons, which sometimes appear as degenerating. Note motor neurons with either low expression (arrowheads) or high expression (arrows) of Stathmins and Golgi SNAREs. Scale bar 20 μm. **e**. Diagram showing immunoreactivities (IR) of Stathmin 1 (x-axis) and GS28 (y-axis) in motor neurons of control non-transgenic mice (in blue) and mutant SOD1^{G85R} mice (in red). Pearson analysis demonstrates significant correlation between both parameters: r = 0.28, p < 0.0066 (ctrl) and r = 0.47, p < 0.0001 (SOD1^{G85R}). The slopes of the regression curves are 0.49 ± 0.18 (ctrl) and 0.68 ± 0.13 (SOD1^{G85R}), n = 91 cells (ctrl) and n = 99 cells (SOD1^{G85R}) analyzed from n = 3 mice per genotype. **f**. Immunoreactivities of Stathmin 2 and GS28 also show significant correlation by Pearson analysis: r = 0.40, p < 0.0047 (ctrl), r = 0.69, p < 0.0001 (SOD1^{G85R}). The slopes of the regression curves are 0.29 ± 0.09 (ctrl) and 0.60 ± 0.09 (SOD1^{G85R}) by linear regression analysis, n = 47 cells and n = 48 cells analyzed respectively from n = 3 mice per genotype

increased at P8 when compared to non-transgenic litter mice (Fig. 4a-b). Their levels continue to rise at P30 and P180 when compared to non-transgenic mice to finally reach >3 fold normal levels at P240 (Fig. 4a-b).

Remarkably, this completely parallels the increase in GS28 protein level with a 1.5 fold increase at P8 and a 4 to 6 fold increase at P240 (Fig. 4a-b). The accumulation of Stathmins 1/2 and GS28 thus precedes by at least five months the first clinical symptoms in two different lines of mutant SOD1 mice. These data confirm that Golgi pathology is an early preclinical sign in mutant SOD1 mice and show that the microtubule-disrupting proteins Stathmin 1 and 2 are progressively up-regulated at kinetics compatible with Golgi fragmentation.

As a second prerequisite, Stathmin up-regulation should specifically occur in motor neurons displaying Golgi SNARE accumulation. To test this, we identified individual motor neurons by choline acetyl transferase (ChAT) expression (Additional file 1: Figure S4A-B) and examined the levels of Stathmins and GS28 by IF on a cell-to-cell basis (Fig. 4c-d). In normal motor neurons, Stathmin 1 is barely detectable, Stathmin 2 is expressed in a faint punctate fashion (Fig. 4c-d, upper left panels) and GS28 levels are also low. In contrast, the increase in Stathmin 1 or 2 labeling intensities seen in numerous motor neurons of mutant SOD1 mice (Fig. 4c-d, upper middle and right panels, arrows) is matched by an increase in GS28 (Fig. 4c-d, lower middle and right panels, arrows, Additional file 1: Figure S4A-B). Interestingly, no up-regulation of GS28 or Stathmins 1/2 was apparent in neighboring ChAT-negative interneurons (Additional file 1: Figure S4A-B).

We also used regression analysis to demonstrate a clear correlation between the immunoreactivities of Stathmin 1 and GS28 (Fig. 4e) and between Stathmin 2 and GS28 (Fig. 4f) in individual mutant SOD1 motor neurons.

As a third prerequisite, Stathmin 1 and 2 should be expressed where microtubules are nucleated or polymerized. In line with earlier reports [9], we find that Stathmin 2 is localized to the MannII-GFP-labelled Golgi in NSC-34 motor neurons whereas Stathmin 1 is mostly cytosolic (Additional file 1: Figure S5).

In summary, the kinetics of Stathmin 1/2 up-regulation and its close temporal and spatial correlation with GS28 accumulation in mutant SOD1 motor neurons all suggest that Stathmin up-regulation may mediate Golgi fragmentation.

Overexpression of Stathmins 1/2 phenocopies expression of mutant SOD1

If Stathmin 1/2 up-regulation is responsible for the Golgi fragmentation observed in mutant SOD1 motor neurons through its effect on the microtubule network, it should lead on its own to the structural and molecular alterations described above, i.e. microtubule disruption, Golgi fragmentation and Golgi SNARE accumulation. We first confirmed that Stathmin 1/2 overexpression in NSC-34 motor neurons leads to the expected microtubule defects. Indeed, we found that the percentage of Stathmin 1 or 2 overexpressing NSC-34 cells with altered microtubules is 3 fold higher than in control-transfected cells (Fig. 5a-b). This is true for microtubules containing α-tubulin or detyrosinated tubulin and similar to that in mutant SOD1-transfected cells (Fig. 3a,b,c,f).

We then tested whether Stathmin 1/2 overexpression in NSC-34 cells triggers Golgi fragmentation and the associated accumulation of Golgi SNAREs GS28 and GS15 (Fig. 1g-i and Fig. 4). We found that it is the case. About 60 % of Stathmin 1 transfected cells exhibit a fragmented Golgi and GS28 dispersal (Fig. 5c-d) and the protein levels of GS28 and GS15 are >2.5 fold higher than in control cells (Fig. 5e). Stathmin 2 transfected cultures show a similar percentage of cells with Golgi fragmentation (Fig. 5c-d) and a similar increase in GS28/GS15 protein levels (Fig. 5e). Taken together, these data show that Stathmin 1 and Stathmin 2 overexpression on its own triggers both microtubule and Golgi alterations that qualitatively and quantitatively resemble those observed in mutant SOD1 motor neurons.

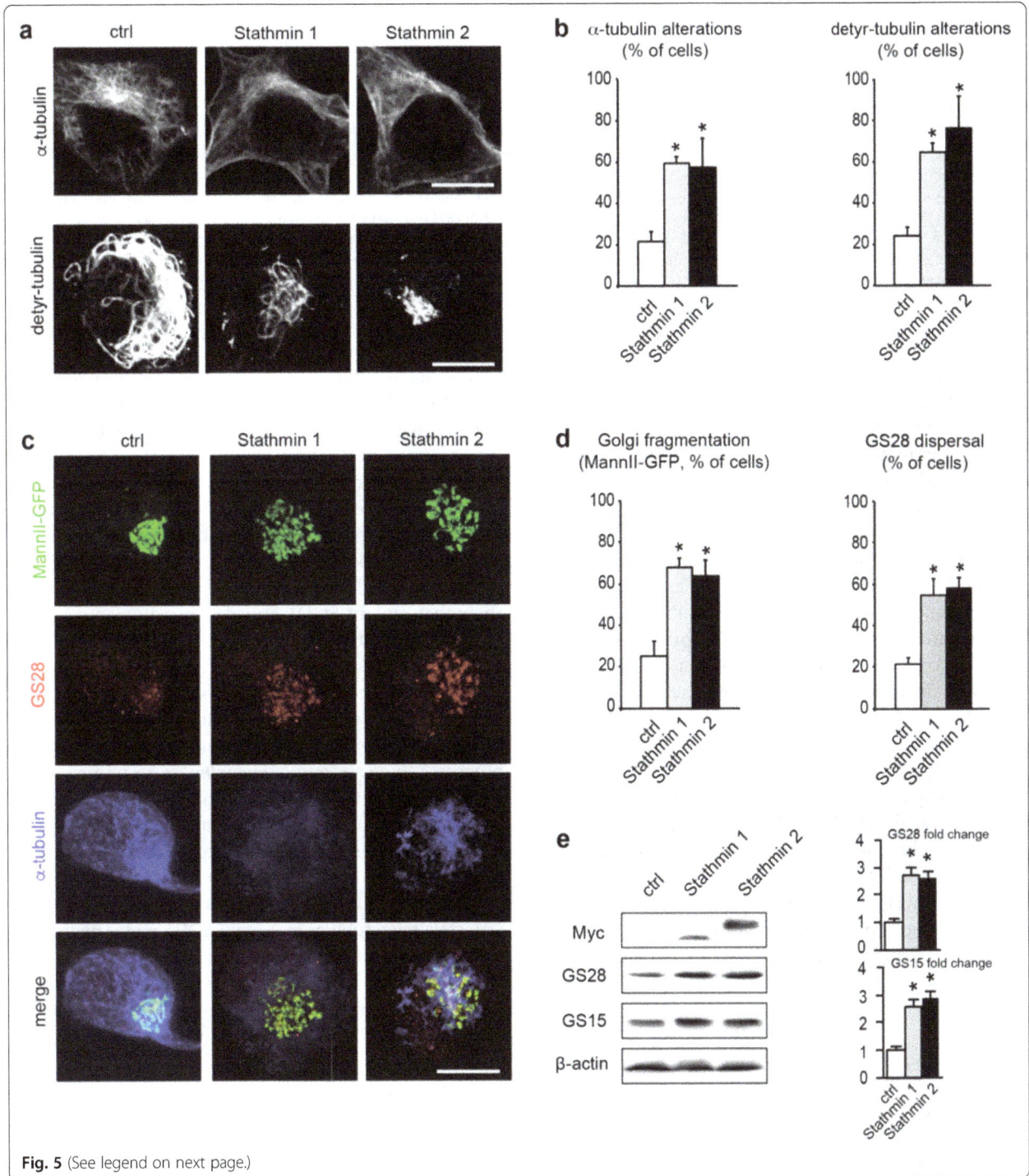

Fig. 5 (See legend on next page.)

(See figure on previous page.)

Fig. 5 Stathmin 1/2 overexpression phenocopies expression of mutant SOD1. **a**. Images showing microtubule alterations in NSC-34 motor neurons transfected with Myc-tagged Stathmin 1 or Stathmin 2, as compared to control cells. Cells were cultured for 2 DIV, fixed with paraformaldehyde and analyzed with antibodies α-tubulin (upper panels), detyrosinated tubulin (lower panels) or Myc (not shown). Scale bar 5 μm. **b**. Quantitative analyses showing percentage of cells with rarefied or broken microtubules (α-tubulin or detyrosinated tubulin). Data represent one typical out of five independent experiments each done in quadruplicate per condition. Number of cells analyzed (ctrl, Stathmin 1, Stathmin 2): α-tubulin (175, 174, 139), detyr-tubulin (184, 146, 152). Statistical significance by Mann–Whitney test: * p < 0.001 as compared to mock. **c**. Images showing Golgi alterations (MannII-GFP, GS28) together with microtubule alterations (α-tubulin) in NSC-34 motor neurons transfected with Stathmin 1 or Stathmin 2 as compared to control cells. Scale bar 5 μm. **d**. Quantitative analyses showing percentage of cells with Golgi alterations (MannII-GFP) or GS28 dispersal). Data represent one typical out of five independent experiments each done in quadruplicate per condition. Number of cells analyzed (ctrl, Stathmin 1, Stathmin 2): MannII-GFP (>500 each). GS28 (482, 434, 526). Statistical significance by Mann–Whitney test: * p < 0.001 as compared to mock. **e**. Western blot analysis of cells transfected with plasmids encoding Myc-tagged Stathmin 1 or Stathmin 2 or with an empty control plasmid (pcDNA). GS15 and GS28 levels are increased after overexpression of Stathmin 1 by 2.7 ± 0.3 and 2.6 ± 0.3 (mean ± sd) respectively. A similar increase in Golgi SNAREs is observed after overexpression of Stathmin 2 (GS15 2.6 ± 0.2, GS28 2.9 ± 0.3). n = 4 blots corresponding to independent experiments, * p < 0.01 by Mann - Whitney test

Knockdown of Stathmins 1 or 2 rescues mutant SOD1-linked Golgi fragmentation

To conclusively validate the role of Stathmin 1/2 up-regulation in mutant SOD1-triggered Golgi fragmentation, we reasoned that removing Stathmins in mutant SOD1-expressing NSC-34 cells should prevent microtubule loss and Golgi fragmentation.

We found that RNAi-mediated knockdown of either Stathmin 1 or Stathmin 2 reduces the percentage of cells with mutant SOD1-triggered microtubule alterations such as rarefied or discontinous microtubules to control values (Fig. 6a-b). We further show that the knockdown of either Stathmin 1 or 2 rescues the morphological Golgi fragmentation evidenced by MannII-GFP (Fig. 6c) and also the vesicular dispersion of GS28-labeled Golgi profiles (Fig. 6c). Quantitative analyses (Fig. 6d-e) demonstrate a complete rescue of both types of alterations.

Finally, we demonstrate that Stathmin 1 knockdown normalizes the pathologically increased levels of GS28 triggered by SOD1^{G85R} or SOD1^{G93A} to those in SOD1^{wt} cultures (Fig. 6f). Stathmin 2 knockdown has a similar effect (Fig. 6g). Taken together, these data indicate that Stathmins 1/2 mediate Golgi alterations in mutant SOD1 motor neurons by triggering microtubule loss.

Discussion

Our study shows that the early Golgi pathology observed in mutant SOD1 motor neurons is triggered by the up-regulation of Stathmins 1/2 that sever the Golgi-nucleated microtubule network. This in turn leads to Golgi fragmentation with tubular/vesicular organelle transformation as its most prominent ultrastructural feature and strong accumulation of Golgi SNAREs GS28 and GS15 as its most striking molecular signature.

Mutant SOD1-linked Golgi fragmentation is due to "somatic microtubulinopathy"

Surprisingly, we find that Golgi fragmentation in mutant SOD1 motor neurons *in vivo* and *in vitro* resembles that described in *pmn* mice mutated in the Golgi-localized

tubulin folding chaperone TBCE, leading to TBCE degradation and defective polymerization of Golgi-derived microtubules in the cell soma [5]. This was unexpected since microtubule alterations in mutant SOD1-linked ALS have so far been only reported in axons, as illustrated by a reduction in axonal tubulin transport [70], an accumulation of β$_{III}$-tubulin in axonal swellings [70] and increases in hyperdynamic microtubules [17] or density of EB3 comets [27] in axons. By contrast, our findings show that mutant SOD1 impedes microtubule dynamics at the Golgi in the motor neuron soma, leading in turn to Golgi fragmentation. Of note, some forms of human ALS are associated with mutations in the α-tubulin gene TUBA4A and these severely disrupt the somatic microtubule network upon overexpression [51]. We therefore propose *"somatic microtubulinopathy"* as a common mechanism triggering Golgi fragmentation in SOD1-linked ALS, progressive motor neuronopathy, human TUBA4A-linked ALS, and similar disorders due to mutations yet to be identified.

Defective microtubules in mutant SOD1 motor neurons via stathmin 1 and 2 up-regulation

How does mutant SOD1 induce somatic microtubulinopathy? We show that mutant SOD1 disrupts the cellular microtubule network through up-regulation of the microtubule-disrupting proteins Stathmin 1 and 2. This up-regulation is specific to mutant SOD1 since wildtype SOD1 has no such effect, and it is independent of SOD1 enzymatic activity since dismutase-inactive SOD1^{G85R} has a similar effect as dismutase active SOD1^{G93A}.

Interestingly, wildtype and mutant forms of SOD1 have been localized to the Golgi by biochemical and imaging methods [63, 64]. We hypothesize that Golgi-localized mutant SOD1 triggers a Golgi stress response to the nucleus, in analogy to the Golgi-disrupting agents Brefeldin A and monensin, which activate the signaling cascades CREB3/ARF4 [45] and TFE3/GASE [59], respectively. According to our bioinformatic analyses, mutant SOD1 does not modulate the gene expression of the transcription

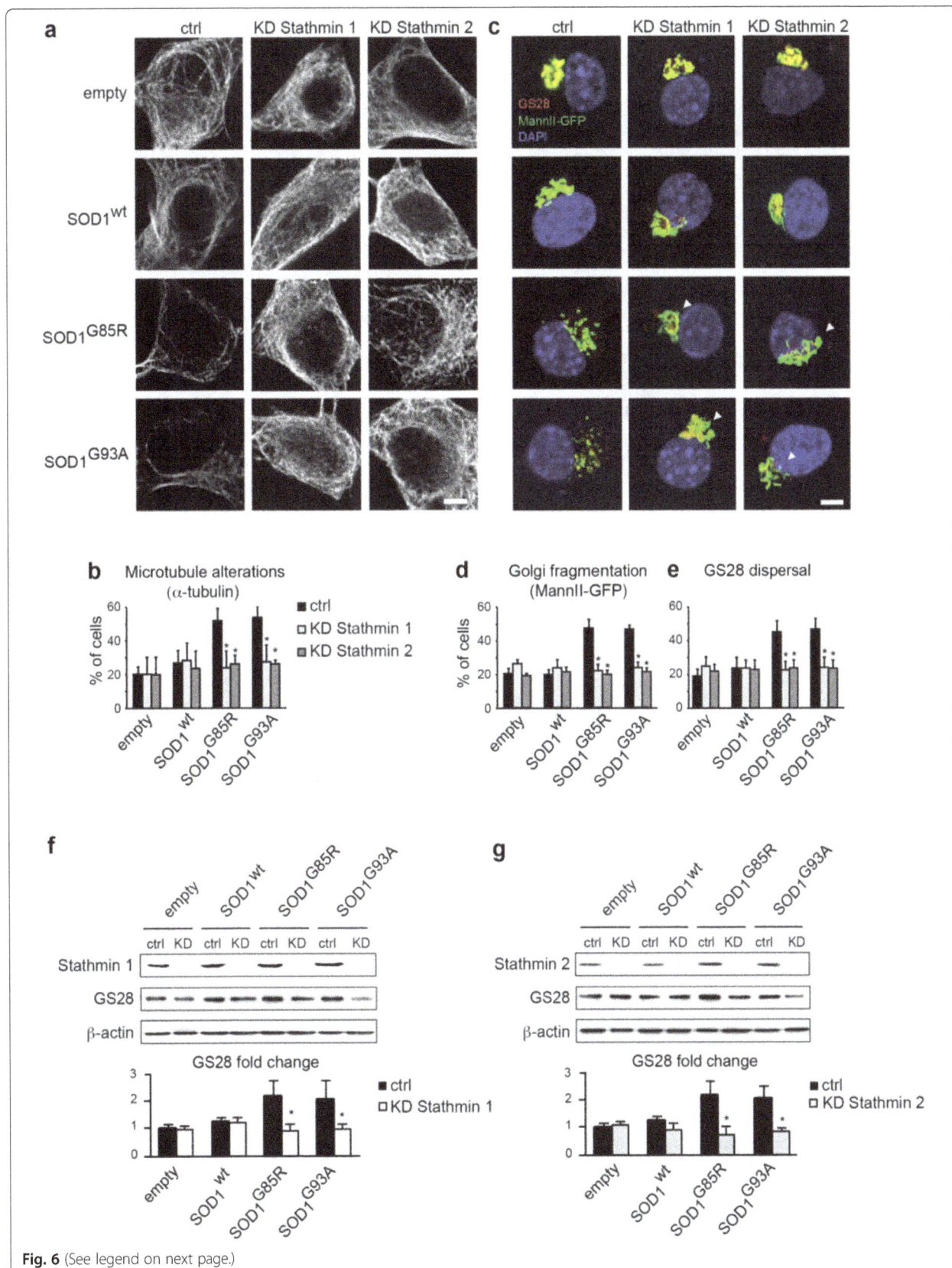

Fig. 6 (See legend on next page.)

Fig. 6 Stathmin 1/2 knockdown rescues microtubule and Golgi alterations triggered by mutant SOD1. **a**. Confocal images showing NSC-34 cells transfected with empty, SOD1^{wt}, SOD1^{G85R} or SOD1^{G93A} plasmids as well as ctrl, Stathmin-1 or Stathmin-2 siRNAs. Cells were immunolabelled for α-tubulin. Note that knockdown of Stathmin 1 or 2 rescues mutant SOD1-triggered microtubule alterations. Transfected cells were identified by expression of co-transfected MannII-GFP (not shown). Scale bar 5 μm. **b**. Diagram showing percentage of microtubule alterations (mean ± sd) under the different conditions. >150 cells were analyzed per condition. Statistical significance * p < 0.01 by Mann–Whitney test. Data are representative of three independent experiments. **c**. Confocal images showing NSC-34 cells transfected as in A and counterstained for GS28. Note rescue (arrowheads) of mutant SOD1-triggered Golgi fragmentation and GS28 dispersal by knockdown of Stathmin 1 or 2. Scale bar 5 μm. **d-e**. Diagram showing percentage (mean ± sd) of Golgi alterations labelled by MannII-GFP (**d**) or GS28 (**e**) under the different conditions. >150 cells were analyzed per condition. Statistical significance * p < 0.01 by Mann–Whitney test. Data are representative of four independent experiments. **f-g**. Western blots show efficient siRNA-mediated knockdown (KD) of Stathmin 1 (**f**) and Stathmin 2 (**g**) in NSC-34 cells transfected with empty, SOD1^{wt}, SOD1^{G85R} or SOD1^{G93A} plasmids as compared to ctrl siRNA (upper blots). Both Stathmin-1 or Stathmin-2 knockdown reduces the GS28 up-regulation triggered by SOD1^{G85R} or SOD1^{G93A} (middle blots). Loading control β-actin (lower blots) indicates reduced protein content in lanes 1 and 2 in F (empty ctrl, empty Stathmin-1 KD). The diagrams below show densitometric quantification of GS28 protein levels each normalized to β-actin (n = 4 blots, mean ± sd, * statistically significant differences between ctrl siRNA and Stathmin 1/2 siRNA as measured by Mann - Whitney test)

factors CREB3 and TFE3 or their respective effectors ARF4 and GCP60 (ACBD3), (data not shown). However, mutant SOD1 enhances gene expression of EZH2 (enhancer of zeste homolog 2), a known de-repressor of the Stathmin 1 gene [11], by 1.65 fold and 1.56 fold in motor neurons of two transgenic lines (p = 0.014 and p = 0.003, dataset GSE46298 [40], providing a potential mechanism for Stathmin 1 up-regulation. In addition, mutant SOD1 may influence the Stathmin 1 activity through posttranslational modification of its isoforms [55]. These findings point to a novel Golgi stress response pathway in ALS that needs to be characterized in further detail.

The respective contribution of Stathmins 1 and 2 to Golgi fragmentation
Our data show that knockdown of Stathmin 1 or 2 completely rescues molecular and morphological Golgi alterations. This rules out that Stathmin 1/2 up-regulation is merely a homeostatic mechanism during Golgi fragmentation, similar to Stathmin up-regulation after axonal injury or during axonal regeneration [25, 32, 49].

We further demonstrate that Stathmin 1 or 2 overexpression has similar effects on Golgi fragmentation and Golgi SNARE accumulation in motor neurons. Yet, Stathmins 1 and 2 differ in their subcellular localization in motor neurons (Additional file 1: Figure S4) and in other cell types [10]. While Stathmin 1 appears mainly cytoplasmic, Stathmin 2 localizes to the Golgi due to its N-terminal domain which is missing in Stathmin 1 [9]. This suggests that these two Stathmins fulfill different functions and potentially act on distinct microtubule subsets. According to recent studies, radial centrosomal microtubules are required for the proper positioning of the Golgi in the cell center whereas microtubules nucleated at the trans-Golgi by CLASPs [14, 34] or at the cis-Golgi by AKAP450/GM130 [46] seem to be required for the lateral continuity of Golgi membranes. It can be speculated that up-regulated Stathmins 1 and 2 cooperatively trigger Golgi fragmentation by regulating interdependent microtubule subsets required for Golgi maintenance.

Are there additional mediators of mutant SOD1-linked Golgi fragmentation?
Our data indicate that Golgi fragmentation in mutant SOD1 motor neurons is associated with displacement of GM130 from intact Golgi membranes to the cytosol (Fig. 1g). A recent study in mitotic cells shows that GM130 stimulates microtubule polymerization by activating the microtubule nucleator TPX2 through sequestration of its inhibitor importin α [67]. Displacement of GM130 to the cytosol with ensuing TPX2/importin α imbalance may thus contribute to mutant SOD1-linked microtubule loss and Golgi fragmentation. Furthermore, mutant SOD1 has been reported to interact aberrantly with chromogranins [64] and the COPII vesicle subunit Sec23 [4], which may impede ER-Golgi and Golgi-plasma membrane transport [4, 54, 64] and further enhance Golgi fragmentation.

Stathmins as potential biomarkers for ALS
Last, this study may contribute to the development of new disease biomarkers. Biomarkers are generally defined as a physiological process, a pathogenic event or a pharmacological response to therapeutic intervention that can be measured. Reliable biomarkers for ALS are currently lacking [41, 62]. In this respect, Stathmins display several interesting features.

First, levels of Stathmins 1 and 2 are already significantly elevated at an early preclinical phase in two lines of mutant SOD1 mice - five months before appearance of clinical symptoms (Fig. 4a-b). Translating this to human ALS patients would help to establish earlier diagnosis and initiate therapies at a more tractable disease phase.

Second, both Stathmins strongly and continuously accumulate during disease course in mutant SOD1 G85R and G93A spinal cords, reaching levels of > 3 fold above normal at endstage (this study, Fig. 4a-b). To our knowledge, this is higher than for any previously reported protein in ALS spinal cord, and may allow sensitive monitoring of disease progression.

Third, Stathmin accumulation represents a patho-logically relevant feature shared between SOD1-linked ALS and mutant SMN-linked spinal muscular atrophy (SMA) [68]. Genetic knockout of Stathmin 1 in *Smn* mice improved neuromuscular function presumably through microtubule stabilization [69], underscoring the pathogenic relevance of Stathmin 1 up-regulation.

Finally, the proteins Stathmin 1 and 2 are both present in normal human blood (Plasma Proteome Database [39]) with Stathmin 1 being measured at a plasma concentration of 3.5 ng/ml [18]. Pathological release of Stathmins from degenerating ALS motor neurons may thus cause a detectable increase in their blood levels.

Stathmins and dys-regulated Golgi proteins should therefore be evaluated as new potential biomarkers for diagnosis, prognosis or therapy response in ALS, SMA and related motor neuron disorders.

Conclusions

This study demonstrates that Stathmin 1/2-triggered microtubule destabilization mediates early presymptom-atic Golgi fragmentation in mutant SOD1 G85R- and G93A-triggered ALS. This may contribute to the development of new blood biomarkers in ALS and related motor neuron diseases.

Methods

Antibodies and reagents

Primary and secondary antibodies are listed in Additional file 1: Table S1. Other reagents were from the following suppliers: PBS, Hbss, trypsin, culture media and supplements (Invitrogen, Carlsbad, CA), taxol, nocodazole (Sigma), OCT (Thermo Scientific, Runcorn, UK), Vecta-shield (Vector laboratories, Burlingame, CA), Complete protease inhibitors (Roche, Basel, Switzerland), Ketamine (Bayer, Leverkusen, Germany) and Xylazine (Mérial, Lyon, France), coverslips and Superfrost Plus glass slides (Menzel, Schwerte, Germany). Plasmid expression vectors contained the following cDNAs: GFP-tagged Mannosidase-II (Dr. M. Bornens, Institut Curie, Paris, France), untagged human SOD1^{wt}, SOD1^{G85R} or SOD1^{G93A} (Dr. D. Borchelt, University of Florida, Gainesville, USA) subcloned in pCAGGS vectors, RFP-tagged human SOD1^{wt}, SOD1^{G85R} or SOD1^{G93A} (Dr. J. Weishaupt, Neurologische Klinik, Ulm, Germany), Myc-tagged human Stathmin 1 or Stathmin 2 (Dr. A. Sobel, Inserm U693, Paris, France).

Animals

Transgenic SOD1^{G93A} mice (line G1del or Tg(SOD1*^{G93Adl})1Gur, http://jaxmice.jax.org/strain/002299.html [1]), SOD1^{G85R} mice (line 148 [6] and SOD1^{wt} mice (line 76 [6]) were maintained as hemizygotes for more than ten generations on a C57/BL6 background and ge-notyped by PCR as described [44]. All experiments with animals were performed in strict compliance with French and European legislation.

Cell culture

NSC-34 cells [7] were cultured in DMEM supplemented with 8 % (v/v) fetal calf serum at 37 °C and 7.5 % CO_2 and differentiated on collagen-coated wells in low fetal calf serum (1 %) for 72 h before transfection. Cells were transfected with plasmids encoding SOD1 (mutant or wildtype, RFP-tagged or not), RFP, Stathmin-1 or Stathmin-2 (0.2 µg/10^4 cells) and/or with siRNAs against Stathmin 1/2 (on target plus, Thermofisher) or luciferase control (Thermofisher) using Lipofectamine 2000 (Invitrogen) as described [48]. Cells were then cultured for 96 h after SOD1 plasmid and/or Stathmin siRNA transfection or for 48 h after Stathmin plasmid transfection.

Immunocytochemistry

Mice deeply anaesthetized with ketamine/xylazine were intracardially perfused with Sorensen buffer followed by 4 % paraformaldehyde. Spinal cords were dissected out, postfixed, cryoprotected in sucrose and frozen in OCT. Cross sections (30 µm) of lumbar spinal cord were cut with a crytotome (Leica) and stained with antibodies as described [5].

Cultured cells were fixed in 4 % formaldehyde (FA), permeabilized with 0.5 % (v/v) Tween in PBS and blocked in a solution containing 2.5 % (v/v) goat serum, 2.5 % (v/v) donkey serum, 1 % (w/v) BSA in PBS. Alternatively, cells were extracted for soluble proteins using MSB (25 mM Hepes, 50 mM Pipes, 10 mM EGTA, 2 mM $MgCl_2$, 1 % formaldehyde in PBS pH 7.0), permeabilized in MSB containing 10 µM Taxol and 0.2 % (v/v) Triton X100 and fixed with 4 % formaldehyde. Cells were stained with antibodies as described [5].

Confocal imaging, morphometry and 3D modeling

Motor neurons in ventral spinal cord were identified by expression of vesicular acetyltransferase (VAChT) or choline acetyltransferase (ChAT), large soma size and faintly DAPI-stained large nucleus [5]. Motor neurons were im-aged with an LSM 510 confocal microscope (Zeiss, Ober-kochen, Germany) using a 63x objective, an xy-resolution of 1024 x 1024 pixel and a z-interval of 0.3 µm.

Morphometric analyses were done with Metamorph soft-ware (Molecular Dynamics) using single confocal cross sections taken at the nuclear midplane. The boundaries of the VAChT-labelled cell soma and the DAPI-stained nucleus were manually delineated with the Metamorph drawing tool. Golgi area was automatically determined with the Meta-morph morphometry tool by applying a fixed threshold to the GM130 signal. Three-dimensional (3D) modelings of the Golgi apparatus were done with Imaris software (Bitplane,

Zurich, Switzerland). Images were processed and Golgi membranes visualized using the IsoSurface mode of the Surpass module. The number of individual Golgi elements per motor neuron was determined in a blinded manner. NSC-34 cells were imaged by confocal microscopy using a z-interval of 0.3 μm and a scan depth of about 10 μm.

The percentage of spinal cord motor neurons displaying Golgi fragmentation (labelled by GM130 or MG160) was determined by conventional microscopy using a Leica DMI 400 fluorescence microscope (63x oil objective). Golgi fragmentation in lumbar spinal cord motor neurons was defined by discontinuous or decreased GM130 or MG160 immunolabeling.

The percentage of transfected NSC-34 cells with subcellular alterations was also quantified by fluorescence microscopy. Golgi dispersal was defined by enlarged area, as compared to neighboring non-transfected cells. A defective microtubule network was defined by less dense or discontinuous microtubules labeled for α-tubulin or detyrosinated tubulin, as compared to neighboring non-transfected cells.

Electron microscopy

Deeply anaesthetized mice were transcardially perfused with Sorensen's phosphate buffer (pH 7.4) followed by glutaraldehyde (2 % v/v in cacodylate). Spinal cords were dissected out, postfixed for 24 h and cut into small segments comprising the ventral spinal cord before processing for resin embedding (epon) following standard protocols. 60 nm ultrathin cross sections were contrasted with uranyl acetate and visualized under a JEOL electron microscope. Two sections each containing up to 30 motor neurons were analyzed per mouse line. Motor neurons were recognized on the basis of their frequency (1:20), large size and pale nucleus with nucleolus.

Immunoblots and subcellular fractionation

Protein extracts from lumbar spinal cords or NSC-34 cells were prepared by homogenization in lysis buffer containing 50 mM Tris HCl pH7.5, 150 mM NaCl, 2 mM EDTA, 1 % Triton X100, protease inhibitors (Complete EDTA-free, Roche). 50 μg protein were subjected to SDS-PAGE and blotted on Immobilon membranes (Millipore) which were processed by standard methods and revealed with Immobilon Western kits (Millipore). Band intensities were quantified by TotalLabQuant software.

Crude fractionation of membranes from lumbar spinal cord was performed after tissue freezing (–80 °C), thawing and homogenization in 50 mM HEPES, pH 7.4, 250 mM sucrose, 1 mM Mg-acetate and protease inhibitors (Complete EDTA-free, Roche). Lysates were homogenized using a Dounce homogenizer (15 passes) and centrifuged at 1.000 g for 10 min. The postnuclear supernatant was centrifuged at 10.000 g for 30 min at 4 °C yielding a P10 pellet

and the supernatant was centrifuged at 100.000 g (Beckman TLA-110) for 1 h at 4 °C yielding an S100 supernatant and a P100 pellet.

Tubulin and microtubule assays

Tubulin polymerization status in NSC-34 cells was analyzed by preparing cell lysates in microtubule stabilization buffer (MSB, 0.1 M PIPES pH 6.75, 1 mM EGTA, 1 mM $MgSO_4$, 30 % glycerol, 5 mM GTP, 5 % DMSO, 1 mM DTT, MiniComplete protease inhibitors). Total tubulin (T) was harvested before fractionation and soluble tubulin (supernatant, S) and precipitable tubulin (pellet, P) were separated by centrifugation for 1 h at 100 000 g in a Beckman Rotor TLA-100.

Cellular microtubule content was determined by flow cytometry using the method of Morrison et al. [35] with some modifications. Briefly, cells were harvested, rinsed with PBS, centrifuged, washed with MSB and treated for 3 min with MSB containing 0.1 % Triton X-100 and 20 μM taxol. Cells were then fixed in formaldehyde, centrifuged, washed, blocked, incubated for 1 h with FITC-coupled antibodies against α-tubulin and washed. 1500 RFP-positive cells per duplicate sample and condition were analyzed with a FACS ARIA SORP cytometer (Becton Dickinson) and FITC signals plotted with FlowJo software. Control experiments with cells that had been treated with Nocodazole or Taxol showed accuracy.

Growth dynamics of Golgi-derived microtubule were determined essentially as described [5]. Briefly, cells cotransfected with MannII-GFP and RFP or RFP-SOD1 plasmids were treated with nocodazole at 5 DIV (10 μM, 5 h, 37 °C). Nocodazole was then washed out, cultures further incubated for up to 12 min, fixed as indicated above, blocked and counterstained for α-tubulin. After confocal imaging of entire cells, length of Golgi-derived microtubules was determined using Metamorph and ImageJ software respectively.

Data mining and bioinformatics

Datasets from [19] and [40] were downloaded from the Gene Omnibus database (GSE10953 and GSE46298 respectively). Analysis and visualization of the corresponding Affymetrix CEL files were made using EASANA® software (GenoSplice technology), which is based on the GenoSplice's FAST DB® annotations [13]. Briefly, microarray data were normalized using RMA and genes were considered significantly differentially expressed when the uncorrected p-value from unpaired Student's t-test was lower or equal to 0.05 and fold-change greater or equal to 1.5. Significant KEGG pathways and Gene Ontology terms were retrieved using DAVID.

Statistical analyses

Each experiment was performed with several biological replicates (see Figure Legends) and repeated at least twice. Data were analysed with Microsoft Excel or Graph-Pad Prism (GraphPad). Data from two groups showing each Gaussian distribution were analysed with student's *t*-test; otherwise the Mann–Whitney *U* test was used. Data from more than two groups showing each Gaussian distribution and equal variance were analyzed with One Way ANOVA and Tukey posthoc test; otherwise Kruskal-Willis test and Dunn posthoc test were used. Cytometry data were tested for significance with the Chi square test using FlowJo software. Immunofluorescence data were tested for Gaussian distribution by D'Agostino & Pearson test and linear regression and correlation quantified with GraphPad Prism. Subcellular co-localization of SOD1 and MannII-GFP was correlated by computing Pearson coefficients with the image processing package Fiji using six independents assays.

Abbreviations
ARF, ADP ribosylation factor; BSA: bovine serum albumine; COPI, coat protein complex I; CREB, cAMP response element-binding protein; DIV, day in vitro; DMSO, dimethylsulfoxide; DTT, dithiotreitol; EB3, end-binding protein 3; EDTA, ethylenediaminetetraacetic acid; EGTA, ethylene glycol tetraacetic acid; EZH2, enhancer of zeste homolog 2; FACS, fluorescent-activated cell sorting; GASE, golgi apparatus stress response element; Hepes, 4-(2-hydroxyethyl)-1-piperazineethanesulfonic acid; MannII, mannosidase II; PBS, phosphate buffered saline; Pipes, piperazine-N,N'-bis(2-ethanesulfonic acid); Rab, ras-related in brain; RFP, red fluorescent protein; SDS, sodium dodecyl sulfate; SMA, spinal muscular atrophy; SMN, survival motor neuron; SNARE, soluble N-ethylmaleimide-sensitive- factor attachment receptor; SOD1, superoxide dismutase 1; TBCE, tubulin-binding cofactor E; TFE3, transcription factor binding to IGHM enhancer 3; TPX2, targeting protein for Xklp2; Tris, tris(hydroxymethyl)aminomethane; VAchT, vesicular acetylcholine transporter

Acknowledgements
We gratefully acknowledge the expert help of Drs. P. Weber, P. Moretti and A. Bernadac (CNRS Marseille, France) in confocal microscopy and membrane modeling and of Tineke Veenendaal (Dept. of Cell Biology, UMC Utrecht, Utrecht, NL) in electron microscopy. We also acknowledge the contribution of N. Cavanne and C. Boudier to an early stage of the project. We thank Drs. A. Andrieux and M.-J. Moutin (CNRS Grenoble, France), M. Bornens (Institut Curie, Paris, France), D. Borchelt (University of Florida, Gainesville, USA), R. Duden (University of Lübeck, Germany), C. Jackson (Institut Jacques Monod, Paris), A. Sobel (INSERM Paris, France) and J. Weishaupt (University of Ulm, Germany) for providing essential reagents and Dr. F. Perrin (University of Montpellier, France) for communicating transcriptomic datasets.
Work in G. Haase's lab is supported by grants from Association Française contre les Myopathies (AFM), Agence Nationale pour la Recherche and ERANET Neuron. S. Bellouze was supported by student fellowships from AFM and Fondation pour la Recherche Médicale (FRM). Dorothée Buttigieg was supported by Agence Nationale pour la Recherche.
Work in C. Rabouille's lab is supported by NWO.

Authors' contributions
SB carried out biochemical, cell biological and histopathological studies in mutant SOD1 motor neurons. GB carried out the Stathmin overexpression and knockdown experiments and analyzed SOD1wt mice. DB performed the flow cytometry, PD performed the bioinformatic analyses. SB, GB, DB and PD performed statistical analyses. CR carried out the electron microscopy analysis. GH conceived and coordinated the study and drafted the manuscript. CR and GH wrote the manuscript. All authors approved the final manuscript.

Competing interests
The authors declare that they have no competing interests.

Author details
[1]Institut de Neurosciences de la Timone, UMR 7289, Centre National de la Recherche Scientifique (CNRS) and Aix-Marseille Université, 27 bd Jean Moulin, 13005 Marseille, France. [2]GenoSplice technology, iPEPS - ICM, Hôpital Pitié Salpêtrière, 47/83, bd de l'Hôpital, 75013 Paris, France. [3]Department of Cell Biology, Hubrecht Institute of the KNAW & UMC Utrecht, Uppsalalaan 8, 3584 CT Utrecht, Netherlands.

References
1. Acevedo-Arozena A, Kalmar B, Essa S, Ricketts T, Joyce P, Kent R, Rowe C, Parker A, Gray A, Hafezparast M, et al. A comprehensive assessment of the SOD1G93A low-copy transgenic mouse, which models human amyotrophic lateral sclerosis. Dis model Mech. 2011;4:686–700. doi:10.1242/dmm.007237.
2. Aguilera-Gomez A, Rabouille C. Intra Golgi transport. In: Bradshaw R, Stahl P (eds) Encyclopedia of Cell Biology. Elsevier; 2015; 354-362. doi:10.1016/B978-0-12-394447-4.20034-5.
3. Amayed P, Pantaloni D, Carlier MF. The effect of stathmin phosphorylation on microtubule assembly depends on tubulin critical concentration. J Biol Chem. 2002;277:22718–24. doi:10.1074/jbc.M111605200.
4. Atkin JD, Farg MA, Soo KY, Walker AK, Halloran M, Turner BJ, Nagley P, Horne MK. Mutant SOD1 inhibits ER-Golgi transport in amyotrophic lateral sclerosis. J Neurochem. 2014;129:190–204. doi:10.1111/jnc.12493.
5. Bellouze S, Schaefer MK, Buttigieg D, Baillat G, Rabouille C, Haase G. Golgi fragmentation in pmn mice is due to a defective ARF1/TBCE cross-talk that coordinates COPI vesicle formation and tubulin polymerization. Hum Mol Genet. 2014;23:5961–75. doi:10.1093/hmg/ddu320.
6. Bruijn LI, Becher MW, Lee MK, Anderson KL, Jenkins NA, Copeland NG, Sisodia SS, Rothstein JD, Borchelt DR, Price DL, et al. ALS-linked SOD1 mutant G85R mediates damage to astrocytes and promotes rapidly progressive disease with SOD1-containing inclusions. Neuron. 1997;18:327–38.
7. Cashman NR, Durham HD, Blusztajn JK, Oda K, Tabira T, Shaw IT, Dahrouge S, Antel JP. Neuroblastoma x spinal cord (NSC) hybrid cell lines resemble developing motor neurons. Dev Dyn. 1992;194:209–21.
8. Chabin-Brion K, Marceiller J, Perez F, Settegrana C, Drechou A, Durand G, Pous C. The Golgi complex is a microtubule-organizing organelle. Mol Biol Cell. 2001;12:2047–60.
9. Chauvin S, Poulain FE, Ozon S, Sobel A. Palmitoylation of stathmin family proteins domain A controls Golgi versus mitochondrial subcellular targeting. Biol Cell. 2008;100:577–89. doi:10.1042/BC20070119.
10. Chauvin S, Sobel A. Neuronal stathmins: a family of phosphoproteins cooperating for neuronal development, plasticity and regeneration. Prog Neurobiol. 2015;126:1–18. doi:10.1016/j.pneurobio.2014.09.002.
11. Chen Y, Lin MC, Yao H, Wang H, Zhang AQ, Yu J, Hui CK, Lau GK, He ML, Sung J, et al. Lentivirus-mediated RNA interference targeting enhancer of zeste homolog 2 inhibits hepatocellular carcinoma growth through down-regulation of stathmin. Hepatology. 2007;46:200–8. doi:10.1002/hep.21668.
12. de la Grange P, Dutertre M, Correa M, Auboeuf D. A new advance in alternative splicing databases: from catalogue to detailed analysis of regulation of expression and function of human alternative splicing variants. BMC Bioinforma. 2007;8:180. doi:10.1186/1471-2105-8-180.
13. de la Grange P, Dutertre M, Martin N, Auboeuf D. FAST DB: a website resource for the study of the expression regulation of human gene products. Nucleic Acids Res. 2005;33:4276–84. doi:10.1093/nar/gki738.
14. Efimov A, Kharitonov A, Efimova N, Loncarek J, Miller PM, Andreyeva N, Gleeson P, Galjart N, Maia AR, McLeod IX, et al. Asymmetric CLASP-dependent nucleation of noncentrosomal microtubules at the trans-Golgi network. Dev Cell. 2007;12:917–30.
15. Ellinger A, Pavelka M. Colchicine-induced tubular, vesicular and cisternal organelle aggregates in absorptive cells of the small intestine of the rat. I. Morphology and phosphatase cytochemistry. Biol Cell. 1984;52:43–52.
16. Fan J, Hu Z, Zeng L, Lu W, Tang X, Zhang J, Li T. Golgi apparatus and neurodegenerative diseases. Int J Dev Neurosci. 2008;26:523–34. doi:10.1016/j.ijdevneu.2008.05.006.

17. Fanara P, Banerjee J, Hueck RV, Harper MR, Awada M, Turner H, Husted KH, Brandt R, Hellerstein MK. Stabilization of hyperdynamic microtubules is neuroprotective in amyotrophic lateral sclerosis. J Biol Chem. 2007;282:23465–72. doi:10.1074/jbc.M703434200.

18. Farrah T, Deutsch EW, Omenn GS, Campbell DS, Sun Z, Bletz JA, Mallick P, Katz JE, Malmstrom J, Ossola R, et al. A high-confidence human plasma proteome reference set with estimated concentrations in PeptideAtlas. Mol Cell Proteomics. 2011;10(M110):006353. doi:10.1074/mcp.M110.006353.

19. Ferraiuolo L, Heath PR, Holden H, Kasher P, Kirby J, Shaw PJ. Microarray analysis of the cellular pathways involved in the adaptation to and progression of motor neuron injury in the SOD1 G93A mouse model of familial ALS. J Neurosci. 2007;27:9201–19. doi:10.1523/JNEUROSCI.1470-07.2007.

20. Fujita Y, Okamoto K, Sakurai A, Amari M, Nakazato Y, Gonatas NK. Fragmentation of the Golgi apparatus of Betz cells in patients with amyotrophic lateral sclerosis. J Neurol Sci. 1999;163:81–5.

21. Fujita Y, Okamoto K, Sakurai A, Gonatas NK, Hirano A. Fragmentation of the Golgi apparatus of the anterior horn cells in patients with familial amyotrophic lateral sclerosis with SOD1 mutations and posterior column involvement. J Neurol Sci. 2000;174:137–40.

22. Gonatas NK, Stieber A, Mourelatos Z, Chen Y, Gonatas JO, Appel SH, Hays AP, Hickey WF, Hauw JJ. Fragmentation of the Golgi apparatus of motor neurons in amyotrophic lateral sclerosis. Am J Pathol. 1992;140:731–7.

23. Haase G, Rabouille C. Golgi Fragmentation in ALS Motor Neurons. New Mechanisms Targeting Microtubules, Tethers, and Transport Vesicles. Front Neurosci. 2015;9:448. doi:10.3389/fnins.2015.00448.

24. Hafezparast M, Klocke R, Ruhrberg C, Marquardt A, Ahmad-Annuar A, Bowen S, Lalli G, Witherden AS, Hummerich H, Nicholson S, et al. Mutations in dynein link motor neuron degeneration to defects in retrograde transport. Science. 2003;300:808–12.

25. Iwata T, Namikawa K, Honma M, Mori N, Yachiku S, Kiyama H. Increased expression of mRNAs for microtubule disassembly molecules during nerve regeneration. Brain Res Mol Brain Res. 2002;102:105–9.

26. Jahn R, Scheller RH. SNAREs–engines for membrane fusion. Nat Rev Mol Cell Biol. 2006;7:631–43. doi:10.1038/nrm2002.

27. Kleele T, Marinkovic P, Williams PR, Stern S, Weigand EE, Engerer P, Naumann R, Hartmann J, Karl RM, Bradke F, et al. An assay to image neuronal microtubule dynamics in mice. Nat Commun. 2014;5:4827. doi: 10.1038/ncomms5827.

28. Lobsiger CS, Boillee S, Cleveland DW. Toxicity from different SOD1 mutants dysregulates the complement system and the neuronal regenerative response in ALS motor neurons. Proc Natl Acad Sci U S A. 2007;104:7319–26.

29. Malsam J, Sollner TH. Organization of SNAREs within the Golgi stack. Cold Spring Harb Perspect Biol. 2011;3:a005249. doi:10.1101/cshperspect.a005249.

30. Marsh BJ, Mastronarde DN, Buttle KF, Howell KE, McIntosh JR. Organellar relationships in the Golgi region of the pancreatic beta cell line, HIT-T15, visualized by high resolution electron tomography. Proc Natl Acad Sci U S A. 2001;98:2399–406.

31. Maruyama H, Morino H, Ito H, Izumi Y, Kato H, Watanabe Y, Kinoshita Y, Kamada M, Nodera H, Suzuki H, et al. Mutations of optineurin in amyotrophic lateral sclerosis. Nature. 2010;465:223–6. doi:10.1038/nature08971.

32. Mason MR, Lieberman AR, Grenningloh G, Anderson PN. Transcriptional upregulation of SCG10 and CAP-23 is correlated with regeneration of the axons of peripheral and central neurons in vivo. Mol Cell Neurosci. 2002;20:595–615.

33. Maximino JR, de Oliveira GP, Alves CJ, Chadi G. Deregulated expression of cytoskeleton related genes in the spinal cord and sciatic nerve of presymptomatic SOD1(G93A) Amyotrophic Lateral Sclerosis mouse model. Front Cell Neurosci. 2014;8:148. doi:10.3389/fncel.2014.00148.

34. Miller PM, Folkmann AW, Maia AR, Efimova N, Efimov A, Kaverina I. Golgi-derived CLASP-dependent microtubules control Golgi organization and polarized trafficking in motile cells. Nat Cell Biol. 2009;11:1069–80. doi:10.1038/ncb1920.

35. Morrison KC, Hergenrother PJ. Whole cell microtubule analysis by flow cytometry. Anal Biochem. 2012;420:26–32. doi:10.1016/j.ab.2011.08.020.

36. Mourelatos Z, Gonatas NK, Stieber A, Gurney ME, Dal Canto MC. The Golgi apparatus of spinal cord motor neurons in transgenic mice expressing mutant Cu, Zn superoxide dismutase becomes fragmented in early, preclinical stages of the disease. Proc Natl Acad Sci U S A. 1996;93:5472–7.

37. Munro S. The golgin coiled-coil proteins of the Golgi apparatus. Cold Spring Harb Perspect Biol. 2011;3: Doi 10.1101/cshperspect.a005256

38. Nakamura N, Lowe M, Levine TP, Rabouille C, Warren G. The vesicle docking protein p115 binds GM130, a cis-Golgi matrix protein, in a mitotically regulated manner. Cell. 1997;89:445–55.

39. Nanjappa V, Thomas JK, Marimuthu A, Muthusamy B, Radhakrishnan A, Sharma R, Ahmad Khan A, Balakrishnan L, Sahasrabuddhe NA, Kumar S, et al. Plasma Proteome Database as a resource for proteomics research: 2014 update. Nucleic Acids Res. 2014;42:D959–965. doi:10.1093/nar/gkt1251.

40. Nardo G, Iennaco R, Fusi N, Heath PR, Marino M, Trolese MC, Ferraiuolo L, Lawrence N, Shaw PJ, Bendotti C. Transcriptomic indices of fast and slow disease progression in two mouse models of amyotrophic lateral sclerosis. Brain. 2013;136:3305–32. doi:10.1093/brain/awt250.

41. Otto M, Bowser R, Turner M, Berry J, Brettschneider J, Connor J, Costa J, Cudkowicz M, Glass J, Jahn O, et al. Roadmap and standard operating procedures for biobanking and discovery of neurochemical markers in ALS. Amyotroph Lateral Scler. 2012;13:1–10. doi:10.3109/17482968.2011.627589.

42. Perrin FE, Boisset G, Docquier M, Schaad O, Descombes P, Kato AC. No widespread induction of cell death genes occurs in pure motoneurons in an amyotrophic lateral sclerosis mouse model. Hum Mol Genet. 2005;14:3309–20. doi:10.1093/hmg/ddi357.

43. Popoff V, Adolf F, Brugger B, Wieland F. COPI budding within the Golgi stack. Cold Spring Harb Perspect Biol. 2011;3:a005231. doi:10.1101/cshperspect.a005231.

44. Raoul C, Estevez AG, Nishimune H, Cleveland DW, deLapeyriere O, Henderson CE, Haase G, Pettmann B. Motoneuron death triggered by a specific pathway downstream of Fas. Potentiation by ALS-linked SOD1 mutations. Neuron. 2002;35:1067–83.

45. Reiling JH, Olive AJ, Sanyal S, Carette JE, Brummelkamp TR, Ploegh HL, Starnbach MN, Sabatini DM. A CREB3-ARF4 signalling pathway mediates the response to Golgi stress and susceptibility to pathogens. Nat Cell Biol. 2013; 15:1473–85. doi:10.1038/ncb2865.

46. Rivero S, Cardenas J, Bornens M, Rios RM. Microtubule nucleation at the cis-side of the Golgi apparatus requires AKAP450 and GM130. Embo J. 2009;28:1016–28. doi:10.1038/emboj.2009.47.

47. Rogalski AA, Singer SJ. Associations of elements of the Golgi apparatus with microtubules. J Cell Biol. 1984;99:1092–100.

48. Schaefer MK, Schmalbruch H, Buhler E, Lopez C, Martin N, Guenet JL, Haase G. Progressive motor neuronopathy: a critical role of the tubulin chaperone TBCE in axonal tubulin routing from the Golgi apparatus. J Neurosci. 2007;27:8779–89.

49. Shin JE, Geisler S, DiAntonio A. Dynamic regulation of SCG10 in regenerating axons after injury. Exp Neurol. 2014;252:1–11. doi:10.1016/j.expneurol.2013.11.007.

50. Skoufias DA, Burgess TL, Wilson L. Spatial and temporal colocalization of the Golgi apparatus and microtubules rich in detyrosinated tubulin. J Cell Biol. 1990;111:1929–37.

51. Smith BN, Ticozzi N, Fallini C, Gkazi AS, Topp S, Kenna KP, Scotter EL, Kost J, Keagle P, Miller JW, et al. Exome-wide rare variant analysis identifies TUBA4A mutations associated with familial ALS. Neuron. 2014;84:324–31. doi:10.1016/j.neuron.2014.09.027.

52. Soo KY, Halloran M, Sundaramoorthy V, Parakh S, Toth RP, Southam KA, McLean CA, Lock P, King A, Farg MA, et al. Rab1-dependent ER-Golgi transport dysfunction is a common pathogenic mechanism in SOD1, TDP-43 and FUS-associated ALS. Acta Neuropathol. 2015;130:679–97. doi:10.1007/s00401-015-1468-2.

53. Stieber A, Chen Y, Wei S, Mourelatos Z, Gonatas J, Okamoto K, Gonatas NK. The fragmented neuronal Golgi apparatus in amyotrophic lateral sclerosis includes the trans-Golgi-network: functional implications. Acta Neuropathol. 1998;95:245–53.

54. Stieber A, Gonatas JO, Moore JS, Bantly A, Yim HS, Yim MB, Gonatas NK. Disruption of the structure of the Golgi apparatus and the function of the secretory pathway by mutants G93A and G85R of Cu, Zn superoxide dismutase (SOD1) of familial amyotrophic lateral sclerosis. J Neurol Sci. 2004; 219:45–53.

55. Strey CW, Spellman D, Stieber A, Gonatas JO, Wang X, Lambris JD, Gonatas NK. Dysregulation of stathmin, a microtubule-destabilizing protein, and up-regulation of Hsp25, Hsp27, and the antioxidant peroxiredoxin 6 in a mouse model of familial amyotrophic lateral sclerosis. Am J Pathol. 2004;165:1701–18.

56. Subramaniam VN, Peter F, Philp R, Wong SH, Hong W. GS28, a 28-kilodalton Golgi SNARE that participates in ER-Golgi transport. Science. 1996;272:1161–3.

57. Sundaramoorthy V, Sultana JM, Atkin JD. Golgi fragmentation in amyotrophic lateral sclerosis. An overview of possible triggers and consequences. Front Neurosci. 2015;9:400. doi:10.3389/fnins.2015.00400.

58. Sundaramoorthy V, Walker AK, Yerbury J, Soo KY, Farg MA, Hoang V, Zeineddine R, Spencer D, Atkin JD. Extracellular wildtype and mutant SOD1 induces ER-Golgi pathology characteristic of amyotrophic lateral sclerosis in neuronal cells. Cell Mol Life Sci. 2013;70:4181–95. doi:10.1007/s00018-013-1385-2.

59. Taniguchi M, Nadanaka S, Tanakura S, Sawaguchi S, Midori S, Kawai Y, Yamaguchi S, Shimada Y, Nakamura Y, Matsumura Y, et al. TFE3 is a bHLH-ZIP-type transcription factor that regulates the mammalian Golgi stress response. Cell Struct Funct. 2015;40:13–30. doi:10.1247/csf.14015.

60. Thyberg J, Moskalewski S. Relationship between the Golgi complex and microtubules enriched in detyrosinated or acetylated alpha-tubulin: studies on cells recovering from nocodazole and cells in the terminal phase of cytokinesis. Cell Tissue Res. 1993;273:457–66.

61. Turner JR, Tartakoff AM. The response of the Golgi complex to microtubule alterations: the roles of metabolic energy and membrane traffic in Golgi complex organization. J Cell Biol. 1989;109:2081–8.

62. Turner MR, Kiernan MC, Leigh PN, Talbot K. Biomarkers in amyotrophic lateral sclerosis. Lancet Neurol. 2009;8:94–109. doi:10.1016/S1474-4422(08)70293-X.

63. Urushitani M, Ezzi SA, Matsuo A, Tooyama I, Julien JP. The endoplasmic reticulum-Golgi pathway is a target for translocation and aggregation of mutant superoxide dismutase linked to ALS. Faseb J. 2008;2:1–12.

64. Urushitani M, Sik A, Sakurai T, Nukina N, Takahashi R, Julien JP. Chromogranin-mediated secretion of mutant superoxide dismutase proteins linked to amyotrophic lateral sclerosis. Nat Neurosci. 2006;9:108–18.

65. van Dis V, Kuijpers M, Haasdijk ED, Teuling E, Oakes SA, Hoogenraad CC, Jaarsma D. Golgi fragmentation precedes neuromuscular denervation and is associated with endosome abnormalities in SOD1-ALS mouse motor neurons. Acta Neuropathol Commun. 2014;2:38. doi:10.1186/2051-5960-2-38.

66. Vlug AS, Teuling E, Haasdijk ED, French P, Hoogenraad CC, Jaarsma D. ATF3 expression precedes death of spinal motoneurons in amyotrophic lateral sclerosis-SOD1 transgenic mice and correlates with c-Jun phosphorylation, CHOP expression, somato-dendritic ubiquitination and Golgi fragmentation. Eur J Neurosci. 2005;22:1881–94.

67. Wei JH, Zhang ZC, Wynn RM, Seemann J. GM130 Regulates Golgi-Derived Spindle Assembly by Activating TPX2 and Capturing Microtubules. Cell. 2015;162:287–99. doi:10.1016/j.cell.2015.06.014.

68. Wen HL, Lin YT, Ting CH, Lin-Chao S, Li H, Hsieh-Li HM. Stathmin, a microtubule-destabilizing protein, is dysregulated in spinal muscular atrophy. Hum Mol Genet. 2010;19:1766–78.

69. Wen HL, Ting CH, Liu HC, Li H, Lin-Chao S. Decreased stathmin expression ameliorates neuromuscular defects but fails to prolong survival in a mouse model of spinal muscular atrophy. Neurobiol Dis. 2013;52:94–103. doi:10.1016/j.nbd.2012.11.015.

70. Williamson TL, Cleveland DW. Slowing of axonal transport is a very early event in the toxicity of ALS-linked SOD1 mutants to motor neurons. Nat Neurosci. 1999;2:50–6.

71. Xu Y, Wong SH, Zhang T, Subramaniam VN, Hong W. GS15, a 15-kilodalton Golgi soluble N-ethylmaleimide-sensitive factor attachment protein receptor (SNARE) homologous to rbet1. J Biol Chem. 1997;272:20162–6.

4

ZNStress: a high-throughput drug screening protocol for identification of compounds modulating neuronal stress in the transgenic mutant sod1G93R zebrafish model of amyotrophic lateral sclerosis

Alexander McGown, Dame Pamela J. Shaw and Tennore Ramesh*

Abstract

Background: Amyotrophic lateral sclerosis (ALS) is a lethal neurodegenerative disease with death on average within 2–3 years of symptom onset. Mutations in superoxide dismutase 1 (SOD1) have been identified to cause ALS. Riluzole, the only neuroprotective drug for ALS provides life extension of only 3 months on average. Thishighlights the need for compound screening in disease models to identify new neuroprotective therapies for this disease. Zebrafish is an emerging model system that is well suited for the study of diseasepathophysiology and also for high throughput (HT) drug screening. The mutant sod1 zebrafish model of ALS mimics the hallmark features of ALS. Using a fluorescence based readout of neuronal stress, we developed a high throughput (HT) screen to identify neuroprotective compounds.

Results: Here we show that the zebrafish screen is a robust system that can be used to rapidly screen thousands ofcompounds and also demonstrate that riluzole is capable of reducing neuronal stress in this model system. The screen shows optimal quality control, maintaining a high sensitivity and specificity withoutcompromising throughput. Most importantly, we demonstrate that many compounds previously failed in human clinical trials, showed no stress reducing activity in the zebrafish assay.

Conclusion: We conclude that HT drug screening using a mutant sod1 zebrafish is a reliable model system which supplemented with secondary assays would be useful in identifying drugs with potential for neuroprotective efficacy in ALS.

Background

Amyotrophic lateral sclerosis (ALS) is a progressive neurodegenerative disorder that leads to death on average within 2–3 years of symptom onset. It is characterised by the progressive loss of upper and lower motor neurons in the motor cortex, brainstem and spinal cord leading to muscle wasting, weakness and eventual paralysis. ALS is predominantly a sporadic disease, but 5–10 % of cases are familial, usually with autosomal dominant inheritance. Over 150 mutations in superoxide dismutase 1 (SOD1) have been identified to cause ALS and several of these mutations have been modelled in multiple species, including mice and zebrafish [1–5]. The only drug currently approved for slowing disease progression in ALS is riluzole, which gives ALS patients a life extension of only 3 months on average [6]. This highlights the need for compound screening in disease models to identify new neuroprotective therapies for this devastating human disease.

High throughput screening (HTS) assays underpin drug discovery efforts as they enable rapid screening of a large library of bioactive molecules in multiple disease models. High throughput screens are typically classified as either target directed drug discovery screens (TDDS) or as phenotypic drug discovery screens (PDDS) [7, 8]. In target based screens manipulation of a known

---
* Correspondence: t.ramesh@sheffield.ac.uk
Sheffield Institute for Translational Neuroscience (SITraN), University of Sheffield, 385A Glossop Road, Sheffield, UK

molecular target is the primary goal, with a main focus on the use of technology for generating throughput. In contrast, phenotypic screens use a top—down approach, where a disease process is manipulated in a screen and the assay uncovers compounds that directly impact on the disease process. Phenotypic screens typically have a lower throughput due to the complexity of the pathways and models used [7, 8]. With advances in genomics and the identification of molecular targets for many diseases, target-based approaches have been the main drivers of drug discovery in the 20th and 21st centuries. However, a recent report indicates that phenotypic screens are still the main providers of new-in-class drugs emerging into the clinic [9]. Among the 45 first-in-class drugs approved by the FDA during the period of 1999 to 2008, 28 drugs were discovered using PDDS, while only 17 were discovered by applying the TDDS method [9]. This occurred despite the fact that the majority of drug discovery efforts during this period were primarily geared towards TDDS based approaches [9].

Neurodegeneration is a field where target based approaches are yet to convincingly demonstrate utility in drug discovery. Furthermore, drug failure rates from bench to clinic in the CNS arena are far higher than in any other disease areas [10]. The lack of understanding in the molecular mechanisms that underlie neurodegeneration, and the lack of clear and specific targets, have played an important role in the poor success rates of drug discovery in neurodegeneration [11]. This highlights a need for new models and carefully designed screens/trials within the neurodegenerative field. The advantages of using PDDS in neurodegeneration are particularly compelling, as the assays developed will be generally unbiased towards a specific target, and may be able to modulate a functional phenotype associated with disease aetiology, multiple molecular pathways and/or symptoms in human patients.

Zebrafish (Danio rerio) are now widely used as in vivo models for many human neurological diseases, including ALS [2, 3, 5, 12–14]. Zebrafish are very useful for modelling human disease and drug screening due to their rapid development, large numbers of offspring, external fertilisation, small size, susceptibility to genetic manipulation and transparency during development, making them an excellent model system for imaging [3, 5]. Zebrafish are an increasingly powerful model in the field of high-throughput in vivo compound screening and have been used to assess both drug efficacy and toxicity [15, 16]. The development of a zebrafish Sod1 G93R model of ALS showed that zebrafish mimic many aspects of the human disease [5]. The mutant Sod1 zebrafish showed hallmark features of ALS that included impaired swimming ability, reduced muscle strength, neuromuscular denervation and loss of motor neurons [5]. Additionally, we have recently shown that inhibitory interneurons are primarily affected at the

embryonic stage in this zebrafish model, long before the motor neurons exhibit pathological changes [3]. This suggests that protection of the inhibitory interneurons at this early embryonic stage may delay the motor neuron degeneration observed in adult zebrafish. These findings are in keeping with recent evidence from human patients indicating that ALS is a disease with a prolonged prodromal stage which may warrant early intervention [17–22].

Heat shock proteins (HSP's) are ubiquitously expressed and found in all organisms. These proteins are upregulated in response to increased temperature as well as other forms of stress, including cellular stress [23, 24]. Heat shock proteins were first identified in 1962 in a Drosophila model where an increase in temperature was seen to induce new RNA synthesis [25]. The main function of the heat shock response is as a protective mechanism involved in the unfolded protein response (UPR), to overcome and promote cell survival in the face of a toxic insult, such as the presence of mutant or misfolded protein species, as is the case in SOD1 mutations. The heat shock response induces the synthesis of a family of heat shock proteins, including hsp70, that act as chaperones, which attempt to refold misfolded proteins or target them for degradation. Therefore heat shock proteins represent an excellent marker of cellular stress and can be used as a readout for mutation driven toxicity. In fact western blotting analysis in the sod1 G93A mouse model of ALS, demonstrated up-regulation of Hsp70 in the brain and spinal cord at 8 months of age [26].

Using an Hsp70-DsRed reporter gene we have developed a neuronal stress readout in a mutant Sod1 zebrafish model of ALS [5]. As the inhibitory interneurons are affected at the early embryonic/larval stages and exhibit activation of a heatshock stress response, we deduced that a readout of hsp70 activation by quantitation of the DsRed fluorescence signal could generate a simple high throughput screen suitable for the identification of modulators of neuronal stress in the zebrafish model. Interestingly, we found that riluzole, the only neuroprotective therapy authorised for the treatment of ALS, was able to reduce the neuronal stress signalled by hsp70 activation. We sought to develop an in vivo high throughput screen based on the identification of compounds which could modulate the quantifiable fluorescent readout of neuronal stress. Our screen utilises a high-capacity liquid handling system and a high-content imaging system to deliver high-throughput drug screening in an in vivo model. By screening for compounds that activate or inhibit the hsp70-DsRed response, we can identify compounds that act upstream or downstream of the mutant Sod1 toxicity pathway (Fig. 1). Thus, this hybrid assay combines a target based approach that can differentiate upstream and downstream pathways and at the same time has the advantages of a phenotypic screen, as it

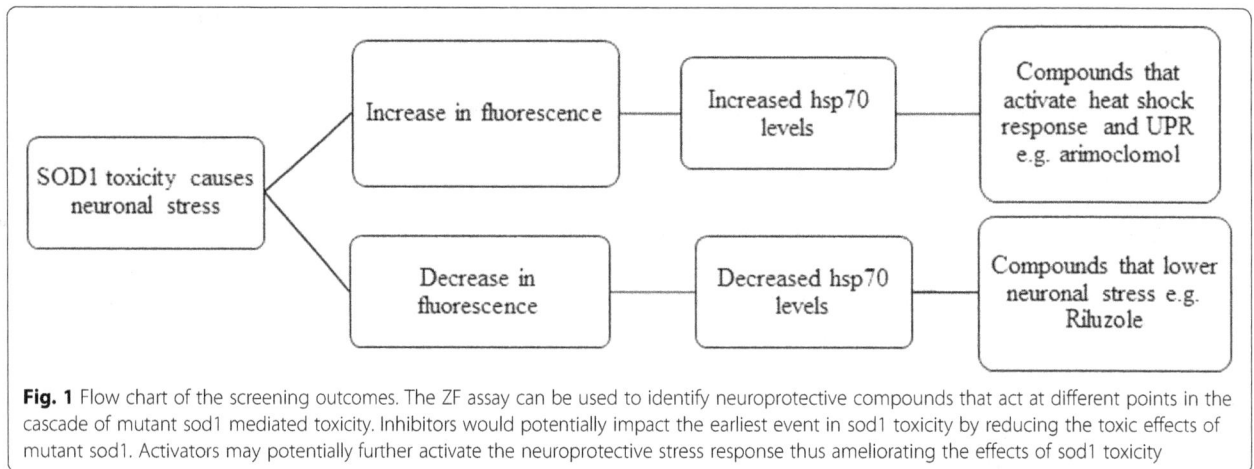

Fig. 1 Flow chart of the screening outcomes. The ZF assay can be used to identify neuroprotective compounds that act at different points in the cascade of mutant sod1 mediated toxicity. Inhibitors would potentially impact the earliest event in sod1 toxicity by reducing the toxic effects of mutant sod1. Activators may potentially further activate the neuroprotective stress response thus ameliorating the effects of sod1 toxicity

involves measuring the pharmacological modulation of a pathophysiological readout. In this study we describe the identification, optimisation, quality control and statistical analysis of the zebrafish neuronal stress (ZNStress) assay using a mutant *Sod1 G93R* zebrafish model of ALS. The Spectrum library of 2000 compounds was screened in the ZNStress assay, to identify modulators of neuronal stress using an *hsp70-DsRed* readout as a marker of neuronal stress. We demonstrate here the reproducibility and throughput of the assay and the ability of a phenotypic in vivo screen to match the statistical robustness of a TDDS.

Methods
Animals
Adult and larvae zebrafish (*Danio Rerio*) were kept at the University of Sheffield Zebrafish Facility, maintained at 28.5 °C and bred according to established procedures [27]. Animal protocols were undertaken in line with a Home Office approved project licence. The care and maintenance of animals were performed under the Home Office project licence as per ASPA regulations. All experiments were performed with embryos generated by out crossing the G93Ros10-SH1 line with the wildtype AB zebrafish strain [3].

Compound library and storage conditions
The spectrum library (Microsource Inc) is a collection of 2000 compounds from the US drug collection, international drug collection and natural plant compounds. The Library is stored in deep well storage plates within the SPOD system (Roylan) to prevent library deterioration. The SPOD system is a specialised drug storage system designed to extend the lifespan of compound libraries by controlling environmental conditions (atmospheric pressure of 0.5PSI, oxygen level <10 %, relative humidity <5 %) and maintaining an inert environment by mixing with N2. To create a screening library, the

stock library was imprinted onto 384 well LDV plates (Labcyte) before dilution to 10 mM to generate a final well volume of 10 µM. All drugs used in the ZNstress assay and spectrum library were solubilized and delivered in DMSO.

ZNStress assay protocol
Embryos were manually dechorinated at 24 h before loading into 96 well plates (Grenier BioOne, µClear) in 70 µl of E3 media and imaged using the Incell Analyser 2000, high-content imaging system (GE healthcare) to genotype the zebrafish prior to initiating the screen for DsRed fluorescence. Only normally developed healthy appearing embryos with expected fluorescence patterns are selected for screening (Additional file 1: Figure S1). All drugs were solubilized in DMSO with a final maximal DMSO concentration of 0.1 % and hence 0.1 % DMSO is used as a negative control. The drugs were loaded onto screening plates using the Echo 550 liquid handling system (Labcyte) to accurately and rapidly transfer the spectrum library of compounds into assay plates at a final drug concentration of 10 µM in 200 µl. The zebrafish transfered into the drug solution at 48hpf and incubated at 28 °C until 6dpf. The plates are monitored each day for death and imaged again at 6 dpf using Incell Analyzer. Wells with dead and defective embryos are noted and excluded. The zebrafish larvae are then terminally anaesthetised using MS-222 (Sigma), transferred individually in 50 µl to V-bottom 96 well plates (Grenier, Bio-One) and each well is then sonicated for 5 s at 25 % amplitude before being centrifuged at 3000 rpm for 15 min. 20 µl of supernatant is then loaded into 384 well plates and the fluorescence measured using the OMEGAstar plate reader system for emission in the DsRed wavelength (BMG Labtech).

In cell and Pherastar imaging
For automated imaging the InCell Analyzer 2000 (GE Healthcare) was used to image embryos before using the

zebrafish segmentation plugin (GE Healthcare) which allows the user to analyse the fluorescence in individual tissues. The software segments the zebrafish based upon the body shape into individual areas such as eye, brain, liver and spinal cord. Unfortunately, the software currently only segments the zebrafish accurately at 4dpf and this limitation introduced variability, making the use of this software unsuitable for the assay. Fluorescence well scanning was performed using the Pherastar FS system (BMG Labtech, 15x15 well scan). This method allows the user to keep the zebrafish alive after the assay. Unfortunately, the well scanning assay is slow for large assays (3–4 h per 96 well plate) and thus drastically reduced the maximum throughput of the assay.

Data analysis and quality control for ZNStress assay

Strictly Standardised Median Difference (SSMD) was used as the criterion for hit selection in the ZNStress assay [28]. In HTS screening an important quality control is to look at how much the positive controls, negative controls and tested compounds differ from one another. Readouts such as the Z-Score, signal to noise (S/N) and signal to background (S/B) are commonly used in HTS as readouts. These readouts work by comparing the values of two different well types in an assay. S/N and S/B only take the variability of one group into account and cannot provide quality control data on an assay with multiple groups. The Z-score takes into account the variability of two groups being analysed but not of the whole plate and so does not control the false positive/negative rate accurately. In addition, these analysis methods do not take into account the strength of difference between a test compound and a negative reference directly, but as a mean value, meaning that weaker hits can be missed. The SSMD calculates the median of differences divided by the standard deviation of the differences between a test compound and a negative reference [29] and therefore represents the average fold change penalised by the variability of the fold change across the plate. SSMD is a more suitable screen readout for in vivo HTS screening as it takes into account the variability across the whole plate, giving each well a readout shown as the magnitude of the difference in fluorescence compared to the whole plate, resulting in a more meaningful biological association. For this assay a threshold of *B* value < -0.5 or >0.5 was taken as the cut-off value to identify hit compounds for further investigation (Additional file 2: Table S1).

Results

Feasibility of Pherastar assay for high throughput fluorescence quantitation

Pherastar is a fluorescence plate reader that can measure fluorescence in a matrix format. This allows quantitation of fluorescence within each well, with high resolution at hundreds of points. We established that, as opposed to an image based quantification system (InCell), a direct high resolution fluorescence detector would be better for quantitating the DsRed fluorescence while still maintaining a degree of anatomical specificity. The Pherastar readout in Additional file 3: Figure S2 demonstrates the reduction in DsRed signalling following exposure to riluzole. The top rows show riluzole treated zebrafish, while the bottom row shows the control zebrafish exposed to DMSO. The data show a large decrease in hsp70-DsRed activation in the riluzole treated zebrafish, particularly in the head/brain region. However, consistent orientation of embryos created a problem in obtaining reproducible results. Also, the system was relatively slow and therefore impacted on the screen throughput capabilities. Hence, although this assay was more sensitive than InCell imaging, as it provided a signal intensity based readout, it was not capable of handling large throughput screening in a reliable fashion.

Use of whole embryonic extract for high throughput fluorescence quantitation

While InCell imaging and the Pherastar system provide an excellent way to measure neuronal stress levels, both of these systems require careful positioning of embryos, sophisticated image analysis software and computation time to analyse the results. We observed that riluzole reduced cellular stress in the CNS, and that the CNS was the primary source of DsRed fluorescence. We decided to determine if whole embryo extracts would be sufficient to measure the change in fluorescence levels. Such an assay, if shown to be robust would be beneficial as a high throughput readout, with enhanced reproducibility and reduced variability. Towards this we homogenised the zebrafish larvae by sonication and measured the fluorescence of the lysate, to determine whether robust inhibition of DsRed fluorescence was observed in the presence of the positive control compound, riluzole. Treatment of embryos from 2dpf to 6dpf with 10 µM riluzole reduced the DsRed fluorescence by approximately 50 % (Fig. 2a).

One important aspect of a screen is the success of identified hit compounds to show a concentration dependent response in the subsequent validation stage. To determine if the embryo extracts could be utilized to measure a dose response to riluzole, embryos were exposed to increasing doses of riluzole and the fluorescence measured. Fluorescence quantitation showed a clear dose-dependent reduction in fluorescence (Fig. 2b), thus confirming the usefulness of this assay in providing a good quantitative method for high throughput screening and drug effect.

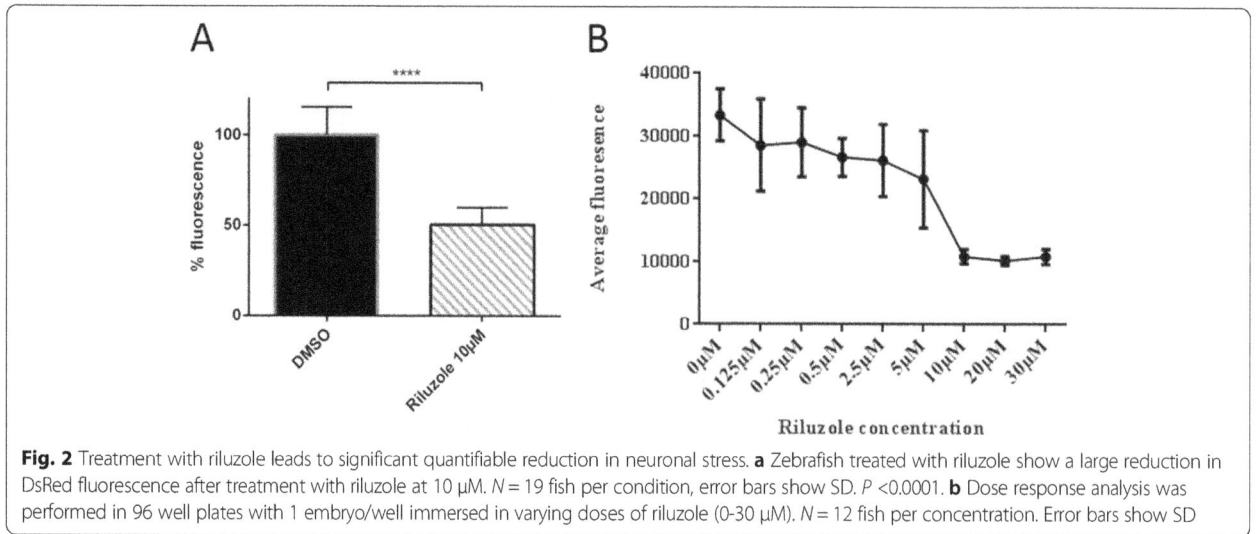

Fig. 2 Treatment with riluzole leads to significant quantifiable reduction in neuronal stress. **a** Zebrafish treated with riluzole show a large reduction in DsRed fluorescence after treatment with riluzole at 10 μM. $N = 19$ fish per condition, error bars show SD. $P < 0.0001$. **b** Dose response analysis was performed in 96 well plates with 1 embryo/well immersed in varying doses of riluzole (0–30 μM). $N = 12$ fish per concentration. Error bars show SD

Reduced between and within plate variability when assessing positive and negative controls using embryonic extract

As the first step prior to increasing throughput, we determined the assay-to-assay variability. The only source of variation observed is the day to day variation, due to the differences in the animals used. To reduce this we measured the variability observed with the positive and negative control compounds, between and within plates (Additional file 4: Figure S3). This variability was found to be minimal, suggesting that biological variation between animals should not greatly impact upon the success of the assay. The quality control analysis of the control compounds within the plate highlighted the applicability of this model to identify compounds such as riluzole that reduce the fluorescence readout of neuronal stress.

Development and optimisation of the high-throughput screen

Optimisation of a high-throughput screen was focused on increasing the number of compounds screened per week without compromising the sensitivity or specificity of the assay. Multiple screen lengths were investigated. The screen was begun at 2dpf as this allows genotyping before the assay begins, reducing the number of compounds per zebrafish, as well as allowing the zebrafish to have a further developed nervous system, compared to 24hpf. Shorter assays of 2 and 3 days of drug exposure showed drug effect, but the reduction in fluorescence was smaller, which reduces the effect window available for hit detection. This led to an increased incidence of false positives and negatives in quality control (QC) experiments. Drug exposure for 4 days gave a large window of drug effect, so that compounds only having a

subtle effect were still detectable, which was not be possible with the shorter drug exposure times.

Multiple endpoint readouts were investigated to identify the readout that reproducibly gave the most accurate results while maintaining a high-throughput. Implementation of robotics systems such as the Echo 550 liquid handling system (Labcyte) and the InCell 2000 (GE healthcare) Analyzer further improved the accuracy and throughput of the screen by automating the genotyping and dosing steps. The schematic of the final optimised screening process is shown in Fig. 3.

The high-throughput screen
Development of HT assay QC: use of strictly standardized median difference with no replicates (SSMD*) in identification of hits

SSMD* is a method described by Zhang et al in an RNAi screen. Screens that have a single well, with no replicates, require a method to identify hits within a plate. In SSMD* analysis, it is assumed that majority of the compounds in the specific plate tested have no efficacy and thus can be potentially considered as negative controls. A hit in the plate will stand out as an outlier and thus can be identified. Hence the median is used to measure the predominantly inert effects of most compounds in the assay. The advantage of this approach is that the whole plate is treated similarly, and hence only wells that are significantly different from the majority of the wells with no effects are identified. Using this method we tested 48 compounds with 12 positive and 12 negative controls in each plate. The layout of the plate is shown in Additional file 5: Figure S4. Thus, if most of the compounds in the plate have no effect at all, only the wells with riluzole should show up as positive hits in the plate. Figure 4a shows the SSMD scores of a representative plate in the screen. As expected, only the wells with

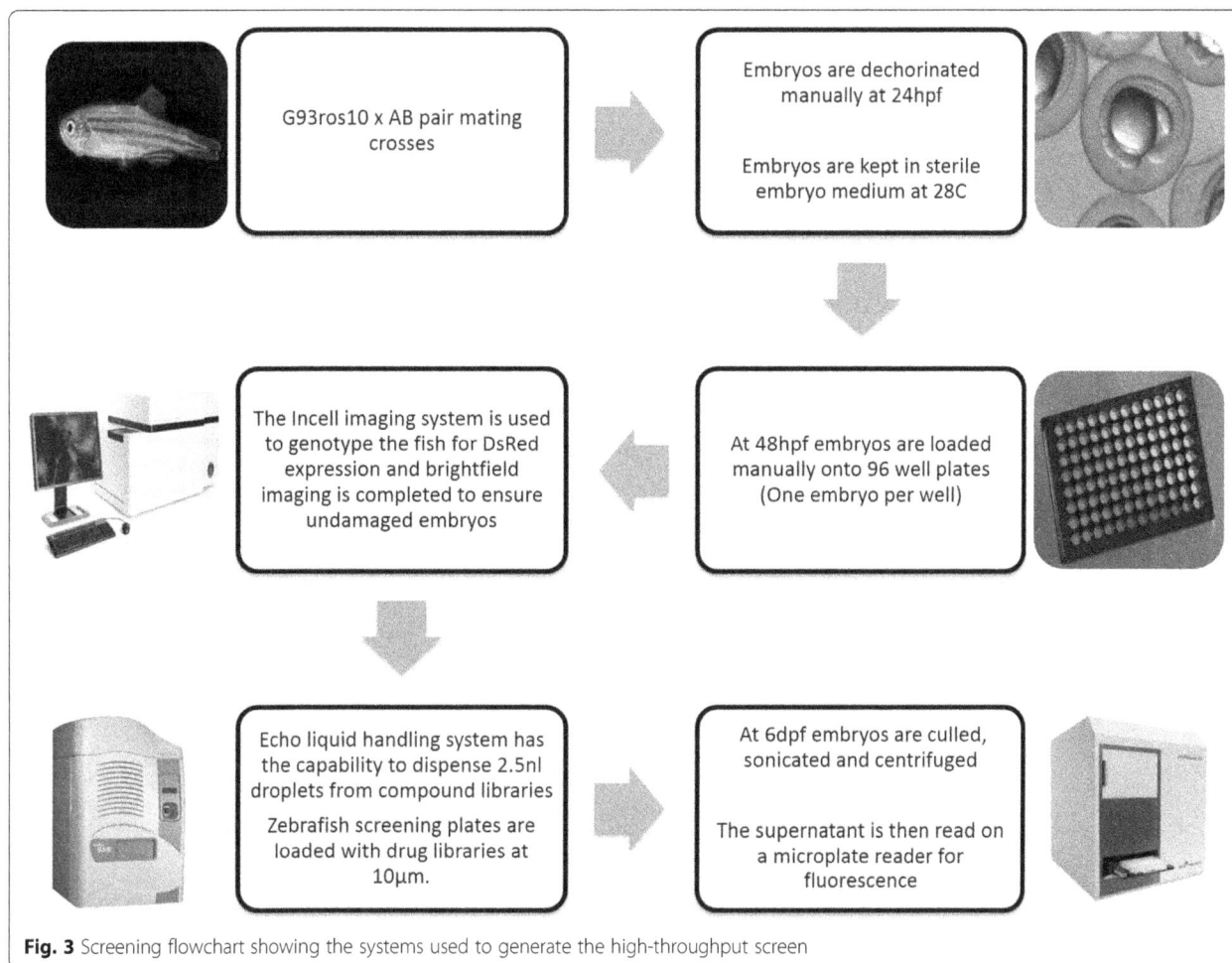

Fig. 3 Screening flowchart showing the systems used to generate the high-throughput screen

riluzole showed an SSMD* score of < -0.5 or more. This step confirmed that legitimate hits can be identified using this methodology.

QC analysis of positive and negative controls within plates and between plates

Using the SSMD* analysis we tested the reproducibility of the assay using riluzole and DMSO controls in each plate in the screen. The screen included 40 plates with 12 positive and 12 negative controls and 48 test compounds in each plate. The whole screen was then repeated a second time. The replicate QC of the screen using positive and negative controls with SSMD* analysis set at a < -0.5 cut-off as hits. The sensitivity of the assay was measured using the formula (#true positive/ (#true positive + #false negative))*100. The specificity of the assay was measured using the formula (#true negative/ (#true negative + #false positive))*100. The assay sensitivity ranged from 94.8–96.8 % and the specificity from 85.2–93.2 % (Table 1). When the SSMD* cut-off for hits was reduced to < -1.0, the sensitivity ranged from

79–81 %, while specificity increased to 96.5–98 % (Table 1).

Hit analysis

Using the cut-off values of < -0.5, <-1.0 (Inhibitors) or >1.0 (Activators) the hits were identified. Figure 4b shows the SSMD* values of all drugs tested in the screen along with positive and negative controls on either side. In all plates screened, riluzole always showed activity. 38 inhibitors of neuronal stress were identified below−0.5 and only 7 below−1.0, which represented 1.9 and 0.35 % of the compounds tested (Table 2). Activators with SSMD* scores above 1.0 were 20 (1 %) and 142 or 7.1 % of the compounds were toxic, causing death of the embryos (Table 2). all toxic compounds were rescreened again at 1 and 0.1 μM concentrations to detect if any had activity at lower concentrations. However, none of the toxic compounds showed any stress modulating activity at lower concentrations. The hits observed in the screen are realistic, with a small fraction of the total pool showing biological activity and

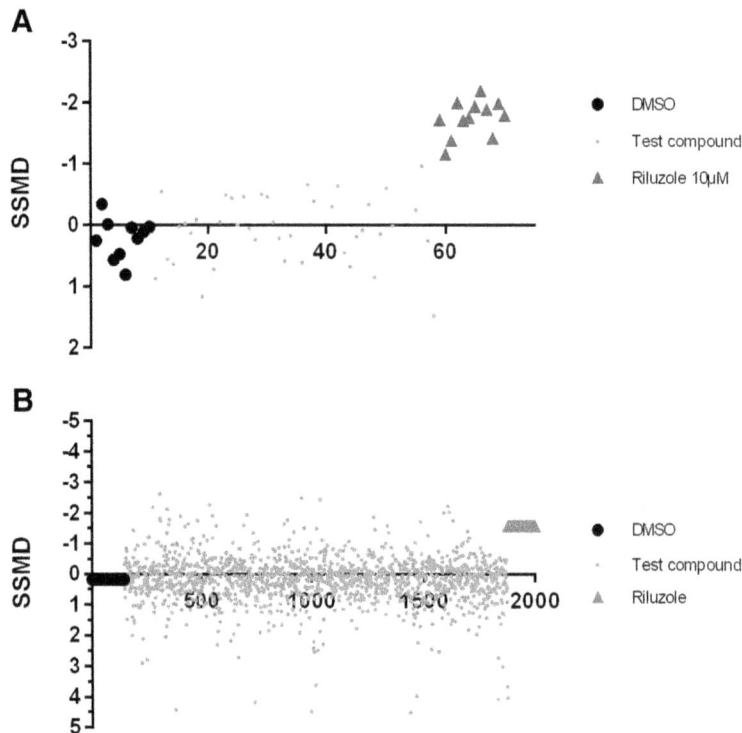

Fig. 4 Representative SSMD* scores of a plate and screen replicate from the ZNStress assay. **a** The plate comprising 12 positive controls (riluzole, black dots) and 12 negative control (DMSO, black triangles) and 48 test compounds (grey squares) were calculated for SSMD*. Riluzole shows a clear inhibitory effect and consistently shows a negative SSMD*, while most test compounds and DMSO controls show very little inhibitory activity. **b** 2000 compounds from the MicroSource Spectrum library were tested over 40 plates. Positive control for inhibitor of neuronal stress (riluzole, grey triangle) and negative DMSO controls (black circle) and test compounds (grey circles). A small fraction of drugs in the screen show biological effects comparable to riluzole and a small fraction of compounds in the library also showed positive SSMD values above 2, indicating that they were activators. Compounds that showed similar efficacy in two trials were classified as hits

with the positive and negative controls showing clear and reproducible effects. The hit compounds were diverse comprising of ion channel regulators, steroids, anti-bacterial, anti-oxidants and anti-inflammatory compounds, although only one compound showed efficacy to similar levels as riluzole.

Efficacy of compounds previously tested in the sod1 mouse model and/or in ALS clinical trials

Many drug trials have been performed in the SOD1 mouse model and multiple compounds have shown efficacy [1]. However, many of these compounds when taken to human clinical trials failed to show efficacy.

Table 1 Specificity and sensitivity of the screening assay based upon an SSMD threshold of < -0.5

	Replicate 1	Replicate 2
Sensitivity in percentage	94.8 % ± 9.85	96.6 % ± 8.8
Specificity in percentage	85.2 % ± 13.2	93.2 % ± 9.0

The assay statistics from 40 plates in each replicate including 12 positive control (riluzole) and 12 negative control wells. The false positive and false negative numbers were utilized to calculate the specificity and sensitivity of the assay expressed as percentage mean and standard deviation

Additionally, several recent publications have cast doubt on the efficacy of compounds previously tested [30–34]. Many of the factors affecting the reproducibility of preclinical testing in the SOD1 mouse model have been standardised and new guidelines have been formulated [32]. In order to examine whether the positive drug effects previously identified in the SOD1 mouse model were reproducible in the mutant Sod1 zebrafish model of neuronal stress, we evaluated 17 drugs which included riluzole. Out of all of these compounds only riluzole

Table 2 Statistics of assay hits from both replicates of the high-throughput screen

SSMD Threshold	Number of replicated hits	Number screened	Percentage hits
Below -0.5	38	2000	1.9 %
Below -1.0	7	2000	0.35 %
Above 1.0	20	2000	1 %
Caused Death	142	2000	7.1 %

Compounds that showed similar activity in both trials were identified as hits using the SSMD* threshold criteria as above. SSMD* below -0.5 are inhibitors of neuronal stress and those above 1.0 are activators of the neuronal heat-shock stress response showed efficacy in reducing neuronal stress (Fig. 5 and Additional file 6: Table S2). These results are in agreement with previously published reports of the lack of efficacy of many of these compounds when tested in follow up pre-clinical studies and/or clinical trials.

Dexpramipexole fails to reduce neuronal stress in the mutant sod1 zebrafish model of ALS

One of the major clinical trials in ALS to fail at phase 3 after promising phase 2 results, was the recent trial of dexpramipexole. Interestingly, prior to the human trial, no pre-clinical mouse data were published. When we tested dexpramipexole using the mutant Sod1 zebrafish model, we observed in the first evaluation a statistically significant effect in the reduction of neuronal stress (Fig. 6a). However, two follow up studies using the same preparation and the same batch of the drug failed to show any reduction in the neuronal stress (Fig. 6b, c). Overall analysis of the pooled data from triplicate experiments showed that dexpramipexole lacked efficacy in reducing neuronal stress in this Zebrafish model system.

Discussion

The ZNStress assay is a step forward in pre-clinical screening for compounds which may exert neuroprotective effects in ALS, as it links the key characteristics of a transgenic zebrafish line with screening techniques, to deliver a truly high-throughput in vivo drug screen. The only true limiting factor relating to this screen is the

number of embryos available each day and the manual pipetting of the zebrafish between plates. In its current format and being run by a single individual, it was comfortably possible to screen 4x96 well plates per day twice per week. This means that a screen of the full library comprising 2000 compounds in duplicate takes 6 weeks to complete. This highlights how suitable zebrafish are for screening and how we are moving towards the ability to screen hundreds of thousands of compounds in vivo to identify potential disease modifiers for human diseases.

Although the primary goal of the reported screen was to identify compounds that reduce neuronal toxicity mediated by mutant Sod1, we were also able to use the same assay to identify compounds that can activate the cellular stress response mediated by up-regulation of the heat-shock protein response, which represents a neuroprotective mechanism [35, 36] (Fig. 1). These compounds act downstream of the initial insult, i.e. the activation of the stress response mediated by mutant Sod1 misfolding and/or its associated toxicity. These compounds are of interest to the ALS field as activation of heat shock proteins has been shown to be neuroprotective and heat shock protein activators, such as arimoclomol, are currently in clinical trials for ALS [35]. Care must be taken as compounds that auto-fluorescence or are toxic also cause an increase in DsRed fluorescence. The compounds that activate the stress response can be further evaluated in secondary screens of efficacy to separate off-target effects from real heat shock protein activation.

The question still remains as to how closely a zebrafish model can mimic a human neurodegenerative disease, especially as this animal model retains the capacity for neuroregeneration. Additionally sod1 mutation is a small sub group comprising of 20 % of familial ALS patients and may not represent the predominant sporadic form of ALS. However, some recent data suggesting wildtype sod1 may be modified to toxic species in a prion like fashion in sporadic ALS [37], warrants the continued utility of sod1 based disease models in ALS research. Nevertheless the wide array of mutations contributing to ALS pathogenesis require additional genetic models to cover a broad spectrum of ALS pathogenesis and warrant the development of a wider net of screening tools. The assay described here is an embryonic/larval screen and hence limits its use to identifying factors involved in early pathogenesis. It is becoming increasingly evident that changes in ALS occur far earlier than clinical manifestation of the disease occur. This poses a challenge in treating the disease. It is also becoming increasingly recognised that potentially clinical stage of disease is too late for therapeutic intervention [19]. Hence, phenotypic identification and early diagnosis are gaining importance

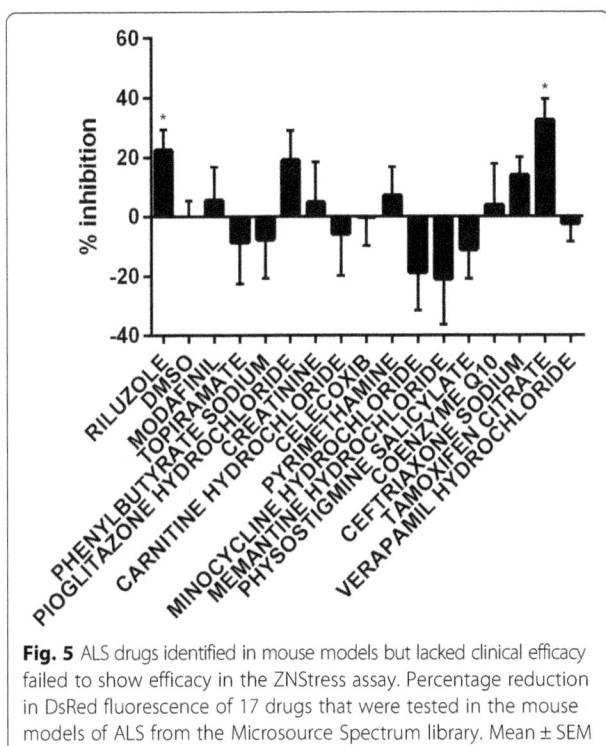

Fig. 5 ALS drugs identified in mouse models but lacked clinical efficacy failed to show efficacy in the ZNStress assay. Percentage reduction in DsRed fluorescence of 17 drugs that were tested in the mouse models of ALS from the Microsource Spectrum library. Mean ± SEM

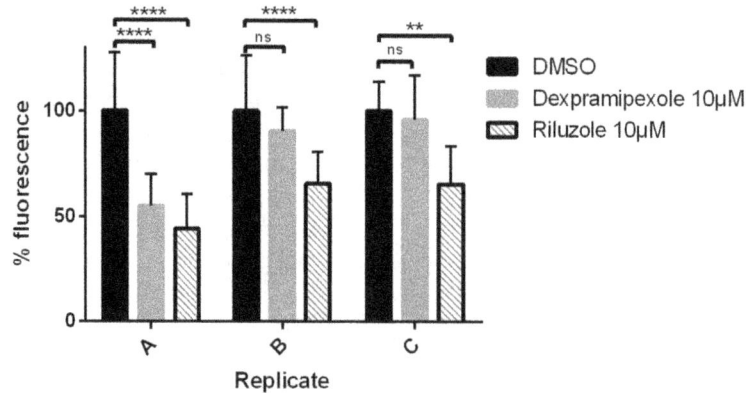

Fig. 6 Experimental variability and occurrence of random efficacy readout in drug trials: Dexpramipexole study. In replicate 1 both riluzole and dexpramipexole (both 10 μM) showed a significant reduction in DsRed fluorescence. However in replicate 2 and 3 only riluzole showed a significant reduction in fluorescence. This highlights the need for stringent assay QC and experimental replicates. $N = >10$ for each replicate, error bars show SD

in therapeutic development for ALS. There is a more focussed push towards biomarker discovery and therapy development bringing in an era of personalized medicine [38].

The utility of the ZNStress zebrafish model is shown by the efficacy of riluzole, the only approved drug used in the treatment of ALS. Riluzole shows robust inhibition of neuronal stress, demonstrates that drugs which are active in human ALS also show similar activity in a zebrafish model. Interestingly, many of the compounds emerging from murine preclinical studies that failed to show efficacy in human ALS clinical trials, also showed no efficacy in the ZNStress assay (Additional file 5: Table S2). The failure to reproduce positive effects of drugs in the SOD1 mouse model was ascribed to poor quality control in pre-clinical studies, necessitating the development of international guidelines for drug studies in rodent ALS models [39]. Low animal numbers, lack of litter matching, transgene copy number variability and lack of clear endpoints contribute to such spurious effects [39]. The need for a high degree of rigour in any pre-clinical evaluation of efficacy is clearly demonstrated by our experience with dexpramipexole. While one trial with dexpramipexole showed efficacy (Fig. 6a), follow up studies showed no efficacy (Fig. 6b, c). Like all HT screens unknown factors can occasionally lead to a spurious false positive result and hence the hits need to be robustly validated subsequently. Thus, high numbers and multiple screening repeats are key in eliminating false positive results. An important advantage of zebrafish is that we can conduct multiple efficacy studies using hundreds of embryos from multiple clutches, thus greatly enhancing the confidence of drug efficacy before testing in rodent models. We believe that zebrafish models are unlikely to replace mouse screens, but they have the ability to identify lead compounds of interest

with high confidence to predict biological activity in a vertebrate system, thus reducing the number of mouse studies required. This approach would be expected to accelerate and reduce the costs of pre-clinical drug discovery.

Future improvement of the screen described here will be to adapt the ZNStress assay readout so that the zebrafish can be kept alive after exposure, allowing genetic modifier and behavioural screens to be performed. An optimal system for this will be the InCell analyser zebrafish plugin as the system can rapidly capture images (96well plate in 2 wavelengths in 10 min at 2x). This will allow a decisive readout on which specific tissues and cell types, show an increase or decrease in fluorescence, alongside the ability to keep the zebrafish alive for downstream evaluation. A further potential improvement to the screen will be the implementation of an automated zebrafish handling system that can selectively genotype and load zebrafish embryos accurately and rapidly into wells, thereby increasing the screen throughput. Unfortunately, these systems are prohibitively expensive currently as they are still in development, but in the future it is likely that these systems will be common place in zebrafish facilities and will further improve the screening throughput.

The ZNStress assay is not limited to this particular zebrafish line, the ALS disease state or the specific field of biology upon which we have focussed in this report. The assay can be used in any fluorescence based zebrafish screen, as it is flexible and can be applied to multiple tissue types. We have developed and utilized the ZNStress assay with transgenic zebrafish carrying *hsp70-DsRed* in the context of *wildtype sod1* to identify neurotoxic genes involved in Parkinson's disease (unpublished data). In the Parkinson's disease model, the neuronal stress produced by specific parkinson mutations activate the DsRed reporter in the WT-sod1 transgenic line. The assay process described here utilized imaging systems that can detect fluorescence at any developmental stage. The assay can be shortened or extended for different lengths of drug exposure and has a readout that can be performed at different wavelengths. In future, the development of additional zebrafish models carrying different ALS mutations is necessary for comprehensive therapeutic screening and enable personalized medicine.

Conclusions
We conclude that HT drug screening using a mutant sod1 zebrafish is a reliable model system which supplemented with secondary assays would be useful in identifying drugs with potential for neuroprotective efficacy in ALS.

Additional files

Additional file 1: Figure S1. Embryonic quality control. Bright field images from Incell Analyzer 2000 of a representative 2 dpf-pre treatment embryo (Top) and 6 dpf embryos treated with DMSO (Middle) and Riluzole (Bottom). The embryos appear normal and undergo normal development. All embryos utilized in the screen were imaged and quality controlled.

Additional file 2: Table S1. Table of SSMD β-value hit selection criteria.

Additional file 3: Figure S2. Pherastar readout showing the ability to detect different drug effects in the screen. G93Ros10xAb zebrafish dosed with riluzole at 10 μM and DMSO. Zebrafish were scanned in a 30x30 point well scan for DsRed fluorescence. The readout is a spectral representation of DsRed expression from purple/blue = low signal to yellow/red = high signal.

Additional file 4: Figure S3. Variability in percent inhibition within and between plates in riluzole and DMSO treated wells. A clear separation of effects of riluzole (black) as compared to the DMSO controls (grey) which is close to zero change. The well to well variability and between plate variability as measured by SEM (error bars) shows that variability does not impact the identification of drug effects compared to DMSO controls.

Additional file 5: Figure S4. Plate layout for ZNStress assay. B – Blank, R - Positive control (riluzole), C- Negative control (DMSO), T- Test compound.

Additional file 6: Table S2. Effects of drugs tested in human ALS in the mutant sod1 ZNSstress assay.

Abbreviations
ALS, amyotrophic lateral sclerosis; DMSO, dimethyl sulfoxide; DsRed, discosoma red fluorescent protein; FDA, food and drug administration; HSP, heat shock protein; HT, high throughput; PDDS, phenotypic drug discovery screen; QC, quality control; SOD, superoxide dismutase; SSMD, strictly standardised median difference; TDDS, target directed drug discovery; UPR, unfolded protein response; ZNStress, zebrafish neuronal stress

Acknowledgements
We thank and acknowledge the support of aquarium staff at the Bateson center zebrafish facility at the University of Sheffield.

Funding
The work was supported by Motor Neurone Disease Association (grant Ramesh Apr11/2011 to T.R. and P.J.S.). AM was supported by a PhD studentship award from Sheffield Hospitals Charitable Trust (grant ref. 101102). PJS is supported as an NIHR Senior Investigator (R135043).

Authors' contributions
A.M, T.R and P.J.S conceived and designed the experiments. A.M performed the experiments. A.M and T.R. analysed the data. A.M and T.R wrote the paper and PJS edited the manuscript. All authors read and approved the final manuscript.

Authors' information
Not applicable.

Competing interests
The authors declare that they have no competing interst.

References
1. Turner BJ, Talbot K. Transgenics, toxicity and therapeutics in rodent models of mutant SOD1-mediated familial ALS. Prog Neurobiol. 2008;85(1):94–134.
2. Da Costa MM, Allen CE, Higginbottom A, Ramesh T, Shaw PJ, McDermott CJ. A new zebrafish model produced by TILLING of SOD1-related amyotrophic lateral sclerosis replicates key features of the disease and represents a tool for in vivo therapeutic screening. Dis Model Mech. 2014;7(1):73–81.
3. McGown A, McDearmid JR, Panagiotaki N, Tong H, Al Mashhadi S, Redhead N, et al. Early interneuron dysfunction in ALS: insights from a mutant sod1 zebrafish model. Ann Neurol. 2013;73(2):246–58.
4. Sakowski SA, Lunn JS, Busta AS, Oh SS, Zamora-Berridi G, Palmer M, et al. Neuromuscular effects of G93A-SOD1 expression in zebrafish. Mol Neurodegener. 2012;7:44.
5. Ramesh T, Lyon AN, Pineda RH, Wang C, Janssen PM, Canan BD, et al. A genetic model of amyotrophic lateral sclerosis in zebrafish displays phenotypic hallmarks of motoneuron disease. Dis Model Mech. 2010;3(9-10):652–62.
6. Miller RG, Mitchell JD, Moore DH. Riluzole for amyotrophic lateral sclerosis (ALS)/motor neuron disease (MND). Cochrane Database Syst Rev. 2012;3:CD001447.
7. Lee JA, Berg EL. Neoclassic drug discovery: the case for lead generation using phenotypic and functional approaches. J Biomol Screen. 2013;18(10):1143–55.
8. Lee JA, Uhlik MT, Moxham CM, Tomandl D, Sall DJ. Modern phenotypic drug discovery is a viable, neoclassic pharma strategy. J Med Chem. 2012;55(10):4527–38.
9. Swinney DC, Anthony J. How were new medicines discovered? Nat Rev Drug Discov. 2011;10(7):507–19.
10. Hurko O, Ryan JL. Translational research in central nervous system drug discovery. NeuroRx. 2005;2(4):671–82.
11. Zhang M, Luo G, Zhou Y, Wang S, Zhong Z. Phenotypic screens targeting neurodegenerative diseases. J Biomol Screen. 2014;19(1):1–16.
12. Patten SA, Armstrong GA, Lissouba A, Kabashi E, Parker JA, Drapeau P. Fishing for causes and cures of motor neuron disorders. Dis Model Mech. 2014;7(7):799–809.
13. Babin PJ, Goizet C, Raldua D. Zebrafish models of human motor neuron diseases: advantages and limitations. Prog Neurobiol. 2014;118:36–58.
14. Xi Y, Noble S, Ekker M. Modeling neurodegeneration in zebrafish. Curr Neurol Neurosci Rep. 2011;11(3):274–82.
15. Jing L, Zon LI. Zebrafish as a model for normal and malignant hematopoiesis. Dis Model Mech. 2011;4(4):433–8.
16. Baxendale S, Holdsworth CJ, Meza Santoscoy PL, Harrison MR, Fox J, Parkin CA, et al. Identification of compounds with anti-convulsant properties in a zebrafish model of epileptic seizures. Dis Model Mech. 2012;5(6):773–84.
17. Ramesh TM, Shaw DP, McDearmid J. A zebrafish model exemplifies the long preclinical period of motor neuron disease. J Neurol Neurosurg Psychiatry. 2014;85(11):1288–9.
18. Eisen A, Kiernan M, Mitsumoto H, Swash M. Amyotrophic lateral sclerosis: a long preclinical period? J Neurol Neurosurg Psychiatry. 2014;85(11):1232–8.
19. Eisen A. Response to a letter by Dr T Ramesh. J Neurol Neurosurg Psychiatry. 2014;85(11):1289.
20. Turner MR, Kiernan MC. Does interneuronal dysfunction contribute to neurodegeneration in amyotrophic lateral sclerosis? Amyotroph Lateral Scler. 2012;13(3):245–50.

21. Carew JD, Nair G, Andersen PM, Wuu J, Gronka S, Hu X, et al. Presymptomatic spinal cord neurometabolic findings in SOD1-positive people at risk for familial ALS. Neurology. 2011;77(14):1370–5.

22. Vucic S, Nicholson GA, Kiernan MC. Cortical hyperexcitability may precede the onset of familial amyotrophic lateral sclerosis. Brain. 2008;131(Pt 6):1540–50.

23. De Maio A. Heat shock proteins: facts, thoughts, and dreams. Shock. 1999;11(1):1–12.

24. Lindquist S. The heat-shock response. Annu Rev Biochem. 1986;55:1151–91.

25. Ritossa F. Discovery of the heat shock response. Cell Stress Chaperones. 1996;1(2):97–8.

26. Liu J, Shinobu LA, Ward CM, Young D, Cleveland DW. Elevation of the Hsp70 chaperone does not effect toxicity in mouse models of familial amyotrophic lateral sclerosis. J Neurochem. 2005;93(4):875–82.

27. Westerfield M. The zebrafish book a guide for the laboratory use of zebrafish Danio (Brachydanio) rerio: Univ. of Oregon Press, Eugene, OR; 2000. Available from: http://zfin.org/zf_info/zfbook/zfbk.html.

28. Zhang XD, Ferrer M, Espeseth AS, Marine SD, Stec EM, Crackower MA, et al. The use of strictly standardized mean difference for hit selection in primary RNA interference high-throughput screening experiments. J Biomol Screen. 2007;12(4):497–509.

29. Zhang XD. Illustration of SSMD, z score, SSMD*, z* score, and t statistic for hit selection in RNAi high-throughput screens. J Biomol Screen. 2011;16(7):775–85.

30. Benatar M. Lost in translation: treatment trials in the SOD1 mouse and in human ALS. Neurobiol Dis. 2007;26(1):1–13.

31. Gill A, Kidd J, Vieira F, Thompson K, Perrin S. No benefit from chronic lithium dosing in a sibling-matched, gender balanced, investigator-blinded trial using a standard mouse model of familial ALS. PLoS One. 2009;4(8):e6489.

32. Ludolph AC, Bendotti C, Blaugrund E, Hengerer B, Loffler JP, Martin J, et al. Guidelines for the preclinical in vivo evaluation of pharmacological active drugs for ALS/MND: report on the 142nd ENMC international workshop. Amyotroph Lateral Scler. 2007;8(4):217–23.

33. Scott S, Kranz JE, Cole J, Lincecum JM, Thompson K, Kelly N, et al. Design, power, and interpretation of studies in the standard murine model of ALS. Amyotroph Lateral Scler. 2008;9(1):4–15.

34. Vieira FG, LaDow E, Moreno A, Kidd JD, Levine B, Thompson K, et al. Dexpramipexole Is Ineffective in Two Models of ALS Related Neurodegeneration. PLoS One. 2014;9(12):e91608.

35. Kalmar B, Novoselov S, Gray A, Cheetham ME, Margulis B, Greensmith L. Late stage treatment with arimoclomol delays disease progression and prevents protein aggregation in the SOD1 mouse model of ALS. J Neurochem. 2008;107(2):339–50.

36. Kieran D, Kalmar B, Dick JR, Riddoch-Contreras J, Burnstock G, Greensmith L. Treatment with arimoclomol, a coinducer of heat shock proteins, delays disease progression in ALS mice. Nat Med. 2004;10(4):402–5.

37. Polymenidou M, Cleveland DW. The seeds of neurodegeneration: prion-like spreading in ALS. Cell. 2011;147(3):498–508.

38. Zou ZY, Liu CY, Che CH, Huang HP. Toward precision medicine in amyotrophic lateral sclerosis. Ann Transl Med. 2016;4(2):27.

39. Ludolph AC, Bendotti C, Blaugrund E, Chio A, Greensmith L, Loeffler JP, et al. Guidelines for preclinical animal research in ALS/MND: A consensus meeting. Amyotroph Lateral Scler. 2010;11(1-2):38–45.

5

Immunochemical characterization on pathological oligomers of mutant Cu/Zn-superoxide dismutase in amyotrophic lateral sclerosis

Eiichi Tokuda[1], Itsuki Anzai[1], Takao Nomura[1], Keisuke Toichi[1], Masahiko Watanabe[2], Shinji Ohara[3], Seiji Watanabe[4], Koji Yamanaka[4], Yuta Morisaki[5], Hidemi Misawa[5] and Yoshiaki Furukawa[1]* 🄳

Abstract

Background: Dominant mutations in Cu/Zn-superoxide dismutase (*SOD1*) gene cause a familial form of amyotrophic lateral sclerosis (*SOD1*-ALS) with accumulation of misfolded SOD1 proteins as intracellular inclusions in spinal motor neurons. Oligomerization of SOD1 *via* abnormal disulfide crosslinks has been proposed as one of the misfolding pathways occurring in mutant SOD1; however, the pathological relevance of such oligomerization in the *SOD1*-ALS cases still remains obscure.

Methods: We prepared antibodies exclusively recognizing the SOD1 oligomers cross-linked *via* disulfide bonds in vitro. By using those antibodies, immunohistochemical examination and ELISA were mainly performed on the tissue samples of transgenic mice expressing mutant SOD1 proteins and also of human *SOD1*-ALS cases.

Results: We showed the recognition specificity of our antibodies exclusively toward the disulfide-crosslinked SOD1 oligomers by ELISA using various forms of purified SOD1 proteins in conformationally distinct states in vitro. Furthermore, the epitope of those antibodies was buried and inaccessible in the natively folded structure of SOD1. The antibodies were then found to specifically detect the pathological SOD1 species in the spinal motor neurons of the *SOD1*-ALS patients as well as the transgenic model mice.

Conclusions: Our findings here suggest that the SOD1 oligomerization through the disulfide-crosslinking associates with exposure of the SOD1 structural interior and is a pathological process occurring in the *SOD1*-ALS cases.

Keywords: Amyotrophic lateral sclerosis, Cu/Zn-superoxide dismutase, Protein misfolding, Disulfide bond

Background

Amyotrophic lateral sclerosis (ALS) is a neurodegenerative disease, which associates with loss of motor neurons in the affected nervous tissues including motor cortex, brainstem, and spinal cords [1]. After several years of disease onset, significant weakness of muscles is usually followed by death due to the failure in respiratory system. While most of the ALS cases are sporadic, dominant mutations in Cu/Zn-superoxide dismutase

(*SOD1*) gene have been shown to cause familial forms of ALS (*SOD1*-ALS) [2]. More than 150 types of pathogenic mutations in *SOD1* gene have been identified [3], but importantly, no ALS-like phenotypes were confirmed in *SOD1*-knockout mice [4]. SOD1 is hence considered to gain toxic properties by pathogenic mutations. A common pathological hallmark in *SOD1*-ALS cases is the abnormal accumulation of mutant SOD1 proteins in motor neurons of affected nervous tissues [5]. Pathogenic mutations have hence been proposed to facilitate "misfolding" of SOD1 into abnormal conformation(s) and thereby exert toxicities causing the disease.

SOD1 is a homodimeric metalloprotein that binds copper and zinc ions and also forms an intramolecular

* Correspondence: furukawa@chem.keio.ac.jp
[1]Laboratory for Mechanistic Chemistry of Biomolecules, Department of Chemistry, Keio University, 3-14-1 Hiyoshi, Kohoku, Yokohama, Kanagawa 223-8522, Japan
Full list of author information is available at the end of the article

disulfide bond [6]. A folded conformation of enzymatically active SOD1 is significantly stabilized through the metal binding and the disulfide formation [7]. Indeed, dissociation of metal ions and reduction of the disulfide bond are known to decrease the conformational stability of SOD1 and thereby facilitate its misfolding in vitro; for example, demetallated (apo) SOD1 forms cross-linked oligomers through the shuffling of the disulfide bond [8], and further reduction of the disulfide bond in apo-SOD1 leads to the formation of the amyloid-like fibrillar aggregates [9]. Abnormal SOD1 trimers have also been recently shown to form in vitro at acidic pH and exhibit toxicities toward cultured cells [10]. Moreover, the structural dynamics of immature SOD1 has been extensively characterized in the atomic level [11–13]. Increasing numbers of recent in vitro studies have revealed various misfolding pathways of SOD1 proteins; however, it still remains obscure how SOD1 changes its conformation under the pathological conditions in vivo.

Actually, quite limited information is available on the biochemical/structural properties of pathological SOD1 species in human SOD1-ALS cases, partly because most of the motor neurons, which are the most affected cell types in ALS, are usually lost at autopsies. Therefore, any changes of SOD1 occurring specifically in affected motor neurons could not become evident in the biochemical experiments using the homogenates of spinal cords. Nonetheless, in transgenic ALS-model mice overexpressing mutant SOD1, the enzymatic activation of SOD1 has been shown to be retarded in spinal cords but not in the control tissues such as kidney and liver [14]. In other words, immature forms of SOD1 are expected to accumulate specifically in the spinal cord as misfolded proteins. Actually, the amyloid-like aggregates, which are composed of SOD1 lacking the disulfide bond, have been detected in the spinal motor neurons of transgenic ALS-model mice [15], while there has been no evidence to support the formation of amyloid-like aggregates in human SOD1-ALS cases [16]. Alternatively, we have previously detected the disulfide-crosslinked SOD1 oligomers in the spinal cord but not in the liver of ALS-model mice [17]. Pathological roles of the disulfide-crosslinked oligomers have been examined mainly in cultured cells [18, 19] but still remain less characterized in the transgenic mice and also in human SOD1-ALS cases.

In this study, we prepared and characterized the antibodies recognizing the disulfide-crosslinked SOD1 oligomers in vitro to test their pathological relevance in SOD1-ALS. Compared to the previous studies, we have more extensively examined the reactivity of our antibodies against purified SOD1 proteins in various metallation/disulfide states and ensured the recognition specificities of our antibodies to the disulfide-crosslinked SOD1 oligomers. In the ALS-model mice, the immunoreactivities

with our antibodies were evident from their presymptomatic stage and also specifically in their spinal cords. More importantly, the immunoreactivities with our antibodies were detected in spinal motor neurons of the human SOD1-ALS cases. We thus propose that the disulfide-crosslinked SOD1 oligomers possess an immunological epitope selective for the SOD1 species with abnormal conformations occurring in the pathological conditions.

Methods
Protein preparation and purification
Introduction of mutations was performed by an Inverse PCR method using a KOD-FX-neo DNA polymerase (TOYOBO) and confirmed by DNA sequencing. *Escherichia coli* SHuffle™ (NEB) was transformed with a pET-15b plasmid (Novagen) containing cDNA of human SOD1, and the protein expression was induced in the shaking culture with 0.1 mM isopropyl β-D-1-thiogalactopyranoside (IPTG) at 20 °C for 20 h. Cells were lysed with ultrasonication in PBS containing 2% Triton X-100, DNase I, and MgSO$_4$, and the supernatant after centrifugation at 20,000 x g for 15 min. was loaded on a HisTrap HP column (1 mL, GE Healthcare). SOD1 proteins were eluted with a buffer containing 50 mM sodium phosphate (Na-Pi), 100 mM NaCl, and 250 mM imidazole at pH 7.0. Metal ions bound to SOD1 proteins were removed by two-step dialysis first against a buffer containing 50 mM sodium acetate, 100 mM NaCl, and 10 mM EDTA at pH 4.0 at 4 °C for 16 h and then against a buffer containing 100 mM Na-Pi, 100 mM NaCl, and 5 mM EDTA at pH 7.4 (called NNE buffer). The proteins were treated with thrombin (GE Healthcare) to remove an N-terminal His-tag and further purified by size-exclusion chromatography using a Cosmosil 5Diol-300-II column (nacalai tesque).

For the epitope mapping of antibodies, we have prepared the following eight peptides as a fusion protein with glutathione-S-transferase, which was further N-terminally tagged with a 6 x His tag: Ala 1 – Lys 23 (Pep^{exon1}), Glu 24 – Ala 55 (Pep^{exon2}), Gly 56 – Arg 79 (Pep^{exon3}), His 80 – Val 118 (Pep^{exon4}), Val 119 – Gln 153 (Pep^{exon5}), Glu 24 – His 43 (Pep1), Ser 34 – Asn 53 (Pep2), and Gly 44 – His 63 (Pep3). All of those fusion proteins were overexpressed in *E. coli* BL21(DE3) with shaking at 20 °C for 20 h in the presence of 0.1 mM IPTG. As described above, the cells were lysed, and the fusion proteins were purified from the soluble supernatant with a HisTrap HP column.

Preparation and purification of anti-SOD1^{olig} antibody
Demetallated SOD1 with A4V mutation as purified above (5 mg/mL) was incubated in the NNE buffer at 37 °C for five days, by which soluble SOD1(A4V) oligomers were prepared. Those SOD1(A4V) oligomers were emulsified with either complete Freund's adjuvant

(DIFCO) in the initial injection or incomplete Freund's adjuvant and injected subcutaneously into a female New Zealand White rabbit at intervals of 2 – 4 weeks. Antisera were sampled at two weeks after the fifth or sixth injection, and immunoglobulins specific to antigen were affinity-purified using CNBr-activated Sepharose 4B (GE Healthcare) conjugated with the SOD1(A4V) oligomers.

To isolate the antibodies recognizing SOD1 oligomers but not the folded proteins, the affinity-purified immunoglobulins were washed with Ni^{2+}-affinity resins that bind His-tagged wild-type $SOD1^{S-S}$ proteins (SOD1-resins). SOD1-resins were prepared by adding 100 μL of His-SELECT nickel affinity gel (Sigma) to 500 μL of 200 μM His-tagged wild-type $SOD1^{S-S}$ in a buffer containing 50 mM Tris and 100 mM NaCl at pH 7.4 and incubated at 4 °C for an hour. The resins were washed with PBS and then incubated with the affinity-purified immunoglobulins in PBS with rotation at 4 °C for an hour. The resins were spun down, and again, the freshly prepared SOD1-resins were added to the supernatant and rotated at 4 °C for an hour. After repeating this absorption procedure four times, Ni^{2+}-affinity resins were added to the supernatant in order to remove His-tagged SOD1 proteins detached from the SOD1-resins. Concentrations of purified antibodies were then determined by Micro BCA Protein Assay kit (Thermo).

Preparation and purification of anti-SOD1^{int} antibody

Production of a polyclonal antibody to a peptide of SOD1 (Gly 44 – Asn 53) was performed by Eurofins Genomics. Briefly, the peptide, H_2N-CG^{44}FHVHEFGDN^{53}-COOH, was conjugated through its N-terminal Cys with keyhole limpet hemocyanin, with which a rabbit was immunized in the 42-day protocol. The sera were then purified using a Sulfo-Link Coupling Resin (Thermo) with the peptide, Gly 44 – Asn 53, Gly 44 – Glu 49, His 46 – Gly 51, or His 48 – Asn 53, by which anti-SOD1$^{44-53}$, anti-SOD1$^{44-49}$, anti-SOD1$^{46-51}$, or anti-SOD1$^{48-53}$ antibody was purified, respectively. All of the peptides have an additional Cys residue at the N-terminus for its conjugation with the resin. For preparation of anti-SOD1^{int} antibody, anti-SOD1$^{44-53}$ antibody was first loaded on a Sulfo-Link Coupling Resin (Thermo) cross-linked with purified apo-SOD1^{S-S} proteins, and the flow-through fraction was collected, concentrated, and then purified using a Sulfo-Link resin conjugated with a His 48 – Asn 53 peptide. Concentrations of purified antibodies were determined by Micro BCA Protein Assay kit (Thermo).

Enzyme-linked immunosorbent assay (ELISA)

To prevent adventitious binding of contaminant metal ions to SOD1 proteins in ELISA, we used Tris-buffered saline (TBS) that was treated with Chelex® 100 Resin (Bio-Rad). For the assay of E,E-SOD1 proteins, a strong chelator for divalent metal ions, EDTA (5 mM), was further included in TBS, by which an artificial supply of divalent metal ions (zinc ions, in particular) from buffers could be prevented. SOD1 variants with distinct metallation and thiol-disulfide status (5 μg/well) were coated on 96-well plates (Nunc-Immuno™ Plate CII, Thermo) overnight at 4 °C. After three washes with TBS containing 0.05% (v/v) Tween 20 (TBS-T), the plates were blocked with TBS containing 0.5% (w/v) BSA for an hour at room temperature. After six washes with TBS-T, either antibody purified in this study, polyclonal anti-human SOD1 (FL-154, Santa Cruz Biotechnology), USOD (#SPC-205, StressMarq Bioscience), or SEDI (#SPC-206, StressMarq Bioscience) antibody was added as a primary antibody (0.2 μg/mL) and incubated for an hour at room temperature, which was then followed by secondary antibody with horseradish peroxidase (goat anti-rabbit IgG, 1:1,000; Thermo Scientific) for an hour at room temperature. As the substrate solution, O-phenylenediamine and 0.012% H_2O_2 in a buffer containing 100 mM sodium citrate at pH 5.0 were used. The absorbance was read at 490 nm using a plate reader (Epoch, BioTek).

For sandwich ELISA, a plate (Nunc-Immuno™ Plate CII, Thermo) was coated with the capture antibodies (0.2 μg/mL anti-SOD1^{int} or 0.02 μg/mL anti-SOD1 (FL-154, Santa Cruz Biotechnology) antibodies) overnight at 4 °C and blocked with 1% BSA for an hour. Soluble extracts of the tissue samples containing 10 μg of total proteins were then applied and incubated at room temperature for an hour. The captured SOD1 proteins were detected by sheep anti-SOD1 (1:2,000, Calbiochem) and HRP-conjugated rabbit anti-sheep (1:1,000, Bio-Rad) antibodies as the detection and secondary antibodies, respectively. As the substrate solution, O-phenylenediamine and 0.012% H_2O_2 in a buffer containing 100 mM sodium citrate at pH 5.0 were used. The absorbance was read at 490 nm using a plate reader (Epoch, BioTek).

Transgenic mice

Transgenic mice carrying human *SOD1* gene with G93A mutation (B6.Cg-Tg(SOD1*G93A)1Gur/J in a C57BL/6 background) and human wild-type *SOD1* gene (B6.Cg-Tg(SOD1)2Gur) were purchased from Jackson Laboratory (Bar Harbor, ME) and maintained heterozygous with a C57BL/6 background. Mice expressing human SOD1 with G37R were described previously [20]. Mice were genotyped for human *SOD1* using tail DNA as described previously [21]. All experiments were reviewed and approved by the Animal Use and Care Committees of Keio University and Nagoya University, and care was taken to minimize suffering and limit the number of animals used.

Mice were deeply anesthetized with sodium pentobarbital and then perfused *via* the aortic cone with PBS, followed by 4% paraformaldehyde in a buffer containing 0.1 M Na-Pi at pH 7.4. The lumbar region of each spinal cord (*ca.* 2 cm) was removed and post-fixed in the same fixative overnight at 4 °C, after which it was immersed in 20% sucrose in 0.1 M Na-Pi, pH 7.4, overnight at 4 °C. The tissue was then frozen in OCT compound (Sakura Finetek) and sectioned at 40 μm on a cryostat. Rabbit anti-SOD1^{olig} (0.02 μg/mL) and mouse monoclonal anti-human SOD1 (0.02 μg/mL, clone 1G2, MBL) antibodies were used for immunohistochemistry as a primary antibody, and biotinylated anti-mouse IgG (H + L) (1:200 dilution, Vector Laboratories, Inc.) was used as a secondary antibody. The immunoreaction was amplified using the VECTASTAIN ABC HRP Kit (Vector Laboratories, Inc.) according to the manufacturer's direction. The free-floating sections were processed using diaminobenzidine (DAB) as the chromogen followed by counter-staining with hematoxylin [22]. Stained sections were then examined using a microscope (BX51, Olympus).

Human cases

The human cases examined in this study included three *SOD1*-ALS cases with C111Y mutation, four sporadic ALS cases with TDP-43-positive inclusions (negative for SOD1 mutations), and three non-ALS controls. All tissues from ALS patients and non-ALS controls were obtained by autopsy with informed consent at Matsumoto Medical Center in Japan, and information on the cases was summarized in Additional file 1: Table S1. The collection of tissues and their use in this study were approved by the institutional review board for research ethics of Matsumoto Medical Center and Keio University, Japan.

For immunohistochemical examination, the spinal cord was fixed in 10% buffered formalin, and multiple tissue blocks were embedded in paraffin. Deparaffinized 4-*μ*m-thick sections were immunostained by the streptavidin-biotin method using rabbit anti-SOD1^{olig} (0.02 μg/mL), rabbit anti-SOD1^{int} (0.3 μg/mL), mouse monoclonal anti-human SOD1 (0.5 μg/mL, clone 1G2, MBL) antibodies, and the corresponding biotin-conjugated secondary antibodies. The sections were processed with HRP-conjugated streptavidin and DAB as the chromogen and further stained for nuclei with hematoxylin. For double immunofluorescence, deparaffinized sections were first incubated with Sudan Black B to suppress auto-fluorescence and then stained with the primary antibodies followed by the corresponding FITC- or Cy3-labeled secondary antibodies (Jackson Labs, Pittsburgh, PA).

Sample preparations for biochemical analysis on human and mouse tissues

For human cases, the ventral and dorsal horns were separately excised from the frozen thoractic spinal cord samples. Frozen mice tissues (lumbar spinal cord,

cervical spinal cord, cerebellum, and brainstem) were also separately prepared. The tissues were then homogenized and ultrasonicated in PBS containing 1% NP-40, 100 mM iodoacetamide, 5 mM EDTA, and EDTA-free Complete Protease inhibitor cocktail (Roche). The homogenates were centrifuged (20,000 x *g*, 30 min. 4 °C) to prepare the soluble supernatants and then examined for their total protein concentrations by using Micro BCA Assay Kit (Thermo Scientific).

Western blotting analysis

Soluble proteins in the tissue extracts (15 μg/lane) were separated using 12.5% polyacrylamide gels and blotted onto a PVDF membrane (0.2 μm, Wako). The membrane was treated with a blocking solution containing 5% (w/v) dried milk and 0.01% (v/v) Tween 20 in PBS at pH 7.4. The blots were probed with rabbit anti-SOD1 antibody (1:10,000; FL-154, Santa Cruz Biotechnology) and HRP-conjugated goat anti-rabbit IgG antibody (1:10,000; Thermo Scientific), visualized using ImmunoStar LD (Wako), and then observed in the LumiCube (Liponics). To validate an equal loading of tissue extracts, glyceraldehyde 3-phosphate dehydrogenase (GAPDH) was used as an internal marker. The membranes were treated with the WB Stripping Solution (nacalai tesque) for 1 h at 37 °C and reprobed with rabbit anti-GAPDH antibody (1:5,000; FL-335, Santa Cruz Biotechnology).

Statistics

All statistical tests were performed using Statcel 3 software (OMS Publishing Inc.). After the determination of normality, multiple group comparisons were performed using a one-way ANOVA followed by the Tukey–Kramer *post-hoc* test.

Results
Preparation of soluble and disulfide-crosslinked oligomers of SOD1 in vitro

Among four Cys residues (Cys 6, 57, 111, and 146) in SOD1, the conserved disulfide bond forms between Cys 57 and 146 within an SOD1 molecule and significantly contributes to structural stabilization of a SOD1 protein [7]. Under destabilizing conditions in vitro, however, the disulfide bond of SOD1 is shuffled among the four Cys residues in inter- as well as intra-molecular fashion, resulting in the formation of SOD1 oligomers crosslinked *via* disulfide bond(s) [8]. In this study, an apo and disulfide form of SOD1 (E,E-SOD1^{S-S}; the first and second E mean empty at copper and zinc sites, respectively; thiol-disulfide status is indicated as superscript.) (Fig. 1a) was first prepared and then incubated at 37 °C for five days without any agitation. SOD1 with ALS-causing mutations formed the high-molecular weight species, which remained in supernatant after centrifugation at 20,000 x *g*

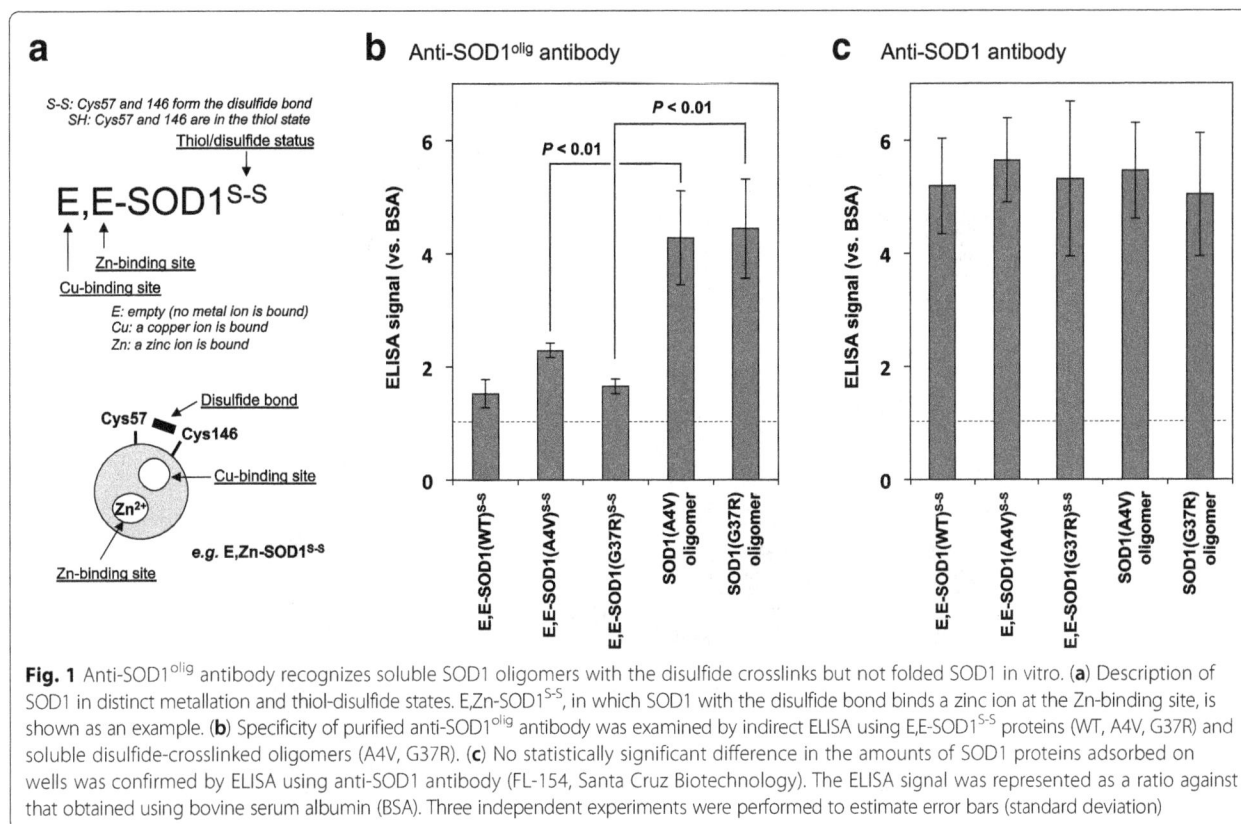

Fig. 1 Anti-SOD1^{olig} antibody recognizes soluble SOD1 oligomers with the disulfide crosslinks but not folded SOD1 in vitro. (**a**) Description of SOD1 in distinct metallation and thiol-disulfide states. E,Zn-SOD1^{S-S}, in which SOD1 with the disulfide bond binds a zinc ion at the Zn-binding site, is shown as an example. (**b**) Specificity of purified anti-SOD1^{olig} antibody was examined by indirect ELISA using E,E-SOD1^{S-S} proteins (WT, A4V, G37R) and soluble disulfide-crosslinked oligomers (A4V, G37R). (**c**) No statistically significant difference in the amounts of SOD1 proteins adsorbed on wells was confirmed by ELISA using anti-SOD1 antibody (FL-154, Santa Cruz Biotechnology). The ELISA signal was represented as a ratio against that obtained using bovine serum albumin (BSA). Three independent experiments were performed to estimate error bars (standard deviation)

and were observed in non-reducing but not in reducing SDS-PAGE (Additional file 2: Figure S1). These results confirm the formation of the soluble SOD1 oligomers cross-linked *via* disulfide bonds.

Purification of an antibody recognizing the disulfide-crosslinked SOD1 oligomers

A rabbit was first immunized with the soluble and disulfide-crosslinked oligomers of A4V-mutant SOD1 prepared in vitro, and then the polyclonal antibodies were affinity-purified using those oligomers. Nonetheless, the purified antibody was not selective to the oligomers; a natively folded SOD1 protein (Cu,Zn-SOD1^{S-S}) significantly reacted with the antibody (data not shown). To increase the specificity of antibodies to the oligomers, the purified antibodies were washed with Ni^{2+}-affinity resins on which wild-type SOD1^{S-S} was immobilized through its N-terminal His tag (see Methods). As shown in Fig. 1b and c, the finally purified antibody (called anti-SOD1^{olig} antibody) exhibited significantly higher ELISA signals to the soluble disulfide-crosslinked SOD1(A4V) oligomer than those to wild-type (WT) and A4V-mutant E,E-SOD1^{S-S} proteins ($P < 0.01$). It is also important to note that anti-SOD1^{olig} antibody can recognize the soluble and disulfide-crosslinked oligomers of G37R-mutant SOD1 but not E,E-SOD1(G37R)$^{S-S}$ ($P < 0.01$: Fig. 1b and c). Our anti-SOD1^{olig} antibody was hence found to exclusively

recognize the soluble and disulfide-crosslinked SOD1 oligomers.

Immunohistochemical detection of pathological SOD1 species by anti-SOD1^{olig} antibody

We previously detected the disulfide-crosslinked SOD1 species by isolating those from the spinal cord homogenates of ALS-model mice [17, 23]. In this study, we attempted to probe the disulfide-crosslinked oligomers during the pathogenesis of *SOD1*-ALS by using our anti-SOD1^{olig} antibody. For that purpose, the ALS-model mice expressing human SOD1 with G93A mutation (G1H mice) on a congenic C57BL/6 background were immunohistochemically examined. As shown in Fig. 2a and b, the species immunoreactive to anti-SOD1^{olig} antibody were observed in the ventral horn of the lumbar spinal cord before the disease onset (at 60 and 100 days of age). No staining with anti-SOD1^{olig} antibody was confirmed in the corresponding area of spinal cords of a non-transgenic mouse (Additional file 3: Figure S2A and B). Also, when anti-SOD1^{olig} antibody was pre-absorbed with the disulfide-crosslinked oligomers of A4V-mutant SOD1, any immunoreactive species were not observed in the spinal cord of a G1H mouse (100 days) (Additional file 3: Figure S2C). Instead, when pre-absorbed with E,Zn-SOD1(A4V)$^{S-S}$, anti-SOD1^{olig} antibody was able to detect the immunoreactive species in the spinal cord of a G1H

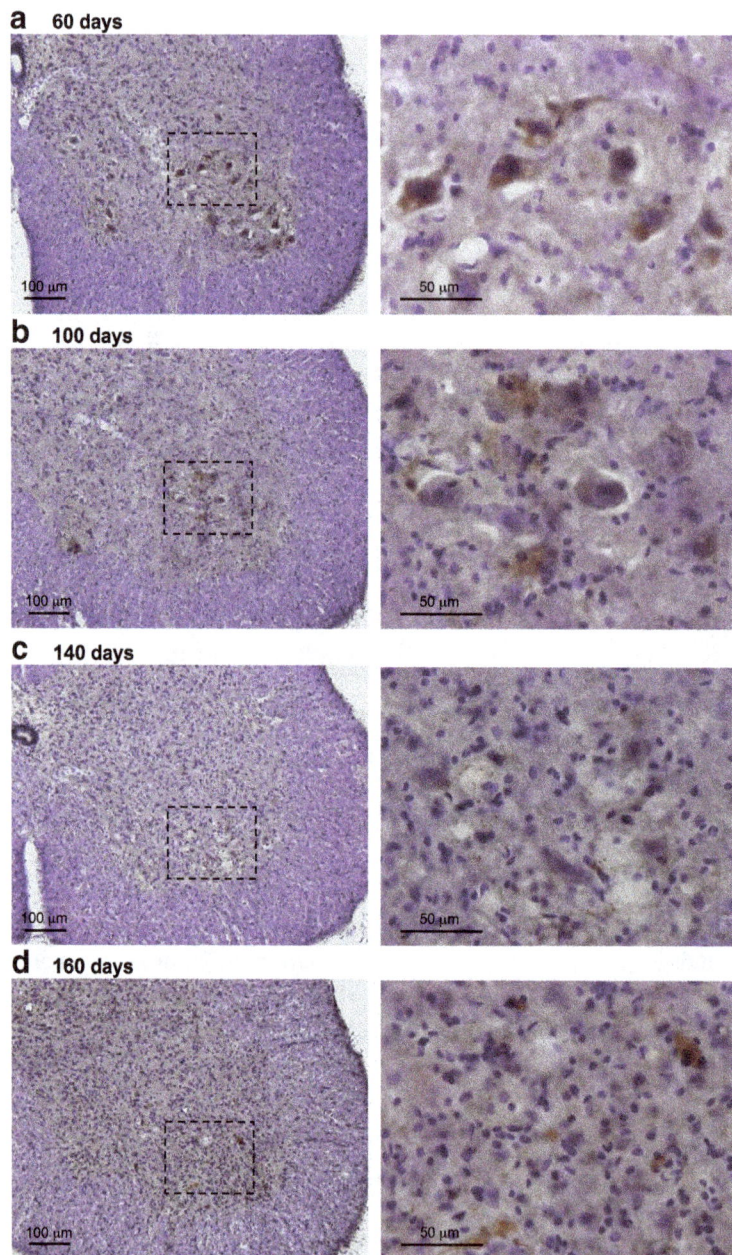

Fig. 2 Immunohistochemical examination on G1H mice with anti-SOD1^{olig} antibody. The sections of lumbar spinal cords (ventral horn) of G1H mice at **a** 60, **b** 100, **c** 140, and **d** 160 days of age were stained with anti-SOD1^{olig} antibody. The images in the low magnification are shown in the left panel, where the region enclosed with a broken line is magnified and shown in the right panel. Nuclei were counterstained with hematoxylin (blue). The bar in each panel represents 100 μm (left panel) and 50 μm (right panel)

mouse (100 days) (Additional file 3: Figure S2D). These control experiments assure the specificity of anti-SOD1^{olig} antibody toward the pathological SOD1 species in the transgenic mice.

At the end stage of the disease (140 and 160 days of age), however, immunostaining with anti-SOD1^{olig} antibody was significantly reduced in the lumbar spinal cord of G1H mice (Fig. 2c and d),. This was not described by the changes in total amounts of soluble SOD1 in the

lumbar spinal cord, which was actually increased during aging ([14]; also see below). We previously showed that the number of the ChAT-positive motor neurons at 140 days of age was reduced down to one third of those at 60 days of age in G1H mice [24]. The reduced immunostaining with anti-SOD1^{olig} antibody might thus indicate loss of motor neurons at the disease end-stage. Nonetheless, mutant SOD1 has been also known to accumulate as inclusions in the surviving motor neurons of diseased G1H mice [25]. Actually, the diffuse staining of SOD1 was observed in the lumbar spinal cord of pre-symptomatic G1H mice (60 and 100 days of age), and the SOD1-positive inclusions became evident in the disease end-stage (140 and 160 days of age) (Additional file 4: Figure S3). Our anti-SOD1^{olig} antibody is hence expected to have little immunoreactivity toward the SOD1-positive inclusions formed in terminally ill G1H mice. Based upon these results, we suggest that anti-SOD1^{olig} antibody specifically detects the pathological SOD1 species occurring in the lumbar spinal cords of the pre-symptomatic G1H mice.

By using anti-SOD1^{olig} antibody, we have further performed immunohistochemical examination on the spinal cords of two SOD1-ALS cases with C111Y mutation. Two cases (III-5 and IV-6 reported in [26]; Additional file 1: Table S1) examined here had the disease duration of 1.2 and 4.0 years, respectively. It has been reported that SOD1-positive inclusions are observed at the cytoplasm and neurites of spinal motor neurons in those SOD1-ALS cases with C111Y mutation [27]. Unlike G1H mice, those SOD1-positive inclusions in the spinal cord of the case IV-6 were immunostained with anti-SOD1^{olig} antibody (Fig. 3a). In the other SOD1-ALS case, III-5, almost no motor neurons were spared due to the intense degeneration of the spinal cord, but sparse immunostaining by anti-SOD1^{olig} antibody was confirmed in the remaining motor neurons of the cervical spinal cord (Fig. 3b). The pathological inclusions in the spinal motor neurons were co-immunostained by anti-SOD1 and anti-SOD1^{olig}

antibodies (Fig. 3c-f), and no immunostaining with anti-SOD1^{olig} antibody was confirmed in non-ALS cases (Additional file 5: Figure S4A). Accordingly, anti-SOD1^{olig} antibody can specifically detect the SOD1 species accumulated as pathological inclusions in spinal motor neurons of SOD1-ALS patients. This appeared to contradict with the declined immunostaining with anti-SOD1^{olig} antibody in the end stage G1H mice (Fig. 2c and d) but actually support the previous reports describing distinct properties of SOD1-positive inclusions between transgenic mice and human cases [15, 16] (also see Discussion).

These results show that our anti-SOD1^{olig} antibody for the disulfide-crosslinked oligomers was able to detect pathological SOD1 species, but a major concern in the preparation of this antibody is a quite low yield (7.5 mL of 0.2 µg/mL antibody from one immunized rabbit) after several purification procedures. Actually, we have little amounts of anti-SOD1^{olig} antibody left, and constant reproduction of anti-SOD1^{olig} antibody would also be quite difficult due to its polyclonal nature. To deal with those troubles on anti-SOD1^{olig} antibody, we attempted to first determine the epitope of anti-SOD1^{olig} antibody and then produce another oligomer-specific antibody by immunizing rabbits with the peptide covering that epitope.

Anti-SOD1^{olig} antibody recognizes interior of the SOD1 folded structure

The epitope mapping of anti-SOD1^{olig} antibody was performed by ELISA using five peptides, Pep$^{exon1-5}$, each of which corresponds to a translated product of five exons

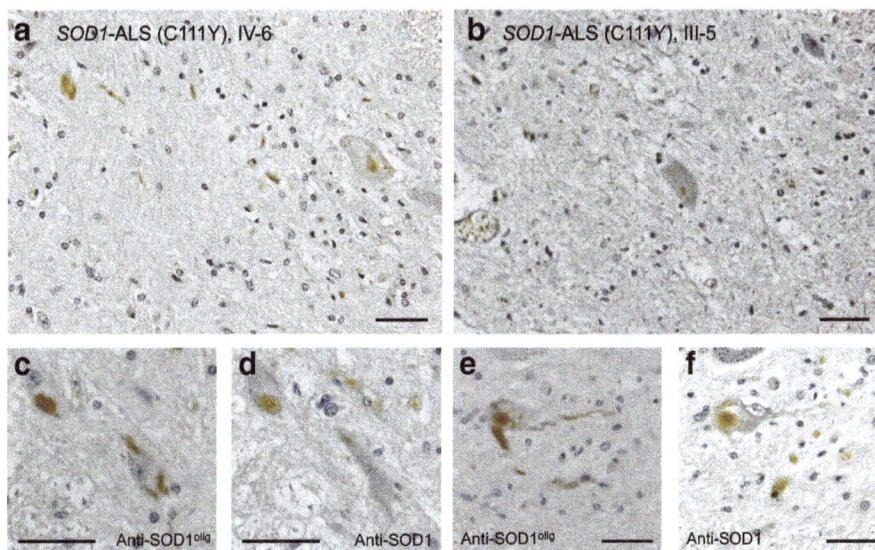

Fig. 3 Immunohistochemical examination of human SOD1-ALS cases (C111Y mutation) with anti-SOD1^{olig} antibody. DAB staining of a a sacral spinal cord (ventral horn) section of the case IV-6 and b a cervical spinal cord (ventral horn) of the case III-5 was performed using anti-SOD1^{olig} antibody. c-f Serial sections of a lumbar spinal cord (ventral horn) of the case IV-6 were immunostained with c, e anti-SOD1^{olig} and d, f anti-SOD1 (clone 1G2, MBL) antibodies. Sections shown in c and d or e and f are serial. Nuclei were also stained by hematoxylin (blue). The bars represent 50 µm

in a *SOD1* gene (Fig. 4a). As shown in the upper panel of Fig. 4b, ELISA signals of anti-SOD1^{olig} antibody were observed exclusively in Pep^{exon2}, suggesting that the antibody recognizes the region between Glu 24 and Ala 55 in SOD1. To further narrow down the epitope region recognized by anti-SOD1^{olig} antibody, Pep^{exon2} was dissected into three peptides, Pep1 – 3 (Fig. 4a), and again examined by ELISA. Pep2 and 3 but not Pep1 gave rise to ELISA signals (the lower panel of Fig. 4b), indicating that anti-SOD1^{olig} antibody recognized the region overlapped between Pep2 and Pep3, *i.e.* from Gly 44 to Asn 53. Quite interestingly, the epitope (Gly 44 – Asn 53) is buried in the folded structure of SOD1 (Fig. 4c), which is consistent with almost no reactivity of anti-SOD1^{olig} antibody toward folded SOD1 proteins (Fig. 1b). These results thus show that the buried region from Gly 44 to Asn 53 becomes exposed upon formation of the disulfide-crosslinked SOD1 oligomers.

Antibody recognizing the structural interior of SOD1 exhibits the specificity to the disulfide-crosslinked oligomers

Polyclonal antibodies were then generated by immunizing a rabbit with the Gly 44 - Asn 53 peptide (Fig. 4c)

and affinity-purified using the same peptide. The resultant antibody (anti-SOD1$^{44-53}$) was found to exhibit the increased immunoreactivity to the soluble and disulfide-crosslinked oligomers over the folded Cu,Zn-SOD1(WT)$^{S-S}$ and E,E-SOD1(A4V)$^{S-S}$ (Fig. 5a and Additional file 6: Figure S5A). We then attempted to increase the specificity of the antibody to the oligomers by further affinity-purification with Gly 44 - Glu 49, His 46 - Gly 51, and His 48 - Asn 53 peptides and prepare anti-SOD1$^{44-49}$, anti-SOD1$^{46-51}$, and anti-SOD1$^{48-53}$ antibody, respectively; however, the specificity to the oligomers was not significantly improved in those three antibody fractions (Fig. 5a, w/o absorption). The antisera were, therefore, first absorbed with His-tagged SOD1(WT)$^{S-S}$ on Ni^{2+}-affinity resins and then affinity-purified with the peptides (44–49, 46–51, and 48–53) covalently immobilized on Sulfo-Link resins. As shown in Fig. 5a (w/ absorption), such an additional absorption procedure was found to increase the specificity of anti-SOD1$^{48-53}$ antibody to the soluble and disulfide-crosslinked oligomers of A4V-mutant SOD1. We hence call this fraction of anti-SOD1$^{48-53}$ as anti-SOD1^{int} antibody in the following section. The yield of anti-SOD1^{int} antibody was high (*ca.* 150 μg from 1 mL of

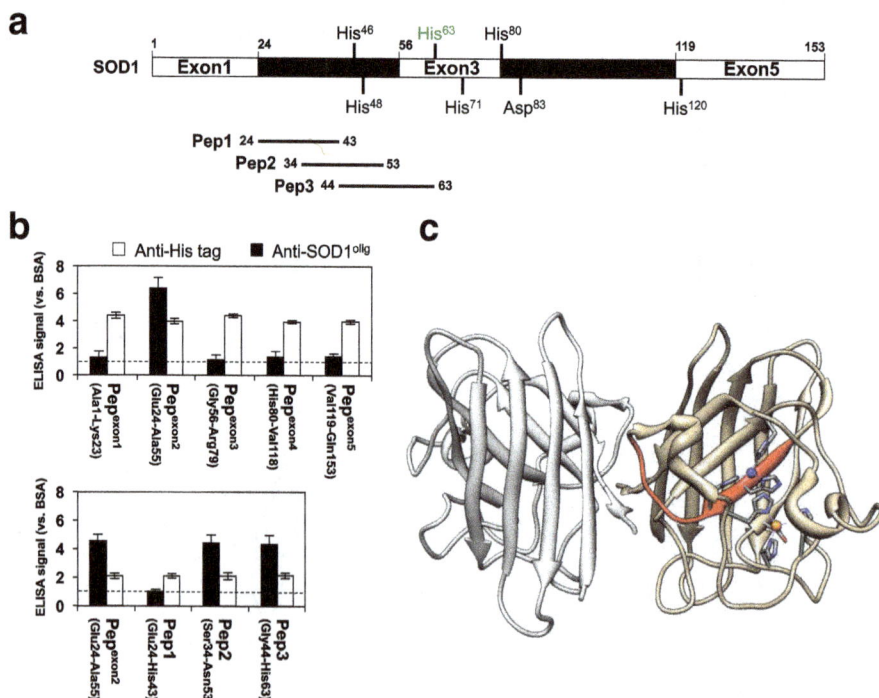

Fig. 4 Anti-SOD1^{olig} antibody reacts with the interior of SOD1 structure. **a** The translated products of five exons in SOD1 and the three peptides, Pep 1, 2, and 3, are shown in schematic representation of the SOD1 primary structure. The ligands for copper and zinc ions are also shown and colored blue and red, respectively. His 63 (colored green) is a ligand for bridging both copper and zinc ions. **b** Identification of the epitope for anti-SOD1^{olig} antibody (filled bars) was performed by indirect ELISA using the dissected peptides of SOD1 shown in (**a**). The peptides were prepared as a fusion protein with an N-terminal 6x His tagged GST. Almost equal amounts of peptides were examined, which was confirmed by ELISA using anti-His tag antibody (sc-8036, Santa Cruz Biotechnology) (open bars). The ELISA signal was represented as a ratio against that obtained using BSA. **c** The region covering the epitope of anti-SOD1^{olig} antibody (Gly44 - Asn53) is shown red in the crystal structure of SOD1 (PDB ID: 2C9V). Copper (blue) and zinc (orange) ions are also indicated with the ligands

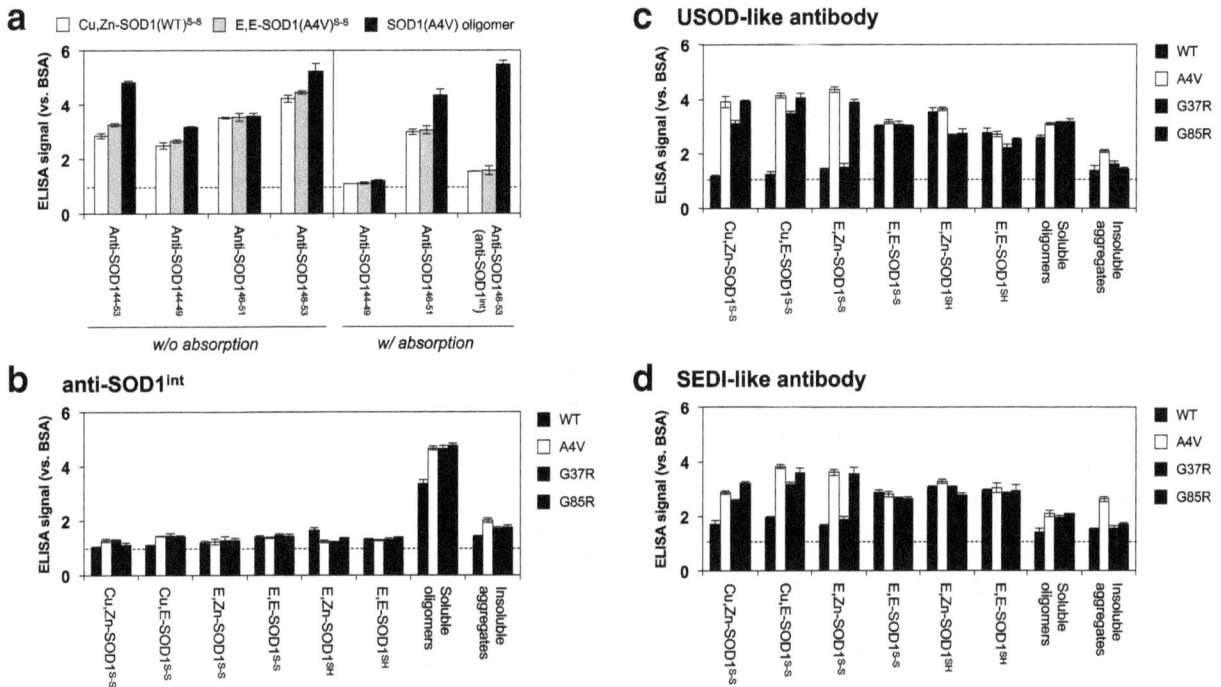

Fig. 5 Anti-SOD1^{int} antibody exclusively recognizes soluble disulfide-crosslinked SOD1 oligomers in vitro. **a** The antibodies were tested for their specific reactivities to soluble disulfide-crosslinked oligomers (black filled bars) over Cu,Zn-SOD1(WT)$^{S-S}$ (open bars) and E,E-SOD1(A4V)$^{S-S}$ (gray filled bars) by indirect ELISA. Antisera were either affinity-purified with the corresponding peptides (w/o absorption) or first absorbed with SOD1(WT)$^{S-S}$ and then affinity-purified with the peptides (w/ absorption). Anti-SOD1$^{48-53}$ antibody obtained after the absorption exclusively reacted with soluble disulfide-crosslinked oligomers and called anti-SOD1^{int} antibody. **b-d** The reactivities of **b** anti-SOD1^{int}, **c** USOD-like, and **d** SEDI-like antibody were examined with indirect ELISA. Several forms of SOD1 (WT, A4V, G37R, G85R) with a distinct metallation/disulfide status, soluble disulfide-crosslinked oligomers and insoluble amyloid-like aggregates were prepared and fixed on an ELISA plate. The ELISA signal was represented as a ratio against that obtained using BSA. Three independent experiments were performed to estimate error bars (standard deviation). Fixation of equal amounts of SOD1 proteins on each well of an ELISA plate was confirmed by ELISA using polyclonal anti-SOD1 antibody (FL-154, Santa Cruz Biotechnology), which is shown in Additional file 6: Figure S5

antisera) enough to conduct its biochemical and immunochemical characterization.

To further check the specificity of our anti-SOD1^{int} antibody in vitro, we prepared various forms of WT and ALS-mutant (A4V, G37R, and G85R) SOD1 proteins including E,E-SOD1^{SH}, E,E-SOD1^{S-S}, E,Zn-SOD1^{SH}, E,Zn-SOD1^{S-S}, Cu,E-SOD1^{S-S}, Cu,Zn-SOD1^{S-S}, and soluble oligomers with disulfide crosslinks (see Fig. 1a). Insoluble and amyloid-like SOD1 aggregates were also prepared by shaking E,E-SOD1^{SH} with 1,200 rpm at 37 °C [9]. Among those, only the soluble and disulfide-crosslinked oligomers but none of the others were recognized by anti-SOD1^{int} antibody (Fig. 5b and Additional file 6: Figure S5B). Based upon these results in vitro, therefore, anti-SOD1^{int} antibody can detect the disulfide-crosslinked SOD1 oligomers, in which the protein interior is significantly exposed to the solvent.

Actually, there are several precedents of the antibodies recognizing the protein interior of SOD1, which include USOD and SEDI polyclonal antibodies raised against the peptides, GG-L^{42}HGFHVH^{48}-GG and GG-R^{143}LACGVIGI^{151}-GG, respectively (also see Discussion) [16, 28]. Unfortunately, canonical USOD and SEDI antibodies reported by Chakrabartty and co-workers were not available, but the polyclonal antibodies raised against the same peptides as above were commercially available. We thus characterized those commercially available "USOD-like" and "SEDI-like" antibodies; indeed, USOD-like and SEDI-like antibodies were confirmed to specifically recognize Pep^{exon2} and Pep^{exon5}, respectively (Additional file 7: Figure S6). As shown in Fig. 5c and d, USOD-like and SEDI-like antibodies exhibited reactivities toward almost all states examined except wild-type SOD1^{S-S} that is fully or partially metallated and would thus be selective to mutant SOD1 proteins. Nonetheless, the recognition specificity of our anti-SOD1^{int} antibody toward the disulfide-crosslinked oligomers was significantly higher than those of USOD/SEDI-like antibodies (Fig. 5b, c and d). These data thus emphasize the unprecedented recognition specificity of our anti-SOD1^{int} antibody toward the disulfide-crosslinked SOD1 oligomers.

Disulfide-crosslinked SOD1 oligomers as an early pathological species in spinal cords of ALS-model mice

To check the availability/specificity of anti-SOD1[int] antibody for the detection of pathological SOD1 in vivo, we first examined the immunohistochemical analysis of G1H mice as well as non-transgenic mice. Unfortunately, however, the lumbar spinal cords of non-transgenic mice were immunostained with anti-SOD1[int] antibody (data not shown). This is in contrast to anti-SOD1[olig] antibody showing no immunostaining in non-transgenic mice (Additional file 3: Figure S2A and B). Those two antibodies hence appear to have distinct specificities in the immunohistochemical examination on mouse tissues. Nonetheless, anti-SOD1[int] as well as anti-SOD1[olig] antibody can exclusively recognize disulfide-crosslinked SOD1 oligomers in vitro in ELISA (Fig. 1b and 5b). We thus further examined homogenates from model mice for disulfide-crosslinked SOD1 oligomers by sandwich ELISA with anti-SOD1[int] antibody.

Briefly, anti-SOD1[int] antibody was first fixed on the surface of an ELISA plate and incubated with soluble fractions of tissue homogenates. The SOD1 species captured by the antibody were then detected with polyclonal anti-SOD1 antibody followed by the corresponding secondary antibody. Significant ELISA signals were observed in the lumbar spinal cords of G1H mice from 30 to 140 days of age (Fig. 6a, red circles) but not in those of non-transgenic mice (Additional file 8: Figure S7A). Compared to G1H mice, moreover, asymptomatic mice overexpressing wild-type human SOD1 (WT mice) contained larger amounts of total soluble SOD1 proteins but exhibited significantly weaker signals with anti-SOD1[int] antibody (Additional file 8: Figure S7A and B). We also observed that the signals with anti-SOD1[int] antibody disappeared upon pre-treatment of the spinal cord samples of G1H mice with a reductant, dithiothreitol (DTT) (Additional file 8: Figure S7C and D). These results thus suggest that anti-SOD1[int] antibody detects disulfide-crosslinked SOD1 oligomers not only in in vitro protein samples but also in the model mice in vivo.

It should also be noted in Fig. 6a (red circles) that the ELISA signals from the lumbar spinal cords increase from 30 to 140 days of age but significantly drop from 140 to 160 days of age ($P < 0.01$). The reduction in the ELISA signals at 160 days of age was not described by the changes in total amounts of soluble SOD1 in the

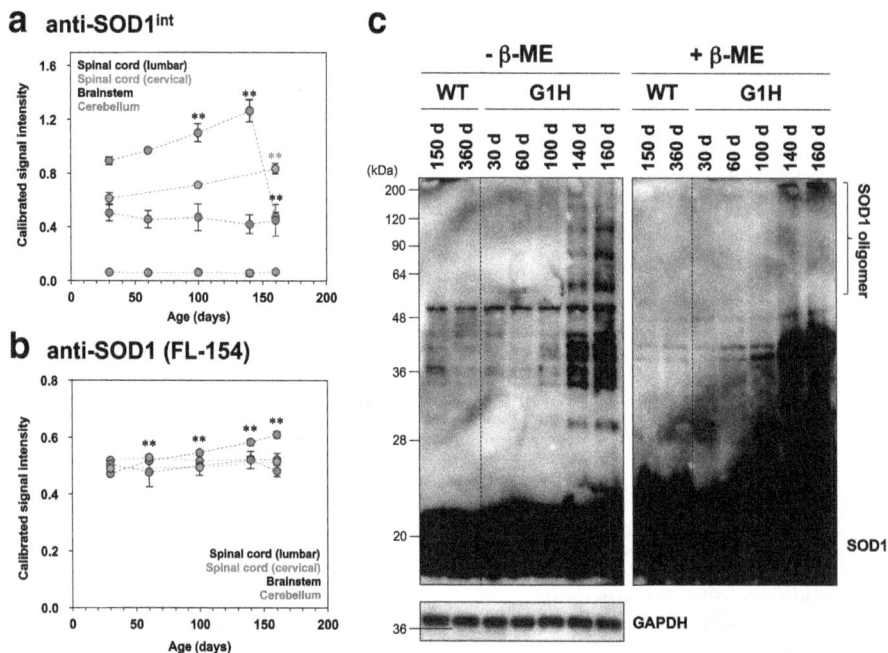

Fig. 6 Anti-SOD1[int] antibody specifically detects pathological SOD1 in spinal cords of ALS-model mice. **a, b** SOD1 species recognized by **a** anti-SOD1[int] and **b** anti-SOD1 (FL-154, Santa Cruz Biotechnology) antibody were quantified in the soluble fraction of the homogenates of lumbar spinal cord (red), cervical spinal cord (green), brainstem (blue), and cerebellum (gray) of G1H mice by sandwich ELISA. Three independent mouse samples at 30, 60, 100, 140, and 160 days of age were examined, and the averages were shown with error bars (standard deviation). ** (red and green) represents the P value less than 0.01 versus the data on lumbar and cervical spinal cords at 30 days of age, respectively. **c** Soluble disulfide-crosslinked SOD1 oligomers in mice were examined by Western blotting. Lumbar spinal cords of WT and G1H mice were homogenized in the presence of 100 mM iodoacetamide and 1% NP-40 and centrifuged at 20,000 x g for 30 min so as to prepare soluble supernatant. In the presence and absence of the reducing reagent, β-ME, the supernatant was then separated in a polyacrylamide gel by SDS-PAGE and probed by Western blot using anti-SOD1 antibody (FL-154, Santa Cruz Biotechnology). GAPDH was used as a protein loading control for Western blot

lumbar spinal cord (Fig. 6b, red circles). This is consistent with the decreased anti-SOD1^{olig} immunostaining of the lumbar spinal cords of G1H mice at 140 and 160 days of age (Fig. 2c and d, Additional file 4: Figure S3C and D), while slightly different age-dependency in immunochemical response between anti-SOD1^{int} and anti-SOD1^{olig} antibodies would reflect their distinct immunological properties. As described later, however, the ELISA signals with anti-SOD1^{int} antibody did not decrease in the other mouse model. The signal reduction in the disease end-stage may thus be a phenomenon specific to the lumbar spinal cord of G1H mice, but an exact reason for this remains obscure. Instead, we would like to emphasize that anti-SOD1^{int} antibody can detect conformationally abnormal SOD1 species in model mice with sandwich ELISA.

To test if SOD1s were oligomerized with disulfide bonds in lumbar spinal cords of ALS-model mice, soluble fractions of the lumbar spinal cord homogenates of G1H mice were separated by non-reducing SDS-PAGE and analyzed by Western blotting. Soluble and disulfide-crosslinked SOD1 oligomers in vitro can be characterized by the reductant-sensitive smears in the high molecular weight region in SDS-PAGE gels (Additional file 2: Figure S1). As shown in Fig. 6c (left panel), smears in the high molecular weight region (>50 kDa) were evident, albeit weak intensity, as early as 60 days of age in G1H mice but not in WT mice (150 and 360 days) and non-transgenic mice (100 days; data not shown). Also importantly, those smears in G1H mice at 60 and 100 days of age disappeared when the soluble fractions were treated with β-mercaptoethanol (β-ME) prior to their loading on an SDS-PAGE gel (Fig. 6c, right panel), supporting the formation of disulfide-crosslinked SOD1 oligomers in the ALS-model mice even before the disease onset.

After the disease onset (at 140 and 160 days of age), in contrast, the reductant-sensitive SOD1 species in lumbar spinal cords of G1H mice were observed as more distinct bands in the high molecular weight region (>50 kDa, Fig. 6c). Also, even in the presence of β-ME, some SOD1-positive species were stuck on top of the separating gel. Therefore, we suppose different molecular properties of SOD1 oligomers between pre- and post-symptomatic stages of G1H mice, which might describe significant reduction of the SOD1 species immunoreactive to anti-SOD1^{int} antibody at 160 days of age (Fig. 6a, red circles). Taken together, we speculate that anti-SOD1^{int} antibody specifically detects the disulfide-crosslinked oligomers formed in the lumbar spinal cords of G1H mice from their pre-symptomatic stages.

We also tested the tissue-specificity in the formation of the disulfide-crosslinked oligomers; soluble supernatants from the homogenates of cervical spinal cord, brainstem and cerebellum of G1H mice were examined by sandwich ELISA using anti-SOD1^{int} antibody. In ALS

cases, the lumbar spinal cord is mainly affected, but the other regions of brains and spinal cords have also been shown to be involved in the pathology [29]. In G1H mice, the lumbar spinal cord is the most severely damaged, and the changes occur later in the cervical spinal cords [30]. Some pathological changes are reported in the brainstem [31], but the cerebellum is relatively spared [32]. As shown in Fig. 6a, the ELISA signal intensities were significantly weaker in cervical spinal cord, brainstem, and cerebellum than those of lumbar spinal cord ($P < 0.01$ within the same age group, except at 160 days of age); in particular, almost no ELISA signals were observed in cerebellum. We confirmed similar levels of total SOD1 proteins among all of those tissues (Fig. 6b). Also, no obvious smears in the high molecular weight region were observed in the Western blots of soluble fractions of the cerebellum, while the brainstem lysates of G1H mice exhibited reductant-sensitive smears at 160 days of age, albeit with weak intensities (Additional file 9: Figure S8A and B). While toxic SOD1 species might appear everywhere but only afflict the spinal cord due to its vulnerability, amounts of SOD1 species probed with anti-SOD1^{int} antibody were well correlated with the intensity of high-molecular-weight smears in the Western blots and also the severity of the damages in tissues (lumbar spinal cord > cervical spinal cord > brainstem > cerebellum) of G1H mice.

We have also examined the ALS model mice expressing human SOD1 with another mutation, G37R (loxG37R mice) [20]. Compared to G1H mice, the expression level of mutant SOD1 is lower, and the disease progression is slower in loxG37R mice (the disease onset: ~350 days of age). The sandwich ELISA showed the age-dependent increase of the anti-SOD1^{int}-positive SOD1 species in lumbar and cervical spinal cords but not in cerebellum of loxG37R mice (Additional file 10: Figure S9A), while amounts of the total soluble SOD1 remained almost constant during aging in loxG37R mice (Additional file 10: Figure S9B). When the spinal cord samples from loxG37R mice were pre-treated with DTT, the ELISA signals with anti-SOD1^{int} antibody disappeared (data not shown). Furthermore, Western blotting analysis on loxG37R mice revealed the reductant-sensitive smears in lumbar spinal cord (Additional file 10: Figure S9C), albeit with significantly weaker intensities compared to those of G1H mice, but not in cerebellum (Additional file 9: Figure S8C). Taken together, these results suggest the formation of the soluble disulfide-crosslinked SOD1 oligomers as pathological changes also in loxG37R mice.

Anti-SOD1^{int} antibody detects pathological SOD1 in SOD1-ALS cases

To test the immunoreactivity of our anti-SOD1^{int} antibody in human cases, the double immunofluorescence staining with anti-SOD1^{int} and anti-SOD1 antibodies was performed on the ventral horn of the lumbar spinal cord section of the *SOD1*-ALS patients with C111Y mutation (the case IV-6 in [26]; Additional file 1: Table S1). As shown in Fig. 7a, abnormally accumulated SOD1 proteins in spinal motor neurons were immunostained by anti-SOD1^{int} antibody. Using serial sections of the primary motor cortex (Fig. 7b), furthermore, the abnormally accumulated SOD1 in cytoplasm and neurites of a Betz cell were also immunostained by anti-SOD1^{int} antibody. In another *SOD1*-ALS case with C111Y mutation (the case III-4 in [26]; Additional file 1: Table S1), the disease duration was exceptionally long (69 years), but

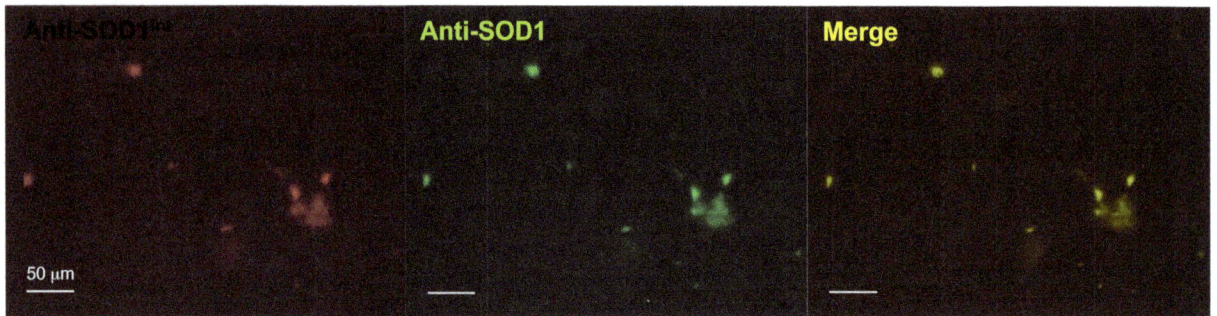

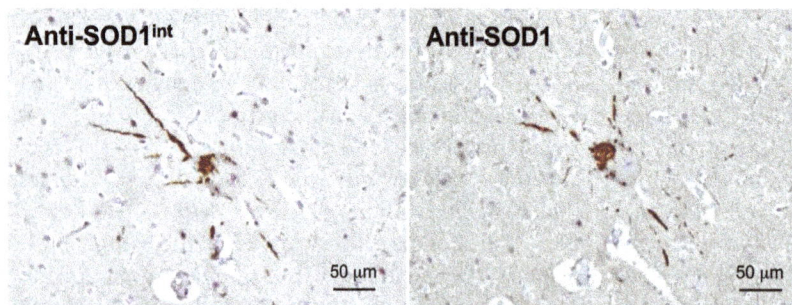

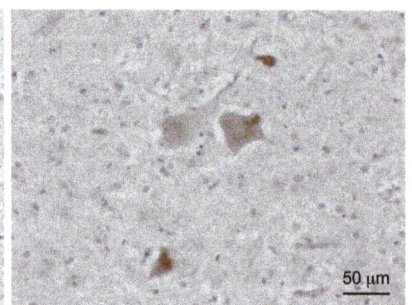

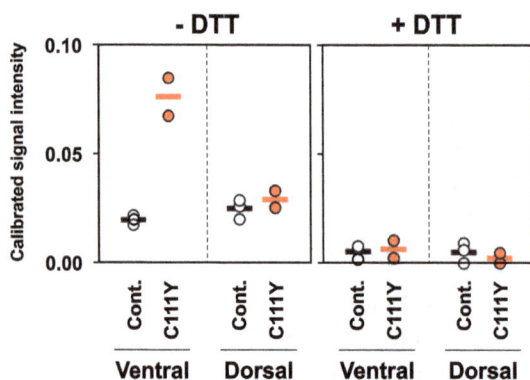

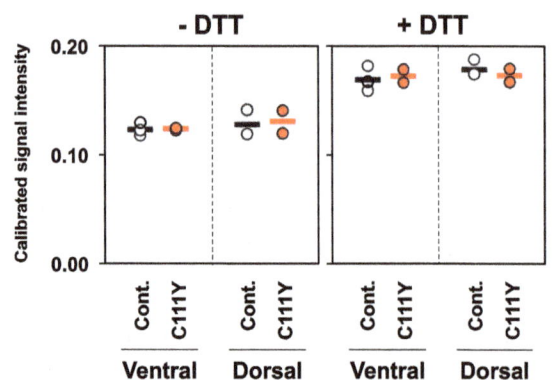

Fig. 7 Immunochemical detection of pathological SOD1 species in the *SOD1*-ALS cases with anti-SOD1^{int} antibody. **a** Double immunofluorescence staining of the lumbar spinal cord section of the *SOD1*-ALS case with C111Y mutation (the case IV-6). The section was stained with rabbit anti-SOD1^{int} and mouse anti-SOD1 (clone 1G2, MBL) antibodies followed by Cy3-modified anti-rabbit (red) and FITC-modified anti-mouse (green) secondary antibodies, respectively. A merged image (yellow) was also shown. **b** Serial sections of the primary motor cortex of the *SOD1*-ALS case (the case IV-6) were immunostained with (left) anti-SOD1^{int} and (right) anti-SOD1 (clone 1G2, MBL) antibodies and visualized with DAB staining. **c** The lumbar spinal cord (ventral horn) of the case III-4, which exhibited exceptionally long disease duration (~69 years), was immunostained with anti-SOD1^{int} antibody. **d, e** SOD1 species recognized by **d** anti-SOD1^{int} and **e** anti-SOD1 (FL-154, Santa Cruz) antibodies were quantified in the soluble fraction of the homogenates of ventral and dorsal horn regions of thoracic spinal cord of human samples by sandwich ELISA. The sandwich ELISA was performed in the absence (–DTT) or presence (+DTT) of pre-treatment of the samples with 10 mM DTT. The *SOD1*-ALS cases III-4 and IV-6 and three non-ALS controls (Additional file 1: Table S1) were examined. The averages were shown as bars

the motor neurons in the ventral horn of the lumbar spinal cord exhibited immunoreactivity to anti-SOD1^{int} antibody (Fig. 7c). Again, no immunoreactivity with anti-SOD1^{int} antibody was observed in the spinal cord/ primary motor cortex of the sporadic ALS cases with TDP-43 pathologies and also of the non-ALS cases (Additional file 5: Figure S4B-D).

To reduce the chance of potential conformational changes of SOD1 during the preparation of sections and their immunostaining procedures, we prepared soluble fractions by centrifugation of the homogenates from either ventral or dorsal horn in the thoracic spinal cords and then examined those by sandwich ELISA using anti-SOD1^{int} antibody. ALS associates with degeneration of motor neurons in the ventral horn with less involvement of sensory neurons in the dorsal horn of the spinal cord [33]. As shown in Fig. 7d, the ventral horn of the SOD1-ALS patients with C111Y mutation (cases III-4 and IV-6; Additional file 1: Table S1) showed higher signal intensities of anti-SOD1^{int} antibody than those of non-ALS controls (three cases). In contrast, weak ELISA signals of anti-SOD1^{int} antibody were detected in the dorsal horn with almost no difference between the controls and the ALS patients (Fig. 7d). Also importantly, the ELISA signals obtained by using anti-SOD1^{int} antibody disappeared upon pre-treatment of the samples with a reductant, DTT, suggesting the involvement of disulfide-crosslinks in the pathological SOD1 species (Fig. 7d). The amounts of total soluble SOD1 proteins in the ventral and dorsal horns were not different between the controls and the ALS patients (Fig. 7e). Collectively, our anti-SOD1^{int} antibody is considered to detect the disulfide-crosslinked SOD1 oligomers as pathological species in SOD1-ALS patients.

Discussion

SOD1-ALS cases are characterized mainly by abnormal accumulation of mutant SOD1 proteins in motor neurons of the affected spinal cords [5], while the pathological involvement of the other types of neurons and glia cells has been reported [20, 29, 34, 35]. The conformational stability of SOD1 is significantly compromised by most of the mutations [36], which triggers the formation of soluble oligomers and insoluble aggregates of SOD1 in vitro. In this study, we successfully prepared anti-SOD1$^{olig/int}$ antibodies exclusively recognizing the disulfide-crosslinked SOD1 oligomers in vitro and then found that those antibodies detect the pathological SOD1 species in spinal cords of the SOD1-ALS patients (C111Y) as well as transgenic model mice (G1H and loxG37R mice).

Several mechanisms for the formation of disulfide-crosslinked SOD1 oligomers have been proposed in vitro [7, 8, 37]. Our epitope analysis of anti-SOD1$^{olig/int}$ antibodies has further revealed the conformation of disulfide-crosslinked SOD1 oligomers, in which the regions

usually buried in the native SOD1 are exposed. More precisely, the epitopes of our antibodies (Gly 44 - Asn 53) were found to include the protein interior (Gly 44 - Glu 49) and the dimer interface (Phe 50 - Asn 53) in SOD1. The protein interior and the dimer interface have been noted as targets for the design of antibodies specifically recognizing misfolded SOD1 proteins [38]. For example, the polyclonal antibodies, USOD [16] and AJ10 [39], were raised against the region covering the protein interior of the natively folded SOD1 (Leu 42 - His 48 and Val 29 - Cys 57, respectively) (Fig. 8a), and both antibodies have been shown to immunostain the pathological inclusions in the spinal motor neurons of SOD1-ALS patients. Also, the monoclonal antibodies, C4F6 and D3H5, have been reported to recognize the conformational epitope buried in the SOD1 native conformation [38, 40–42] and detect pathological inclusions in SOD1-ALS patients [43, 44]. Because SOD1 forms a very tight homodimer ($K_d \sim$ 0.1 nM) [45], furthermore, the dimer interface in the natively folded conformation is also buried. The polyclonal antibodies called SEDI and 131–153 Ra-ab were raised against the peptides containing the dimer-interface region (SEDI, Arg 143 - Ile 151; 131–153 Ra-ab, Asn 131 - Gln 153; Fig. 8a and b) [28, 46] and again exclusively immunostained the inclusions in the affected spinal motor neurons of SOD1-ALS patients [16, 28, 47–50]. In the pathological conditions, therefore, SOD1 is supposed to misfold into a conformation with the exposed structural interior and the disrupted interface for dimerization.

Depending upon experimental conditions in vitro and in vivo, nonetheless, SOD1 is known to misfold in distinct pathways [8–10, 51–54]. Therefore, we could not exclude the possibility that our antibodies detect certain misfolded species other than the disulfide-crosslinked oligomer. It has been known that several misfolded conformations of SOD1 can be reproduced in vitro simply by metal dissociation and/or disulfide reduction. Actually, we have shown that reduction of the disulfide bond drastically increases fluctuation of the loops IV and VII (Fig. 8b), temporarily "peels" those loops off from the β-barrel scaffold, and thus potentially exposes the epitope of anti-SOD1^{int} antibody [55]. As shown in Fig. 5b, however, disulfide-reduced and/or demetallated forms of SOD1 were not recognized by our anti-SOD1^{int} antibody. Therefore, the reversible conformational fluctuation increased by disulfide reduction/demetallation is probably not sufficient to allow the antibody to access the epitope buried inside the protein. The disulfide-reduced and demetallated SOD1 has been shown to irreversibly form the amyloid-like aggregates [56], which were again not recognized by anti-SOD1^{int} antibody (Fig. 5b). We further examined ELISA to test the reactivities of anti-SOD1^{int} antibody toward E,E-SOD1^{S-S} and E,E-SOD1^{SH} that were misfolded/unfolded with either

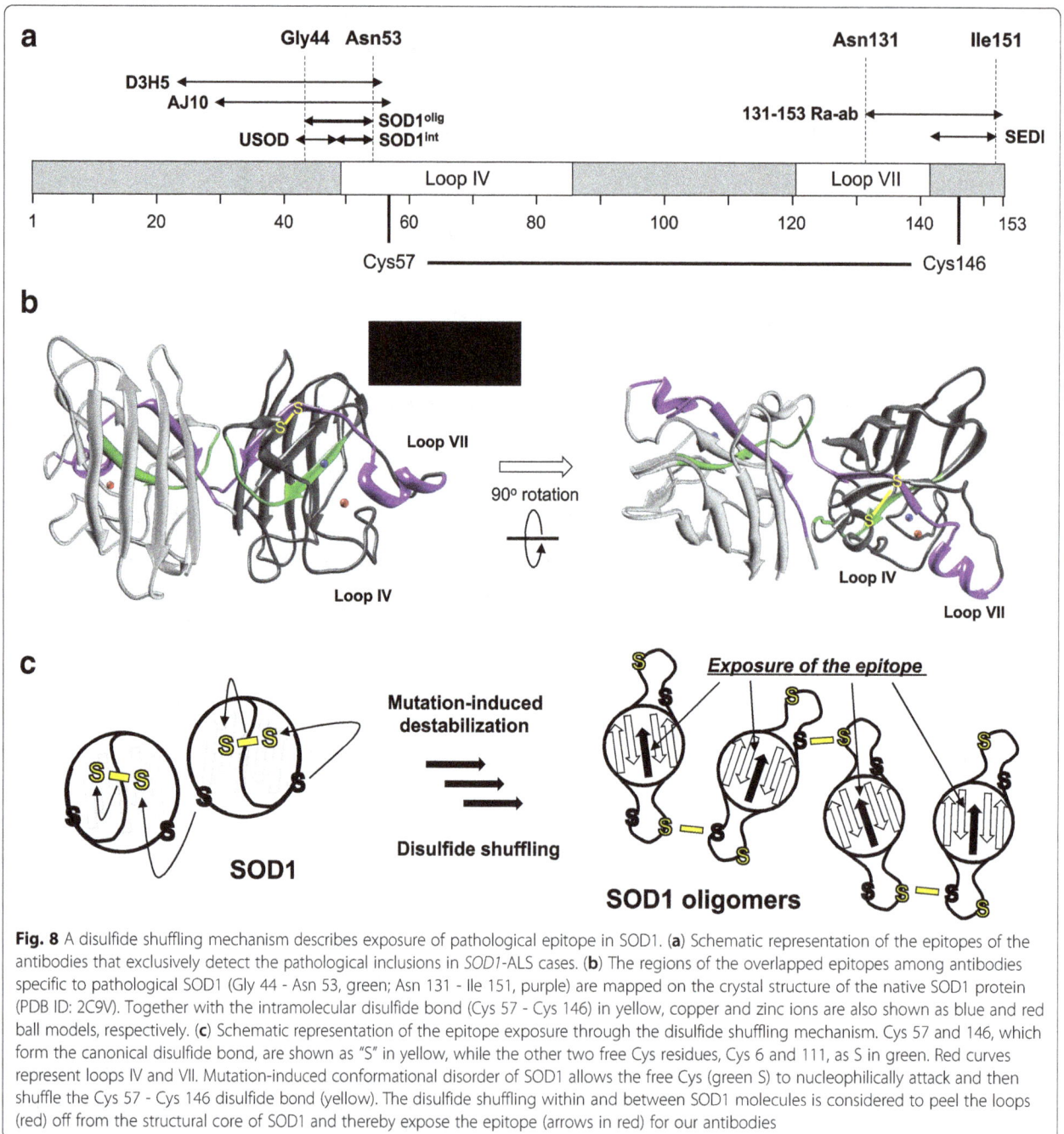

Fig. 8 A disulfide shuffling mechanism describes exposure of pathological epitope in SOD1. (**a**) Schematic representation of the epitopes of the antibodies that exclusively detect the pathological inclusions in *SOD1*-ALS cases. (**b**) The regions of the overlapped epitopes among antibodies specific to pathological SOD1 (Gly 44 - Asn 53, green; Asn 131 - Ile 151, purple) are mapped on the crystal structure of the native SOD1 protein (PDB ID: 2C9V). Together with the intramolecular disulfide bond (Cys 57 - Cys 146) in yellow, copper and zinc ions are also shown as blue and red ball models, respectively. (**c**) Schematic representation of the epitope exposure through the disulfide shuffling mechanism. Cys 57 and 146, which form the canonical disulfide bond, are shown as "S" in yellow, while the other two free Cys residues, Cys 6 and 111, as S in green. Red curves represent loops IV and VII. Mutation-induced conformational disorder of SOD1 allows the free Cys (green S) to nucleophilically attack and then shuffle the Cys 57 - Cys 146 disulfide bond (yellow). The disulfide shuffling within and between SOD1 molecules is considered to peel the loops (red) off from the structural core of SOD1 and thereby expose the epitope (arrows in red) for our antibodies

guanidine hydrochloride (6 M) or acidic buffer (pH 3.0) in vitro, but no signals were observed (Additional file 11: Figure S10A). In sharp contrast, USOD-like and SEDI-like antibodies were found to react with various non-native forms of SOD1 proteins (Fig. 5c and d, Additional file 11: Figure S10B, C, and D). Taken together, those extensive tests reveal quite high recognition specificity of our anti-SOD1^{int} antibody toward the disulfide-crosslinked SOD1 oligomer.

Anti-SOD1^{int} antibody detected pathological SOD1 species in vivo, and also, the reductant-sensitive smears

of SOD1 were observed in the Western blots of the affected tissues of model mice (Fig. 6, Additional file 10: Figure S9). We hence speculate that the disulfide-crosslinked SOD1 oligomer is involved in the pathology of *SOD1*-ALS. Actually, disulfide-crosslinked oligomers of SOD1 have been reproduced in cultured cells [18, 57]. While the reducing environment of the cytoplasm might be unfavorable for crosslinking proteins *via* disulfide bonds, our preliminary in vitro experiments confirmed the formation of disulfide-crosslinked SOD1 oligomers in the presence of 5 mM reduced glutathione with 0.5 mM oxidized glutathione (data not shown), which is a feasible redox condition of the cytoplasm [58]. In our proposed mechanism for the formation of SOD1 oligomers [8], the disulfide bond is not newly introduced but rather shuffled among the Cys residues in SOD1 (Fig. 8c). More specifically, the disulfide shuffling will break the canonical Cys 57 - Cys 146 disulfide bond and detain SOD1 in the misfolded conformation where the loops IV and VII are peeled off from the β-barrel scaffold with the persistent exposure of the epitope region (Fig. 8c). Such a disulfide shuffling may be more robust against reducing environment than *de novo* formation of disulfide bonds.

We have also shown here that immunoreactivities of our anti-SOD1$^{olig/int}$ antibodies are quite exclusive to the human *SOD1*-ALS cases as well as the transgenic mice (G1H and loxG37R mice) but not to the controls without *SOD1* mutations. Their immunoreactivities were, furthermore, well correlated with the severity of degeneration in the model mice (lumbar spinal cord > cervical spinal cord > brainstem > cerebellum; Fig. 6a, Additional file 10: Figure S9A) and in the *SOD1*-ALS cases (ventral horn > dorsal horn; Fig. 7d). As described in the Results section, nonetheless, we should note significant reduction in the immunoreactivities of anti-SOD1$^{olig/int}$ antibodies toward the G1H mice in the disease end stage (Figs. 2 and 6a). While such decline will be partly because of the concomitant loss of motor neurons [24], mutant SOD1 is also known to accumulate as amyloid-like aggregates in the spinal cord of the model mice after the appearance of motor symptoms [9, 15]. Given that our anti-SOD1^{int} antibody was not able to react with the amyloid-like SOD1 aggregates in vitro (Fig. 5b), the declined immunoreactivity of anti-SOD1$^{olig/int}$ antibodies at the end-stage might indicate the formation of amyloid-like SOD1 aggregates due to quite high expression of G93A SOD1 proteins in G1H mice.

In contrast, the spinal motor neurons of the *SOD1*-ALS patients in their disease end-stage were immunostained with anti-SOD1$^{olig/int}$ antibodies (Figs. 3 and 7), suggesting distinct properties of pathological SOD1 species between G1H mice and the patients. Because the inclusions in *SOD1*-ALS patients exhibited no reactivity to an amyloid-diagnostic dye, Thioflavin-S [16], the amyloid-like SOD1 aggregates would form only in the end-stage G1H mice but not in human *SOD1*-ALS cases. While it needs to be tested whether the SOD1 species detected by our antibodies was an on-pathway intermediate for the formation of amyloid-like SOD1 aggregates, the pathologies in the autopsied human cases might not proceed into the terminal stage as in the G1H mice at 160 days of age. Compared to the amyloid-like SOD1 aggregates in the end stage of G1H mice, we speculate that SOD1 species detected by anti-SOD1$^{olig/int}$ antibodies in the pre-symptomatic G1H mice have more significance in the pathogenicity of *SOD1*-ALS.

It is also important to note moderate immunoreactivities of anti-SOD1^{int} antibody in the spinal cords of WT mice at 360 days but not at 150 days of age (Additional file 8: Figure S7A). WT mice do not develop severe motor phenotypes but show several neuropathological and symptomatic changes in their advanced age including mitochondrial vacuolization in spinal cords (>210 days), impaired motor performance (>410 days), and motor neuron death (~2 years) [59]. No immunoreactivities of C4F6 and SEDI antibodies were reported in the spinal cords of WT mice at 215 and 100 days of age, respectively [28, 43]. Instead, the immunoreactivity of anti-SOD1^{int} antibody appears to match with the neuropathological changes in WT mice and would hence probe the misfolded SOD1 proteins with toxicity toward motor neurons. Involvement of wild-type SOD1 proteins in the ALS pathogenesis still remains controversial [60], and no immunostaining by anti-SOD1^{int} antibody was confirmed in our sporadic ALS cases without *SOD1* mutations (Additional file 5: Figure S4C and D). Nonetheless, we speculate that SOD1 could become toxic to motor neurons by assuming the anti-SOD1$^{olig/int}$ antibody-positive conformation such as the disulfide-crosslinked oligomers even in the absence of any pathogenic mutations.

Conclusions

In summary, we successfully prepared the antibodies exclusively recognizing the disulfide-crosslinked SOD1 oligomers in vitro. Pathological SOD1 species in the affected tissues of *SOD1*-ALS patients as well as transgenic mice provided the immunological epitope to those antibodies. While it is possible that the epitope of our antibodies becomes available upon misfolding of SOD1 through some other mechanisms, we propose that the oligomerization *via* shuffling of the disulfide bond has pathological significance in *SOD1*-ALS.

Additional files

Additional file 1: Table S1. Information on human cases examined in this study.

Additional file 2: Figure S1. Preparation of soluble disulfide-crosslinked SOD1 oligomers in vitro. E,E-SOD1^{S-S} (100 μM) was incubated in the NNE buffer at 37 °C for five days and then centrifuged at 20,000 x g for 10 min. to remove any insoluble materials. The samples were further reacted with 100 mM iodoacetamide in the presence of 2% SDS and analyzed by (left) non-reducing and (right) reducing SDS-PAGE. The electrophoretic mobility of monomeric SOD1(G85R) has been known to be faster than those of the other SOD1 proteins (WT, A4V, and G37R).

Additional file 3: Figure S2. Specificity of anti-SOD1^{olig} antibody for immunohistochemical examination of mouse spinal cords. The sections of lumbar spinal cords of (A, B) a non-transgenic mouse (C57BL/6) at 200 days of age and (C, D) a G1H mouse at 100 days of age were stained with anti-SOD1^{olig} antibody. For the absorption experiments shown in (C, D), the anti-SOD1^{olig} antibody was pre-absorbed on ice for 5 h with either (C) soluble disulfide-crosslinked SOD1(A4V) oligomers (6.7 μM in monomer base) or (D) E,Zn-SOD1^{S-S} (6.7 μM). Nuclei were also counter-stained with hematoxylin (blue).

Additional file 4: Figure S3. Immunohistochemical examination on lumbar spinal cords of G1H mice with anti-SOD1 antibody. The sections of lumbar spinal cords of G1H mice at (A) 60, (B) 100, (C) 140, and (D) 160 days of age were stained with monoclonal anti-SOD1 (clone 1G2, MBL) antibody. The images in the low magnification are shown in the left panel, where the region enclosed with a broken line is magnified and shown in the right panel. Nuclei were counterstained with hematoxylin (blue). The bar in each panel represents 100 μm (left panel) and 50 μm (right panel).

Additional file 5: Figure S4. Representative images for immunohistochemical examination of non *SOD1*-ALS cases. Spinal cord sections of (A) non-ALS (C1 in Additional file 1: Table S1), (B) non-ALS (C3 in Additional file 1: Table S1), (C) sporadic ALS (sALS3 in Additional file 1: Table S1), and (D) sporadic ALS (sALS4 in Additional file 1: Table S1) cases were immunostained with either (A) anti-SOD1^{olig} or (B-D) anti-SOD1^{int} antibody. Nuclei were also stained by hematoxylin (blue). The bars represent 50 μm.

Additional file 6: Figure S5. Equal fixation of various forms of SOD1 proteins on the ELISA plate. Amounts of SOD1 proteins fixed on the ELISA plates for the experiments in Fig. 5 were quantified by indirect ELISA with polyclonal anti-SOD1 antibody (FL-154, Santa Cruz Biotechnology). Amounts of SOD1 in the plates for experiments in Fig. 5a were shown in the panel (A), while those in Fig. 5b, c, and d were in the panel (B). The ELISA signal was represented as a ratio against that obtained using BSA. Three independent experiments were performed to estimate error bars (standard deviation). No statistically significant difference in the ELISA signal was confirmed among the in vitro samples examined.

Additional file 7: Figure S6. Epitope analysis on USOD-like and SEDI-like antibodies by indirect ELISA. The peptides were prepared as a fusion protein with an N-terminal 6x His tagged GST and adsorbed on an ELISA plate. SOD1 species recognized by (A) USOD-like and (B) SEDI-like antibodies were quantified as ELISA signals that were represented as a ratio against those of BSA. Almost equal amounts of peptides were adsorbed on the plate, which was confirmed by an ELISA using anti-GST antibody (C). Three independent experiments were performed to estimate error bars (standard deviation).

Additional file 8: Figure S7. Anti-SOD1^{int} antibody specifically detects pathological SOD1 in spinal cords of ALS-model mice. (A, B) SOD1 species recognized by (A) anti-SOD1^{int} and (B) anti-SOD1 (FL-154, Santa Cruz Biotechnology) antibody were quantified in the soluble fraction of the homogenates of lumbar spinal cords of non-transgenic (nonTG), WT, and G1H mice by sandwich ELISA. The data on G1H mice at 30 days of age are the same with those in Fig. 6a and b and shown here again for comparison. (C, D) Sandwich ELISA with (C) anti-SOD1^{int} and (D) anti-SOD1 (FL-154, Santa Cruz Biotechnology) antibody was examined by using the soluble fraction of the homogenates of lumbar spinal cords of G1H mice. The samples were pre-treated with 10 mM DTT for reducing disulfide bonds. In all panels, three independent mouse samples were examined to estimate error bars (standard deviation), and the statistical analysis has been performed to obtain the *P* values indicated in the figures.

Additional file 9: Figure S8. Examination of soluble SOD1 disulfide-crosslinked oligomers in cerebellum and brainstem of ALS-model mice. (A) Cerebellum and (B) brainstem of non-transgenic (NTG) and G1H mice and (C) cerebellum of loxG37R mice were homogenized in the presence of 100 mM iodoacetamide and 1% NP-40 and centrifuged at 20,000 x *g* for 30 min so as to prepare soluble supernatant. The supernatant was then separated in a polyacrylamide gel by non-reducing SDS-PAGE and probed by Western blot using anti-SOD1 antibody (FL-154, Santa Cruz Biotechnology). For comparison, the soluble fraction of the lumbar spinal cord homogenates of G1H mice at 160 days of age was also loaded on the same gel. GAPDH was used as a protein loading control for Western blot.

Additional file 10: Figure S9. Anti-SOD1^{int} antibody specifically detects pathological SOD1 in spinal cords of loxG37R mice. (A, B) SOD1 species

recognized by (A) anti-SOD1^{int} and (B) anti-SOD1 (FL-154, Santa Cruz Biotechnology) antibody were quantified in the soluble fraction of the homogenates of lumbar spinal cord (red), cervical spinal cord (green), brainstem (blue), and cerebellum (gray) of loxG37R mice by sandwich ELISA. Ages of the mouse samples examined are as follows; 100 (three independent mice), 174 (two independent mice), 188, 374 (three independent mice), 386, 392, and 445 days of age. The data were divided into two groups before and after the onset of the disease (350 days of age) and statistically analyzed by two-tailed student's *t* test. The difference in the signal intensity before and after the disease onset was statistically significant in lumbar and cervical spinal cords (**: *P* < 0.01). (C) Soluble disulfide-crosslinked SOD1 oligomers in loxG37R mice were examined by Western blotting. Lumbar spinal cords of loxG37R and G1H mice at indicated days of ages were homogenized in the presence of 100 mM iodoacetamide and 1% NP-40 and centrifuged at 20,000 x *g* for 30 min so as to prepare soluble supernatant. In the presence and absence of the reducing reagent, β-ME, the supernatant was then separated in a polyacrylamide gel by SDS-PAGE and probed by Western blot using anti-SOD1 antibody (FL-154, Santa Cruz Biotechnology). GAPDH was used as a protein loading control for Western blot. (PDF 870 kb)

Additional file 11: Figure S10. Reactivity of the antibodies toward chemically misfolded/unfolded forms of SOD1. E,E-SOD1^{SH} and E,E-SOD1^{S-S} (100 μM; WT, A4V, G37R, and G85R) were first incubated at room temperature for two hours either in 50 mM Tris/100 mM NaCl/5 mM EDTA/6 M guanidine hydrochloride (GdnHCl) at pH 7.4 or in 50 mM sodium acetate buffer at pH 3.0 and then fixed on an ELISA plate. ELISA was performed using (A) anti-SOD1^{int}, (B) USOD-like, (C) SEDI-like, and (D) anti-SOD1 (FL-154, Santa Cruz Biotechnology) antibodies. The ELISA signal was represented as a ratio against that obtained using BSA. Three independent experiments were performed to estimate error bars (standard deviation). (PDF 49 kb)

Abbreviations
ALS: Amyotrophic lateral sclerosis; G1H mouse: A transgenic mouse carrying human *SOD1* gene with G93A mutation; loxG37R mouse: A transgenic mouse carrying SOD1 gene with G37R mutation; SOD1: Cu/Zn-superoxide dismutase; *SOD1*-ALS: ALS with mutations in SOD1 gene; WT mouse: A transgenic mouse carrying human wild-type *SOD1* gene.

Acknowledgements
Not applicable.

Funding
This work was supported by Grants-in-Aid 16H04768 for Scientific Research (B) (to YF), 15H01566 for Scientific Research on Innovative Areas (to YF), 15 K14480 for Challenging Exploratory Research (to YF), 15H06588 for Young Scientists (Start-up) (to ET) from the Ministry of Education, Culture, Sports, Science and Technology of Japan. Preparation of anti-SOD1^{olig} antibody was supported by Comprehensive Brain Science Network (CBSN), Japan.

Authors' contributions
YF directed the project, analyzed the data and wrote the manuscript. ET, IA, TN, and KT prepared the purified protein samples and purified the antibodies. ET and TN performed Western blotting experiments and ELISA. MW prepared the anti-SOD1^{olig} antibody, and immunohistochemical examination on mice was performed by SW, KY, YM and HM. Clinical data collection as well as immunohistochemical examination on human cases was performed by SO. All authors read and approved the manuscript.

Competing interests
The authors declare that they have no competing interests.

Author details
[1]Laboratory for Mechanistic Chemistry of Biomolecules, Department of Chemistry, Keio University, 3-14-1 Hiyoshi, Kohoku, Yokohama, Kanagawa

223-8522, Japan. [2]Department of Anatomy, Hokkaido University Graduate School of Medicine, Sapporo 060-8638, Japan. [3]Department of Neurology, Matsumoto Medical Center, Matsumoto 399-0021, Japan. [4]Department of Neuroscience and Pathobiology, Research Institute of Environmental Medicine, Nagoya University, Nagoya 464-8601, Japan. [5]Division of Pharmacology, Faculty of Pharmacy, Keio University, Tokyo 105-8512, Japan.

References

1. Andersen PM, Al-Chalabi A. Clinical genetics of amyotrophic lateral sclerosis: what do we really know? Nat Rev Neurol. 2011;7:603–15.
2. Rosen DR, Siddique T, Patterson D, Figlewicz DA, Sapp P, Hentati A, et al. Mutations in Cu/Zn superoxide dismutase gene are associated with familial amyotrophic lateral sclerosis. Nature. 1993;362:59–62.
3. Abel O, Powell JF, Andersen PM, Al-Chalabi A. ALSoD: A user-friendly online bioinformatics tool for amyotrophic lateral sclerosis genetics. Hum Mutat. 2012;33:1345–51.
4. Reaume AG, Elliott JL, Hoffman EK, Kowall NW, Ferrante RJ, Siwek DF, et al. Motor neurons in Cu/Zn superoxide dismutase-deficient mice develop normally but exhibit enhanced cell death after axonal injury. Nat Genet. 1996;13:43–7.
5. Bruijn LI, Houseweart MK, Kato S, Anderson KL, Anderson SD, Ohama E, et al. Aggregation and motor neuron toxicity of an ALS-linked SOD1 mutant independent from wild-type SOD1. Science. 1998;281:1851–4.
6. McCord JM, Fridovich I. Superoxide dismutase. An enzymic function for erythrocuprein (hemocuprein). J Biol Chem. 1969;244:6049–55.
7. Furukawa Y, O'Halloran TV. Amyotrophic lateral sclerosis mutations have the greatest destabilizing effect on the apo, reduced form of SOD1, leading to unfolding and oxidative aggregation. J Biol Chem. 2005;280:17266–74.
8. Toichi K, Yamanaka K, Furukawa Y. Disulfide scrambling describes the oligomer formation of superoxide dismutase (SOD1) proteins in the familial form of amyotrophic lateral sclerosis. J Biol Chem. 2013;288:4970–80.
9. Furukawa Y, Kaneko K, Yamanaka K, O'Halloran TV, Nukina N. Complete loss of post-translational modifications triggers fibrillar aggregation of SOD1 in familial form of ALS. J Biol Chem. 2008;283:24167–76.
10. Proctor EA, Fee L, Tao Y, Redler RL, Fay JM, Zhang Y, et al. Nonnative SOD1 trimer is toxic to motor neurons in a model of amyotrophic lateral sclerosis. Proc Natl Acad Sci USA. 2016;113:614–9.
11. Banci L, Bertini I, Boca M, Calderone V, Cantini F, Girotto S, et al. Structural and dynamic aspects related to oligomerization of apo SOD1 and its mutants. Proc Natl Acad Sci USA. 2009;106:6980–5.
12. Luchinat E, Barbieri L, Rubino JT, Kozyreva T, Cantini F, Banci L. In-cell NMR reveals potential precursor of toxic species from SOD1 fALS mutants. Nat Commun. 2014;5:5502.
13. Sekhar A, Rumfeldt JA, Broom HR, Doyle CM, Bouvignies G, Meiering EM, et al. Thermal fluctuations of immature SOD1 lead to separate folding and misfolding pathways. eLife. 2015;4:e07296.
14. Jonsson PA, Graffmo KS, Andersen PM, Brannstrom T, Lindberg M, Oliveberg M, et al. Disulphide-reduced superoxide dismutase-1 in CNS of transgenic amyotrophic lateral sclerosis models. Brain. 2006;129:451–64.
15. Wang J, Xu G, Gonzales V, Coonfield M, Fromholt D, Copeland NG, et al. Fibrillar inclusions and motor neuron degeneration in transgenic mice expressing superoxide dismutase 1 with a disrupted copper-binding site. Neurobiol Dis. 2002;10:128–38.
16. Kerman A, Liu HN, Croul S, Bilbao J, Rogaeva E, Zinman L, et al. Amyotrophic lateral sclerosis is a non-amyloid disease in which extensive misfolding of SOD1 is unique to the familial form. Acta Neuropathol. 2010;119:335–44.
17. Furukawa Y, Fu R, Deng HX, Siddique T, O'Halloran TV. Disulfide cross-linked protein represents a significant fraction of ALS-associated Cu, Zn-superoxide dismutase aggregates in spinal cords of model mice. Proc Natl Acad Sci USA. 2006;103:7148–53.
18. Karch CM, Borchelt DR. A limited role for disulfide cross-linking in the aggregation of mutant SOD1 linked to familial amyotrophic lateral sclerosis. J Biol Chem. 2008;283:13528–37.
19. Niwa J, Yamada S, Ishigaki S, Sone J, Takahashi M, Katsuno M, et al. Disulfide bond mediates aggregation, toxicity, and ubiquitylation of familial amyotrophic lateral sclerosis-linked mutant SOD1. J Biol Chem. 2007;282:28087–95.
20. Yamanaka K, Chun SJ, Boillee S, Fujimori-Tonou N, Yamashita H, Gutmann DH, et al. Astrocytes as determinants of disease progression in inherited amyotrophic lateral sclerosis. Nat Neurosci. 2008;11:251–3.
21. Williamson TL, Cleveland DW. Slowing of axonal transport is a very early event in the toxicity of ALS-linked SOD1 mutants to motor neurons. Nat Neurosci. 1999;2:50–6.
22. Ichikawa T, Ajiki K, Matsuura J, Misawa H. Localization of two cholinergic markers, choline acetyltransferase and vesicular acetylcholine transporter in the central nervous system of the rat: in situ hybridization histochemistry and immunohistochemistry. J Chem Neuroanat. 1997;13:23–39.
23. Deng HX, Shi Y, Furukawa Y, Zhai H, Fu R, Liu E, et al. Conversion to the amyotrophic lateral sclerosis phenotype is associated with intermolecular linked insoluble aggregates of SOD1 in mitochondria. Proc Natl Acad Sci USA. 2006;103:7142–7.
24. Morisaki Y, Niikura M, Watanabe M, Onishi K, Tanabe S, Moriwaki Y, et al. Selective Expression of Osteopontin in ALS-resistant Motor Neurons is a Critical Determinant of Late Phase Neurodegeneration Mediated by Matrix Metalloproteinase-9. Sci Rep. 2016;6:27354.
25. Watanabe M, Dykes-Hoberg M, Culotta VC, Price DL, Wong PC, Rothstein JD. Histological evidence of protein aggregation in mutant SOD1 transgenic mice and in amyotrophic lateral sclerosis neural tissues. Neurobiol Dis. 2001;8:933–41.
26. Nakamura A, Hineno A, Yoshida K, Sekijima Y, Hanaoka-Tachibana N, Takei Y, et al. Marked intrafamilial phenotypic variation in a family with SOD1 C111Y mutation. Amyotroph Lateral Scler. 2012;13:479–86.
27. Takei Y, Oguchi K, Koshihara H, Hineno A, Nakamura A, Ohara S. alpha-Synuclein coaggregation in familial amyotrophic lateral sclerosis with SOD1 gene mutation. Hum Pathol. 2013;44:1171–6.
28. Rakhit R, Robertson J, Vande Velde C, Horne P, Ruth DM, Griffin J, et al. An immunological epitope selective for pathological monomer-misfolded SOD1 in ALS. Nat Med. 2007;13:754–9.
29. Swinnen B, Robberecht W. The phenotypic variability of amyotrophic lateral sclerosis. Nat Rev Neurol. 2014;10:661–70.
30. Garbuzova-Davis S, Saporta S, Haller E, Kolomey I, Bennett SP, Potter H, et al. Evidence of compromised blood-spinal cord barrier in early and late symptomatic SOD1 mice modeling ALS. PLoS One. 2007;2:e1205.
31. Zang DW, Cheema SS. Degeneration of corticospinal and bulbospinal systems in the superoxide dismutase 1(G93A G1H) transgenic mouse model of familial amyotrophic lateral sclerosis. Neurosci Lett. 2002;332:99–102.
32. Dal Canto MC, Gurney ME. Neuropathological changes in two lines of mice carrying a transgene for mutant human Cu, Zn SOD, and in mice overexpressing wild type human SOD: a model of familial amyotrophic lateral sclerosis (FALS). Brain Res. 1995;676:25–40.
33. Metcalf CW, Hirano A. Amyotrophic lateral sclerosis. Clinicopathological studies of a family. Arch Neurol. 1971;24:518–23.
34. Boillee S, Yamanaka K, Lobsiger CS, Copeland NG, Jenkins NA, Kassiotis G, et al. Onset and progression in inherited ALS determined by motor neurons and microglia. Science. 2006;312:1389–92.
35. Kang SH, Li Y, Fukaya M, Lorenzini I, Cleveland DW, Ostrow LW, et al. Degeneration and impaired regeneration of gray matter oligodendrocytes in amyotrophic lateral sclerosis. Nat Neurosci. 2013;16:571–9.
36. Rodriguez JA, Shaw BF, Durazo A, Sohn SH, Doucette PA, Nersissian AM, et al. Destabilization of apoprotein is insufficient to explain Cu, Zn-superoxide dismutase-linked ALS pathogenesis. Proc Natl Acad Sci USA. 2005;102:10516–21.
37. Banci L, Bertini I, Durazo A, Girotto S, Gralla EB, Martinelli M, et al. Metal-free superoxide dismutase forms soluble oligomers under physiological conditions: a possible general mechanism for familial ALS. Proc Natl Acad Sci USA. 2007;104:11263–7.
38. Rotunno MS, Bosco DA. An emerging role for misfolded wild-type SOD1 in sporadic ALS pathogenesis. Front Cell Neurosci. 2013;7:253.
39. Sabado J, Casanovas A, Hernandez S, Piedrafita L, Hereu M, Esquerda JE. Immunodetection of disease-associated conformers of mutant cu/zn superoxide dismutase 1 selectively expressed in degenerating neurons in amyotrophic lateral sclerosis. J Neuropathol Exp Neurol. 2013;72:646–61.
40. Gros-Louis F, Soucy G, Lariviere R, Julien JP. Intracerebroventricular infusion of monoclonal antibody or its derived Fab fragment against misfolded forms of SOD1 mutant delays mortality in a mouse model of ALS. J Neurochem. 2010;113:1188–99.
41. Rotunno MS, Auclair JR, Maniatis S, Shaffer SA, Agar J, Bosco DA. Identification of a misfolded region in superoxide dismutase 1 that is exposed in amyotrophic lateral sclerosis. J Biol Chem. 2014;289:28527–38.

42. Urushitani M, Ezzi SA, Julien JP. Therapeutic effects of immunization with mutant superoxide dismutase in mice models of amyotrophic lateral sclerosis. Proc Natl Acad Sci USA. 2007;104:2495–500.

43. Brotherton TE, Li Y, Cooper D, Gearing M, Julien JP, Rothstein JD, et al. Localization of a toxic form of superoxide dismutase 1 protein to pathologically affected tissues in familial ALS. Proc Natl Acad Sci USA. 2012;109:5505–10.

44. Okamoto Y, Ihara M, Urushitani M, Yamashita H, Kondo T, Tanigaki A, et al. An autopsy case of SOD1-related ALS with TDP-43 positive inclusions. Neurology. 2011;77:1993–5.

45. Khare SD, Caplow M, Dokholyan NV. The rate and equilibrium constants for a multistep reaction sequence for the aggregation of superoxide dismutase in amyotrophic lateral sclerosis. Proc Natl Acad Sci USA. 2004;101:15094–9.

46. Jonsson PA, Ernhill K, Andersen PM, Bergemalm D, Brannstrom T, Gredal O, et al. Minute quantities of misfolded mutant superoxide dismutase-1 cause amyotrophic lateral sclerosis. Brain. 2004;127:73–88.

47. Forsberg K, Andersen PM, Marklund SL, Brannstrom T. Glial nuclear aggregates of superoxide dismutase-1 are regularly present in patients with amyotrophic lateral sclerosis. Acta Neuropathol. 2011;121:623–34.

48. Forsberg K, Jonsson PA, Andersen PM, Bergemalm D, Graffmo KS, Hultdin M, et al. Novel antibodies reveal inclusions containing non-native SOD1 in sporadic ALS patients. PLoS One. 2010;5:e11552.

49. Liu HN, Sanelli T, Horne P, Pioro EP, Strong MJ, Rogaeva E, et al. Lack of evidence of monomer/misfolded superoxide dismutase-1 in sporadic amyotrophic lateral sclerosis. Ann Neurol. 2009;66:75–80.

50. Stewart HG, Mackenzie IR, Eisen A, Brannstrom T, Marklund SL, Andersen PM. Clinicopathological phenotype of ALS with a novel G72C SOD1 gene mutation mimicking a myopathy. Muscle Nerve. 2006;33:701–6.

51. Chattopadhyay M, Durazo A, Sohn SH, Strong CD, Gralla EB, Whitelegge JP, et al. Initiation and elongation in fibrillation of ALS-linked superoxide dismutase. Proc Natl Acad Sci USA. 2008;105:18663–8.

52. Oztug Durer ZA, Cohlberg JA, Dinh P, Padua S, Ehrenclou K, Downes S, et al. Loss of metal ions, disulfide reduction and mutations related to familial ALS promote formation of amyloid-like aggregates from superoxide dismutase. PLoS One. 2009;4:e5004.

53. Rakhit R, Cunningham P, Furtos-Matei A, Dahan S, Qi XF, Crow JP, et al. Oxidation-induced misfolding and aggregation of superoxide dismutase and its implications for amyotrophic lateral sclerosis. J Biol Chem. 2002;277: 47551–6.

54. Stathopulos PB, Rumfeldt JA, Scholz GA, Irani RA, Frey HE, Hallewell RA, et al. Cu/Zn superoxide dismutase mutants associated with amyotrophic lateral sclerosis show enhanced formation of aggregates in vitro. Proc Natl Acad Sci USA. 2003;100:7021–6.

55. Furukawa Y, Anzai I, Akiyama S, Imai M, Cruz FJ, Saio T, et al. Conformational Disorder of the Most Immature Cu, Zn-Superoxide Dismutase Leading to Amyotrophic Lateral Sclerosis. J Biol Chem. 2016;291:4144–55.

56. Furukawa Y, Kaneko K, Yamanaka K, Nukina N. Mutation-dependent polymorphism of Cu, Zn-superoxide dismutase aggregates in the familial form of amyotrophic lateral sclerosis. J Biol Chem. 2010;285:22221–31.

57. Niwa J, Ishigaki S, Hishikawa N, Yamamoto M, Doyu M, Murata S, et al. Dorfin ubiquitylates mutant SOD1 and prevents mutant SOD1-mediated neurotoxicity. J Biol Chem. 2002;277:36793–8.

58. Ferri A, Cozzolino M, Crosio C, Nencini M, Casciati A, Gralla EB, et al. Familial ALS-superoxide dismutases associate with mitochondria and shift their redox potentials. Proc Natl Acad Sci USA. 2006;103:13860–5.

59. Jaarsma D, Haasdijk ED, Grashorn JA, Hawkins R, van Duijn W, Verspaget HW, et al. Human Cu/Zn superoxide dismutase (SOD1) overexpression in mice causes mitochondrial vacuolization, axonal degeneration, and premature motoneuron death and accelerates motoneuron disease in mice expressing a familial amyotrophic lateral sclerosis mutant SOD1. Neurobiol Dis. 2000;7:623–43.

60. Furukawa Y. Pathological roles of wild-type cu, zn-superoxide dismutase in amyotrophic lateral sclerosis. Neurol Res Int. 2012;2012:323261.

6

Dioxins and related environmental contaminants increase TDP-43 levels

Peter E. A. Ash[1], Elizabeth A. Stanford[2], Ali Al Abdulatif[1], Alejandra Ramirez-Cardenas[2], Heather I. Ballance[1], Samantha Boudeau[1], Amanda Jeh[1], James M. Murithi[3], Yorghos Tripodis[4], George J. Murphy[3], David H. Sherr[2] and Benjamin Wolozin[1,5]* ⓘ

Abstract

Background: Amyotrophic lateral sclerosis (ALS) is a debilitating neurodegenerative condition that is characterized by progressive loss of motor neurons and the accumulation of aggregated TAR DNA Binding Protein-43 (TDP-43, gene: *TARDBP*). Increasing evidence indicates that environmental factors contribute to the risk of ALS. Dioxins, related planar polychlorinated biphenyls (PCBs), and polycyclic aromatic hydrocarbons (PAHs) are environmental contaminants that activate the aryl hydrocarbon receptor (AHR), a ligand-activated, PAS family transcription factor. Recently, exposure to these toxicants was identified as a risk factor for ALS.

Methods: We examined levels of TDP-43 reporter activity, transcript and protein. Quantification was done using cell lines, induced pluripotent stem cells (iPSCs) and mouse brain. The target samples were treated with AHR agonists, including 6-Formylindolo[3,2-b]carbazole (FICZ, a potential endogenous ligand, 2,3,7,8-tetrachlorodibenzo(p)dioxin, and benzo(a)pyrene, an abundant carcinogen in cigarette smoke). The action of the agonists was inhibited by concomitant addition of AHR antagonists or by AHR-specific shRNA.

Results: We now report that AHR agonists induce up to a 3-fold increase in TDP-43 protein in human neuronal cell lines (BE-M17 cells), motor neuron differentiated iPSCs, and in murine brain. Chronic treatment with AHR agonists elicits over 2-fold accumulation of soluble and insoluble TDP-43, primarily because of reduced TDP-43 catabolism. AHR antagonists or AHR knockdown inhibits agonist-induced increases in TDP-43 protein *and TARDBP* transcription demonstrating that the ligands act through the AHR.

Conclusions: These results provide the first evidence that environmental AHR ligands increase TDP-43, which is the principle pathological protein associated with ALS. These results suggest novel molecular mechanisms through which a variety of prevalent environmental factors might directly contribute to ALS. The widespread distribution of dioxins, PCBs and PAHs is considered to be a risk factor for cancer and autoimmune diseases, but could also be a significant public health concern for ALS.

Keywords: Neurodegeneration, ALS, Protein aggregation, Promoter, Transcription, Gene regulation, Toxicants, Alpha-synuclein, Ataxin-2, Fus

* Correspondence: bwolozin@bu.edu
[1]Department of Pharmacology, Boston University School of Medicine, 72 East Concord St., R614, Boston, MA 02118-2526, USA
[5]Department of Neurology, Boston University School of Medicine, 72 East Concord St., R614, Boston, MA 02118-2526, USA
Full list of author information is available at the end of the article

Background

Amyotrophic lateral sclerosis (ALS) is a debilitating condition characterized by relentless, progressive loss of motor function that typically leads to death within 3–6 years after onset [1]. The causes of ALS are poorly understood, but environmental factors are established contributors to the risk of ALS [2]. Increasing age, gender, smoking [3–5] and diet [6] are often cited environmental risks of ALS. Military veterans are at an increased risk of developing ALS [7, 8]. Dietary exposure to toxins is also associated with ALS. For instance, ingestion of the amino acid β-Methylamino-L-alanine (BMAA) is associated with ~100X increased risk of a complex of neurological disorders consisting of Parkinsonism, dementia and ALS [9]. Exposure to organophosphates in agricultural herbicides and pesticides [5, 7], or heavy metals (including lead, mercury and selenium) [10] also increase odds ratios of developing ALS.

The aryl hydrocarbon receptor (AHR) is a ligand-activated transcription factor that is responsive to a variety of endogenous ligands [11, 12] and potent environmental chemicals including polycyclic aromatic hydrocarbons (PAHs), polychlorinated biphenyls (PCBs) and dioxins. These environmental AHR ligands are common by-products of industrial processing (e.g., smelting, chlorine bleaching, pesticide manufacturing) and/or combustion of any carbon source (e.g. fossil fuels and tobacco). PCBs and PAHs have been previously associated with increased cancer risk [13, 14], and epidemiological studies indicate an association of dioxins with neurodegenerative diseases. PCB and airborne aromatic exposures are linked to an increased risk of ALS [15, 16]. Elevated serum levels of the pesticide DDT [17] is a risk of Alzheimer's disease; DDT is metabolized to DDE, which is also an activator of the AHR [18]. Thus, multiple studies suggest an association between environmental AHR ligands, ALS and possibly other neurodegenerative diseases. Taken together, these data point to an important role for environmental toxicants in the risk of ALS, but also raise the possibility that there are other environmental factors contributing to the risk of ALS that have yet to be identified.

Recent advances in human genetics and molecular pathology have dramatically increased our understanding of the genetics and pathophysiology of ALS. The most prevalent pathology that develops in ALS is the accumulation of phosphorylated insoluble aggregates of TAR DNA binding protein 43 kDa (protein TDP-43; gene *TARDBP*) [19, 20]. Mutations in the *TARDBP* gene cause familial ALS and drive pathological deposition of TDP-43 [21–23]. TDP-43 pathology is also a consistent feature of essentially all of the 90–95% of sporadic ALS cases [24], which are cases that occur with no family history of the disease. The accumulation of insoluble TDP-43 is also observable post-mortem in other neurological and systematic pathologies including in 19–57% of Alzheimer's disease patients [25], 85% of cases of chronic traumatic encephalopathy [26] and in Lewy body-related dementias [27]. Transgenic approaches that increase TDP-43 expression in model organisms (rodents, *C. elegans* and *Drosophila*) are sufficient to drive neurodegeneration, suggesting that increased levels of TDP-43 protein can accelerate progression of ALS and possibly other neurodegenerative conditions [28, 29]. It is clear, therefore, that accumulation of TDP-43 is a key component in the pathological progression of ALS and possibly other neurodegenerative conditions.

Given the importance of TDP-43 for the pathophysiology of ALS, we hypothesized that AHR ligands might affect the risk of ALS by increasing TDP-43 expression in the central nervous system. We now report that disparate AHR ligands lead to the accumulation of soluble and insoluble TDP-43 in a time-dependent manner. AHR-mediated increases in TDP-43 are evident in human cell lines and in iPSC-derived neuronal cells, as well as in murine brain. These increases are blocked with a well-characterized AHR competitive inhibitor or by shRNA against the AHR. Mechanistic studies indicate that the increases in TDP-43 result from slower degradation of TDP-43 protein, rather than an increase in *TARDBP* transcript. These data provide the first lines of evidence that AHR ligands can increase levels of proteins related to ALS in neurons, suggesting a mechanism through which at least some environmental chemicals might contribute to the risk or progression of ALS. They also suggest the possibility of targeting the AHR with competitive inhibitors to either prevent or ameliorate ALS.

Methods

Cell culture

BE-M17 (M17) neuroblastoma and H4 glioblastoma cell lines were maintained using standard cell culture techniques in DMEM/F12 50/50 supplemented with 10% FBS, Pen/Strep, NEAA and 10 mM HEPES (Gibco). M17 were differentiated for up to 7 days in media containing reduced (3%) FBS and 10 μM Retinoic Acid (RA; Sigma). M17.shAHR stable cell lines were generated by transduction (in 8 μg/ml Polybrene) with lentiviral-vectored doxycycline (Dox)-inducible human targeted *TurboRFP-shAHR TRIPZ* (Open Biosystems), selection with 2 μg/ml Puromycin (Gibco) and isolation of individual clonal colonies. M17.shAHR lines were then maintained in 10% tet-free FBS and 0.5 μg/ml Puromycin. AHR knockdown was achieved by addition of 1 μg/ml Doxycycline. Stable lines were assessed for efficiency of knock down by qPCR. 6-Formylindolo[3,2-b]carbazole (FICZ; Santa Cruz sc-300,019) and CB7993113 (2-((2-(5-

bromofuran-2-yl)-4-oxo-4H-chromen-3-yl)oxy)acetamide; synthesized by Dr. M. Pollastri, Northeastern University [30, 31]) were resuspended in DMSO. M17 cells were treated with vehicle (DMSO), 0.5 μM FICZ or FICZ plus 10 μM CB7993113. In further experiments, M17 cells were treated with vehicle (DMSO), 10 μM Benzo(a)pyrene (B(a)P) or B(a)P plus 10 μM CB7993113.

Blotting and qPCR

Pelleted cells were lysed in RIPA buffer (50 mM Tris pH 7.4; 150 mM NaCl; 1 mM EDTA; 1% NP-40; 0.1% SDS; 0.1% sodium deoxycholate; 1 mM PMSF; PhosSTOP and cOmplete PIC (Roche)) sonicated, and quantified by BCA assay. Equal sample amounts were then immunoblotted using Bolt gels and buffers (Thermo Fisher). Blots were blocked in 5% non-fat dry milk in TBSt (0.05% tween), washed in TBSt and incubated overnight at 4 °C with the following antibodies: anti-TDP-43 (ProteinTech; 12,892–1-AP; 10,782–2-AP); anti-Actin (Millipore; MAB1501); anti-α-synuclein (BD 610787); anti-ATXN2 (BD Biosciences; 611,378); anti-VCP (Thermo.; MA3–004); anti-AHR (Thermo.; MA1–514); anti-α-tubulin (Sigma-Aldrich; T5168). After washing, HRP-conjugated secondary antibodies (Jackson) were incubated with the blots the following day. Blots were activated with Pierce ECL chemiluminescent substrates (Thermo Fisher) and imaged using a ChemiDoc XRS+ Imager (BioRad). Band densitometries were assessed using Image Lab Software (BioRad).

RNA was collected from cultured cells by RNeasy minikit (Qiagen). cDNA was generated using High-Capacity cDNA Reverse Transcriptase (ABI). qPCR was performed using iQ SYBR green Supermix (Bio-Rad) on a 7900HT Fast Real-Time PCR system and the data was analyzed on SDS software. qPCR primer sequences are available in Additional file 1: Table S1.

Exposure of mice to 7,12-Dimethylbenz(a)anthracene (DMBA) and Benzo(a)pyrene

Male, 4–5 month old C57Bl/6 J mice were treated by intraperitoneal (i.p.) injection. Three groups of 11 individuals were treated with: 1) vegetable/sesame oil (control); 2) 100 mg/kg AHR-agonist 7,12-Dimethylbenz(a)anthracene (DMBA) in sesame oil; or 3) DMBA (in sesame oil) and 100 mg/kg AHR-antagonist CB7993113 in vegetable oil. Three groups of 4 individuals were treated with: 1) vegetable/sesame oil (control); 2) 100 mg/kg AHR-agonist Benzo(a)pyrene (B(a)P) in sesame oil; or 3) B(a)P (in sesame oil) and 100 mg/kg AHR-antagonist CB7993113 in vegetable oil. Mice receiving CB7993113 were pre-treated 30 min before DMBA/B(a)P injection with 100 mg/kg CB7993113 (200 mg/kg CB7993113 total for the experiment). Mice were euthanized 30 h after DMBA treatment. The brains were extracted,

rinsed in ice-cold DPBS and dissected on ice to collect from each hemisphere a 20-30 mg section of the somatomotor/sensory cortex, the remaining cortical tissue, the hippocampus, the striatum and the cerebellum. Tissue sections (20-30 mg) of liver and spleen were dissected, rinsed in ice-cold DPBS and collected from each mouse. Tissue samples were stored at −80 °C. Lysates of the somatomotor/sensory cortex were prepared in RIPA buffer for immunoblotting (as above). RNA was extracted from frozen tissue samples using QIAzol Lysis Reagent following the Lipid tissue RNeasy minikit protocol (Qiagen). qPCR on reverse transcribed total RNA was performed as above. Primer sets are indicated in Additional file 1: Table S1. Immunoblotting was performed as described above.

Induced pluripotent stem cell (iPSC) maintenance, generation of neuronal-lineage and treatment

iPSCs were generated from a 64 year old male patient heterozygous for the G298S mutation in *TARDBP* [36] as previously described in Sommer et al. [33]. iPSCs were differentiated into a neuronal-lineage as described previously by Chambers et al. [34] and Hu et al. [35] and cultured for 15 days before treatment every 48 h with DMSO, 0.125 μM FICZ or FICZ with 5 μM CB7993113 for a further 10 days. Cells were then washed in DPBS, collected and lysed in RIPA buffer (50 mM Tris pH 8, 150 mM NaCl, 0.5 mM EDTA, 1% NP-40, 0.1% sodium deoxycholate and 0.1% SDS) containing 1 mM PMSF, Complete PIC and PhosSTOP (Roche). After determining protein concentration, 150 μg of each sample was spun at 100,000 rcf 30 mins at 4 °C, the RIPA soluble fraction was removed before the pellets were washed and re-sonicated in RIPA buffer and spun again as before. The final pellets were dissolved in Urea buffer (8 M Urea; 2 M Thiourea; 4% CHAPS; 30 mM Tris HCl pH 8.5) [32, 36]. Total lysate and insoluble protein fractions were analyzed by immunoblot as above.

AHR-responsive luciferase reporters

AHR-responsive luciferase reporters were constructed by PCR amplification (iProof HF, BioRad) of the genomic promoter sequences directly upstream of the translation start site (or nucleotide "Tsl + 1") of the human *CYP1B1* and *TARDBP* genes. Primer sequences for amplification are listed in Additional file 2: Table S2. Amplicons were blunt TOPO cloned into pCR-Blunt-II vector and screened, then subcloned into pGL4.17[*luc2*/Neo] in which the cloning site from *Xho*I to *Hind*III was edited to include the restriction site *Pme*I using the annealed oligos "pGL4.17_MCS_F":"pGL4.17_MCS_R". Ligations were transformed into NEB Stable *E.coli* (NEB) and grown at 30 °C. "*Acc65I.CYP1B1*_Tsc-3kb_F":"*CYP1B1*_Tsc-628_R" and "*CYP1B1*_Tsc-765_F":"*PmeI.CYP1B1*_Tsl-

1_R" fragments were then sequentially recombined by subcloning (using NEB enzymes and Zymo DNA purification columns) into the *Acc65I/NheI* and *NheI/PmeI* sites of pGL4.17[*luc2*/Neo] (Promega) to construct pGL4.17[*CYP1B1*_-3.8 kb/*luc2*] containing 3792 nucleotides of the promoter (corresponding to human chr2:38,075,389–38,079,181; UCSC hg38).

The fragment "*Acc65I.TARDBP*_Tsc-3.1kb_F":"*TARDBP*_Tsc-816_R" was amplified using KOD Hot Start Master Mix (EMD). The fragment "*TARDBP*_Tsc-888_F":"*PmeI.TARDBP*_Tsl-1_R" was amplified using iProof polymerase. These sequences were then sequentially recombined by subcloning (using NEB enzymes and Zymo DNA purification columns) into the *Acc65I/XhoI* and *XhoI/PmeI* sites of pGL4.17[*luc2*/ Neo] (Promega) to construct pGL4.17[*TARDBP*_-4.1 kb/ *luc2*] containing 4138 nucleotides of the promoter (corresponding to human chr1:11,009,590–11,013,727; UCSC hg38). Plasmid DNA was sequenced to confirm accuracy using amplification primers and primers pGL4.17_pA_F and *luc2*_R.

M17 and the tet-inducible M17.shAHR_11 stable lines were plated (day 0) at 5×10^5 cells per well of 6wps and transfected the following day (day 1) using Lipofectamine 2000 (Thermo Fisher) with 200 ng pGL4.74 [*hRluc*/TK] (Promega) renilla transfection control plasmid and 2000 ng per well of pGL4.17 [*luc2*/Neo] (Promega; empty vector control), pGL4.17 [*CYP1B1*_-3.8 kb/ *luc2*] or pGL4.17 [*TARDBP*_-4.1 kb/*luc2*] for 3 h before replacing with growth media overnight at 37 °C. On day 2 wells were trypsinized, counted, and plated at 5×10^4 cells per well in 0.1 mg/ml Poly-L-lysine-coated 96 well culture plates. Doxycycline (1 μg/ml) was added to half the wells for the M17.shAHR_11 line. From days 3–5 cells were treated daily by replacing the media containing compounds as indicated. On day 6 cells were harvested by aspiration, washed 2× with PBS, and lysed with 30 μl passive lysis buffer before luminescence detection with Dual-Luciferase Reporter Assay System (Promega; E1960).

The more robust H4 cell line was used for assessing responses to toxic AHR ligands. H4 cells (3.5×10^5) were plated and transfected with AHR-responsive luciferase reporters in 6 well plates as above, then replated the following day at 2×10^4 cells per well of 96 well culture plates. Cultures were then treated daily for 3 days with 0.01 μM 2,3,7,8-Tetrachlorodibenzo-p-dioxin (TCDD), 10 μM Benzo[a]pyrene (B(a)P), or its non-toxic congener benzo[e]pyrene (B(e)P) or 5 μM pyocyanin. All compound from Sigma-Aldrich were dissolved in DMSO.

Click-iT labelling of nascent proteins in M17

M17 cells were maintained as described above, plated in 10 cm dishes (4.0×10^6 cells/dish) and differentiated 7 days in 3% FBS media with 10 μM RA. On Day 7, cultures were treated with vehicle (DMSO) or 0.5 μM FICZ. On Day 8 plates were washed with pre-warmed PBS. The PBS was then removed and replaced with pre-warmed serum-free, methionine-free RPMI (Thermo A1451701) and cultures maintained at 37 °C for 1 H. *media* was then removed and replaced with pre-warmed serum-free, methionine-free RPMI containing 3% FBS, PS, NEAA and 10 mM HEPES and 50 μM Click-iT AHA (L-Azidohomoalanine; Thermo C10102). This media was also supplemented with DMSO or 0.5 μM FICZ according to the previous pattern of treatment from Day 7. This treatment defines the start time point for the Click-iT AHA pulse-labelling of nascent protein. After 2 h at 37 °C, the Click-iT AHA pulse media was removed and replaced with maintenance media for the remainder of the experiment. At this same time point, '2 h from Start of Pulse', the M17 cells from three DMSO- and three FICZ-treated plates were washed in PBS, collected and lysed in 300 μl 50 mM HEPES-KOH pH 7.5, 150 mM NaCl, 0.2% NP-40, 0.05% Sodium Deoxycholate, 0.1% SDS, PMSF, cOmplete PIC and PhosSTOP. The samples were incubated on ice for 15 mins, sonicated and frozen. At the following time points, the M17 cells from three DMSO-treated and three FICZ-treated cultures were similarly harvested: '4 h from Start of Pulse' (representing 2 h in Click-iT AHA media, 2 h off); '6 h from Start of Pulse' (representing 2 h in Click-iT AHA media, 4 h off); '12 h from Start of Pulse' (representing 2 h in Click-iT AHA media, 10 h off); and '24 h from Start of Pulse' (representing 2 h in Click-iT AHA media, 22 h off).

M17 samples with AHA-labelled nascent proteins were thawed on ice, re-sonicated and spun down at 13,000 rcf for 5 min. The protein concentrations of the clarified lysates were determined by BCA assay. Then, from 200 μg total clarified lysate, the AHA-labelled nascent proteins were biotinylated using Click-iT Protein Reaction buffer kit protocol (Thermo; C10276) and 40 μM Biotin Alkyne (PEG4 carboxamide-Propargyl Biotin; Thermo; B10185). As a negative control, a representative sample from each time point was included in which the Click-iT chemistry was performed without the addition of Biotin Alkyne. Protein from samples was precipitated using Methanol/Chloroform and then pelleted by centrifugation. Protein pellets were washed twice in ice cold acetone and allowed to completely air dry. Protein pellets were resuspended in 30 μl 50 mM HEPES-KOH pH 7.5, 150 mM NaCl, 0.2% NP-40, 0.05% Sodium Deoxycholate, 2% SDS, PMSF, PIC, PhosSTOP by incubating at 55 °C for 1 h and then sonicating to homogenize the protein. 3 μl "clicked" lysates (representing approximately 20 μg of protein) were saved for immunoblot analysis. The remaining resuspended "clicked" lysates were then brought up to 300 µl in affinity purification buffer: 50 mM HEPES-KOH pH 7.5, 150 mM NaC, 0.2% NP-40, 0.05% Sodium Deoxycholate, 0.1% SDS, PMSF, PIC, PhosSTOP.

The resuspended "clicked" lysates were pre-cleared against affinity purification buffer washed control agarose resin (Pierce; 26,150), then affinity purified using 5% BSA blocked, affinity purification buffer washed avidin-agarose resin (Pierce; 20,228). The non-biotinylated negative control (above) was affinity purified against avidin-agarose resin. As an additional negative control, a representative "clicked" lysate sample from each time point was affinity purified using control agarose resin. All incubation and wash steps were performed using Pierce spin columns (69705). Flow through from affinity purifications were collected, then the columns were washed before eluting precipitated proteins by boiling 10mins at 98 °C in 60 µl 50 mM Tris pH 7.4, 2× LDS buffer, 1× reducing agent (Thermo). Clicked lysates, avidin-agarose affinity purified lysates and the flow throughs from those purifications were immunoblotted as above. Blots were probed using antibodies to TARDBP (Abnova; M01) and Actin (Millipore; MAB1501), and Streptavidin-HRP. The 3 µl affinity purified lysates and 5 µl flow throughs were also dot blotted to compare signal strength across samples. Densitometry was performed from dot blots using Image Studio (Licor). Signal intensities were normalized to the means of DMSO-treated samples from the "2 h from Start of Pulse" group and then plotted using GraphPad Prism. A non-linear regression curve was fit to the mean TDP-43 signals of both the DMSO- and FICZ-treated sample across the time points (one phase exponential decay;

GraphPad). Statistical significance was calculated by comparison of fit (with the null hypothesis that one curve is descriptive of both data sets).

Results

AHR agonism increases levels of endogenous TDP-43 protein

Because regulation of TDP-43 protein levels plays a key role in the pathophysiology of ALS, we investigated whether AHR agonists increased TDP-43 protein as well as mRNA. Human neuroblastoma M17 cells were differentiated for 7 days in 3% FBS media with 10 µM retinoic acid and treated for a further 7 days with vehicle, AHR agonist 6-formylindolo[3,2-b]carbazole (FICZ) or with agonist and antagonist; FICZ is a non-toxic, high-affinity AHR agonist and putative endogenous AHR ligand [30, 31]. FICZ (0.5 µM) treatment upregulated the expression of monomeric TDP-43 (3.1 fold) (Fig. 1a and b; control = 1.00 arbitrary units (AU), s.d. 0.072; FICZ = 3.10 AU, s.d. 0.859; n = 3; $P < 0.01$ ANOVA with Dunnett's multiple comparison test versus control). Treatment with the AHR antagonist, CB7993113 (10 µM), reduced the 35 KD band, but not the 43 KD TDP-43 band (Fig. 1) [30, 31]. The reasons why CB7993113 does not inhibit the TDP-43 full-length protein catabolism are unknown and might reflect differential responsiveness of the particular AHR heterodimers present in the M17 line. AhR acts in concert with the aryl hydrocarbon receptor nuclear translocator (ARNT) to stimulate transcription, but expression of ARNT varies by condition, tissue or cell line, and with this variation comes variations in responses to agonists and antagonists [37]. How ligands regulate

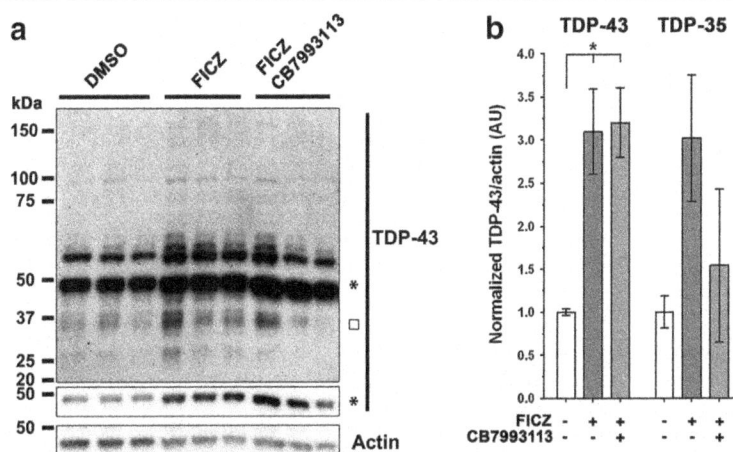

Fig. 1 FICZ treatment of M17 cells increases endogenous TDP-43 expression. a Immunoblots of total lysates of M17 neuroblastoma cells, differentiated for 7 days in 10 µM RA, then treated for 7 days with AHR agonist FICZ (0.5 µM) or with FICZ and CB7993113, the antagonist (10 µM). Densitometry of monomeric TDP-43 (*) and the C-terminal fragment TDP-35 (□) shown in panel A immunoblots were quantified in b (N = 3; mean ± SEM, ANOVA w/ Tukey's; ** P < 0.01, * P < 0.05). FICZ agonism increases these TDP-43 entities and higher molecular weight species (# in panel a)

the varied states of this complex is unknown. The low efficacy of CB7993113 in M17 cells contrasts with the robust inhibition by CB7993113 observed in human motor neuron derived iPSCs shown below in Figs. 2, 3 and 4, which could reflect differential regulation of AhR as it interacts with other binding partners, such as ARNT. Regardless, these data demonstrate that agonist-mediated activation of AHR elicits robust increases in TDP-43 protein.

The differential sensitivity of the 43 and 35 KD TPD-43 bands to CB7993113 inhibition prompted us to investigate the requirement for AHR further. We proceeded to use knockdown of the AHR as a genetic means to test whether the actions of FICZ were mediated by AHR. The additional shAHR-mediated knockdown experiments clearly demonstrated that the response to FICZ was AHR-dependent. We generated

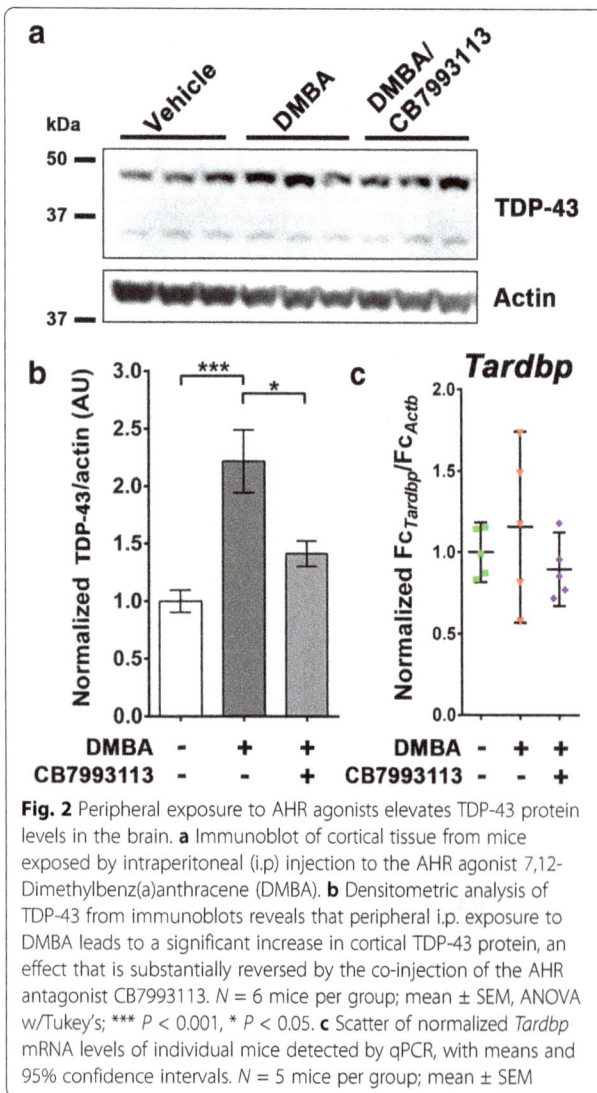

Fig. 3 Benzo(a)pyrene treatment increases endogenous TDP-43 levels in M17 cells and in the murine brain. **a** Immunoblot of total lysates of M17 neuroblastoma cells, differentiated for 7 days in 10 μM RA, then treated for 7 days with vehicle, the AHR-activating toxin Benzo(a)pyrene (B(a)P; 10 μM), or with B(a)P and CB7993113, the AHR antagonist (10 μM). **b** Immunoblot of cortical tissue from mice exposed by intraperitoneal (i.p) injection to the AHR agonist Benzo(a)pyrene. Densitometry of monomeric TDP-43 bands shown in the immunoblots were quantified in **c** for the M17 cell samples ($N = 3$; mean ± SEM, ANOVA w/ Tukey's; ** $P < 0.01$) and in **d** (for the murine cortical tissue ($N = 4$; mean ± SEM, ANOVA w/Tukey's; ** $P < 0.01$, * $P < 0.05$). The environmental toxin, B(a)P, increases levels of endogenous TDP-43 protein in both cultured human cells and in the brains of mice exposure by intraperitoneal injection. This increase is substantially reversed in each model system by co-treatment with the AHR antagonist CB7993113

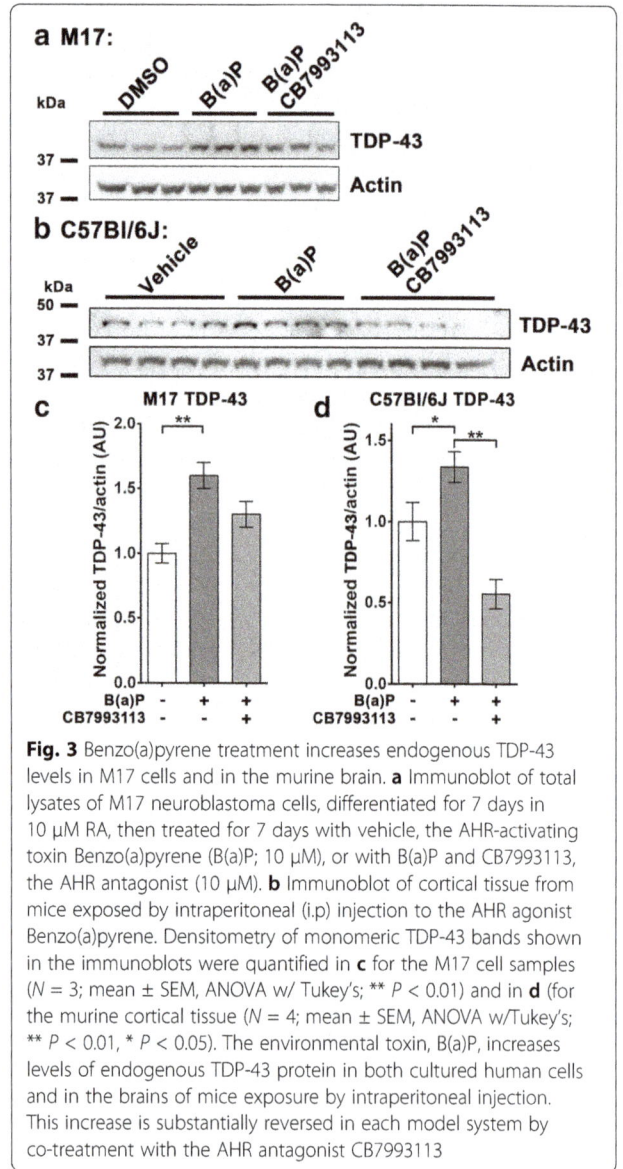

Fig. 2 Peripheral exposure to AHR agonists elevates TDP-43 protein levels in the brain. **a** Immunoblot of cortical tissue from mice exposed by intraperitoneal (i.p) injection to the AHR agonist 7,12-Dimethylbenz(a)anthracene (DMBA). **b** Densitometric analysis of TDP-43 from immunoblots reveals that peripheral i.p. exposure to DMBA leads to a significant increase in cortical TDP-43 protein, an effect that is substantially reversed by the co-injection of the AHR antagonist CB7993113. $N = 6$ mice per group; mean ± SEM, ANOVA w/Tukey's; *** $P < 0.001$, * $P < 0.05$. **c** Scatter of normalized *Tardbp* mRNA levels of individual mice detected by qPCR, with means and 95% confidence intervals. $N = 5$ mice per group; mean ± SEM

a line of M17 neuroblastoma cells that stably expressed doxycycline-inducible shAHR (Additional file 3: Figure S1). Under basal conditions, these cells responded to treatment with 0.5 μM FICZ treatment with a significant increase in endogenous TDP-43 protein (DMSO = 1.00 AU, s.d. 0.280; FICZ = 2.00 AU, s.d. 0.063; $n = 3$; $P < 0.001$, ANOVA with Tukey's posthoc test). Induction of the shAHR by addition of doxycycline (1 μg/ml) for 72 h significantly reduced the FICZ-mediated increase in TDP-43 (Additional file 3: Figure S1; FICZ/Dox = 1.52 AU, s.d. 0.036 $n = 3$, $P < 0.05$, ANOVA with Tukey's posthoc versus FICZ only). This data further confirm that TDP-43 expression is responsive to AHR agonists and that the observed increase in TDP-43 is AHR dependent.

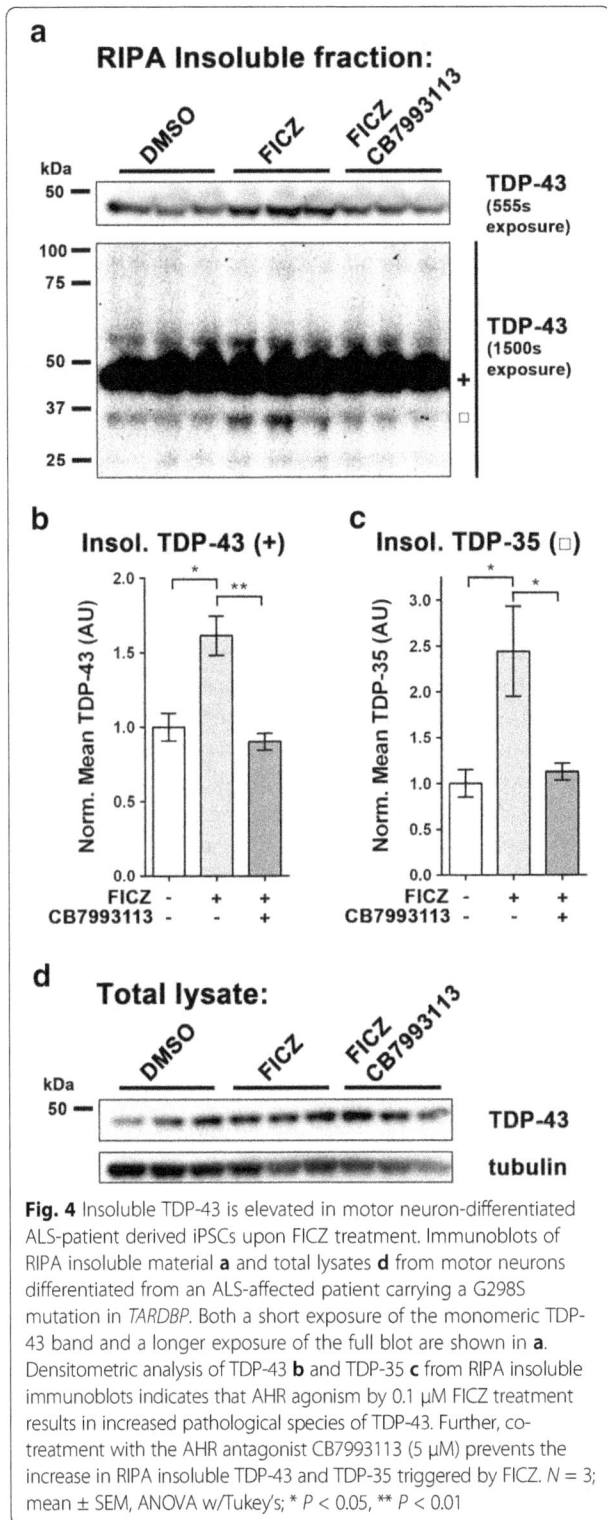

Fig. 4 Insoluble TDP-43 is elevated in motor neuron-differentiated ALS-patient derived iPSCs upon FICZ treatment. Immunoblots of RIPA insoluble material **a** and total lysates **d** from motor neurons differentiated from an ALS-affected patient carrying a G298S mutation in *TARDBP*. Both a short exposure of the monomeric TDP-43 band and a longer exposure of the full blot are shown in **a**. Densitometric analysis of TDP-43 **b** and TDP-35 **c** from RIPA insoluble immunoblots indicates that AHR agonism by 0.1 μM FICZ treatment results in increased pathological species of TDP-43. Further, co-treatment with the AHR antagonist CB7993113 (5 μM) prevents the increase in RIPA insoluble TDP-43 and TDP-35 triggered by FICZ. $N = 3$; mean ± SEM, ANOVA w/Tukey's; * $P < 0.05$, ** $P < 0.01$

when administered to mice by intra-peritoneal (i.p.) injection [38]. We used this prior study as a guide to investigate whether a similar peripheral administration of DMBA could lead to the induction of TDP-43 in the CNS of mice. Male C57Bl/6 J mice were treated in three groups ($n = 11$ per group) with i.p. injection of: 1) vehicle, 2) 100 mg/kg DMBA or 3) DMBA together with 200 mg/kg CB7993113 (split into two doses). The brains were harvested after 30 h and dissected; 20-30 mg tissue sections of liver and spleen were also collected. Cortical protein levels were determined by immunoblotting of total tissue lysates followed by densitometric analysis. Cortical TDP-43 protein was significantly increased upon exposure to DMBA (Fig. 2a, b; vehicle = 1.00 AU, s.d. 0.238; DMBA = 2.22 AU, s.d. 0.669; $n = 6$; $P < 0.001$, ANOVA with Tukey's posthoc test) and co-treatment with CB7993113 significantly reduced this increase (Fig. 2a, b; DMBA/CB = 1.41 AU, s.d. 0.267; $n = 6$; $P < 0.05$, ANOVA with Tukey's posthoc test versus DMBA). qPCR analysis of transcript changes of the somatosensory cortex of these mice revealed increased *Cyp1a1* and *Cyp1b1* upon exposure to DMBA (data not shown).

DMBA also elicited a trend towards increased *Tardbp* transcription (Fig. 2c). Further investigations into transcriptional mechanisms are described below. Interestingly, DMBA treatment greatly increased subject variability compared to the vehicle only group (vehicle range = 0.836–1.153, s.d. = 0.147, DMSO range = 0.578–1.734, s.d = 0.473, DMSO/CB range = 0.720–1.179, s.d = 0.182; $n = 5$). The Brown-Forsythe test indicates the standard deviations of the treatment groups are significantly different ($P = 0.0495$). Comparing variance in the DMBA group to that in the vehicle group (F-test) indicates significantly unequal variation ($P = 0.0442$). The increased variance is consistent with DMBA priming (and in some cases inducing) *Tardbp* transcription, making it more responsive to potentially concurrent stimuli. Co-treating mice with DMBA and the antagonist CB7993113 reduced the variability between the individual animals (Fig. 2c), with the f-test detecting no difference in standard deviation between the vehicle and DMBA/CB7993113 treated groups.

C57BL/6 mice treated with DMBA did not show significantly increased levels of α-synuclein, Ataxin-2 or VCP protein in the cortex (Additional file 3: Figure S2A-D). These data suggest that TDP-43 exhibits a selective response to AHR activation.

B(a)P, a representative environmental PAH class toxicant also increases cortical TDP-43 in vivo

Having demonstrated the in vivo activity of DMBA, we proceeded to test whether a AHR agonist that is a documented environmental contaminant also increases levels

DMBA, a prototypic PAH, increases cortical TDP-43 in vivo

Previous reports demonstrate that the polycyclic aromatic hydrocarbon, 7,12-Dimethylbenz(a)anthracene (DMBA), increases expression of *Cyp1a1* in the brain of TDP-43. We examined the actions of benzo(a)pyrene (B(a)P), which is a representative environmental PAH and AHR agonist found in cigarette smoke, (54). We began by examining the effects of B(a)P on human neuroblastoma M17 cells, using the same protocol as described above for FICZ. The cells were differentiated for 7 days in 3% FBS media with 10 μM retinoic acid and treated for a further 7 days with vehicle, B(a)P (10 μM) or B(a)P plus CB7993113 (10 μM). The cells were then harvested and TDP-43 immunoblotted (Fig. 3). Exposure to B(a)P increased levels of TDP-43 by >50% (Fig. 3a, c; control = 1.00 AU, s.d. 0.132; B(a)P = 1.60 AU, s.d. 0.174 n = 3; $P < 0.01$, ANOVA with Tukey's posthoc test), while TDP-43 levels did not show a statistically significant increase when co-treated with B(a)P and CB7993113 (Fig. 3a, c; B(a)P/CB = 1.30 AU, s.d. 0.171;).

Next we investigated whether a similar peripheral administration of B(a)P could lead to the induction of TDP-43 in the CNS of mice, similar to that observed for DMBA. Male C57Bl/6 J mice were treated in three groups (n = 4 per group) with i.p. injection of: 1) vehicle, 2) 100 mg/kg B(a)P or 3) B(a)P together with 200 mg/kg CB7993113 (split into two doses). The brains were harvested after 30 h and dissected. Cortical protein levels were determined by immunoblotting of total tissue lysates followed by densitometric analysis. Cortical TDP-43 protein was significantly increased upon exposure to B(a)P (Fig. 3b, d; vehicle = 1.00 AU, s.d. 0.234; B(a)P = 1.34 AU, s.d. 0.189 n = 4; $P < 0.05$, ANOVA with Tukey's posthoc test) while co-treatment with CB7993113 greatly reduced this increase (Fig. 2a, b; B(a)P/CB = 0.55 AU, s.d. 0.181; n = 4; $P < 0.001$, ANOVA with Tukey's posthoc test versus B(a)P). These data indicate that peripheral exposure to two different PAHs are able to significantly increase levels of TDP-43 in the CNS.

Neuronally differentiated ALS-patient derived iPSCs accumulate insoluble TDP-43 when treated with AHR agonist

We have previously established an induced pluripotent stem cell line (iPSC) from an ALS-affected individual carrying a G298S mutation in the *TARDBP* gene and a protocol for differentiating them into class III β-tubulin, DLX/HB9 positive motor neurons [32]. Over an extended (25 days) culture period, these iPSC-derived motor neurons (MN-iPSCs) progressively accumulate insoluble TDP-43 as well as high-molecular weight and proteolytically cleaved species of TDP-43. We used this protocol to test the effects of an AHR agonist on MN-iPSCs. The human G298S TDP-43 MN-iPSCs were grown for 15 days and then treated with 0.1 μM FICZ for a period of 10 days. Cells were harvested and fractionated to yield total and RIPA insoluble protein

fractions. Each fraction was immunoblotted and bands quantified by densitometry. Treatment with the AHR ligand FICZ led to a significant elevation of monomeric TDP-43 and the 35 kDa TDP-43 cleavage product (Fig. 4a-d; DMSO = 1.00 AU, s.d. 0.1610; FICZ = 1.62, s.d. 0.229; n = 3; $P < 0.05$ ANOVA with Tukey's multiple comparison test) (Fig. 4a-d). Concurrently treating with FICZ and 5 μM CB793113 prevented the increase in TDP-43 land TDP-35 demonstrating the contribution of the AHR for these increases. These data demonstrate that exposure of human motor neurons to AHR agonists increases total and insoluble TDP-43 pools.

AHR activates the TARDBP promoter

Next we sought to determine the mechanism through which AHR agonists might increase levels of TDP-43 protein. The AHR acts as a ligand-dependent, PER/ARNT/SIM (PAS) family transcription factor. Upon ligand binding, the AHR translocates to the nucleus and recruits co-factors to the appropriate AHR responsive elements (AHREs) to effect gene expression [39, 40]. Alternative AHR signaling pathways, not mediated through AHRE binding or transcriptional regulation, have also been described [31, 41–43] and suggest a larger constellation of AHR-mediated biologic outcomes than previously appreciated. The canonical action of AHR is described by induction of the cytochrome P450 enzymes, including CYP1A1 and CYP1B1, which are responsible for metabolizing some, but not all, AHR ligands. AHR is expressed throughout the brain (Allen brain atlas, mouse.brain-map.org/experiment/show/71380375). In addition, previous reports demonstrate that intra-peritoneal delivery of AHR ligands increases *Cyp1a1* and *Cyp1b1* transcript levels in the brain [38].

Bioinformatic analysis identified multiple AHR responsive elements (AHREs) in the promoter regions of the ALS-relevant gene *TARDBP*. Clusters of the consensus sequence "5′-GCGTG-3′" [44, 45], similar to those observed in the canonically AHR targeted metabolic genes *CYP1A1* and *CYP1B1*, are present within 5000 base pairs of the transcription start sites (Fig. 5a). The presence of canonical AHR consensus sequences in the *TARDBP* promoter raised the possibility that AHR was directly increasing *TARDBP* transcription.

To test this possibility, we first generated a *TARDBP*-promoter luciferase reporter to determine whether the AHR could actively stimulate transcription through binding sites in the *TARDBP* promoter (Fig. 5a). The luciferase reporter, "*TARDBP*_-4.1 kb/*luc2*", was generated with 4.1 kb of the human *TARDBP* promoter sequence upstream of the translation start site fused to *luc2*. Luciferase reporters containing known AHR-responsive promoters were used as positive controls for AHR

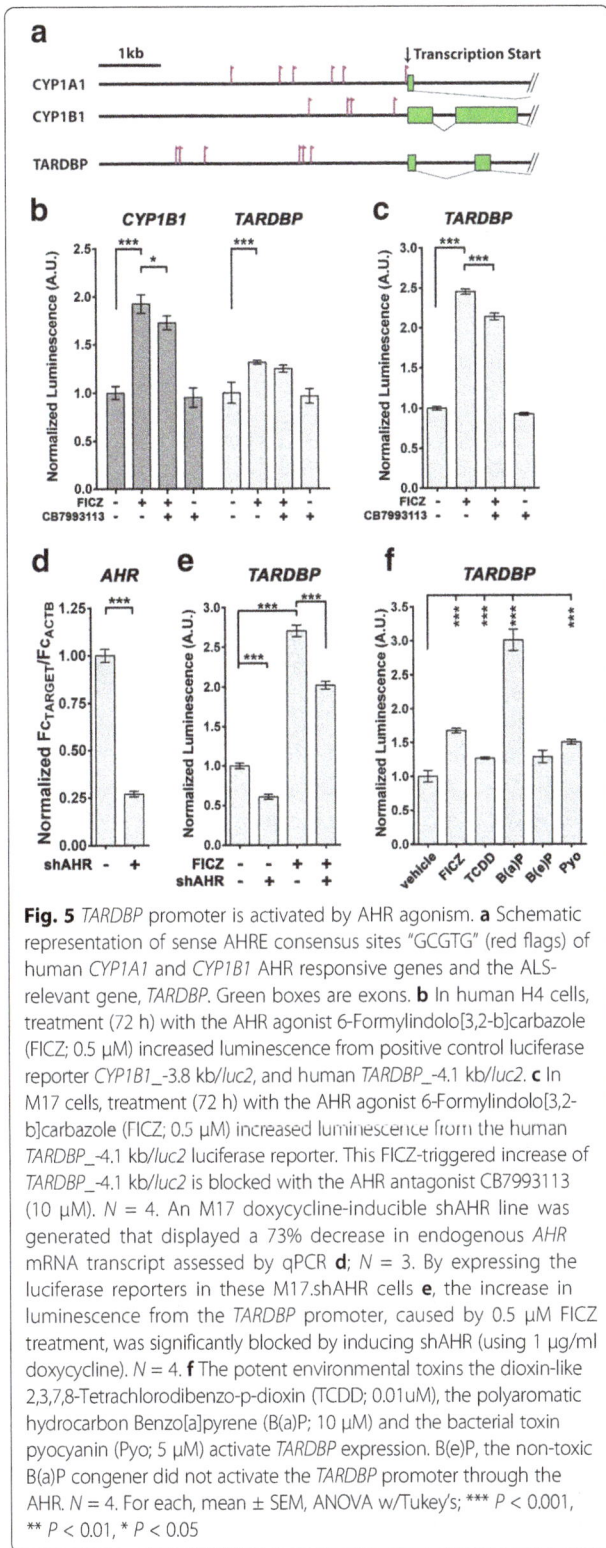

Fig. 5 *TARDBP* promoter is activated by AHR agonism. **a** Schematic representation of sense AHRE consensus sites "GCGTG" (red flags) of human *CYP1A1* and *CYP1B1* AHR responsive genes and the ALS-relevant gene, *TARDBP*. Green boxes are exons. **b** In human H4 cells, treatment (72 h) with the AHR agonist 6-Formylindolo[3,2-b]carbazole (FICZ; 0.5 μM) increased luminescence from positive control luciferase reporter *CYP1B1*_-3.8 kb/*luc2*, and human *TARDBP*_-4.1 kb/*luc2*. **c** In M17 cells, treatment (72 h) with the AHR agonist 6-Formylindolo[3,2-b]carbazole (FICZ; 0.5 μM) increased luminescence from the human *TARDBP*_-4.1 kb/*luc2* luciferase reporter. This FICZ-triggered increase of *TARDBP*_-4.1 kb/*luc2* is blocked with the AHR antagonist CB7993113 (10 μM). N = 4. An M17 doxycycline-inducible shAHR line was generated that displayed a 73% decrease in endogenous *AHR* mRNA transcript assessed by qPCR **d**; N = 3. By expressing the luciferase reporters in these M17.shAHR cells **e**, the increase in luminescence from the *TARDBP* promoter, caused by 0.5 μM FICZ treatment, was significantly blocked by inducing shAHR (using 1 μg/ml doxycycline). N = 4. **f** The potent environmental toxins the dioxin-like 2,3,7,8-Tetrachlorodibenzo-p-dioxin (TCDD; 0.01uM), the polyaromatic hydrocarbon Benzo[a]pyrene (B(a)P; 10 μM) and the bacterial toxin pyocyanin (Pyo; 5 μM) activate *TARDBP* expression. B(e)P, the non-toxic B(a)P congener did not activate the *TARDBP* promoter through the AHR. N = 4. For each, mean ± SEM, ANOVA w/Tukey's; *** $P < 0.001$, ** $P < 0.01$, * $P < 0.05$

described dioxin-responsive *pGudLuc1.1* reporter, consisting of the putative AHREs of the mouse *Cyp1a1* gene [46], was also used as a positive control (data not shown).

Human H4 neuroglioma cells (Fig. 5b) and M17 neuroblasmtoma cells (Fig. 5c) were transfected with these reporters and treated for 72 h with the AHR agonist FICZ (0.5 μM) with or without the previously described competitive AHR inhibitor, CB7993113 (10 μM), with DMSO as a vehicle control [30, 31]. As expected, the *CYP1B1*_-3.8 kb/*luc2* reporter responded to the presence of FICZ with significantly increased luciferase expression (Fig. 5b). FICZ treatment of H4 cells expressing the *TARDBP*_-4.1 kb/*luc2* reporter also lead to a significant increase in luciferase luminescence (Fig. 5b; DMSO vehicle control = 1.00 AU, s.d. 0.107; FICZ = 1.32 AU, s.d. 0.019; n = 4; P < 0.001). Similarly, M17 cells expressing the *TARDBP*_-4.1 kb/*luc2* reporter showed a significant increase in luciferase in response to treatment with FICZ (Fig. 5c; DMSO vehicle control = 1.00 AU, s.d. 0.024; FICZ = 2.46 AU, s.d. 0.033; n = 4; P < 0.001). Further, in the M17 cells, CB7993113 significantly blocked FICZ-induced upregulation of *TARDBP*_-4.1 kb/*luc2* transcription (FIZC/CB = 2.143 AU, s.d. 0.044; n = 4; P < 0.001 versus FICZ alone, ANOVA with Tukey's multiple comparison test). CB7993113 tended to decrease the induction of TARDBP in H4 cells, although statistical significance was not reached in this series of experiments (Fig. 5a).

To confirm AHR regulation of the *TARDBP* promoter reporter construct, we generated M17 lines stably expressing a tetracycline-inducible shAHR construct. Addition of doxycycline (1 μg/ml) to M17.shAHR cells for 72 h resulted in a significant 73% reduction of *AHR* mRNA (Fig. 5d; s.d. 0.026; n = 3; p < 0.001 t-test). Interestingly, AHR knockdown significantly reduced the TARDBP reporter activity suggesting that the more efficient decrease in AHR activity see with shAHR, as compared with CB7993113, may be enough to reduce baseline levels of AHR-driven TARDBP transcription. Treatment with 0.5 μM FICZ significantly increased reporter activity as compared to vehicle controls (Fig. 5e, DMSO = 1.00 AU, s.d. 0.036; FICZ = 2.71 AU, s.d. 0.073 n = 4; p < 0.001, ANOVA with Tukey's posthoc test) and shAHR-induction with doxycycline significantly blocked FICZ-mediated *TARDBP* reporter activity (FICZ/Dox = 2.02 AU, s.d. 0.049 n = 4, P < 0.001 ANOVA with Tukey's posthoc versus FICZ only). These data demonstrate that the *TARDBP* promoter is responsive to the FICZ in an AHR-dependent manner.

Potent environmental toxicants activate the TARDBP promoter

The studies above demonstrate that AHR activates the *TARDBP* promoter and contributes to expression of

activation. A positive control luciferase reporter, "*CYP1B1*_-3.8 kb/*luc2*", was generated with 3.8 kb of the human *CYP1B1* promoter sequence upstream of the translation start site fused to *luc2*. The previously baseline levels of *TARDBP* transcript. Next, we used the *CYP1B1*-specific and *TARDBP*_-4.1 kb/*luc2* luciferase reporters to screen a number of potent environmental AHR ligands for their ability to induce reporter activity. H4 cells were used because the M17 cells were highly susceptible to these toxicants and few survived. As before, transfected cells were treated for 72 h with 0.5 μM FICZ, 0.01 μM TCDD, the most potent and persistent environmental AHR ligand, 10 μM benzo(a)pyrene (B(a)P), a representative environmental PAH and AHR agonist found in cigarette smoke, 10 μM benzo(e)pyrene (B(e)P), a non-toxic B(a)P congener that does not active the AHR, and 5 μM pyocyanin, a microbiome-derived AHR ligand (54). FICZ, TCDD, B(a)P, and pyocyanin all increased *CYP1B1*- and *TARDBP* promoter-driven reporter activity as compared with vehicle (DMSO) controls (Fig. 5f; $P < 0.001$, Additional file 3: Figure S3).

Interestingly, *TARDBP* promoter usage was significantly upregulated by 26.6% by 0.01 μM TCDD (Fig. 5f; s.d. 0.016; $n = 4$; $P < 0.001$), even more robustly by 10 μM B(a)P (300.9%, s.d. 0.157; $n = 4$; $P < 0.001$) and by 5 μM pyocyanin (50.3%, s.d. 0.035; $n = 4$; $P < 0.001$) suggesting that environmentally relevant toxins can upregulate TDP-43 expression. Importantly, Benzo(e)pyrene, the non-toxic congener of B(a)P, had no effect on the *TARDBP* promoter driven luciferase reporter (Fig. 5f, Additional file 3: Figure S3). These data indicate that classic environmental toxicants, a putative endogenous ligand, and, to a lesser extent, a microbiome-derived ligand, activate the AHR in neuronal-derived cells and are able to stimulate *TARDBP* expression.

AHR agonism modestly increases levels of endogenous TARDBP, SOD1, PON2 and C9ORF72 transcripts

Many promoters of genes linked to ALS contain multiple AHR-responsive elements (AHREs)(Additional file 3: Figure S5). To determine whether these promoters are AHR-responsive, we investigated whether AHR agonists increase expression of endogenous *TARDBP* transcript and other transcripts related to ALS, including *SOD1, PON2, C9ORF72, FUS* and *ATXN-2*.

H4 cells were treated for 48 h with vehicle or 0.5 μM FICZ and the levels of *TARDBP, SOD1, PON2, C9ORF72, FUS* and *ATXN2* and *PON2* transcripts were measured by quantitative PCR (qPCR). FICZ treatment led to a substantial increase in transcription of *CYP1B1* ($P < 0.001$), *TARDBP* ($P < 0.05$), *SOD1* ($P < 0.05$), *PON2* ($P < 0.01$) and *C9ORF72* ($P < 0.05$) compared to vehicle-treated control samples (Fig. 6). While *FUS* expression tended to increase, statistical significance was not reached. FICZ had no significant effect on *ATXN-2* expression. These data indicate that AHR agonists can increase transcription of a variety of genes linked to ALS. However, the relatively small change in *TARDBP*

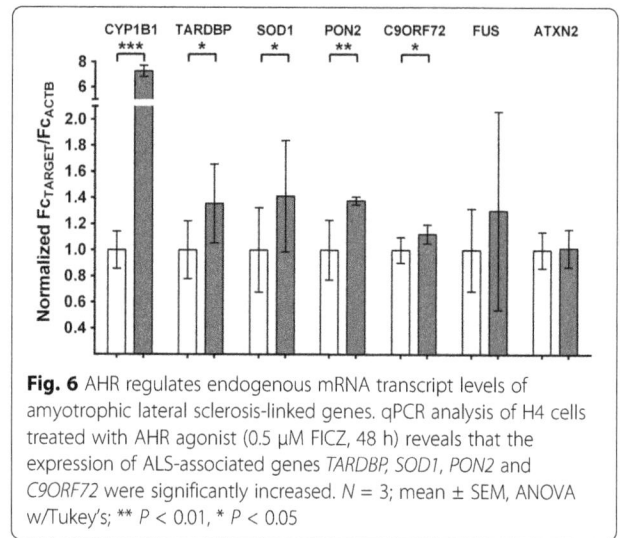

Fig. 6 AHR regulates endogenous mRNA transcript levels of amyotrophic lateral sclerosis-linked genes. qPCR analysis of H4 cells treated with AHR agonist (0.5 μM FICZ, 48 h) reveals that the expression of ALS-associated genes *TARDBP, SOD1, PON2* and *C9ORF72* were significantly increased. $N = 3$; mean ± SEM, ANOVA w/Tukey's; ** $P < 0.01$, * $P < 0.05$

transcript (~35%) (Fig. 6) stands in stark contrast to the 2–3-fold increase in TDP-43 protein observed upon treatment with FICZ or DMBA (e.g., Fig. 1).

AHR agonism increases stability of endogenous TDP-43

The ability of AHR agonists to increase TDP-43 protein more than *TARDBP* transcript expression raised the possibility that AHR agonists increase TDP-43 levels through post-transcriptional mechanisms. To investigate this question, the synthesis and degradation of nascent TDP-43 protein was measured using Click-iT labeling ±0.5 μM FICZ. Click-iT chemistry utilizes a 2 h pulse of L-Azidohomoalanine (AHA) in methionine-starved cells to incorporate this azide tagged metabolite into nascent proteins. The AHA-labeled proteins in the cell lysates were subsequently chemoselectively ligated to a Biotin alkyne, and the labeled proteins selectively isolated using avidin-agarose affinity purification.

Biotinylated-nascent proteins ("clicked" input lysates shown in Additional file 3: Figure S4A) were affinity purified in triplicate from differentiated M17 cells pulsed for 2 h with Click-iT AHA metabolite then chased for 0 h (2 h from Start of Pulse), 2 h (4 h from Start of Pulse), 4 h (6 h from Start of Pulse), 10 h (12 h from Start of Pulse), and 22 h (24 h from Start of Pulse). Immunoblots of affinity purified material revealed that, while the rate of translation of TDP-43 in 0.5 μM FICZ-treated cells during the 2 h pulse was not significantly elevated, the stability of labeled TDP-43 across the 24 h chase period was significantly increased (Fig. 7a). To facilitate quantification of labeled TP-43 across the time points, affinity purified material was analyzed by dot blot using a highly specific TDP-43 antibody (Additional file 3: Figure S4C, D and E). Mean signal intensities were normalized to the mean of DMSO-treated samples from

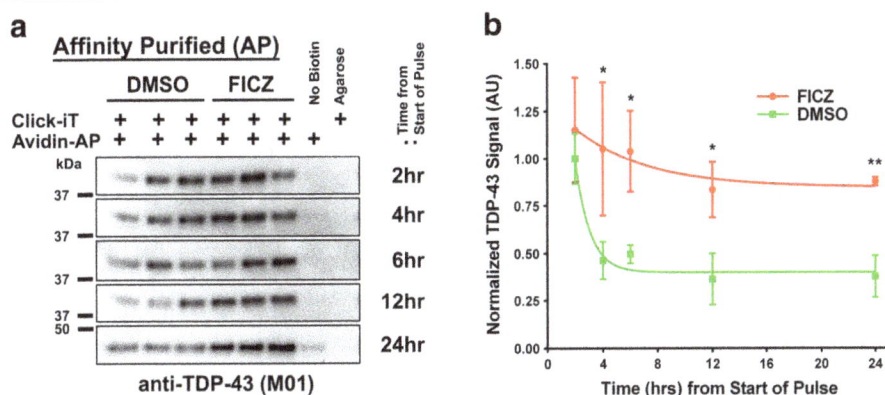

Fig. 7 FICZ treatment of M17 cells increases endogenous TDP-43 stability. **a** Immunoblots of Avidin-agarose affinity purified (Avidin-AP) Click-iT AHA-labelled nascent proteins from lysates treated with DMSO vehicle or 0.5 μM FICZ, with a 2 h pulse of Click-iT AHA-labeling of endogenous nascent proteins then (by row) periods of culture in the absence of the Click-iT metabolite to observe degradation of AHA labelled nascent proteins. Blots are probed with anti-TARDBP antibody (see Additional file 3: Figure S4C). As negative controls for Avidin-AP, a representative sample from each time point, processed using the Click-iT chemistry but in the absence of the Biotin-alkyne chemoselective ligation tag, was also affinity purified against avidin-agarose (lanes 7: "No Biotin"). A further representative sample ligated using the Biotin-alkyne was affinity purified against control agarose resin as an additional negative control (lanes 8: "Agarose"). Densitometry of TDP-43 signal from dot blots (Additional file 3: Figure S4D) were quantified in **b** (*n* = 3; mean ± sd, curves fit by non-linear regression; t-tests were also performed for each data time point DMSO vs FICZ, ** *P* < 0.01, * *P* < 0.05). FICZ agonism of AHR increases the stability of TDP-43

the "2 h from Start of Pulse" group then plotted. A non-linear regression curve (one phase exponential decay; GraphPad) was fit to the mean TDP-43 signals of both the DMSO- and FICZ-treated sample across the time points (Fig. 7b). A comparison of fit (with the null hypothesis that one curve is descriptive of both data sets) revealed a statistical significance (*P* < 0.001) difference between the rate of degradation of TDP-43 in DMSO- and FICZ-treated M17 cells. Thus, treatment of M17 cells with 0.5 μM FICZ led to an increase in the stability of TDP-43 as compared to vehicle controls.

Discussion

AHR agonists constitute some of the most dangerous environmental contaminants, including dioxins and PCBs. The Environmental Protection Agency (EPA) and World Health Organization (WHO) indicate that exposure to dioxin and other AHR ligands is widespread. These toxins have long half-lives when absorbed in fatty tissues and can bio-accumulate in the food chain [47]. Importantly, PCB and airborne aromatic exposures are linked to an increased risk of ALS, but the mechanism underlying the risk is unknown [15, 16]. Our results demonstrate that AHR agonists increase levels of TDP-43 protein. We demonstrate this phenomenon through multiple independent methods and approaches, examining transcript and/or protein in human MN iPSCs, human cell lines and mouse brain. For levels of TDP-43 protein, longer exposure to AHR ligands leads to stronger effects, with increases in insoluble TDP-43 strongly evident after chronic exposure. Although dioxins and

PAHs can increase the levels of *TARDBP* transcript modestly, the predominant mechanism of action appears to occur through reduced TDP-43 turnover.

The ability of AHR agonists to increase levels of TDP-43 RNA and protein is notable, because TDP-43 expression is tightly regulated. The TDP-43 protein binds and auto-regulates the stability of its own transcript through a mechanism dependent upon the 3'UTR [48]. For instance, over-expressing transgenic TDP-43 without 3' UTR leads to compensatory decreases in endogenous TDP-43, apparently through nonsense-mediated RNA decay. Perhaps because of this, few other genes have been noted to modulate TDP-43 transcript levels.

The control of TDP-43 protein levels, though, is more nuanced. TDP-43 protein can be regulated at the level of protein synthesis or degradation. In addition, TDP-43 protein can increase in the soluble pool, accumulate in an insoluble pool and/or can be cleaved to produce smaller fragments that also have a tendency to aggregate [36]. Because the increases in TDP-43 protein were greater than the increases in *TARDP* transcript, we directly measured TDP-43 translation, using pulse labeling with Click-IT technology. The results demonstrated no change in TDP-43 production following AHR ligand treatment, but greatly reduced TDP-43 catabolism (Fig. 7b). In contrast, neither α-synuclein, ataxin-2 nor VCP showed changes in protein levels in response to AHR agonists. The differential sensitivity of TDP-43 to AHR agonists compared to these other proteins suggests that the mechanism through which AHR agonists regulate TDP-43 turnover is specific to

TDP-43 and does not reflect a generalized increase in activity of the autolysosomal or ubiquitin-proteasomal systems.

Many prior experiments show that increasing expression levels of genes linked to neurodegenerative diseases accelerates the pathophysiology of disease. Increased TDP-43 expression by transgenic over-expression induces disease in animal models [49]; the relationship between expression level and disease is also apparent for genes linked to other diseases including α-synuclein (Parkinson's disease, amyloid precursor protein (Alzheimer's disease) and microtubule associated protein tau (frontotemporal dementia) [50]. In addition, genetic factors that increase expression of α-synuclein (gene duplication, triplication or polymorphisms) or β-amyloid (mutations in amyloid precursor protein or presenilins) explicitly cause disease in humans. The ability of AHR agonists to increase insoluble TDP-43 raises the possibility that they could potentiate the pathophysiology of ALS since the accumulation of insoluble TDP-43 is the predominant aggregating species in ALS, and mutations in TDP-43 that increase accumulation of insoluble TDP-43 are sufficient to cause disease in humans. It is notable that FICZ also increased expression of SOD1 and showed a trend for FUS, which raises the possibility that environmental AHR ligands might impact on a variety of genes linked to ALS and be an important environmental modifier of disease incidence or progression.

Increasing evidence suggests that cases of neurodegenerative disease labeled as sporadic might reflect the accumulated effects of multiple risk factors [51]. Each risk factor would contribute incrementally to the risk of ALS with the convergence of multiple risk factors achieving a threshold sufficient to initiate the pathophysiology of ALS. In this context, the increase in TDP-43 associated with exposure to AHR ligands could contribute to a cumulative risk score, overcoming the threshold for initiation of disease.

Conclusions

Epidemiological studies suggest that dioxins are associated with increased risk of ALS. Demonstration that dioxin/PCB family environmental toxicants increase the accumulation of TARDBP transcript and TDP-43 protein provides a mechanism for this epidemiological observation, and supports the hypothesis that compounds in the dioxin/PCB family are able to increase the expression and accumulation of TDP-43, which in turn potentiates the pathophysiology of ALS. Taken together, these studies suggest a new public health risk associated with dioxins, PCBs and other ubiquitous AHR ligands, which could represent risk factors that act alone or interact with other genetic, viral or behavioral risk factors to increase the risk of ALS.

Additional files

Additional file 1: Table S1.

Additional file 2: Table S2.

Additional file 3: Figure S1. Elevation of endogenous TDP-43 is dependent upon AHR expression. Figure S2. The effect on TDP-43 protein levels in the brain of peripheral exposure to AHR agonists is not observed with other disease related proteins. Figure S3. TARDBP promoter is activated by AHR agonism. Figure S4. Click-iT pulse-chase labelling of nascent proteins in differentiated M17 cells. Figure S5. Schematic representation of sense AHRE consensus sites "GCGTG" (red flags) of human CYP1A1 and CYP1B1 AHR responsive genes and the ALS-relevant genes TARDBP, SOD1, PON2, C9ORF72, FUS and ATXN2, assayed for changes in transcript levels in Fig. 2. Green boxes are exons.

Abbreviations
AHR: Aryl hydrocarbon receptor; AHRE: Consensus AHR response element; ALS: Amyotrophic lateral sclerosis; B(a)P: Benzo(a)pyrene; BMAA: β-Methylamino-L-alanine; DMBA: 7,12-dimethylbenz(a)anthracene; EPA: Environmental Protection Agency; FICZ: 6-Formylindolo[3,2-b]carbazole; PAHs: Polycyclic aromatic hydrocarbons; PCBs: Polychlorinated biphenyls; PAS: PER/ARNT/SIM family transcription factor; TDP-43, gene: TARDBP; TAR: DNA Binding Protein-43; WHO: World Health Organization.

Acknowledgements
Not applicable

Funding
Was provided by the following agencies and foundations: PA: American Parkinson Disease Association Post-Doctoral Fellowship. BW: NIEHS (ES020395), NINDS (NS089544), NIA (AG050471), Alzheimer Association, Brightfocus Foundation, and the CureAlzheimer Foundation.

Authors' contributions
PEAA designed experiments, performed most of the experiments, wrote the manuscript and analyzed the data. EAS, AAA, SB, AR-C, HIB, AJ, JMM contributed to experiments. YT provided statistical oversight. GJM directed experiments related to the iPSC work. DHS, BW conceived of the project, designed experiments, co-wrote and edited the manuscript, and helped to analyze the data. All authors read and approved the final manuscript.

Competing interests
Benjamin Wolozin is a co-founder and chief scientific officer for Aquinnah Pharmaceuticals Inc.

Author details
[1]Department of Pharmacology, Boston University School of Medicine, 72 East Concord St., R614, Boston, MA 02118-2526, USA. [2]Department of Environmental Health, Boston University School of Public Health, Boston, MA 02118, USA. [3]Center for Regenerative Medicine, Boston University, Boston, MA 02118, USA. [4]Department of Biostatistics, Boston University School of Public Health, Boston, MA 02118, USA. [5]Department of Neurology, Boston University School of Medicine, 72 East Concord St., R614, Boston, MA 02118-2526, USA.

References
1. Ling SC, Polymenidou M, Cleveland DW. Converging mechanisms in ALS and FTD: disrupted RNA and protein homeostasis. Neuron. 2013;79:416–38.
2. Oskarsson B, Horton DK, Mitsumoto H. Potential environmental factors in amyotrophic lateral sclerosis. Neurol Clin. 2015;33:877–88.

3. de Jong SW, Huisman MH, Sutedja NA, van der Kooi AJ, de Visser M, Schelhaas HJ, Fischer K, Veldink JH, van den Berg LH. Smoking, alcohol consumption, and the risk of amyotrophic lateral sclerosis: a population-based study. Am J Epidemiol. 2012;176:233–9.

4. Wang H, O'Reilly EJ, Weisskopf MG, Logroscino G, McCullough ML, Thun MJ, Schatzkin A, Kolonel LN, Ascherio A. Smoking and risk of amyotrophic lateral sclerosis: a pooled analysis of 5 prospective cohorts. Arch Neurol. 2011;68:207–13.

5. Das K, Nag C, Ghosh M. Familial, environmental, and occupational risk factors in development of amyotrophic lateral sclerosis. N Am J Med Sci. 2012;4:350–5.

6. Morozova N, Weisskopf MG, McCullough ML, Munger KL, Calle EE, Thun MJ, Ascherio A. Diet and amyotrophic lateral sclerosis. Epidemiology. 2008; 19:324–37.

7. Weisskopf MG, Morozova N, O'Reilly EJ, McCullough ML, Calle EE, Thun MJ, Ascherio A. Prospective study of chemical exposures and amyotrophic lateral sclerosis. J Neurol Neurosurg Psychiatry. 2009;80:558–61.

8. Weisskopf MG, O'Reilly EJ, McCullough ML, Calle EE, Thun MJ, Cudkowicz M, Ascherio A. Prospective study of military service and mortality from ALS. Neurology. 2005;64:32–7.

9. Munoz-Saez E, de Munck GE, Arahuetes Portero RM, Martinez A, Solas Alados MT, Miguel BG. Analysis of beta-N-methylamino-L-alanine (L-BMAA) neurotoxicity in rat cerebellum. Neurotoxicology. 2015;48:192–205.

10. Beghi E, Logroscino G, Chio A, Hardiman O, Mitchell D, Swingler R, Traynor BJ, Consortium E. The epidemiology of ALS and the role of population-based registries. Biochim Biophys Acta. 2006;1762:1150–7.

11. Quintana FJ, Sherr DH. Aryl hydrocarbon receptor control of adaptive immunity. Pharmacol Rev. 2013;65:1148–61.

12. Murray IA, Patterson AD, Perdew GH. Aryl hydrocarbon receptor ligands in cancer: friend and foe. Nat Rev Cancer. 2014;14:801–14.

13. Gammon MD, Neugut AI, Santella RM, Teitelbaum SL, Britton JA, Terry MB, Eng SM, Wolff MS, Stellman SD, Kabat GC, et al. The Long Island breast cancer study project: description of a multi-institutional collaboration to identify environmental risk factors for breast cancer. Breast Cancer Res Treat. 2002;74:235–54.

14. Mordukhovich I, Rossner P Jr, Terry MB, Santella R, Zhang YJ, Hibshoosh H, Memeo L, Mansukhani M, Long CM, Garbowski G, et al. Associations between polycyclic aromatic hydrocarbon-related exposures and p53 mutations in breast tumors. Environ Health Perspect. 2010;118:511–8.

15. Ruder AM, Hein MJ, Hopf NB, Waters MA. Mortality among 24,865 workers exposed to polychlorinated biphenyls (PCBs) in three electrical capacitor manufacturing plants: a ten-year update. Int J Hyg Environ Health. 2014; 217(2-3):176–87. doi:10.1016/j.ijheh.2013.04.006.

16. Malek AM, Barchowsky A, Bowser R, Heiman-Patterson T, Lacomis D, Rana S, Ada Y, Talbott EO. Exposure to hazardous air pollutants and the risk of amyotrophic lateral sclerosis. Environ Pollut. 2015;197:181–6.

17. Richardson JR, Roy A, Shalat SL, von Stein RT, Hossain MM, Buckley B, Gearing M, Levey AI, German DC: Elevated Serum Pesticide Levels and Risk for Alzheimer Disease. JAMA Neurol 2014.

18. Wojtowicz AK, Honkisz E, Zieba-Przybylska D, Milewicz T, Kajta M. Effects of two isomers of DDT and their metabolite DDE on CYP1A1 and AhR function in human placental cells. Pharmacol Rep. 2011;63:1460–8.

19. Neumann M, Sampathu DM, Kwong LK, Truax AC, Micsenyi MC, Chou TT, Bruce J, Schuck T, Grossman M, Clark CM, et al. Ubiquitinated TDP-43 in frontotemporal lobar degeneration and amyotrophic lateral sclerosis. Science. 2006;314:130–3.

20. Arai T, Hasegawa M, Akiyama H, Ikeda K, Nonaka T, Mori H, Mann D, Tsuchiya K, Yoshida M, Hashizume Y, Oda T. TDP-43 is a component of ubiquitin-positive tau-negative inclusions in frontotemporal lobar degeneration and amyotrophic lateral sclerosis. Biochem Biophys Res Commun. 2006;351:602–11.

21. Mackenzie IR, Rademakers R, Neumann M. TDP-43 and FUS in amyotrophic lateral sclerosis and frontotemporal dementia. Lancet Neurol. 2010;9:995–1007.

22. Rutherford NJ, Zhang YJ, Baker M, Gass JM, Finch NA, Xu YF, Stewart H, Kelley BJ, Kuntz K, Crook RJ, et al. Novel mutations in TARDBP (TDP-43) in patients with familial amyotrophic lateral sclerosis. PLoS Genet. 2008;4:e1000193.

23. Sreedharan J, Blair IP, Tripathi VB, Hu X, Vance C, Rogelj B, Ackerley S, Durnall JC, Williams KL, Buratti E, et al. TDP-43 mutations in familial and sporadic amyotrophic lateral sclerosis. Science. 2008;319:1668–72.

24. Mackenzie IR, Bigio EH, Ince PG, Geser F, Neumann M, Cairns NJ, Kwong LK, Forman MS, Ravits J, Stewart H, et al. Pathological TDP-43 distinguishes sporadic amyotrophic lateral sclerosis from amyotrophic lateral sclerosis with SOD1 mutations. Ann Neurol. 2007;61:427–34.

25. Josephs KA, Murray ME, Whitwell JL, Parisi JE, Petrucelli L, Jack CR, Petersen RC, Dickson DW. Staging TDP-43 pathology in Alzheimer's disease. Acta Neuropathol. 2014;127:441–50.

26. McKee AC, Stein TD, Nowinski CJ, Stern RA, Daneshvar DH, Alvarez VE, Lee HS, Hall G, Wojtowicz SM, Baugh CM, et al. The spectrum of disease in chronic traumatic encephalopathy. Brain. 2013;136:43–64.

27. Nakashima-Yasuda H, Uryu K, Robinson J, Xie SX, Hurtig H, Duda JE, Arnold SE, Siderowf A, Grossman M, Leverenz JB, et al. Co-morbidity of TDP-43 proteinopathy in Lewy body related diseases. Acta Neuropathol. 2007;114:221–9.

28. Ash PE, Zhang YJ, Roberts CM, Saldi T, Hutter H, Buratti E, Petrucelli L, Link CD. Neurotoxic effects of TDP-43 overexpression in C. elegans. Hum Mol Genet. 2010; ePub

29. Wegorzewska I, Baloh RH. TDP-43-based animal models of neurodegeneration: new insights into ALS pathology and pathophysiology. Neurodegener Dis. 2011;8:262–74.

30. Parks AJ, Pollastri MP, Hahn ME, Stanford EA, Novikov O, Franks DG, Haigh SE, Narasimhan S, Ashton TD, Hopper TG, et al. In silico identification of an aryl hydrocarbon receptor antagonist with biological activity in vitro and in vivo. Mol Pharmacol. 2014;86:593–608.

31. Shivanna S, Kolandaivelu K, Shashar M, Belghasim M, Al-Rabadi L, Balcells M, Zhang A, Weinberg J, Francis J, Pollastri MP, et al. The aryl hydrocarbon receptor is a critical regulator of tissue factor stability and an antithrombotic target in uremia. J Am Soc Nephrol. 2016;27:189–201.

32. Liu-Yesucevitz L, Lin AY, Ebata A, Boon JY, Reid W, Xu YF, Kobrin K, Murphy GJ, Petrucelli L, Wolozin B. ALS-linked mutations enlarge TDP-43-enriched neuronal RNA granules in the Dendritic arbor. J Neurosci. 2014;34:4167–74.

33. Sommer CA, Stadtfeld M, Murphy GJ, Hochedlinger K, Kotton DN, Mostoslavsky G. Induced pluripotent stem cell generation using a single lentiviral stem cell cassette. Stem Cells. 2009;27:543–9.

34. Chambers SM, Fasano CA, Papapetrou EP, Tomishima M, Sadelain M, Studer L. Highly efficient neural conversion of human ES and iPS cells by dual inhibition of SMAD signaling. Nat Biotechnol. 2009;27:275–80.

35. Hu BY, Du ZW, Li XJ, Ayala M, Zhang SC. Human oligodendrocytes from embryonic stem cells: conserved SHH signaling networks and divergent FGF effects. Development. 2009;136:1443–52.

36. Liu-Yesucevitz L, Bilgutay A, Zhang YJ, Vanderweyde T, Citro A, Mehta T, Zaarur N, McKee A, Bowser R, Sherman M, et al. Tar DNA binding protein-43 (TDP-43) associates with stress granules: analysis of cultured cells and pathological brain tissue. PLoS One. 2010;5:e13250.

37. Vorrink SU, Domann FE. Regulatory crosstalk and interference between the xenobiotic and hypoxia sensing pathways at the AhR-ARNT-HIF1alpha signaling node. Chem Biol Interact. 2014;218:82–8.

38. Shimada T, Sugie A, Shindo M, Nakajima T, Azuma E, Hashimoto M, Inoue K. Tissue-specific induction of cytochromes P450 1A1 and 1B1 by polycyclic aromatic hydrocarbons and polychlorinated biphenyls in engineered C57BL/6J mice of arylhydrocarbon receptor gene. Toxicol Appl Pharmacol. 2003;187:1–10.

39. Beischlag TV, Wang S, Rose DW, Torchia J, Reisz-Porszasz S, Muhammad K, Nelson WE, Probst MR, Rosenfeld MG, Hankinson O. Recruitment of the NCoA/SRC-1/p160 family of transcriptional coactivators by the aryl hydrocarbon receptor/aryl hydrocarbon receptor nuclear translocator complex. Mol Cell Biol. 2002;22:4319–33.

40. Wang S, Ge K, Roeder RG, Hankinson O. Role of mediator in transcriptional activation by the aryl hydrocarbon receptor. J Biol Chem. 2004;279:13593–600.

41. Tian Y, Ke S, Denison MS, Rabson AB, Gallo MA. Ah receptor and NF-kappaB interactions, a potential mechanism for dioxin toxicity. J Biol Chem. 1999;274:510–5.

42. Kim DW, Gazourian L, Quadri SA, Romieu-Mourez R, Sherr DH, Sonenshein GE. The RelA NF-kappaB subunit and the aryl hydrocarbon receptor (AhR) cooperate to transactivate the c-myc promoter in mammary cells. Oncogene. 2000;19:5498–506.

43. Wilson SR, Joshi AD, Elferink CJ. The tumor suppressor Kruppel-like factor 6 is a novel aryl hydrocarbon receptor DNA binding partner. J Pharmacol Exp Ther. 2013;345:419–29.

44. Swanson HI, Chan WK, Bradfield CA. DNA binding specificities and pairing rules of the ah receptor, ARNT, and SIM proteins. J Biol Chem. 1995;270: 26292–302.

45. Zhang L, Savas U, Alexander DL, Jefcoate CR. Characterization of the mouse Cyp1B1 gene. Identification of an enhancer region that directs aryl

hydrocarbon receptor-mediated constitutive and induced expression. J Biol Chem. 1998;273:5174–83.

46. Garrison PM, Tullis K, Aarts JM, Brouwer A, Giesy JP, Denison MS. Species-specific recombinant cell lines as bioassay systems for the detection of 2,3,7,8-tetrachlorodibenzo-p-dioxin-like chemicals. Fundam Appl Toxicol. 1996;30:194–203.

47. Mrema EJ, Rubino FM, Brambilla G, Moretto A, Tsatsakis AM, Colosio C. Persistent organochlorinated pesticides and mechanisms of their toxicity. Toxicology. 2013;307:74–88.

48. Ayala YM, De Conti L, Avendano-Vazquez SE, Dhir A, Romano M, D'Ambrogio A, Tollervey J, Ule J, Baralle M, Buratti E, Baralle FE. TDP-43 regulates its mRNA levels through a negative feedback loop. EMBO J. 2011; 30:277–88.

49. Tsao W, Jeong YH, Lin S, Ling J, Price DL, Chiang PM, Wong PC. Rodent models of TDP-43: recent advances. Brain Res. 2012;1462:26–39.

50. LaFerla FM, Green KN. Animal models of Alzheimer disease. Cold Spring Harb Perspect Med. 2012;2(11). doi:10.1101/cshperspect.a006320. PMID: 23002015.

51. Renton AE, Chio A, Traynor BJ. State of play in amyotrophic lateral sclerosis genetics. Nat Neurosci. 2014;17:17–23.

7

Blood hemoglobin A1c levels and amyotrophic lateral sclerosis survival

Qian-Qian Wei[1], Yongping Chen[1], Bei Cao[1], Ru Wei Ou[1], Lingyu Zhang[1], Yanbing Hou[1], Xiang Gao[2*] and Huifang Shang[1*]

Abstract

Background: There are inconsistences regarding the correlation between diabetes or fasting blood glucose concentrations and the risk and survival of amyotrophic lateral sclerosis (ALS) in the previous studies. Moreover, the association between hemoglobin A1c (HbA1c) levels, which reflect long-term glycemic status, and ALS survival was not examined.

Methods: A prospective cohort study including 450 Chinese sporadic ALS patients (254 men and 196 women; mean age: 55.4 y). We identified 223 deaths during average 1.6 years of follow-up. We assessed levels of fasting HbA1c (primary exposure) and glucose (secondary exposure) via ion exchange high-performance liquid chromatography and hexokinase/glucose-6-pgosphate dehydrogenase methods, respectively. Multivariate Cox proportional hazards regression model was used to calculate hazard ratios (HRs) and 95% confidence intervals (CIs) of ALS mortality across the exposures.

Results: Our results indicated that, higher levels of HbA1c, but not fasting blood glucose concentrations, were significantly associated with higher risks of mortality. The adjusted HR was 1.40 (95% confidence interval (95% CI): 1.02–1.99) for HbA1c of 5.7–6.4%, and 2.06 (95% CI: 1.07–3.96) for HbA1c $\geq$6.5%, relative to HbA1c <5.7% (P trend =0.01), after adjustment for age, smoking, obesity, disease severity, site of onset, lifestyle, and other potential confounders. The adjusted HR was 1.38 (95% CI: 0.81–2.35, P trend =0.13) for fasting glucose concentrations $\geq$7.0 mmol/L vs <5.6 mmol/L. We did not observe any significant interactions between HbA1c levels and age, sex, smoking, body mass index, rate of disease progression of ALS, and site of onset (P-interactions >0.05 for all).

Conclusion: In this prospective study, we observed that individuals with higher HbA1c levels at the baseline had higher risk of mortality, which is independent of other known risk factors.

Keywords: Amyotrophic lateral sclerosis, HbA1c, Fasting glucose, Survival, Body mass index

Background

Amyotrophic lateral sclerosis (ALS) is an incurable neurodegenerative disorder characterized by degeneration of both upper and lower motor neurons, with a median survival of 3–5 years after symptoms onset [1]. Several modifiable vascular factors and comorbidities have recently been studied as potential therapeutic targets for ALS. Interestingly, the presence of vascular risk factors (e.g., higher body mass index (BMI) and hypercholesterolemia) was reported to be associated with a lower risk and mortality of ALS [2–4].

In contrast, results regarding the association between diabetes mellitus (DM) and the risk, progression and survival of ALS were inconsistent or even contradictory [5–12]. DM was associated with a higher risk of ALS in a population-based cohort study from Taiwan [6] and a lower risk of ALS in studies conducted in western countries [7, 8]. Studies examined DM/ impaired glucose tolerance (IGT) status and ALS progression/survival failed to generate significant results [9–12]. However, some of these studies lacked information on obesity index and life style factors such as smoking that could confound the association between DM and ALS. Furthermore, status of DM and IGT was dominantly diagnosed by fasting blood glucose (FBG) concentrations in these studies, which only represented short-term glycemic

* Correspondence: xxg14@psu.edu; hfshang2002@163.com
[2]Department of Nutritional Science, The Pennsylvania State University, 109 Chandlee Lab, University Park, PA 16802, USA
[1]Department of Neurology, West China Hospital, Sichuan University, 37 Guoxue Xiang, Chengdu, Sichuan 610041, China

status. Hemoglobin A1c (HbA1c) levels, which can reflect the cumulative glycemic history of the preceding 2 to 3 months, has recently been recommended as a possible substitute to FBG for the diagnosis of diabetes by the American Diabetes Association [13]. It provided a reliable measurement of chronic hyperglycemia and correlates well with the risk of developing long-term diabetes complications [13]. Elevated HbA1c levels have been regarded as an independent risk factor for cardiovascular diseases in individuals with or without diabetes [14]. However, the associations between HbA1c levels and the mortality and survival of ALS remain unknown.

Therefore, a large prospective study was conducted to examine the association between HbA1c and the mortality among 450 Chinese adults with ALS, adjusting for BMI, lipid profiles, disease status and lifestyle factors. We also explored potential interactions between HbA1c levels and these factors, in relation to ALS mortality. As a secondary exposure, the association between FBG concentrations and the mortality of ALS were also studied.

Methods
Participants and fellow-up
The study was conducted in the Department of Neurology, West China Hospital of Sichuan University in the southwest of China. Patients who were diagnosed with definite or probable ALS according to the El Escorial revised criteria [15] were recruited into our study at their first visit to our tertiary referral center from March 2009 to September 2014 (referred to as "baseline" in the current manuscript). Patients with progressive muscular atrophy, progressive bulbar paralysis, primary lateral sclerosis, and familial and juvenile ALS were excluded in the current analyses. There was a total of 558 sporadic ALS (SALS) patients met our inclusion criteria and 450 (80.6%) had complete hematological data. All 450 eligible patients were followed up with telephone or face-to-face interview in 3 or 6 months interval by neurologists (QQW, LYZ and YBH). Death information was collected from provincial public security bureau records and family reports. The institutional ethics committee of West China Hospital approved this study. All the participants were informed with the study and signed written informed consents. All methods were performed in accordance with the relevant guidelines and regulations.

Assessment of HbA1c levels, FBG concentrations, and covariates
Blood samples after an overnight fasting (> 8 h) were collected at the baseline. HbA1c levels were assessed by ion exchange high-pressure liquid chromatography on a Tosoh G7 standard mode (Tosoh Corporation, Japan) using reagents according to the manufacturer's instructions in the clinical laboratory, West China Hospital.

Intralaboratory analytical coefficients of variation were <2%. Participants were categorized into three groups based on their HbA1c levels (<5.7% (38 mmol/mol), 5.7–6.4% (38–46 mmol/mol), and ≥6.5% (48 mmol/mol)) and the lowest group was used as the reference [16]. Participants who were treated with insulin or oral hypoglycemic agents were assigned into the group of HbA1c ≥6.5% regardless their actual HbA1c values.

FBG concentrations were measured with the hexokinase/glucose-6-pgosphate dehydrogenase method. The coefficient of variation using blind quality control specimens was <2.0%. Participants were identified as having DM if they had a FBG ≥7.0 mmol/L, or were treated with insulin or oral hypoglycemic agents [17]. And IGT was defined as FBG concentration between 5.6 and 6.9 mmol/L.

Assessment of potential covariates
Baseline concentrations of fasting serum total cholesterol (TC), and triglyceride (TG) were measured by an enzymatic colorimetric method using an automatic analyzer (Olympus AU400; Olympus, Japan). Automatic hematology analyzer (Sysmex XE 5000, Kobe, Japan) completed blood counts. It performs hematology analysis according to the sheath flow DC detection method for erythrocytes and platelets and flow cytometry method using a semiconductor laser and fluorescent measurement for leukocytes and differential. Body height was measured, without wearing shoes, with an accuracy of 0.5 cm, using a stadiometer at the baseline. Body weight was measured to the nearest 0.1 kg with a steelyard scale, with underwear and no shoes. BMI was calculated as weight in kilograms divided by height in meters squared, and it was categorized according to the World Health Organization [18]. Blood pressure was also measured at the baseline and hypertension was defined as systolic BP ≥140 mmHg or diastolic ≥90 mmHg or use of antihypertensive medications in past 2 weeks. Information on lifestyle and personal history, including cigarette smoking status and drinking status, were collected via questionnaires [19]. Our previous studies have used the Chinese version of Addenbrooke's Cognitive Examination-revised (ACE-R) and the Chinese version of the frontal assessment battery (FAB) to evaluate cognitive function and frontal lobe function in sporadic ALS patients and healthy controls [20, 21]. The ACE-R score less than 75 was defined as cognitive impairment and FAB score less than 16 was defined as frontal lobe dysfunction according to the previous studies [20, 21].

All the clinical data were collected at the baseline and during the follow-up evaluations, including age of onset, the region of symptom onset (upper limb, lower limb or bulbar), disease duration at baseline, diagnostic delay, the ALS Functional Rating Scale-Revised (ALSFRS-R) score, and the use of riluzole, gastrostomy percutaneous endoscopy (PEG) and noninvasive positive pressure ventilation

(NIPPV). The rate of disease progression was assessed by the changes of ALSFRS-R per month (Formula: (48 − ALSFRS-R score at the baseline visit)/ month intervals between first symptom onset and the baseline visit).

Statistical analysis

Person-years for each participant were calculated from the date of recruitment to the date of death or tracheotomy which was taken as equivalent to death, or September 1st, 2015, whichever came first. Continuous variables were expressed as the mean ± standard deviation (SD). The Student's t tests were performed for between-group comparisons of continuous variables. Chi-Square tests were used to determine the differences of categorical variables between groups. The multivariate Cox proportional hazards regression model was performed to calculate hazard ratios (HRs) and their 95% confidence intervals (CIs) of ALS mortality across the exposure (i.e., HbA1c and FBG) categories as the proportional hazards assumption was satisfied. We adjusted for potential confounders, including age, sex, site of onset, rate of disease progression, smoking, alcohol drinking, BMI, TC concentrations, anemia, hypertension, and use of riluzole, NIPPV and PEG (because the treatments were associated with ALS mortality, as suggested in previous studies [22, 23]. Tests for linear trend in effect across HbA1c and FBG categories were performed using the median value in each category and treating this value as continuous variables. Because the use of hypoglycemic agents impacted levels of HbA1c and FBG, we conducted a sensitivity analysis by excluding individuals who used any hypoglycemic agents. We also tested the interactions between HbA1c levels and age, sex, BMI, anemia, hypertension, smoking status, site of onset and the rate of disease progression on ALS mortality. All the data were analyzed using SPSS18.0 statistical software (SPSS Inc., Chicago, IL, USA). A P-value less than 0.05 were considered as statistical significance.

Results

Clinical features

The mean age of enrolled patients was 55.4 ± 13.9 years, including 254 (56.4%) men and 196 (43.6%) women. The mean age of onset was 54.5 ± 12.2 years. The mean diagnostic delay was 15.7 ± 15.3 months. The ALSFRS-R total score was 39.1 ± 6.0 at the baseline (ranging from 12 to 48). For the site of onset, 244 (54.2%) patients had upper limb onset, 108 (24.0%) patients had lower limb onset, and 98 (21.8%) patients had bulbar onset. The average rate of disease progression was 0.77.

Demographic and clinical characteristics of ALS patients among different HbA1c status are shown in Table 1. Compared with ALS patients with lower HbA1c levels, those with higher HbA1c levels were more likely to be older. The results of other potential

Table 1 Demographic and Clinical Characteristics of ALS patients in different HbA1c status (N = 450)

HbA1c, %	<5.7	5.7–6.4	≥6.5	P-trend
Number	263	152	35	
Age of onset, years	52.7(12.6)	57.0(11.2)	57.7(10.0)	<0.001
Age, years	53.1(15.3)	58.5(11.2)	59.4(9.8)	<0.001
Gender				
Male, %	57.4	53.3	62.9	0.52
Female, %	42.6	46.7	37.1	
Onset form				
Upper limb, %	54.8	51.9	62.9	0.20
Lower limb, %	20.9	29.6	22.9	
Bulbar, %	24.3	19.1	14.3	
ALS disease duration, months	16.0(15.5)	17.7(16.9)	19.7(16.4)	0.33
ALS diagnostic delay, months	14.9(14.8)	16.2(15.9)	19.1(16.6)	0.29
Education, years	7.9(4.3)	7.6(4.5)	6.2(2.9)	0.28
ALSFRS-R total score	39.3(5.7)	38.6(6.1)	38.3(7.5)	0.35
Rate of disease progression	0.75(0.65)	0.78(0.65)	0.84(0.71)	0.79
FAB (N = 195)				
<16 score, %	37.7	35.1	54.5	0.48
≥ 16 score, %	62.3	64.9	45.5	
ACE-R (N = 195)				
<75, %	38.0	40.7	33.3	0.86
≥ 75, %	62.0	59.3	66.7	

Abbreviations: *ALS* amyotrophic lateral sclerosis, *HbA1c* Hemoglobin A1c, *ALSFRS-R* amyotrophic lateral sclerosis functional rating scale-revised, *FAB* frontal assessment battery, *ACE-R* Addenbrooke's Cognitive Examination-revised

covariates in regards to HbA1c levels are reported in Table 2. Compared with ALS patients with lower HbA1c levels, those with higher HbA1c levels were more likely to have higher blood cell counts of erythrocytes, platelets, total leukocytes, neutrophils, lymphocytes, and monocytes, and blood concentrations of TG and TC. Other parameters, such as the frequencies of cognitive deficits and frontal lobe dysfunction, and the history of smoking and drinking, were not significantly associated with HbA1c levels. We did not find significant association between HbA1C levels and ALS severity — HbA1c levels were similar when compared participants with low and high ALSFRS-R scores, based on median value (data not shown).

Some patients also underwent an extensive genetic assessment using standard procedures. Four patients (2.07%, 4/193) had *SOD1* mutations, 3 patients (0.95%, 3/316) carried a *C9ORF72* GGGGCC repeat expansion, 1 patient carried a *FUS* mutation (0.47%, 1/212), 1 patient (0.53%, 1/187) carried a *CHCHD10* mutation, and no patient had *TARDBP* mutation (0/165). The frequencies of these ALS causative genes mutations were very low.

Table 2 Results of other potential covariates in ALS patients between different HbA1c status (N = 450)

HbA1c, %	<5.7	5.7–6.4	≥6.5	P-trend
Number	263	152	35	
BMI, kg/m^2	22.3(3.3)	22.0(3.0)	22.7(3.1)	0.57
BMI status				
Normal, %	84.8	86.2	82.9	0.79
Overweight, %	14.4	13.8	17.1	
Obesity, %	0.8	0.0	0.0	
Smoking, %	32.3	29.6	31.4	0.85
Alcohol drinking, %	32.7	26.3	25.7	0.33
Hypertension, %	11.8	19.7	17.1	0.08
Anemia, %	7.2	5.3	8.6	0.67
Erythrocytes, 10^{12}/L	4.5(0.5)	4.6(0.5)	4.7(0.5)	0.003
Platelets, 10^9/L	164.1(54.9)	171.8(55.9)	193.6(58.0)	0.01
Total leukocytes, 10^9/L	5.6(1.4)	5.9(2.0)	7.0(2.9)	<0.001
Neutrophils, 10^9/L	3.4(1.2)	3.7(1.8)	4.5(2.2)	0.001
Lymphocytes, 10^9/L	1.6(0.5)	1.7(0.5)	2.0(0.8)	0.001
Monocytes, 10^9/L	0.3(0.1)	0.4(0.1)	0.4(0.2)	<0.001
Triglyceride, mmol/L	1.4(0.9)	1.4(0.7)	2.2(1.8)	<0.001
Total Cholesterol, mmol/L	4.5(0.8)	4.8(0.9)	5.0(1.2)	<0.001
Use of hypoglycemic agents, %	0.0	0.0	60.0	<0.001

Abbreviations: ALS amyotrophic lateral sclerosis, *HbA1c* Hemoglobin A1c, *BMI* body mass index

Multivariate Cox proportional hazards regression model

During average 19.2 months of follow-up, 223 participants were deceased (Fig. 1). Survival time was not significant different between patients with limb onset and with bulbar onset (P = 0.20, HR =1.23), between patients with and without cognitive deficits (P = 0.88, HR = 0.97), and between patients with and without frontal lobe dysfunction (P = 0.79, HR = 0.95). As expected, higher BMI was associated with lower risks of mortality (adjusted HR =0.92 for each kg/m^2 increment; 95% CI: 0.86–0.99; P trend =0.02) after adjustment for potential confounders. In contrast, higher baseline HbA1c levels were associated with a higher risk of mortality during the follow-up (Fig. 2a). The adjusted HR was 1.40 (95% CI: 1.02–1.99) for HbA1c of 5.7–6.4%, and 2.06 (95% CI: 1.07–3.96) for HbA1c ≥6.5%, relative to HbA1c <5.7% after adjustment for age, sex, site of onset, the rate of disease progression, BMI and other covariates. Each additional increased unit (%) of HbA1c was associated with a 50% (95% CI: 9%–107%, P trend =0.01) increased risk of mortality. We did not observe any significant interactions between HbA1c and other variables, in relation to survival of ALS patients (P-interaction >0.05 for all). In contrast, although there was a similar trend between higher FBG concentrations and a higher mortality risk, the association was not statistically significant (adjusted HR =1.37 for each mmol/L increment; P trend =0.13; Fig. 2b).

Sensitivity analyses

Sensitivity analyses generated similar results. After we excluded 21 participants who were using hypoglycemic agents, higher baseline HbA1c levels, but not FBG concentrations were associated with a higher risk of mortality.

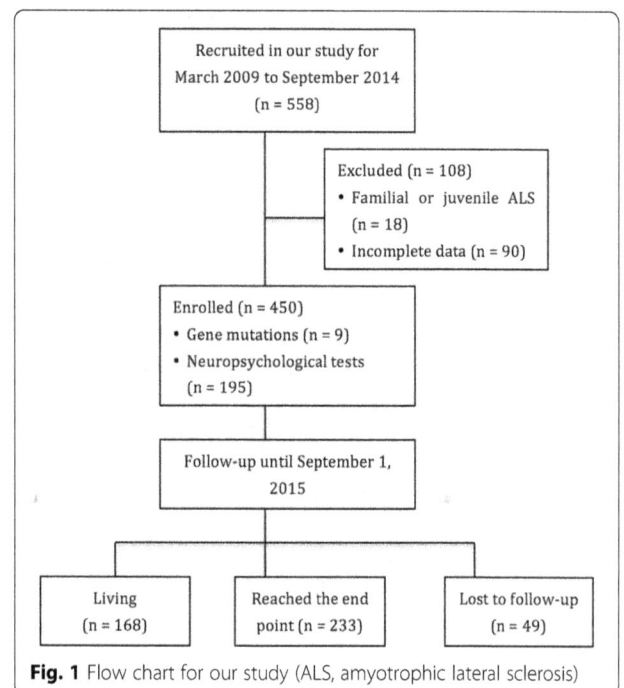

Fig. 1 Flow chart for our study (ALS, amyotrophic lateral sclerosis)

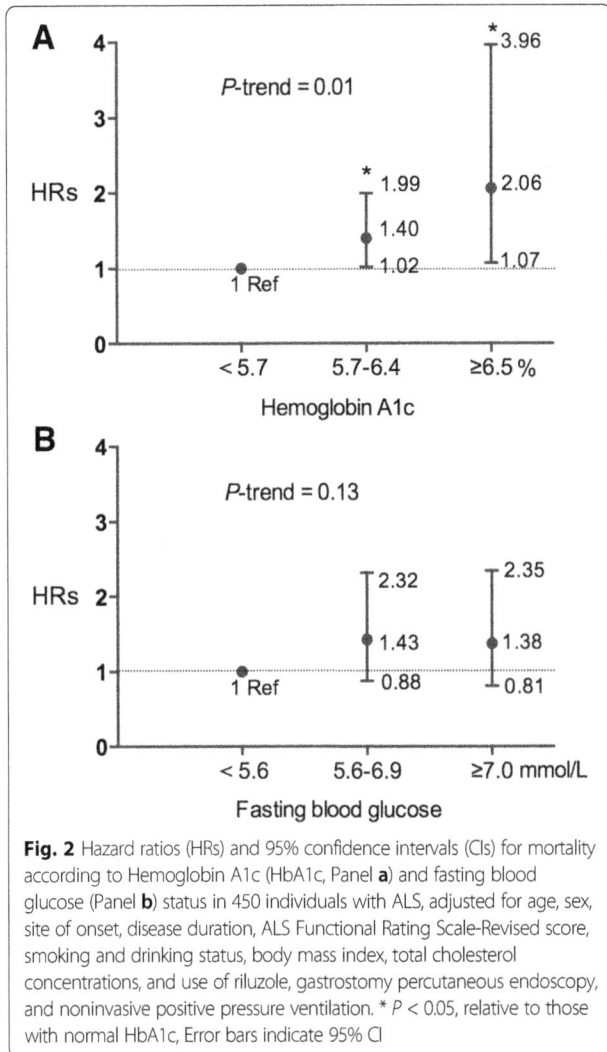

Fig. 2 Hazard ratios (HRs) and 95% confidence intervals (CIs) for mortality according to Hemoglobin A1c (HbA1c, Panel **a**) and fasting blood glucose (Panel **b**) status in 450 individuals with ALS, adjusted for age, sex, site of onset, disease duration, ALS Functional Rating Scale-Revised score, smoking and drinking status, body mass index, total cholesterol concentrations, and use of riluzole, gastrostomy percutaneous endoscopy, and noninvasive positive pressure ventilation. * $P < 0.05$, relative to those with normal HbA1c, Error bars indicate 95% CI

(Adjusted HR =1.43 for each unit increment, P trend =0.02 vs. adjusted HR =1.29 for each unit increment, P trend =0.12, respectively). Excluding participants who carried *SOD1, C9ORF72, FUS,* or *CHCHD10* mutations did not change the results materially (data not shown).

Discussion

In this prospective study, we found that the risk of mortality was doubled for individuals with HbA1c ≥6.5% at the baseline, compared to those with normal HbA1c level (<5.7%). Pre-diabetes status, as defined by HbA1c of 5.7–6.4%, was also significantly associated with higher risk of mortality. The significant association between HbA1c and ALS mortality was independent of known risk factors, including BMI, blood cholesterol concentrations, and disease severity. Interestingly, no significant association was found between FBG and ALS mortality.

A previous systematic review including 5 case-control and 2 cross-sectional studies [10] and a following pooled analysis including 6 ALS clinical trials [9] suggested that a

history of pre-morbid DM2 was not an independent prognostic predictor for ALS progression and survival. It is worth noting that, all studies included in this review, except for one (conducted during 2006–2012) [24], were conducted in or prior to 2010 when HbA1c was recommended to be included in the DM diagnosis criteria [25].

Consistent with previous study [26], FBG was not associated with ALS mortality in our cohort. The FBG test is an excellent test for "in the moment" glucose levels, but it provided limited information about the time-course trend of the glucose levels. Analysis of HbA1c in blood provides evidence about an individual's average blood glucose levels during the previous 2 to 3 months and has been recommended as a standard of testing and monitoring DM recently [13, 25]. There is a direct association between HbA1c and insulin resistance, where HbA1c has been shown to be more strongly associated with the insulin sensitivity in healthy individuals with normal glucose tolerance [27]. The value of HbA1c was found to have minimal overlap between subjects with normal glucose tolerances and subjects with DM2 when studying on glycemic spectrum for insulin resistance. Therefore, HbA1c is a reliable biomarker of insulin resistance for testing individuals for DM and pre-diabetes [28].

Several potential mechanistic pathways including mitochondrial dysfunction, oxidative stress, and insulin resistance could underlie the observed relation between HbA1c and the mortality of ALS. On the one hand, mitochondria, which plays a crucial role in cell apoptosis, has shown to be an early target in ALS pathogenesis and contribute to disease progression [29] and its dysfunction has a critical role in the pathogenesis of mutant superoxide dismutase 1 (SOD1) mediated familial ALS. On the other hand, previous studies have demonstrated a mitochondrial function defect in substrate oxidation with a decrease in mitochondrial density in disorders of insulin resistance [30]. And as a result of fuel oxidation, mitochondria generate considerable amounts of reactive oxygen species, which are implicated in the pathophysiology of DM and its complications [31]. Besides, oxidative stress is also associated with both insulin resistance [32] and motor neuron degeneration in ALS patients [33]. These studies suggest a potential link between the HbA1c, oxidative stress, mitochondrial dysfunction of insulin resistance, and the pathogenesis of ALS.

Systematic review study have demonstrated that the presence of iron deficiency with or without anemia (IDA) can lead to an increase in HbA1c values compared with controls, with no concomitant rise in glucose indices [34], which means HbA1c is likely to show a spurious increase due to iron deficiency and IDA. And, non-iron deficiency forms of anemia may lead to a decreased HbA1c [34]. This may lead to confusion when diagnosing DM using HbA1c. But in our study, no significant interaction was found between HbA1c and anemia (P-interaction >0.05). Anemia had no associated with the risk of mortality in ALS after adjustment in the Cox model without enough information on the iron levels. So, it clearly identifies the need for further investigation, especially in focusing on the associations between types and degrees of anemia, HbA1c and ALS. Although it is suggested that respiratory insufficiency that occurs with loss of respiratory muscle function may influence HbA1c values, the mean scores of ALSFRS-R subscale (respiratory function) were no significant difference in the subgroups regarding to the HbA1c values.

Our current study was included in a Chinese population to find out that higher baseline HbA1c levels but not FBG concentrations were associated with a higher risk of mortality. Interestingly, there were some previous studies exploring DM and the risk of ALS in different ethnicity generated conflicting results: in Europe-based studies, presence of DM was associated with a lower risk of developing ALS [8, 35], but in Asia-based study [6], participants with DM had a higher risk of developing ALS, relative to those without DM [5]. Previous studies reported DM associated with a higher risk of ALS in younger individuals [8, 36]. The inconsistent findings could be partially explained by the various confounders and ethnic variations across these studies. Firstly, Chinese ALS patients appeared to have a younger age at onset compared to Caucasians, as suggested by these studies [5, 6], Consistently, the mean age of onset in our current study was 54.5 years, relative to 65–68 years in aforementioned studies in Europe. Second, with different ethnic background, the impact of genetic factors on ALS might be different. For example, nearly 20% of familial Caucasian ALS patients had the repeat expansions in chromosome 9 open reading frame 72 (C9orf72) gene, but the prevalence of the expansions was very low or absent in Chinese ALS patients [37] and patients from Japan and Iran [38–40]. Further, Asian populations are prone to insulin resistant states at much lower BMI categories than Caucasian counterparts [41]. In our previous study based on 100,000 Chinese adults, we found that even individuals traditionally considered to be "thin" or "non-overweight" (BMI <20 kg/m^2 or <23 kg/m^2, respectively) exhibited steady increases in fasting blood glucose over time.

Several limitations of the present study should be noted. First, all the participants were solely recruited through a tertiary referral center in China; thus our results may not be generalized to other populations. However, the mean ALSFRS-R scores were similar (39.0 ± 6.0) between the current study and previous studies on this topic (39.0 ± 5.7) [9]. Second, we did not collect information on diabetes duration. A recent case-control study reported that DM duration might modify the association between DM and the risk of ALS [35]. Further exclusion of participants who used hypoglycemic agents (a surrogate for a longer DM duration) did not

change results materially. Consistently, pre-diabetes, as suggested by HbA1c of 5.7–6.4%, was also significantly associated with higher ALS mortality. Finally, not all of enrolled patients in the current study were screened all of ALS causative genes mutations. This was one of the limitations of the current study.

Conclusions

In this Chinese ALS cohort, we observed a strong dose-response relation between higher baseline HbA1c levels and higher future risks of mortality. Further studies performed in ALS patients with different ethnic backgrounds are needed to verify, whether higher HbA1c levels are also associated with increased ALS risks.

Abbreviations
ALS: Amyotrophic lateral sclerosis; ALSFRS-R: ALS Functional rating scale-revised; BMI: Body mass index; C9orf72: Chromosome 9 open reading frame 72; CIs: Confidence intervals; DM: Diabetes mellitus; FBG: Fasting blood glucose; HbA1c: Hemoglobin A1c; HRs: Hazard ratios; IDA: Iron deficiency anemia; IGT: Impaired glucose tolerance; NIPPV: Noninvasive positive pressure ventilation; PEG: Percutaneous endoscopy gastrostomy; SD: Standard deviation; SOD1: Superoxide dismutase 1; TC: Total cholesterol; TG: Triglyceride

Acknowledgements
The authors thank the ALS patients for participation.

Funding
This study was supported by the funding of the National Natural Science Foundation of China (Grant No. 81371394 and No. 81511140101), the National Key Research and Development Program of China (No. 2016YFC0901504) and the Science and Technology Bureau Fund of Sichuan Province (2014FZ0072).

Authors' contributions
QW wrote the manuscript and collected data and interpretation data. YC analyzed and critically reviewed the manuscript. BC critically reviewed the manuscript. RO critically reviewed the manuscript and collected data. LZ critically reviewed the manuscript and collected data. YH critically reviewed the manuscript and collected data. HS supervised the study, study design, and critically reviewed and edited the manuscript. XG supervised the study, and critically reviewed and edited the manuscript. All authors read and approved the final manuscript.

Competing interests
The authors declare that they have no competing interests.

References
1. Mitchell JD, Borasio GD. Amyotrophic lateral sclerosis. Lancet. 2007; 369(9578):2031–41.
2. Dupuis L, Corcia P, Fergani A, Gonzalez De Aguilar JL, Bonnefont-Rousselot D, Bittar R, et al. Dyslipidemia is a protective factor in amyotrophic lateral sclerosis. Neurology. 2008;70:1004–9.
3. O'Reilly EJ, Wang H, Weisskopf MG, Fitzgerald KC, Falcone G, McCullough ML, et al. Premorbid body mass index and risk of amyotrophic lateral

sclerosis. Amyotroph Lateral Scler Frontotemporal Degener. 2013;14:205–11.

4. Scarmeas N, Shih T, Stern Y, Ottman R, Rowland LP. Premorbid weight, body mass, and varsity athletics in ALS. Neurology. 2002;59:773–5.

5. Logroscino G. Motor neuron disease: Are diabetes and amyotrophic lateral sclerosis related? Nat Rev Neurol. 2015;11:488–90.

6. Sun Y, Lu CJ, Chen RC, Hou WH, Li CY. Risk of Amyotrophic Lateral Sclerosis in Patients With Diabetes: A Nationwide Population-Based Cohort Study. J Epidemiol. 2015;25:445–51.

7. Jawaid A, Salamone AR, Strutt AM, Murthy SB, Wheaton M, McDowell EJ, et al. ALS disease onset may occur later in patients with pre-morbid diabetes mellitus. Eur J Neurol. 2010;17:733–9.

8. Kioumourtzoglou MA, Rotem RS, Seals RM, Gredal O, Hansen J, Weisskopf MG. Diabetes Mellitus, Obesity, and Diagnosis of Amyotrophic Lateral Sclerosis: A Population-Based Study. JAMA Neurol. 2015;72:905–11.

9. Paganoni S, Hyman T, Shui A, Allred P, Harms M, Liu J, et al. Pre-morbid type 2 diabetes mellitus is not a prognostic factor in amyotrophic lateral sclerosis. Muscle Nerve. 2015;52:339–43.

10. Lekoubou A, Matsha TE, Sobngwi E, Kengne AP. Effects of diabetes mellitus on amyotrophic lateral sclerosis: a systematic review. BMC Res Notes. 2014;7:171.

11. Korner S, Kollewe K, Ilsemann J, Muller-Heine A, Dengler R, Krampfl K, et al. Prevalence and prognostic impact of comorbidities in amyotrophic lateral sclerosis. Eur J Neurol. 2013;20:647–54.

12. Pradat PF, Bruneteau G, Gordon PH, Dupuis L, Bonnefont-Rousselot D, Simon D, et al. Impaired glucose tolerance in patients with amyotrophic lateral sclerosis. Amyotroph Lateral Scler. 2010;11:166–71.

13. Sherwani SI, Khan HA, Ekhzaimy A, Masood A, Sakharkar MK. Significance of HbA1c Test in Diagnosis and Prognosis of Diabetic Patients. Biomark Insights. 2016;11:95–104.

14. Martin-Timon I, Sevillano-Collantes C, Segura-Galindo A, Del Canizo-Gomez FJ. Type 2 diabetes and cardiovascular disease: Have all risk factors the same strength? World J Diabetes. 2014;5:444–70.

15. Brooks BR, Miller RG, Swash M, Munsat TL. El Escorial revisited: revised criteria for the diagnosis of amyotrophic lateral sclerosis. Amyotroph Lateral Scler Other Motor Neuron Disord. 2000;1:293–9.

16. American Diabetes Association (ADA). Diagnosis and classification of diabetes mellitus. Diabetes Care. 2011;34(Suppl 1):S62–9.

17. Diabetes, Chinese Medical Association (CMA). The guidelines for the diagnosis and treatment of diabetes in China. Chin J Diabetes. 2014;8:2–42.

18. Youngquist ST, McIntosh SE, Swanson ER, Barton ED. Air ambulance transport times and advanced cardiac life support interventions during the interfacility transfer of patients with acute ST-segment elevation myocardial infarction. Prehosp Emerg Care. 2010;14:292–9.

19. Weisskopf MG, McCullough ML, Calle EE, Thun MJ, Cudkowicz M, Ascherio A. Prospective study of cigarette smoking and amyotrophic lateral sclerosis. Am J Epidemiol. 2004;160:26–33.

20. Wei Q, Chen X, Zheng Z, Huang R, Guo X, Cao B, et al. Frontal lobe function and behavioral changes in amyotrophic lateral sclerosis: a study from Southwest China. J Neurol. 2014;261:2393–400.

21. Wei Q, Chen X, Zheng Z, Huang R, Guo X, Cao B, et al. Screening for cognitive impairment in a Chinese ALS population. Amyotroph Lateral Scler Frontotemporal Degener. 2015;16:40–5.

22. Chio A, Logroscino G, Hardiman O, Swingler R, Mitchell D, Beghi E, et al. Prognostic factors in ALS: A critical review. Amyotroph Lateral Scler. 2009;10:310–23.

23. Zoccolella S, Beghi E, Palagano G, Fraddosio A, Guerra V, Samarelli V, et al. Riluzole and amyotrophic lateral sclerosis survival: a population-based study in southern Italy. Eur J Neurol. 2007;14:262–8.

24. Cudkowicz ME, Titus S, Kearney M, Yu H, Sherman A, Schoenfeld D, et al. Safety and efficacy of ceftriaxone for amyotrophic lateral sclerosis: a multi-stage, randomised, double-blind, placebo-controlled trial. Lancet Neurol. 2014;13:1083–91.

25. Committee IE. International Expert Committee report on the role of the A1C assay in the diagnosis of diabetes. Diabetes Care. 2009;32:1327–34.

26. Dorst J, Kuhnlein P, Hendrich C, Kassubek J, Sperfeld AD, Ludolph AC. Patients with elevated triglyceride and cholesterol serum levels have a prolonged survival in amyotrophic lateral sclerosis. J Neurol. 2011;258:613–7.

27. Lin JD, Chang JB, Wu CZ, Pei D, Hsieh CH, Hsieh AT, et al. Identification of insulin resistance in subjects with normal glucose tolerance. Ann Acad Med Singap. 2014;43:113–9.

28. Borai A, Livingstone C, Abdelaal F, Bawazeer A, Keti V, Ferns G. The relationship between glycosylated haemoglobin (HbA1c) and measures of insulin resistance across a range of glucose tolerance. Scand J Clin Lab Invest. 2011;71:168–72.

29. Shi P, Wei Y, Zhang J, Gal J, Zhu H. Mitochondrial dysfunction is a converging point of multiple pathological pathways in amyotrophic lateral sclerosis. J Alzheimers Dis. 2010;20(Suppl 2):S311–24.

30. Abdul-Ghani MA, DeFronzo RA. Mitochondrial dysfunction, insulin resistance, and type 2 diabetes mellitus. Curr Diabetes Rep. 2008;8:173–8.

31. Sivitz WI, Yorek MA. Mitochondrial dysfunction in diabetes: from molecular mechanisms to functional significance and therapeutic opportunities. Antioxid Redox Sign. 2010;12:537–77.

32. Park K, Gross M, Lee DH, Holvoet P, Himes JH, Shikany JM, et al. Oxidative stress and insulin resistance: the coronary artery risk development in young adults study. Diabetes Care. 2009;32:1302–7.

33. Barber SC, Shaw PJ. Oxidative stress in ALS: key role in motor neuron injury and therapeutic target. Free Radical Bio Med. 2010;48:629–41.

34. English E, Idris I, Smith G, Dhatariya K, Kilpatrick ES, John WG. The effect of anaemia and abnormalities of erythrocyte indices on HbA1c analysis: a systematic review. Diabetologia. 2015;58:1409–21.

35. Mariosa D, Kamel F, Bellocco R, Ye W, Fang F. Association between diabetes and amyotrophic lateral sclerosis in Sweden. Eur J Neurol. 2015;22:1436–42.

36. Turner MR, Goldacre R, Ramagopalan S, Talbot K, Goldacre MJ. Autoimmune disease preceding amyotrophic lateral sclerosis: an epidemiologic study. Neurology. 2013;81(14):1222–5.

37. Chen Y, Lin Z, Chen X, Cao B, Wei Q, Ou R, et al. Large C9orf72 repeat expansions are seen in Chinese patients with sporadic amyotrophic lateral sclerosis. Neurobiol Aging. 2016;38(217):e15–22.

38. Williams KL, McCann EP, Fifita JA, Zhang K, Duncan EL, Leo PJ, et al. Novel TBK1 truncating mutation in a familial amyotrophic lateral sclerosis patient of Chinese origin. Neurobiol Aging. 2015;36(3334):e1–5.

39. Konno T, Shiga A, Tsujino A, Sugai A, Kato T, Kanai K, et al. Japanese amyotrophic lateral sclerosis patients with GGGGCC hexanucleotide repeat expansion in C9ORF72. J Neurol Neurosurg Psychiatry. 2013;84:398–401.

40. Alavi A, Nafissi S, Rohani M, Shahidi G, Zamani B, Shamshiri H, et al. Repeat expansion in C9ORF72 is not a major cause of amyotrophic lateral sclerosis among Iranian patients. Neurobiol Aging. 2014;35(267):e1–7.

41. Consultation. WE. Appropriate body-mass index for Asian populations and its implications for policy and intervention strategies. Lancet. 2004;363:157–63.

8

Fibroblast bioenergetics to classify amyotrophic lateral sclerosis patients

Csaba Konrad[1], Hibiki Kawamata[1], Kirsten G. Bredvik[1], Andrea J. Arreguin[1], Steven A. Cajamarca[1], Jonathan C. Hupf[2], John M. Ravits[3], Timothy M. Miller[4], Nicholas J. Maragakis[5], Chadwick M. Hales[6], Jonathan D. Glass[6], Steven Gross[7], Hiroshi Mitsumoto[2] and Giovanni Manfredi[1]*

Abstract

Background: The objective of this study was to investigate cellular bioenergetics in primary skin fibroblasts derived from patients with amyotrophic lateral sclerosis (ALS) and to determine if they can be used as classifiers for patient stratification.

Methods: We assembled a collection of unprecedented size of fibroblasts from patients with sporadic ALS (sALS, $n = 171$), primary lateral sclerosis (PLS, $n = 34$), ALS/PLS with *C9orf72* mutations ($n = 13$), and healthy controls ($n = 91$). In search for novel ALS classifiers, we performed extensive studies of fibroblast bioenergetics, including mitochondrial membrane potential, respiration, glycolysis, and ATP content. Next, we developed a machine learning approach to determine whether fibroblast bioenergetic features could be used to stratify patients.

Results: Compared to controls, sALS and PLS fibroblasts had higher average mitochondrial membrane potential, respiration, and glycolysis, suggesting that they were in a hypermetabolic state. Only membrane potential was elevated in *C9Orf72* lines. ATP steady state levels did not correlate with respiration and glycolysis in sALS and PLS lines. Based on bioenergetic profiles, a support vector machine (SVM) was trained to classify sALS and PLS with 99% specificity and 70% sensitivity.

Conclusions: sALS, PLS, and *C9Orf72* fibroblasts share hypermetabolic features, while presenting differences of bioenergetics. The absence of correlation between energy metabolism activation and ATP levels in sALS and PLS fibroblasts suggests that in these cells hypermetabolism is a mechanism to adapt to energy dissipation. Results from SVM support the use of metabolic characteristics of ALS fibroblasts and multivariate analysis to develop classifiers for patient stratification.

Keywords: Bioenergetics, Mitochondria, ALS, Fibroblasts, PLS, Machine learning

Background

Amyotrophic lateral sclerosis (ALS) is the most common form of adult onset motor neuron disease, with a yearly incidence rate of 1–2.6 cases per 100,000. ALS leads to death within 3–5 years from disease onset [1]. Typical ALS is characterized by a rapidly progressive loss of upper and lower motor neurons. However, milder forms of the disease, such as primary lateral sclerosis (PLS), cause only upper motor neuron degeneration [2]. Unfortunately, most ALS clinical trials have been unsuccessful [3], and as a

result there are only two currently approved drugs for ALS, Riluzole and Edaravone, both of which only prolong life by a few months. The ineffectiveness of candidate therapies, the heterogeneity of the disease phenotype, and the diversity of ALS-linked genes support the emerging concept that distinct pathogenic mechanisms may participate in the development of ALS. For this reason, research efforts are increasingly concentrated on finding biomarkers that allow stratifying patients into groups better suited for targeted clinical trials.

Recently, a number of candidate biomarkers have been proposed, including some obtained by neuroimaging [4, 5], electrical impedance myography [6], and proteomics of cerebrospinal fluid [7–10]. However, despite their potential

---

* Correspondence: gim2004@med.cornell.edu
[1]Feil Family Brain and Mind Research Institute, Weill Cornell Medicine, 407 East 61st Street, RR507, New York, NY 10065, USA
Full list of author information is available at the end of the article

link to disease pathogenesis, complex cellular functions have not yet been explored as ALS biomarkers. Clearly, functional measures in living cells from affected tissues, such as the spinal cord, could be problematic, but one could envision that more accessible cell types could serve as surrogate samples. In ALS, skin fibroblasts display numerous abnormalities [11–14], many of which are shared with motor neurons [15–27]. This suggests that these apparently unaffected cells may share common pathogenic pathways with motor neurons. Furthermore, fibroblasts can be propagated in culture, frozen, and stored almost indefinitely, and transformed in cell types that are severely affected by the disease, such as motor neurons and astrocytes [28]. Furthermore, fibroblasts derived from ALS patients were used to generate a tissue-engineered skin model, which recapitulated many of the skin alterations found in ALS [29, 30]. Therefore, studying complex functional measures in fibroblasts from ALS patients could provide a promising source of new classifiers.

Here, we have investigated a large cohort of ALS fibroblasts and characterized their bioenergetic properties. We used a battery of assays to study cellular energy metabolism, and found a hypermetabolic phenotype in ALS, involving both oxidative phosphorylation and glycolysis. Importantly, using a machine learning approach on bioenergetic profiles, we provide a proof of concept that fibroblast bioenergetic markers could differentiate between ALS and PLS, and could therefore be proposed as tools for discriminating among different forms of ALS.

Methods
Chemicals
All chemicals used were form Sigma (St. Louis, MO), unless otherwise specified.

Skin biopsy and fibroblast cultures
After informed consent, a punch skin biopsy was obtained from the volar part of the forearm. Skin biopsies were de-identified to protect patients' identity. Fibroblast samples were provided to our laboratory as coded samples. Some lines were obtained from the NINDS catalog of motor neuron disease fibroblasts. Skin fibroblasts were cultured as described previously [31] in Dulbecco's modified Eagle medium (DMEM) (Thermo Fisher Scientific, Waltham, MA) supplemented with 25 mM glucose, 4 mM glutamine, 1 mM pyruvate, and 10% fetal bovine serum (hereafter growth medium). All cultured fibroblast lines were studied at passages ranging between 5 and 10. We have not observed loss of contact inhibition in any of the lines or apparent differences in growth between any of the groups.

Measurements of TMRM and MTG fluorescence
Skin fibroblasts were seeded at the density of 1.5×10^4 cells/well in replicates of eights in 96-well tissue culture plates in growth medium and incubated at 37 °C in 5% CO_2. The following day, cells were washed and loaded with 50 nM of the potentiometric dye Tetramethylrhodamine-methyl-ester (TMRM, 544ex, 590em; Thermo Fisher Scientific) and 450 nM MitoTracker Green (MTG, 490ex, 516em; Thermo Fisher Scientific) for 30 min at 37 °C in phenol-free DMEM containing 5 mM glucose, 4 mM glutamine, and 1 mM pyruvate. Samples were incubated in the absence or the presence of 2 μM cyanide p-trifluoromethoxyphenylhydrazone (FCCP) to completely depolarize mitochondria and obtain background TMRM and MTG fluorescence. After washing with DMEM, MTG and TMRM fluorescence were simultaneously recorded in a plate reader equipped with a polychromator (Spectramax M5; Molecular Devices Sunnyvale, CA). Background fluorescence was subtracted from the total fluorescence. MTG and TMRM fluorescence values were expressed as relative fluorescence units per milligram of total cellular proteins measured with the DC Protein Assay (BioRad, Hercules, CA).

Measurement of ATP content
Fibroblasts were seeded at the density of 1.5×10^4 cells/well in replicates of nines in 96-well tissue culture plates in growth medium incubated at 37 °C in 5% CO_2. The next day cells were incubated in triplicates in DMEM containing 5 mM glucose, 4 mM glutamine, and 1 mM pyruvate (ATP baseline), or DMEM containing 4 mM glutamine, 1 mM pyruvate, and 5 mM 2-deoxy-D-glucose (2DG) to bock glycolysis (ATP 2DG), or DMEM containing 5 mM glucose, 4 mM glutamine, 1 mM pyruvate, and 1 μM oligomycin to block the mitochondrial ATPase (ATP Oligo). After 90 min incubation, cells were washed with phosphate buffered saline (PBS) and lysed in 30 μl tichloroacetic acid (2.5% W/V) on ice for 30 min. Following lysis, 20 μl aliquots were transferred into a separate plate for protein determination (DC Protein Assay). 45 μl Tris-acetate buffer (400 mM, pH = 8.0) was added to the remaining lysate. Cellular ATP content was measured after addition of 20 μl of luciferase reagent (Promega, Madison, WI) in a luminescence plate reader (Spectramax M5). Luminescence values were normalized against an ATP standard.

Measurements of oxygen consumption and extracellular acidification
Oxygen consumption rate (OCR) and extracellular acidification rate (ECAR) were measured with a XF96 Extracellular Flux Analyzer (Agilent, Santa Clara, CA). Cell lines were seeded in 12 wells of a XF 96-well cell culture microplate (Agilent) at a density of 1×10^4 cells/well (cells reach confluency on the experimental day) in 200 μL of growth medium and incubated for 24 h at 37 °

C in 5% CO_2. After replacing the growth medium with 200 μL of XF Assay Medium (Agilent) supplemented with 5 mM glucose, 1 mM pyruvate and 4 mM glutamine, pre-warmed at 37 °C, cells were degassed for 1 h before starting the assay procedure, in a non-CO_2 incubator. OCR and ECAR were recorded at baseline followed by sequential additions of 1 μM oligomycin, 2 μM FCCP and 0.5 μM Antimycin A plus 0.5 μM Rotenone. Non-mitochondrial oxygen consumption (in the presence of AA + Rot) was subtracted from all OCR values and technical replicates outside of two standard deviations of the means were discarded for both ECAR and OCR. Values were normalized by the mean protein value of each line. The measurement of OCR and ECAR in galactose medium was performed as described above, with the exception that the growth medium and assay medium contained no glucose and was supplemented with 5 mM galactose.

Lactate excretion rate measurement

Lactate production was measured using a kit (Enzy-FluoTM L-lactate Assay Kit (EFLLC-100), BioAssay Systems) based on a fluorescent probe linked to NADH generated from lactate. Cell lines were seeded in XF 96-well cell culture microplates as described for OCR and ECAR measurements. On the experimental day, the growth medium was replaced with 200 μL of XF Assay Medium supplemented with 5 mM glucose, 1 mM pyruvate and 4 mM glutamine, pre-warmed at 37 °C. Cells were allowed to excrete lactate by incubation for 210 min at 37 °C in 5% CO_2. Aliquots of the medium were then collected, and diluted 5 fold for the assay. Lactate standards diluted in Assay medium were used for quantification.

Statistical analyses

Bioenergetic features were tested for normality by D'Agostino-Pearson test (scipy v0.15.1; www.scipy.org), which combines skewness and kurtosis to produce an omnibus test of normality. Since none of the parameters passed the normality test, we used non-parametric tests. Differences amongst groups were compared using Kruskal–Wallis one-way ANOVA, followed by Dunn's multiple comparison test, as post hoc analysis (scipy v0.15.1). Correlations amongst bioenergetic features were tested using Spearman rank-order correlation coefficient. The p-values of correlations were adjusted for multiple comparisons by Benjamini-Hochberg correction with a false discovery rate set to <0.05. Data in the text are presented as % average (±95% confidence intervals of the differences). There were no correlations between any of the measured bioenergetics parameters and patient age, sex, or cell line passage number. Therefore, no adjustment for these parameters was necessary.

Support vector machines

The complexity and performance of the SVM model is controlled by tunable parameters (class weights, kernels, penalties and gamma values). For each classification problem (i.e., control vs. disease, sALS vs. PLS), we tested an array of 1120 different sets of model parameters (grid search). A less complex model would have lower performance, but a more complex one would "overfit" the data, and the resulting decision boundary would follow the noise of the samples rather than inherent patterns that generalize well to the population. To find the best performing SVM that does not overfit, we used the well-established metod of k-fold cross-validation as a measure model performance: first the data was randomly divided into 10 sets, then for each set of model parameters the SVM was trained on 9 and validated on one set of the data. This step was repeated 10 times, using a different set as the validation set each time. Model performance was calculated as the average of the 10 validation performances (% accuracy). Fitting SVMs and generating receiver operating characteristic (ROC) curves were performed using scikit-learn v0.18 (www.scikit-learn.org). ROC curves are the averages of the 10 cross-validation sets.

Results
Clinical features of study subjects

Table 1 summarizes the clinical characteristics of the sALS, PLS, C9Orf72, and control subjects whose de-identified fibroblasts were utilized for this study. sALS patients ($n = 171$) were clinically defined based on definite or probable ALS diagnosis. sALS patients did not have family history of ALS are were negative for SOD1 and C9orf72 mutations. PLS patients ($n = 34$) were clinically defined on the basis of pure upper motor neuron disease, >5 years after symptom onset, normal electromyogram, and no definable causes. As expected, there were more males in both the sALS and PLS groups, consistent with higher frequency of the disease in males [32]. Also predictably, the rate of progression (i.e., the rate at which the ALS Functional Rating Scale, ALSFRS, worsens) and the forced vital capacity (FVC) decline were significantly less severe in the PLS group than in sALS (mean: 17.7%, CI: 7.2 to 27.7%, $p = 1.9E-18$ and mean: 117.8%, CI: 107.1 to 128.1%, $p = 2.9E-4$ respectively), consistent with the milder phenotype in PLS. The age of disease onset was significantly earlier in the PLS group (mean: 89.6%, CI: 84.2 to 95.0%, $p = 6.1E-05$). We included in the study fibroblasts from patients with C9orf72 expansion who had ALS ($n = 12$) or PLS ($n = 1$). However, we did not compare the clinical features of the genetically defined C9orf72 group, because of the relatively low number of samples available.

Table 1 Clinical characteristics of study subjects

	n	Sex F/M	Age at onset	Age at biopsy	ALSFRS	Rate of progression	FVC (%)	BMI	Onset S/B
Controls	91	0.88	–	60.3 (47–83)	–	–	–	NA	–
sALS	171	0.67	58.3 (26–79)	59.7 (27–80)	34.2 (8–47)	1.0 (0.06–3.4)	76.1 (6–138)	26.4 (16.2–39.7)	1.98
PLS	34	0.79	51.7* (32–74)	59.2 (41–81)	33.2 (14–44)	0.2* (0.07–0.37)	89.6* (31–143)	26.9 (19–34.6)	2.67
C9Orf72	13	1.50	56.3 (40–70)	58.3 (38–72)	34.9 (30–41)	0.9 (0.24–2.0)	79.3 (38–115)	27.8 (20.5–50.4)	3.00

Values indicate averages and values in brackets indicate ranges. Sex F/M, is the female to male ratio; ALSFRS, is the ALS functional rating scale at time of skin biopsy; Rate of progression is the % of ALSFRS decline per month; FVC is the forced vital capacity at time of skin biopsy expressed as % of normal; BMI is the body mass index at time of skin biopsy; Onset S/B is the ratio of site of disease onset, spinal (S) or bulbar (B). *NA* not available

*$p < 0.005$ PLS vs. ALS, based on Mann-Whitney U test

Bioenergetic characterization of sALS, PLS, and C9Orf72 fibroblasts

To generate a comprehensive bioenergetic profile of fibroblast lines in disease and control groups we measured the following parameters: mitochondrial membrane potential, cellular ATP content, cell respiration, and glycolysis. The fluorescence intensity of tetramethylrhodamine methyl ester (TMRM), an indicator of mitochondrial membrane potential, was significantly higher in all disease groups relative to controls (sALS mean: 127.6%, CI: 112.5 to 142.8%; PLS mean: 165.1%, CI: 142.1 to 189.3%; C9Orf72 mean: 155.1%, CI: 125.5 to 191.5%, Fig. 1a). To determine whether increased mitochondrial membrane potential could be attributed to differences in mitochondrial content, we measured the fluorescence of MitoTrackerGreen (MTG), a dye that is trapped and enriched in mitochondria, with minimal dependence on membrane potential [31], and can therefore be used as a readout of mitochondrial content. sALS and C9Orf72 lines showed no differences in MTG fluorescence relative to controls (Fig. 1b), whereas PLS had a significant decrease in MTG fluorescence (mean: 62.1%, CI: 36.3 to 88.8%). Since increased TMRM fluorescence in sALS and PLS was not matched by proportional increases in MTG fluorescence, we inferred that higher TMRM fluorescence was attributable to increased mitochondrial membrane potential, and not to mitochondrial content. Note that the number of samples tested for TMRM and MTG fluorescence was smaller than the total number of sALS lines available, because a subset of them were assessed for these two bioenergetic parameters in a previous study, which also indicated higher TMRM values in a smaller cohort of sALS and PLS lines [31].

Next, we measured mitochondrial OCR (Fig. 2a, blue curve) using flux analysis. In this experiment, baseline OCR is first measured, followed by the addition of the ATPase inhibitor oligomycin, which decreases OCR, as the proton motive force cannot be used for ATP production. The oligomycin sensitive OCR is calculated by subtracting oligomycin OCR rate from baseline. Then, the proton motive force is dissipated using the uncoupler FCCP, which allows the respiratory chain to consume oxygen at its fastest rate. The FCCP OCR rate is

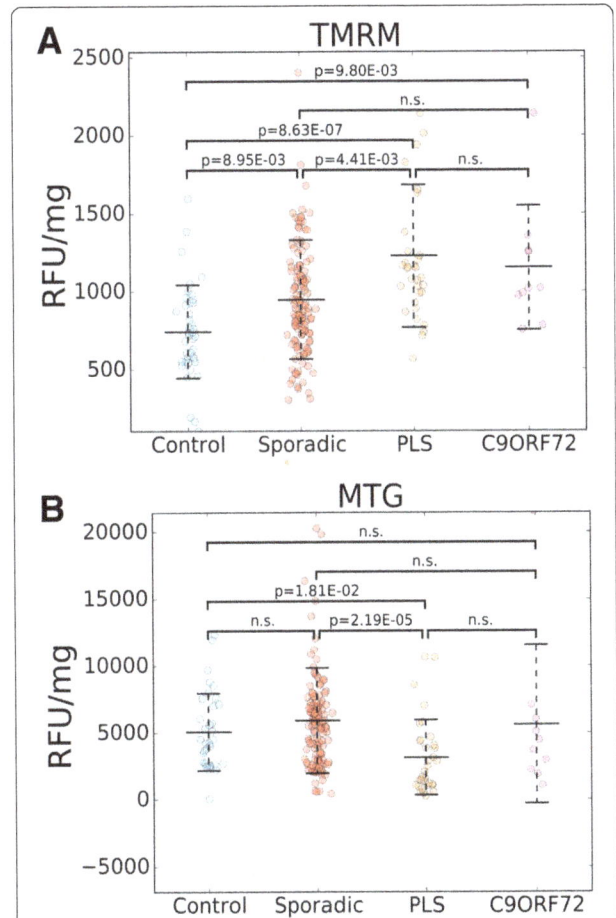

Fig. 1 Higher mitochondrial membrane potential in fibroblasts from patients with motor neuron disease. Scatter plots of TMRM **a** Control mean: 743.4, SD: 298.5; sALS mean: 948.3, SD: 380.3, PLS mean: 1227.3, SD: 456.7, C9Orf72 mean: 1153.0, SD: 397.5) and MTG **b** Control mean: 5080.9, SD: 2886.7, sALS mean: 5918.7, SD: 3939.6, PLS mean: 3153.6, SD: 2813.2; C9Orf72 mean: 5616.9, SD: 5911.8) values in sALS, PLS, C9Orf72, and control fibroblast lines. Middle bars represent the average values and error bars show standard deviations. RFU: relative fluorescence units. *p*-values are indicated where there was a significant difference between two groups. n.s.: no significant difference. n = 127 sALS, n = 33 PLS, n = 10 C9Orf72, n = 41 controls

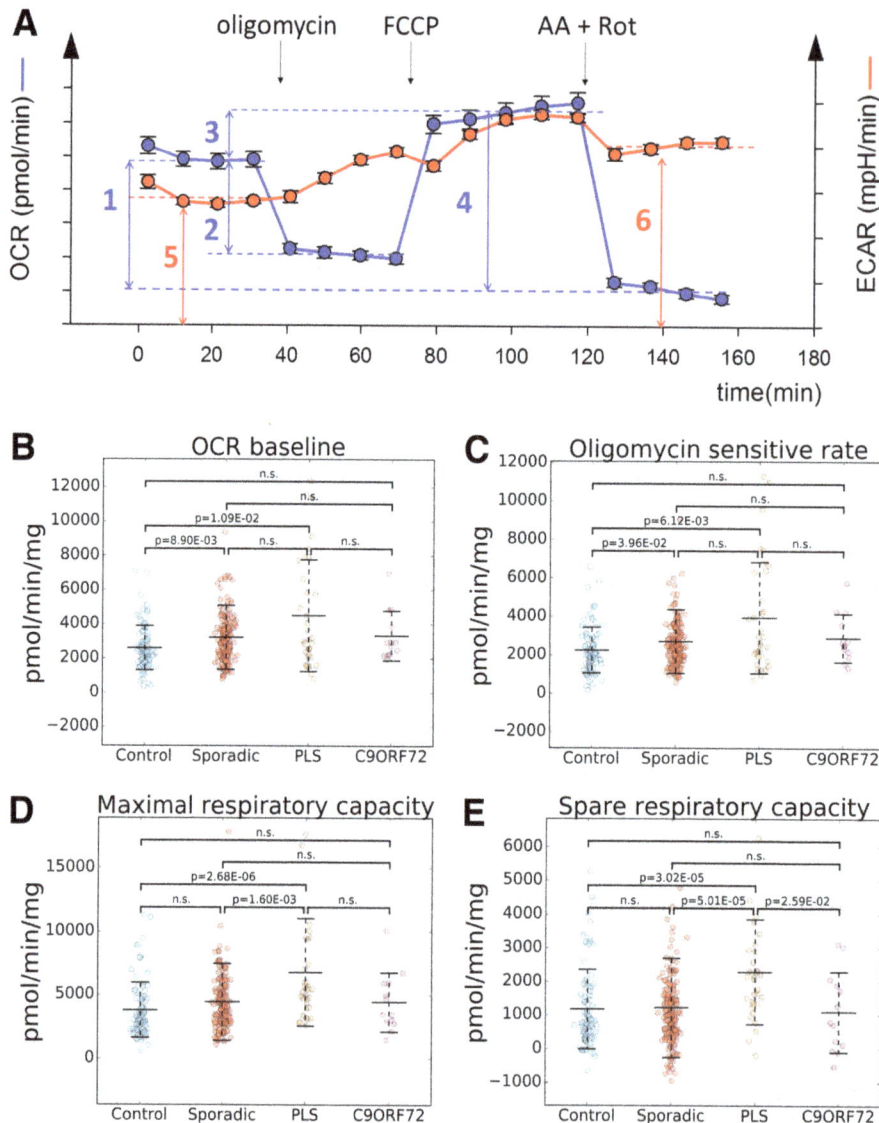

Fig. 2 Higher oxygen consumption rates in sALS and PLS fibroblasts. **a** Schematic illustration of a typical flux experiment and the calculated metrics (1: OCR baseline, 2: oligomycin sensitive rate, 3: spare respiratory capacity, 4: maximal respiratory capacity, 5: ECAR baseline, 6: ECAR AA-Rot). B-E: scatter plots of OCR baseline **b** Control mean: 2606.9, SD: 1290.5; sALS mean: 3224.0, SD: 1864.5; PLS mean: 4504.6, SD: 3259.3; *C9orf72* mean: 3338.2, SD: 1450.7), oligomycin sensitive rate **c** Control mean: 2248.2, SD: 1193.9; sALS mean: 2707.6, SD: 1656.9; PLS mean: 3947.9, SD: 2892.3; *C9Orf72* mean: 2900.4, SD: 1251.4), maximal respiratory capacity **d** Control mean: 3784.6, SD: 2166.9; sALS mean: 4445.7, SD: 3048.2; PLS mean: 6797.1, SD: 4247.2; *C9orf72* mean: 4443.5, SD: 2339.5), spare respiratory capacity **e** Control mean: 1177.7, SD: 1187.2; sALS mean: 1221.7, SD: 1476.5; PLS mean: 2292.5, SD: 1563.6; *C9orf72* mean: 1105.3, SD: 1195.8). Values are shown comparing sALS, PLS, *C9orf72*, and control lines. Middle bars represent the average values and error bars show standard deviations. *p*-values are indicated where there was a significant difference between two groups. n.s.: no significant difference. *n* = 171 sALS; *n* = 34 PLS, *n* = 13 *C9Orf72*, *n* = 91 controls

considered as maximal respiratory capacity, and the spare respiratory capacity is calculated as the difference between maximal and baseline OCR. Lastly, a mixture of the respiratory chain complex III and I inhibitors (Antimycin A and Rotenone, AA + Rot, respectively) are added to assess non-mitochondrial respiration, which is considered as background.

Relative to controls, sALS and PLS had elevated baseline OCR (sALS mean: 123.7%, CI: 109.1 to 138.9%; PLS mean: 172.8%, CI: 131.6 to 216.4%, Fig. 2b), oligomycin sensitive OCR (sALS mean: 120.4%, CI: 105.3 to 136.0%; PLS mean: 175.6%, CI: 134.5 to 220.5%, Fig. 2c), and maximal respiratory capacity (sALS mean: 117.5%, CI: 100.8 to 135.0%; PLS mean: 179.6%, CI: 142.0 to 220.4%, Fig. 2d). Spare respiratory capacity was only significantly elevated in PLS lines (mean: 194.7%, CI: 149.4 to 243.7%, Fig. 2e). Comparing sALS, PLS and *C9orf72*, there was no difference in baseline OCR and oligomycin sensitive respiration, but relative to PLS sALS had lower maximal capacity (mean: 65.4%, CI: 43.0 to 85.8%), and both sALS and *C9Orf72* had lower spare respiratory capacity (sALS: mean: 53.3%, CI: 27.7 to 76.9%; C9Orf72: mean: 48.2%, CI: 12.9 to 83.3% Fig. 2e).

In parallel to OCR, the flux analyzer allows for measurement of ECAR (Fig. 2a, red curve). Relative to controls, both sALS and PLS cells had higher baseline ECAR (sALS: mean: 124.6%, CI: 111.0 to 138.0%; PLS: mean: 192.0%, CI: 157.4 to 230.5%, Fig. 3a). ECAR AA + Rot (i.e., maximal ECAR when the respiratory chain is fully inhibited) was also higher (sALS: mean: 118.8%, CI: 17.0 to 130.5%; PLS: mean: 186.1%, CI: 153.5 to 222.9%, Fig. 3b). Moreover, PLS had higher ECAR baseline (mean: 154.1%, CI: 126.5 to 185.1%, Fig. 3a) and ECAR AA + Rot (mean: 156.6%, CI: 129.9 to 187.3%, Fig. 3b) than sALS.

Taken together, these results showed that sALS and PLS fibroblasts upregulate both oxidative phosphorylation and glycolysis. Furthermore, the extent of relative OCR and ECAR increase was similar in the two groups, suggesting that both bioenergetic pathways are similarly upregulated. This was confirmed by calculating the ratio between OCR baseline and ECAR baseline, which was not different among the groups (Fig. 3c), indicating that there was no metabolic shift towards either glycolysis or oxidative phosphorylation. Of note, in highly aerobic states, CO_2 production from mitochondria can contribute to ECAR. However, it was empirically determined that in cells with low baseline OCR/ECAR ratio (e.g., < 4) CO_2 has a negligible contribution to ECAR [33]. Since in fibroblasts the average OCR/ECAR ratio was approximately 1.5, the CO_2 contribution to ECAR was likely not significant, suggesting that glycolysis was the major contributor to ECAR. Furthermore, since under conditions of full respiratory chain inhibition CO_2 production in the Krebs cycle is strongly attenuated, the interpretation of higher glycolysis is also supported by the higher ECAR values in sALS and PLS after AA + Rot addition. To test experimentally the assumption that ECAR reflects lactate excretion we measured lactate production rates in a subset of 12 sALS, 12 PLS, and 12 control lines, under baseline conditions. Lactate production rate and ECAR baseline were significantly correlated ($p = 0.02$, data not shown), indicating that medium acidification reflects lactate excretion. Collectively, these results suggest that sALS and PLS fibroblasts have a hypermetabolic phenotype involving both oxidative phosphorylation and anaerobic glycolysis.

Next, we measured cellular steady-state ATP levels at baseline and after 90 min treatment with either 2DG to inhibit glycolysis or oligomycin to inhibit mitochondrial ATP production. In sALS, we found higher baseline ATP content compared to controls (mean: 114.9%, CI:

13.6 to 125.8%, Fig. 4a). Interestingly, PLS fibroblasts did not show higher ATP content, despite having the highest average respiration and glycolytic fluxes among all groups. The decline in ATP content after 2DG (ATP 2DG delta) was greater in sALS relative to controls (mean: 117.5%, CI: 106.4 to 128.7%, Fig. 4b). However, neither PLS nor *C9Orf72* lines had ATP 2DG delta greater than controls. When oxidative phosphorylation was inhibited (ATP Oligo delta), we observed no significant decline in ATP content in controls or sALS, while PLS showed a small but significant decline (−8.9%, Fig. 4c). Overall, these results suggest that sALS lines are more dependent on glucose utilization for ATP maintenance than controls, PLS or *C9Orf72*. Additionally, PLS is the only group that exhibits dependency on oxidative phosphorylation for ATP maintenance.

We performed correlation analyses of bioenergetic parameters of fibroblasts to assess if the interdependence of the parameters differed among groups (Table 2). The underlying assumption was that parameters would correlate when they were co-regulated. First, these analyses confirmed that all groups were dependent on glycolysis for energy production, as baseline ATP and sensitivity to 2DG (ATP 2DG delta) were strongly correlated. Second, the maximal glycolytic rate (ECAR AA-Rot) significantly correlated with the maximal OCR rate (OCR Max) in both sALS and PLS. Similarly, there was a direct correlation between OCR baseline and ECAR baseline in sALS and PLS, but not in controls. Taken together, these correlations suggest that in sALS and PLS lines glycolytic and oxidative fluxes are co-regulated. Despite these similarities, there were also differences between sALS and PLS. For example, only in PLS there was a negative correlation between the OCR/ECAR ratio and ATP content. Furthermore, only PLS cells showed a negative correlation between OCR/ECAR ratio and ATP 2DG delta.

To test the ability of fibroblasts to respond to forced oxidative metabolism we grew a subset of lines in medium containing galactose instead of glucose for 24 h. In these conditions, fibroblasts are forced to oxidize glycolysis-derived pyruvate for energy production, because galactose is not converted to glucose-6P as efficiently as glucose [34]. We tested the 12 controls, 12 sALS, and 12 PLS lines that had ECAR and OCR values closest to the average of their respective groups. As expected, in galactose medium baseline OCR was faster than in glucose medium (compare Additional file 1: Figure S1A and Figure 2B), while ECAR was lower (compare Additional file 1: Figure S1E and Figure 3A). This was also apparent from the increase of the OCR/ECAR ratio from approximately 1.5 in glucose to 3.5 in galactose (compare Additional file 1: Figure S1F and Figure 3C). The differences in baseline OCR and ECAR between sALS and controls, PLS and controls, and sALS

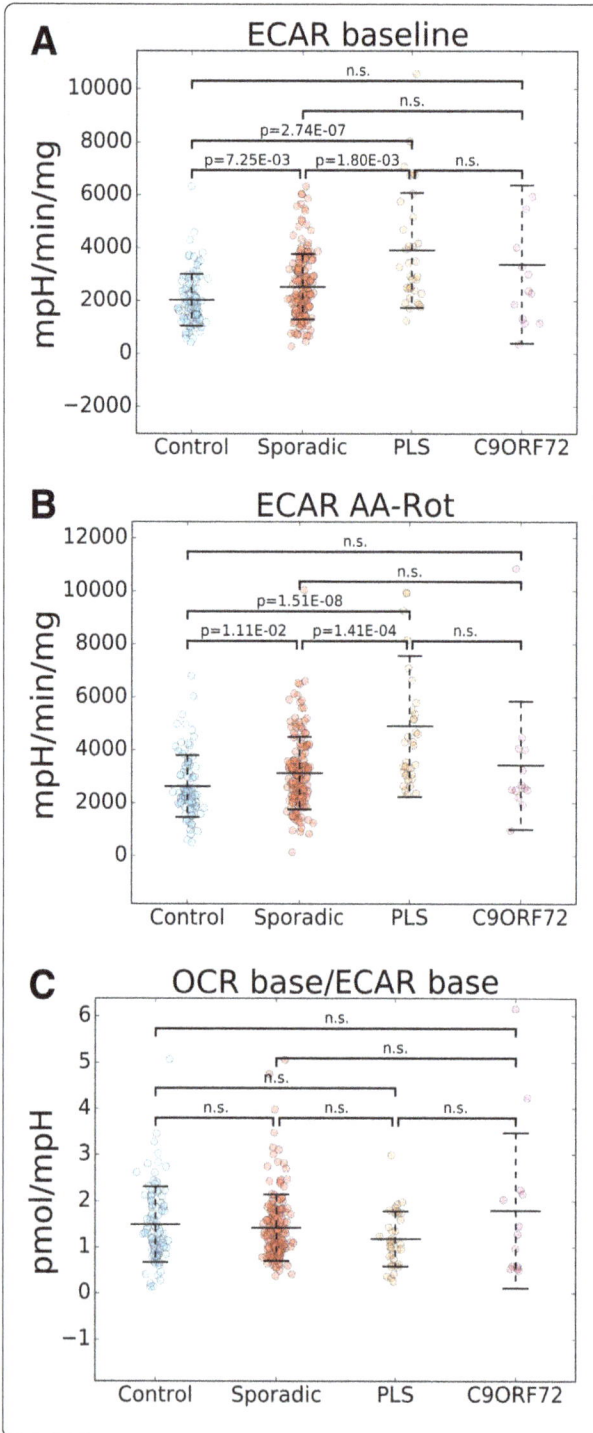

Fig. 3 Higher extracellular acidification rates in sALS and PLS fibroblasts. Scatter plots of ECAR baseline **a** Control mean: 2035.9, SD: 987.4; sALS mean: 2536.0, SD: 1237.8; PLS mean: 3909.1, SD: 2175.4; C9Orf72 mean: 3381.9, SD: 2988.0), ECAR AA-Rot **b** Control mean: 2631.1, SD: 1164.4; sALS mean: 3126.2, SD: 1366.6; PLS mean: 4895.2, SD: 2661.5; C9Orf72 mean: 3426.1, SD: 2425.9), and OCR base/ECAR base **c** Control mean: 1.5, SD: 0.8; sALS mean: 1.4, SD: 0.7; PLS mean: 1.2, SD: 0.6; C9Orf72 mean: 1.8, SD: 1.7) values are shown comparing sALS, PLS, C9Orf72, and control lines. The method by which features were calculated is illustrated in Fig. 2a. Middle bars represent the average values and error bars show standard deviations. p-values are indicated where there was a significant difference between two groups. n.s.: no significant difference. n = 171 sALS; n = 34 PLS, n = 13 C9Orf72, n = 91 controls

and PLS that was observed in glucose was not detected in galactose (Additional file 1: Figure S1A and S1E). These results suggest that control cells can upregulate OCR in galactose to match sALS and PLS. Interestingly, in galactose, the spare respiratory capacity was significantly lower in sALS than controls (Additional file 1: Figure D), while in PLS it was similar to controls. Since in glucose the spare respiratory capacity was higher in sALS and PLS than control (Fig. 2e), we interpret the result in galactose as an indication that ALS and PLS fibroblasts have respiration closer to maximal in glucose and cannot upregulate it much more when placed in galactose.

Stratification of ALS patients based on individual bioenergetic features

We separated our cohort of sALS fibroblast in two equally sized groups by the median values of key bioenergetic parameters: TMRM fluorescence (mitochondrial membrane potential), ECAR AA + Rot (maximal glycolytic activity), and oligomycin sensitive OCR (ATP synthesizing respiration). We then compared the two groups (i.e., with above median and below median values) for key clinical parameters: sex, age of disease onset, site of onset (i.e., bulbar vs. spinal), rate of disease progression, FVC at time of biopsy. We found that patients with high ECAR AA + Rot had significantly higher FVC (14%, $p = 0.01$) and more frequent spinal onset (25%, $p = 0.02$). We also found that patients with high TMRM had a faster rate of decline (18%, $p = 0.04$). Similar analyses were not performed for PLS or C9Orf72 lines, because the number of samples was too small to obtain adequately sized groups. Indeed, although interesting, the significant differences between upper and lower halves of the sALS lines were not large. Furthermore, significant liner correlations between individual key bioenergetic and clinical parameters, after correction for multiple correlations, were not found (not shown). Therefore, based on the available samples, we suggest that individual bioenergetic parameters in fibroblast lines may not be adequate to provide definite clinical classifications.

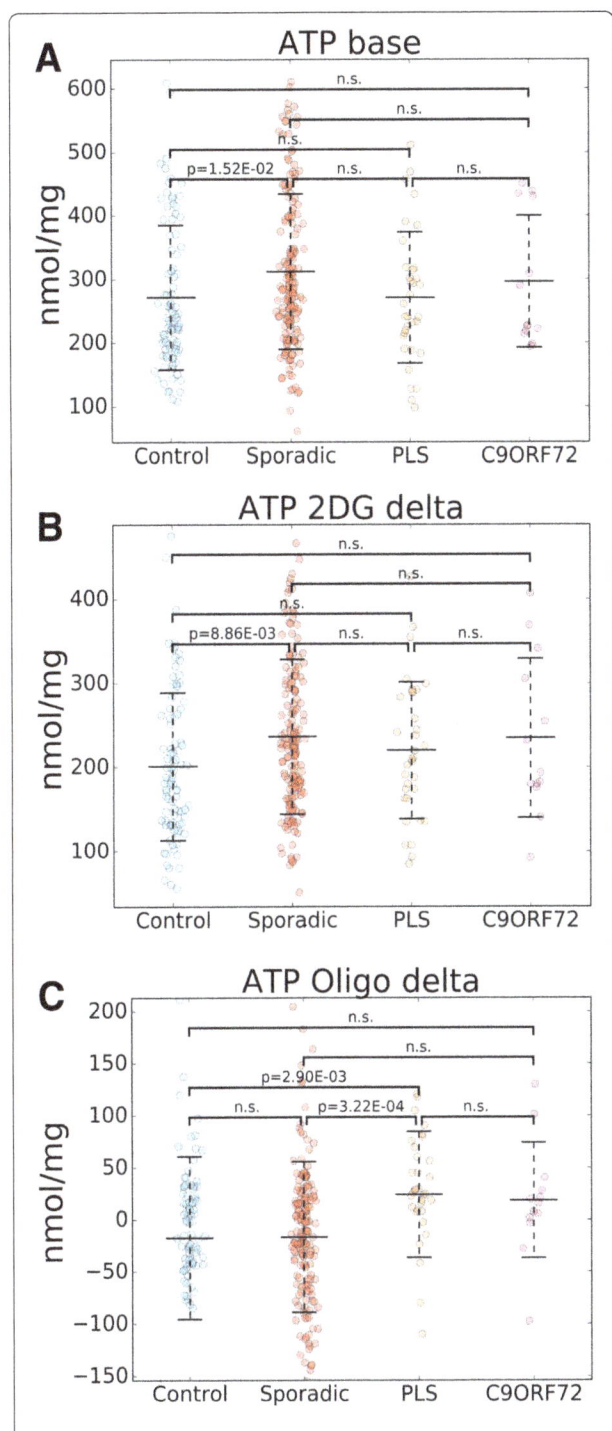

Fig. 4 ATP content in sALS and PLS fibroblasts. Scatter plots of baseline ATP content **a** Control mean: 271.6, SD: 113.7; sALS mean: 312.1, SD: 122.2; PLS mean: 271.1, SD: 103.2; *C9Orf72* mean: 296.1, SD: 103.8), ATP content lost after 2DG treatment **b** Control mean: 201.2, SD: 87.8; sALS mean: 236.4, SD: 92.1; PLS mean: 220.1, SD: 81.4; *C9Orf72* mean: 234.7, SD: 94.6), and ATP content lost after oligomycin treatment **c** Control mean: -17.3, SD: 78.1; sALS mean: -16.6, SD: 72.4; PLS mean: 24.1, SD: 60.2; *C9Orf72* mean: 18.6, SD: 55.1) are shown comparing sALS, PLS, *C9Orf72*, and control lines. Groups were compared using Kruskal–Wallis one-way analysis of variance followed by Dunn's post hoc analysis. Middle bars represent the average values and error bars show standard deviations. *p*-values are indicated where there was a significant difference between two groups. n.s.: no significant difference. n = 171 sALS; n = 34 PLS, n = 13 *C9Orf72*, n = 91 controls

Supervised machine learning on bioenergetic profiles classifies sALS and PLS fibroblasts with high specificity

As no individual bioenergetic measure had sufficient sensitivity or specificity to be used as a tool for classification by itself (data not shown), we took advantage of the high dimensionality of the data gathered and performed multivariate analysis. The following 12 features from 301 records (control, sALS, PLS, and *C9Orf72* combined) were used: TMRM, MTG, ECAR base, ECAR AA-Rot, OCR baseline, oligomycin sensitive respiration, spare respiratory capacity, maximal respiration, OCR baseline/ECAR baseline, ATP baseline, ATP 2DG delta and ATP Oligo delta. The goal was to determine if fibroblast groups could be clustered and predicted based purely on their bioenergetic features. Importantly, considering that such tool could have translational applications in helping to stratify patients, we wanted to establish proof of principle that multivariate analyses could distinguish between sALS and PLS. To this end, we utilized support vector machines (SVM), which are trained to fit non-linear decision boundaries to high dimensional data.

First we sought to classify control fibroblasts versus all disease groups combined (i.e., sALS, PLS and *C9Orf72*). Receiver operating characteristics (ROC) curves were generated based on the SVM classifier that yielded the highest accuracy (probability of correct assignment of samples to their respective groups). The best performing SVM yielded good sensitivity (88.5%, CI: 84.2 to 92.7%), but low specificity (38.1%, CI: 27.7 to 48.5%) (Fig. 5a). Other parameters of the performance of this SVM classifier included, positive predictive value (78.7%, CI: 73.6 to 83.8%), negative predictive value (56.1%, CI: 43.3 to 69.0%), false positive rate (61.9%, CI: 51.5 to 72.3%), false negative rate (11.5%, CI: 7.3 to 15.8%), and false discovery rate (21.3%, CI: 16.2 to 26.4%). Interestingly, our best performing SVM to classify sALS versus PLS (Fig. 5b) yielded good sensitivity (70.6%, CI: 55.3 to 85.9%), and high specificity (98.8%, CI: 97.2 to 100.0%), with a

Table 2 Correlations among bioenergetics features

Feature 1	Feature 2	Control		sALS		PLS		C9Orf72	
		R	p value	R	p value	R	p value	R	p value
ATP baseline	ATP 2DG delta	0.922	6.45E-37	0.924	7.07E-71	0.941	4.61E-15	0.648	n.s.
ECAR AA-Rot	OCR Max	0.638	9.62E-11	0.683	6.00E-24	0.826	2.07E-08	0.489	n.s.
ECAR baseline	OCR baseline	0.234	n.s.	0.574	1.49E-15	0.551	3.01E-03	0.170	n.s.
OCR base/ECAR base	ATP baseline	0.211	n.s.	−0.017	n.s.	−0.508	7.45E-03	0.384	n.s.
OCR base/ECAR base	ATP 2DG delta	0.248	n.s.	0.012	n.s.	−0.491	9.53E-03	0.264	n.s.
OCR baseline	ATP baseline	0.182	n.s.	0.155	n.s.	−0.434	2.42E-02	0.445	n.s.
ECAR baseline	ATP baseline	0.012	n.s.	0.124	n.s.	0.005	n.s.	−0.148	n.s.

Values indicate Spearman's correlation coefficients (R) and p-values (corrected by the Benjamini-Hochberg method with a false discovery rate set to <0.05). n.s., not significant

positive predictive value of 92.3%, CI: 82.1 to 100.0%, negative predictive value of 94.4%, CI: 91.0 to 97.8%, false positive rate of 1.2%, CI: 0.0 to 2.8%, false negative rate of 29.4%, CI: 14.1 to 44.7%, and false discovery rate of 7.7%, CI: 0.0 to 17.9%. In summary, the SVM analysis of fibroblast bioenergetic features was most effective in classifying the two forms of motor neurons disease, sALS and PLS, as indicated by the high area under the curve value (0.94) and the steep rise of true positive rate of the mean ROC curve (Fig 5b).

Discussion

In this study, we characterized the bioenergetics of a large number of sALS and PLS primary skin fibroblast lines with the goal of finding disease classifiers. In addition, we studied the bioenergetics of a smaller cohort of fibroblast lines from the most common genetic form of fALS, C9orf72, to assess if bioenergetic features generalized to this form of the disease. We found that compared to healthy controls, sALS, PLS, and C9orf72 shared higher mitochondrial membrane potential, and that sALS and PLS also shared features indicative of hypermetabolism, characterized by higher mitochondrial respiration and glycolytic fluxes.

So far, studies on metabolic function in sALS and fALS fibroblasts have been conducted in much smaller cohorts. In a study of 6 sALS and 10 control fibroblast lines, it was reported that sALS had a lower average OCR baseline [34]. However, the number of the samples was thirty-fold smaller than the one studied here. We think that the sample size is important in this case, because of the variability observed among individual lines in all bioenergetic assays. Importantly, when they looked selectively at the older (≥70 years of age at onset) patients, they found that ECAR was significantly higher than controls. This is in agreement with our results showing increased ECAR in sALS, PLS. Therefore, except for the OCR baseline result, which could differ because of the difference in sample sizes, glycolytic flux increase appears to be a common finding in the two studies. Furthermore, mitochondrial function measurements performed in 3 sALS fibroblast lines and 10 controls identified a defect of cytochrome c oxidase in sALS, which correlated with a lower respiratory activity, but only when cells were forced to respire with succinate as substrate after blocking complex I with rotenone [35]. In this study, we did not assess individual respiratory chain complexes, and since fibroblasts do not naturally utilize succinate as a major respiratory substrate, we did not analyze this pathway because of relatively low physiological significance. Instead, we performed measurements of respiration in intact cells allowed to utilize glucose and NADH-generating substrates, such as glutamine and pyruvate. Therefore, the differences in the findings may be attributable to the different sample size, but also to the different approaches utilized. Lastly, a recent study of 4 C9orf72 and 4 control fibroblast lines found increased mitochondrial membrane potential in the C9orf72 lines [36] similar to that found in our C9orf72 cohort.

In our sALS and PLS fibroblast cohorts hypermetabolism was not accompanied by an increase in mitochondrial content or by a proportional increase in ATP content. Taken together, the data could be best interpreted as an adaptation to higher ATP demands, involving both oxidative and glycolytic pathways of energy generation. When cells were forced to maximize oxidative phosphorylation in galactose medium, the sALS and PLS were not capable of maintaining a faster respiratory rate than controls, suggesting that their capacity was close to maximal under glucose.

Further studies will be needed to dissect the mechanisms leading to hypermetabolism in ALS fibroblasts. However, we could hypothesize that several pathways may contribute to high ATP expenditure, including anabolic reactions, such as RNA and protein synthesis, catabolic reactions, such as protein degradation, vesicle acidification by V-ATPases, and ion homeostasis. The average values of several bioenergetic features were significantly different in PLS and sALS compared to controls, but also between sALS and PLS. The latter is a less

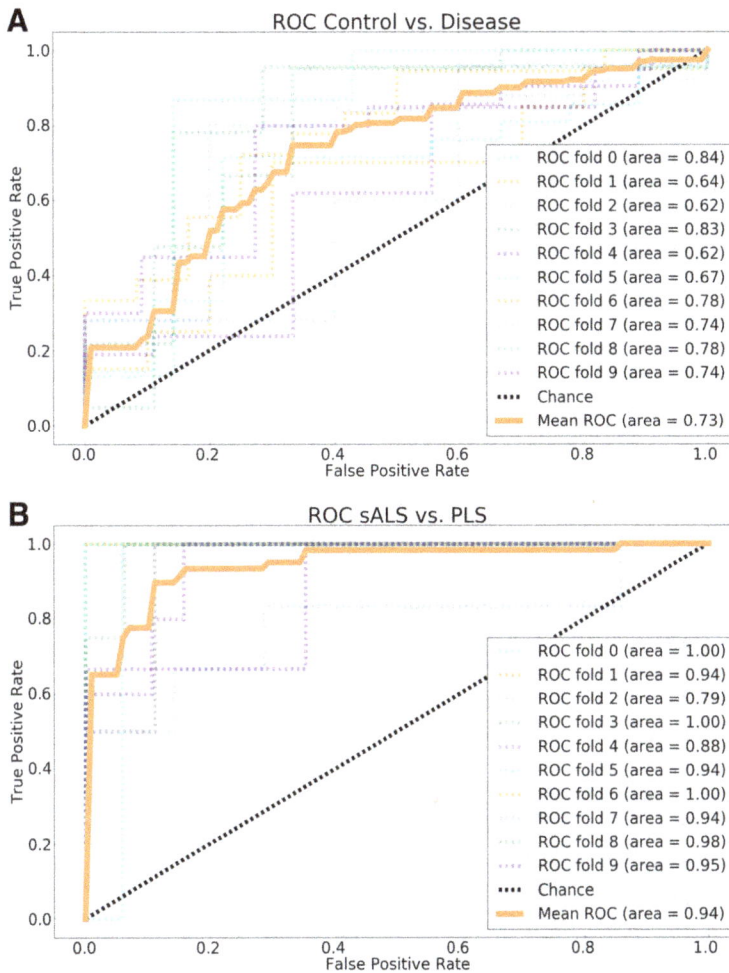

Fig. 5 Receiver operating characteristic (ROC) curves of SVM classifiers distinguishes lines with motor neuron disease from controls (**a**), and sALS from PLS (**b**). SVMs were trained to distinguish between two groups, based on 12 bioenergetics features. Each continuous orange ROC curve represents the mean of 10 cross-validation curves, each shown as a dotted line. Values of the area under the curve for each ROC curve (0–9 fold ROC and mean ROC) are indicated in the boxes

aggressive form of motor neuron disease as compared to sALS, since it only affects the upper motor neurons and progresses more slowly. In light of these findings, it could be speculated that hypermetabolism could be a functional adaptation to increased ATP demands common to fibroblasts and neurons. Future studies utilizing neurons differentiated from fibroblast derived induced pluripotent cells or directly derived from fibroblasts will test the hypothesis that hypermetabolism is shared by fibroblasts and neurons.

We deemed that we could exploit the metabolic differences between disease and control lines and between sALS and PLS to identify disease classifiers. Despite the significant differences among groups in bioenergetic parameters, because of the large variability of the values, no single metric performed well enough to be used individually as a predictive classifier (e.g., to discriminate between controls, sALS and PLS). To overcome the constraints associated with single parameters, we opted to use multivariate analyses. We implemented a widely employed machine learning method of supervised multivariate analysis, the SVM, which takes all bioenergetics parameters from each cell line as input to make a prediction. This system generates its own hypothesis based on a learning process and produces a model for a decision boundary. The model was able to distinguish control and disease lines (sALS, PLS and *C9Orf72* combined) with moderate accuracy, likely because the variability among the disease groups. Importantly, we found that sALS and PLS fibroblasts could be distinguished with high specificity using the machine learning model.

This result suggests that a machine learning model based on fibroblast bioenergetics may serve as a classifier to predict, prior to a definite clinical diagnosis, whether a patient will develop sALS or the milder motor neuron disease PLS, a prediction that would have clear prognostic implications. Admittedly, machine learning works best with high number of examples and more diverse features than the ones currently available to us. Although our collection of ALS fibroblast lines is likely one of the largest in existence, we predict that expanding the database with additional lines and features will increase the performance of the classification model. In addition, since in this work we did not have enough *C9orf72* lines to be able to analyze them as a separate group, in the future it will be important increase the *C9orf72* cohort. This would allow us to include them in the multivariate analyses of disease groups, for example to predict whether a *C9orf72* patient will develop frontotemporal dementia, ALS, or both. Another development could include patients with different neuropathies, such as spinal muscular atrophy and hereditary spastic paraplegia, to assess whether the model's power of distinction between sALS from PLS can be also extended to other forms of lower and upper motor neuron degeneration.

Conclusions

We have identified bioenergetic markers of hypermetabolism in ALS fibroblasts. These findings will open new avenues of investigation of the molecular and biochemical mechanisms responsible for the bioenergetic modifications and their relationship to disease pathogenesis. We have also devised a novel approach that utilizes bioenergetic features to distinguish between fibroblast groups, which performed well in discriminating between sALS and PLS. Therefore, it is conceivable that analyses of fibroblasts bioenergetic features will help to stratify ALS patients into well-defined classes (e.g., hypermetabolic vs. normometabolic), to preselect patients entering clinical trials or to be used as post hoc criteria to interpret trial results. They could also help developing makers of prognosis and response to therapy, by implementing longitudinal studies on ALS fibroblast bioenergetics on subsequent skin biopsies obtained during disease progression and during the course of treatments.

Additional file

Additional file 1: Figure S1. *Flux analysis of control, sALS and PLS fibroblasts under forced oxidative metabolism in galactose medium.* Scatter plots of OCR baseline (A; Control mean: 3850.0, SD: 1936.7; sALS mean: 3307.5, SD: 1430.7; PLS mean: 2989.2, SD: 1164.7), oligomycin sensitive rate (B; Control mean: 3630.0, SD: 1772.0; sALS mean: 2835.0, SD: 1135.4; PLS mean: 2707.5, SD: 1138.9), maximal respiratory capacity (C; Control mean: 5325.8, SD: 2993.3; sALS mean: 3613.3, SD: 1662.5; PLS mean: 3741.7, SD: 2102.3), spare respiratory capacity (D; Control mean: 1478.8, SD: 1385.2; sALS mean: 306.8, SD: 589.2; PLS mean: 754.5, SD: 1120.1), ECAR baseline (E; Control mean: 1114.8, SD: 349.3; sALS mean: 1063.3, SD: 573.2; PLS mean: 1007.8, SD: 351.7), and OCR base/ECAR base (F; Control mean: 3.6, SD: 1.3; sALS mean: 3.5, SD: 1.4; PLS mean: 3.3, SD: 1.4). Values are shown comparing sALS, PLS, and control lines. Middle bars represent the average values and error bars show standard deviations. *p*-values are indicated where there was a significant difference between groups. n.s.: no significant difference. *n* = 12 sALS; n = 12 PLS, n = 12 controls.

Abbreviations

2DG: 2-Deoxy-D-glucose; AA + Rot: Antimycin A + Rotenone; ALS: Amyotrophic lateral sclerosis; ALSFRS: ALS Functional Rating Scale; BMI: Body mass index; DMEM: Dulbecco modified Eagle medium; ECAR: Extracellular acidification rate; FCCP: Cyanide p-trifluoromethoxyphenylhydrazone; FVC: Forced vital capacity; MTG: MitoTracker Green; OCR: Oxygen consumption rate; PBS: Phosphate buffered saline; PLS: Primary lateral sclerosis; ROC: Receiver operating characteristic; sALS: Sporadic ALS; SVM: Support vector machine; TMRM: Tetramethylrhodamine-methyl-ester

Acknowledgments

This study used fibroblast samples from the NINDS Repository, as well as clinical data related to the samples. NINDS Repository sample numbers corresponding to the samples used are: (ND39022, ND39023, ND29422, ND29774, ND29149, AG13244, AG12598, AG13285, AG14284, AG11482, AG13150, AG13968, AG12657, AG12597, AG12851, AG11489, AG12964, AG12850, AG13144, AG13994, AG14048, AG13348, AG13990).

Funding

This work was funded by NIH R01NS062055 and by ALS Association grant 15-IIP-195 to GM.

Authors' contributions

Key contributors: CK, HK, KGB, AJA, SAC, MS, SG, HM, GM. Data acquisition contributors: JCH, JMR, TMM, NJM, CMH, JDG. All authors read and approved the final manuscript.

Competing interests

The authors declare that they have no competing interests.

Author details

[1]Feil Family Brain and Mind Research Institute, Weill Cornell Medicine, 407 East 61st Street, RR507, New York, NY 10065, USA. [2]Department of Neurology, Columbia University, New York, NY, USA. [3]Department of Neuroscience, University of California San Diego, La Jolla, CA, USA. [4]Department of Neurology, Washington University School of Medicine, St. Louis, MO, USA. [5]Department of Neurology, Johns Hopkins University School of Medicine, Baltimore, MD, USA. [6]Department of Neurology, Emory School of Medicine, Atlanta, GA, USA. [7]Department of Pharmacology, Weill Cornell Medicine, New York, NY, USA.

References

1. Talbott EO, Malek AM, Lacomis D. The epidemiology of amyotrophic lateral sclerosis. Handb Clin Neurol. 2016;138:225–38.
2. Chio A, Calvo A, Moglia C, Mazzini L, Mora G, group Ps. Phenotypic heterogeneity of amyotrophic lateral sclerosis: a population based study. J Neurol Neurosurg Psychiatry. 2011;82:740–6.
3. Katz JS, Barohn RJ, Dimachkie MM, Mitsumoto H. The dilemma of the clinical trialist in amyotrophic lateral sclerosis: the hurdles to finding a cure. Neurol Clin. 2015;33:937–47.
4. Menke RA, Agosta F, Grosskreutz J, Filippi M, Turner MR. Neuroimaging endpoints in amyotrophic lateral sclerosis. Neurotherapeutics. 2016;14(1):11–23.
5. Grolez G, Moreau C, Danel-Brunaud V, Delmaire C, Lopes R, Pradat PF, El Mendili MM, Defebvre L, Devos D. The value of magnetic resonance imaging as a biomarker for amyotrophic lateral sclerosis: a systematic review. BMC Neurol. 2016;16:155.
6. Rutkove SB, Caress JB, Cartwright MS, Burns TM, Warder J, David WS, Goyal N, Maragakis NJ, Clawson L, Benatar M, et al. Electrical impedance myography as a biomarker to assess ALS progression. Amyotroph Lateral Scler. 2012;13:439–45.

7. Chen Y, Liu XH, Wu JJ, Ren HM, Wang J, Ding ZT, Jiang YP. Proteomic analysis of cerebrospinal fluid in amyotrophic lateral sclerosis. Exp Ther Med. 2016;11:2095–106.

8. Oeckl PP, Jardel CPP, Salachas FM, Lamari FM, Andersen PMMP, Bowser RP, de Carvalho MP, Costa JP, van Damme PMP, Gray EP, et al. Multicenter validation of CSF neurofilaments as diagnostic biomarkers for ALS. Amyotroph Lateral Scler Frontotemporal Degener. 2016;17:404–13.

9. Lehnert S, Costa J, de Carvalho M, Kirby J, Kuzma-Kozakiewicz M, Morelli C, Robberecht W, Shaw P, Silani V, Steinacker P, et al. Multicentre quality control evaluation of different biomarker candidates for amyotrophic lateral sclerosis. Amyotroph Lateral Scler Frontotemporal Degener. 2014;15:344–50.

10. Steinacker P, Feneberg E, Weishaupt J, Brettschneider J, Tumani H, Andersen PM, von Arnim CA, Bohm S, Kassubek J, Kubisch C, et al. Neurofilaments in the diagnosis of motoneuron diseases: a prospective study on 455 patients. J Neurol Neurosurg Psychiatry. 2016;87:12–20.

11. Tsukie T, Masaki H, Yoshida S, Fujikura M, Ono S. Decreased amount of collagen in the skin of amyotrophic lateral sclerosis in the Kii peninsula of Japan. Acta Neurol Taiwanica. 2014;23:82–9.

12. Ono S, Toyokura Y, Mannen T, Ishibashi Y. Increased dermal collagen density in amyotrophic lateral sclerosis. J Neurol Sci. 1988;83:81–92.

13. Ono S, Imai T, Tsumura M, Takahashi K, Jinnai K, Suzuki M, Tagawa A, Shimizu N. Increased serum hyaluronic acid in amyotrophic lateral sclerosis: relation to its skin content. Amyotroph Lateral Scler Other Motor Neuron Disord. 2000;1:213–8.

14. Beach RL, Rao JS, Festoff BW, Reyes ET, Yanagihara R, Gajdusek DC. Collagenase activity in skin fibroblasts of patients with amyotrophic lateral sclerosis. J Neurol Sci. 1986;72:49–60.

15. Fang L, Huber-Abel F, Teuchert M, Hendrich C, Dorst J, Schattauer D, Zettlmeissel H, Wlaschek M, Scharffetter-Kochanek K, Tumani H, et al. Linking neuron and skin: matrix metalloproteinases in amyotrophic lateral sclerosis (ALS). J Neurol Sci. 2009;285:62–6.

16. Fang L, Teuchert M, Huber-Abel F, Schattauer D, Hendrich C, Dorst J, Zettlmeissel H, Wlaschek M, Scharffetter-Kochanek K, Kapfer T, et al. MMP-2 and MMP-9 are elevated in spinal cord and skin in a mouse model of ALS. J Neurol Sci. 2010;294:51–6.

17. Fukazawa H, Tsukie T, Higashida K, Fujikura M, Ono S. An immunohistochemical study of increased tumor necrosis factor-alpha in the skin of patients with amyotrophic lateral sclerosis. J Clin Neurosci. 2013;20:1371–6.

18. Higashida K, Tsukie T, Fukazawa H, Fujikura M, Ono S. Immunohistochemical studies of angiogenin in the skin of patients with amyotrophic lateral sclerosis. J Neurol Sci. 2013;326:18–23.

19. Ishikawa H, Yasui K, Oketa Y, Suzuki M, Ono S. Increased expression of valosin-containing protein in the skin of patients with amyotrophic lateral sclerosis. J Clin Neurosci. 2012;19:522–6.

20. Liu WC, Liu T, Liu ZH, Deng M. Detection the mutated protein aggregation and mitochondrial function in fibroblasts from amyotrophic lateral sclerosis patients with SOD1 gene mutations. Zhonghua Yi Xue Za Zhi. 2016;96:1982–6.

21. Oketa Y, Higashida K, Fukasawa H, Tsukie T, Ono S. Abundant FUS-immunoreactive pathology in the skin of sporadic amyotrophic lateral sclerosis. Acta Neurol Scand. 2013;128:257–64.

22. Ono S, Hu J, Shimizu N, Imai T, Nakagawa H. Increased interleukin-6 of skin and serum in amyotrophic lateral sclerosis. J Neurol Sci. 2001;187:27–34.

23. Suzuki M, Mikami H, Watanabe T, Yamano T, Yamazaki T, Nomura M, Yasui K, Ishikawa H, Ono S. Increased expression of TDP-43 in the skin of amyotrophic lateral sclerosis. Acta Neurol Scand. 2010;122:367–72.

24. Suzuki M, Watanabe T, Mikami H, Nomura M, Yamazaki T, Irie T, Ishikawa H, Yasui K, Ono S. Immunohistochemical studies of vascular endothelial growth factor in skin of patients with amyotrophic lateral sclerosis. J Neurol Sci. 2009;285:125–9.

25. Wang X, Zhou S, Ding X, Ma M, Zhang J, Zhou Y, Wu E, Teng J. Activation of ER stress and autophagy induced by TDP-43 A315T as pathogenic mechanism and the corresponding histological changes in skin as potential biomarker for ALS with the mutation. Int J Biol Sci. 2015;11:1140–9.

26. Watanabe T, Okeda Y, Yamano T, Ono S. An immunohistochemical study of ubiquitin in the skin of sporadic amyotrophic lateral sclerosis. J Neurol Sci. 2010;298:52–6.

27. Yang S, Zhang KY, Kariawasam R, Bax M, Fifita JA, Ooi L, Yerbury JJ, Nicholson GA, Blair IP. Evaluation of skin fibroblasts from amyotrophic lateral sclerosis patients for the rapid study of pathological features. Neurotox Res. 2015;28:138–46.

28. Sances S, Bruijn LI, Chandran S, Eggan K, Ho R, Klim JR, Livesey MR, Lowry E, Macklis JD, Rushton D, et al. Modeling ALS with motor neurons derived from human induced pluripotent stem cells. Nat Neurosci. 2016;19:542–53.

29. Pare B, Gros-Louis F. Potential skin involvement in ALS: revisiting Charcot's observation - a review of skin abnormalities in ALS. Rev Neurosci. 2017;28:551–72.

30. Pare B, Touzel-Deschenes L, Lamontagne R, Lamarre MS, Scott FD, Khuong HT, Dion PA, Bouchard JP, Gould P, Rouleau GA, et al. Early detection of structural abnormalities and cytoplasmic accumulation of TDP-43 in tissue-engineered skins derived from ALS patients. Acta Neuropathol Commun. 2015;3:5.

31. Kirk K, Gennings C, Hupf JC, Tadesse S, D'Aurelio M, Kawamata H, Valsecchi F, Mitsumoto H, Groups APCS, Manfredi G. Bioenergetic markers in skin fibroblasts of sporadic amyotrophic lateral sclerosis and progressive lateral sclerosis patients. Ann Neurol. 2014;76:620–4.

32. McCombe PA, Henderson RD. Effects of gender in amyotrophic lateral sclerosis. Gend Med. 2010;7:557–70.

33. Divakaruni AS, Paradyse A, Ferrick DA, Murphy AN, Jastroch M. Analysis and interpretation of microplate-based oxygen consumption and pH data. Methods Enzymol. 2014;547:309–54.

34. Allen SP, Duffy LM, Shaw PJ, Grierson AJ. Altered age-related changes in bioenergetic properties and mitochondrial morphology in fibroblasts from sporadic amyotrophic lateral sclerosis patients. Neurobiol Aging. 2015;36:2893–903.

35. Vielhaber S, Winkler K, Kirches E, Kunz D, Buchner M, Feistner H, Elger CE, Ludolph AC, Riepe MW, Kunz WS. Visualization of defective mitochondrial function in skeletal muscle fibers of patients with sporadic amyotrophic lateral sclerosis. J Neurol Sci. 1999;169:133–9.

36. Onesto E, Colombrita C, Gumina V, Borghi MO, Dusi S, Doretti A, Fagiolari G, Invernizzi F, Moggio M, Tiranti V, et al. Gene-specific mitochondria dysfunctions in human TARDBP and C9ORF72 fibroblasts. Acta Neuropathol Commun. 2016;4:47.

9

Advances, challenges and future directions for stem cell therapy in amyotrophic lateral sclerosis

Yuri Ciervo[1,2], Ke Ning[1,2], Xu Jun[2], Pamela J. Shaw[1] and Richard J. Mead[1*]

Abstract: Amyotrophic lateral sclerosis (ALS) is a rapidly progressive neurodegenerative condition where loss of motor neurons within the brain and spinal cord leads to muscle atrophy, weakness, paralysis and ultimately death within 3–5 years from onset of symptoms. The specific molecular mechanisms underlying the disease pathology are not fully understood and neuroprotective treatment options are minimally effective.

In recent years, stem cell transplantation as a new therapy for ALS patients has been extensively investigated, becoming an intense and debated field of study. In several preclinical studies using the SOD1^{G93A} mouse model of ALS, stem cells were demonstrated to be neuroprotective, effectively delayed disease onset and extended survival. Despite substantial improvements in stem cell technology and promising results in preclinical studies, several questions still remain unanswered, such as the identification of the most suitable and beneficial cell source, cell dose, route of delivery and therapeutic mechanisms. This review will cover publications in this field and comprehensively discuss advances, challenges and future direction regarding the therapeutic potential of stem cells in ALS, with a focus on mesenchymal stem cells. In summary, given their high proliferation activity, immunomodulation, multi-differentiation potential, and the capacity to secrete neuroprotective factors, adult mesenchymal stem cells represent a promising candidate for clinical translation. However, technical hurdles such as optimal dose, differentiation state, route of administration, and the underlying potential therapeutic mechanisms still need to be assessed.

Keywords: Neurodegeneration, Amyotrophic lateral sclerosis, Stem cell transplantation, Adipose derived stem cells

Background

Amyotrophic lateral sclerosis (ALS), also known as Lou Gehrig's disease, is a rapidly progressive neurodegenerative condition characterized by selective degeneration of both upper motor neurons (MNs) in the motor cortex, and lower motor neurons in the brainstem and ventral horn of the spinal cord [1]. The estimated incidence of ALS across the world is 2/100,000, with a prevalence of up to 7.4/100000 [2].

The disease typically manifests during the sixth to seventh decade of life leading to progressive muscle atrophy, weakness and paralysis. Affected individuals usually die within 2 to 5 years after diagnosis due to respiratory failure [2]. ALS is mainly sporadic in origin (SALS) but a family history of the disorder can be found in ~10% of cases. Hereditary forms of the disease (familial ALS or FALS), are predominantly autosomal dominant and rarely X-linked or recessive [2].

More than 20 mutated genes have been found to cause FALS including SOD1 [3], TARDBP [4, 5], FUS [6, 7], OPTN [8], VCP [9, 10], UBQLN2 [11], C9orf72 [12, 13] and very recently TBK1 [14, 15]. SALS and FALS are clinically indistinguishable, and since mutations in FALS genes are also present in sporadic or isolated cases of ALS, the disease can be interpreted as complex and multi-factorial [16]. Nevertheless, clinical variability such as rate of progression, site of onset (limb or bulbar) and survival within patients and even relatives who carry the same gene mutation highlight the importance of external factors which may play a role in the susceptibility and age of onset of the disease [16].

The specific molecular mechanisms behind ALS onset, development and progression are not fully understood. However, the discovery of causative inherited and de novo gene mutations, together with the generation of

---

* Correspondence: r.j.mead@sheffield.ac.uk
[1]Sheffield Institute for Translational Neuroscience (SITraN), Department of Neuroscience, Faculty of Medicine, Dentistry and Health, University of Sheffield, 385a Glossop Rd S10 2HQ, Sheffield, UK
Full list of author information is available at the end of the article

the SOD1^{G93A} transgenic mouse model uncovered important pathological mechanisms in ALS [17, 18]. The SOD1^{G93A} mice demonstrate many of the features seen in human ALS pathology and represent the most widely used in vivo model for the study of ALS. Indeed, axon retraction, selective spinal motor neuron death, loss of innervation of motor end-plates, muscular atrophy and progressive motor deficit with terminal paralysis of hind limbs are observed in this murine model [17, 18].

Several pathophysiological mechanisms have been proposed including: cytoplasmic protein mis-localization and aggregation [19], aberrant protein homeostasis [20], RNA toxicity [13], dysregulation of RNA processing [21], excitotoxicity mediated by excessive glutamate receptor activation [22], mitochondrial dysfunction [23], endoplasmic reticulum stress response and microglial activation [24], abnormal rearrangement of the cytoskeleton with impaired axonal transport [25], and oxidative stress [26]. Moreover, the contribution of microglial cells, oligodendrocytes and astrocytes seems to be critical for the development of the disease influencing significantly the speed of disease progression after onset [27–31]. Indeed, ALS is considered as a non-cell autonomous disease, where the start and progression of motor neuron degeneration seems to be influenced by complex interaction among different kinds of cells, together with the development of a sustained inflammatory milieu [32]. Figure 1 summarizes the major pathological mechanisms contributing to motor neuron injury in ALS.

The complex heterogeneity of ALS, where several molecular mechanisms contribute to the pathology, enables various opportunities for therapeutic intervention. However, the complexity of the disease and clinical variability within patients inevitably makes the identification of a universal single drug or therapy capable of correcting the pathophysiology of ALS in its totality, very difficult. Various therapeutic strategies are being experimentally evaluated such as immunomodulation, approaches to improve mitochondrial function, induction of autophagy and anti-oxidant agents [16]. However, after over twenty years of encouraging results in preclinical studies, no efficacious treatment has been developed so far and riluzole, the only recognised neuroprotective agent in ALS, prolongs life expectancy by only approximately 3–4 months [16].

During the last decade, progress in stem cell biology has paved the way for potential cellular based therapy in neurological diseases. Albeit still at an early stage and with several issues to be solved, stem cell therapy holds great promise for the treatment of ALS. Stem cells are a population of cells which are defined by functional characteristics. They are undifferentiated cells capable of self-renewal, able to form clones in vitro and capable of differentiation into mature cell lines of various tissues.

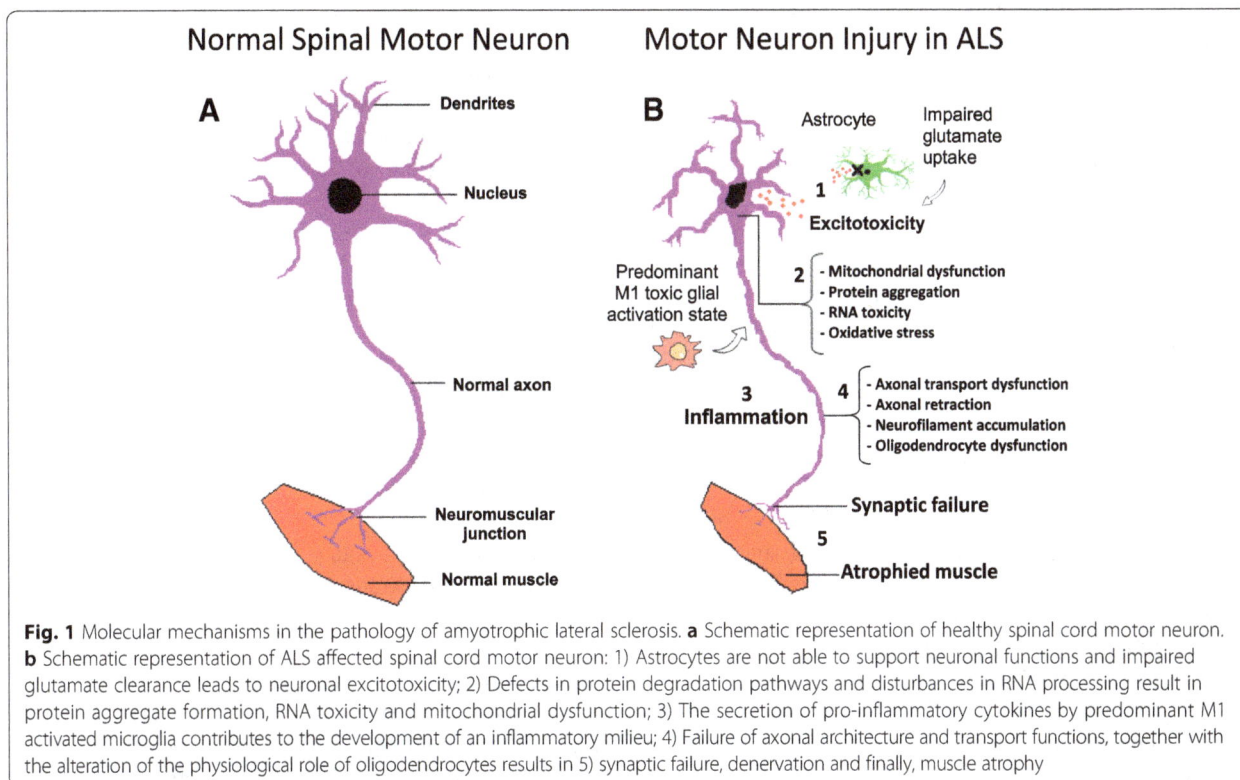

Fig. 1 Molecular mechanisms in the pathology of amyotrophic lateral sclerosis. a Schematic representation of healthy spinal cord motor neuron. b Schematic representation of ALS affected spinal cord motor neuron: 1) Astrocytes are not able to support neuronal functions and impaired glutamate clearance leads to neuronal excitotoxicity; 2) Defects in protein degradation pathways and disturbances in RNA processing result in protein aggregate formation, RNA toxicity and mitochondrial dysfunction; 3) The secretion of pro-inflammatory cytokines by predominant M1 activated microglia contributes to the development of an inflammatory milieu; 4) Failure of axonal architecture and transport functions, together with the alteration of the physiological role of oligodendrocytes results in 5) synaptic failure, denervation and finally, muscle atrophy

There are several potential advantages to the use of stem cells in ALS:

1) The complexity of ALS pathology may not allow the use of a single drug or targeted treatment;

2) The capability of stem cells to differentiate into neuron-like cells and potentially replace the neuronal population lost in ALS;

3) The degeneration of existing motor neurons could be prevented by the release of neuroprotective trophic factors and the immunomodulatory properties of transplanted stem cells, thus modifying the toxic microenvironment in ALS.

This review will outline the recent progress relevant to stem cell-based therapies in general in ALS, and will focus on the therapeutic potential of mesenchymal stem cells by discussing the major technical issues, challenges and future directions.

Stem cell therapy in ALS

There are different types of stem cells which differ according to the source, clonogenic capacity, differentiation potential and availability.

Human embryonic stem cells (hESC)

Human embryonic stem cells (hESC) are derived from the inner cell mass of the blastocyst and can indefinitely propagate in vitro, preserving the capacity to differentiate into any cell type of the three embryonic germ layers (endoderm, mesoderm and ectoderm) [33]. For the first time in 2005, Shin and colleagues obtained motor neuron-like cells expressing markers such as islet1 and choline acetyltransferase from hESC using conditioned media containing basic fibroblast growth factor (bFGF), retinoic acid (RA) and sonic hedgehog (Shh) [34]. The survival, differentiation and beneficial neurotrophic support of motor neuron progenitors (MNP) derived from hESC has also been demonstrated after lumbar intraspinal transplantation into $SOD1^{G93A}$ mice and other MND models [35, 36]. Wyatt et al., transplanted hESC derived MNPs directly into the spinal cord of immunosuppressed $SOD1^{G93A}$ mice, spinal muscular atrophy (SMA) $\Delta7SMN$ pups and rats with spinal cord injury (SCI), demonstrating the in vivo differentiation of the engrafted cells into a mixed population of mature and immature motor neuron cells [36]. The axons of the differentiated cells did not reach the periphery, and the authors did not prove the integration of the differentiated cells into the existing neural circuit. However, the transplanted cells were able to reduce motor neuron loss in proximity to the injection site by actively releasing neurotrophic factors such as neurotrophin-3 (NT-3) and nerve growth factor (NGF) [36]. In particular, in $SOD1^{G93A}$ mice that received MNPs, 43 ± 5 endogenous neurons cranial to the injection site survived until the end of the study (110 days old), in comparison to the vehicle control group in which 27 ± 3 neurons were counted [36]. Yet, the use of hESCs in the clinic is hindered because of ethical concerns, potential tumorigenicity in vivo and the potential for graft rejection [37].

Foetal neural progenitors (NSC)

Foetal neural progenitors (NSC) are multipotent stem cells derived from foetal spinal cord or brain, capable of in vitro self-renewal and able to differentiate into astrocytes, neurons and oligodendrocytes. Given their partial maturation state they have less propensity to form teratomas in vivo [38]. Several studies investigated the safety and therapeutic potential of spinal, intrathecal or intracranial transplantation of hNSC in ALS rodent models [39–41]. In particular, a well-characterized hNSC cell line (NSI-566RSC) derived from an 8-week human foetal spinal cord showed very promising results in transplanted $SOD1^{G93A}$ rodents [42, 43].

In 2006, Yan et al. performed spinal cord injections of NSI-566RSC cells in the ventral horn of 8-week-old $SOD1^{G93A}$ mice at the lumbar level L4-L5, under combined immunosuppression or CD4 antibodies [42]. Four separate injections were carried out per mouse, with a total of 8×10^4 cells. The authors showed that the graft survived for more than two months after transplantation, with most of the engrafted NSCs showing differentiation into $TUJ1^+$ neurons, and evidence of synaptic contacts with host neurons [42]. Moreover, in mice injected with live NSCs cells, disease onset was delayed by 15 days and life span extended by 12 days in comparison to the control group that received injections of dead cells. A statistically significant later onset and a slowing of disease progression, was also confirmed by analysis of motor performance [42]. The same group of authors, investigated the therapeutic potential of the NSCs-566RSC cell line after injection of around 8×10^5 cells into the lumbar spinal cord of $SOD1^{G93A}$ rats at a pre-symptomatic disease stage [43]. In this study, rats that received live NSCs showed an increase in survival of around 11 days and a delay in disease onset of 7 days when compared to the control placebo group. The beneficial effect could be associated with the release of neurotrophins such as glial-derived neurotrophic factor (GDNF) and brain-derived neurotrophic factor (BDNF), which in turn delayed the death of α-motor neurons in the lumbar region [43].

Despite these encouraging data, the restricted number of cells available for transplantation represents a potential limitation for obtaining therapeutic efficacy in humans.

Induced pluripotent stem cells (iPSCs)

Induced pluripotent stem cells (iPSC) are an adult source of pluripotent stem cells derived from somatic cells (e.g. dermal fibroblasts) by forced genetic induction of four factors that preserve pluripotency in ESCs (KLF4, SOX2, OCT4 and c-MYC) [44, 45]. The differentiation of human iPSCs into electrically active motor neurons has been accomplished by several groups both in vitro and in vivo [46, 47].

Interestingly, Popescu et al. demonstrated in vivo differentiation of human iPSC-derived neural progenitors (NPs) in presymptomatic SOD1^{G93A} rats following stem cell injection into the ventral horns of the lumbar spinal cord [48]. At 30 days post-transplantation human mitochondria positive cells displayed expression of the neuronal precursor marker doublecortin (DCX), indicating the presence of undifferentiated progenitors. Substantial differentiation into mature motor neurons could be observed only after 60 days, with the majority of engrafted cells expressing the neuronal marker MAP2 [48]. This relatively long time is something to bear in mind, considering that transplantation was performed before disease onset and NPs could survive and differentiate within a less toxic environment in comparison to the symptomatic stage. If cells were transplanted during disease progression, as would occur in the clinic, NPs may not have a permissive environment and/or the necessary time to differentiate into mature motor neurons. The therapeutic potential of iPSC-derived NPs has also been investigated in the SOD1^{G93A} mouse model of ALS [49]. iPSC-derived neural stem cells (NSCs), further selected for the expression of the integrin VLA4$^+$, were transplanted either by repeated ($n = 3$) intrathecal or weekly intravenous injections. Intrathecal injection of cells extended survival by 10 days, while systemic delivery increased survival by 23 days, compared to control PBS injected mice [49]. The molecular protective mechanism of iPSC-derived NSCs may be attributed to the capacity of these cells to secrete trophic factors such as GDNF, BDNF, NT-3 and TGF-α, which in turn protects resident motor neurons and reduces astrogliosis [49].

The opportunity for reprogramming somatic cells into neural stem cells (NSCs) could overcome the immune rejection problem by autologous transplantation, and bypass the ethical problems related to the use of ESCs and foetal cells. However, several issues need to be addressed, such as reprogramming efficiency, epigenetic memory and safety before translation of the use of iPSCs into clinical practice.

Mesenchymal stem cells (MSCs)

Adult mesenchymal stem cells (MSCs) are stromal multipotent stem cells that can be derived from umbilical cord, bone marrow, adipose tissue and peripheral blood and have the capacity to differentiate into different components of mesodermal origin (cartilage, bone, fat, muscle and stroma) [50]. These cells can be expanded and maintained by several passages in plastic-adherent tissue culture. MSCs show fibroblast-like morphology, they do not differentiate spontaneously and are characterized by the expression of specific surface markers [50]. In addition to mesodermal commitment, several authors showed the potential of bone marrow-derived MSCs (BM-MSC) to differentiate into neuron-like cells, oligodendrocytes and astrocytes [51–59].

Several characteristics make the use of MSCs very attractive in ALS cell therapy. MSCs can be obtained and expanded from adults relatively easily, bypassing the ethical constraints related to the use of embryonic and human foetal derived stem cells. Also, they are less immunogenic and can be harvested from ALS patients so allowing both allogenic and autologous transplantation [50]. Moreover, these cells are capable of homing to areas of insult, possess immunomodulation and anti-apoptotic properties, and are capable of secreting several cytokines, extracellular matrix proteins and growth factors relevant in neuroprotection and tissue repair [60]. Because of these properties, mesenchymal stem cells are receiving significant attention amongst researchers.

Proof-of-concept for MSCs therapy in the SOD1^{G93A} model of ALS

Several studies were performed in ALS rodent models in order to investigate the potential of either human (hMSC) or murine (mMSC) bone marrow-derived MSCs (BM-MSCs) for cell therapy in ALS. Different approaches have been tested by varying the delivery method, the amount of injected cells, the timing of intervention, and the differentiation state. Table 1 shows a summary of preclinical studies described in the literature with injection of BM-MSCs in ALS models.

Intravenous delivery

In 2007, Zhao and colleagues delivered 3 million hBM-MSCs into 60 day pre-irradiated SOD1^{G93A} mice by intravenous infusion [61]. The recipient mice showed about 14 days delay in disease onset, and prolonged survival of about 18 days in comparison to untreated mice. Moreover, the decrease in motor performance (rotarod test) was delayed by 3 weeks [61]. However, immunostaining experiments showed that only a few transplanted cells migrated and penetrated into the grey and white spinal cord matter, surviving for no more than 20 days [61].

In another study, 1 million engineered hBM-MSCs overexpressing neurogenin1 (Ngn1) were injected in the tail vein of pre-symptomatic SOD1^{G93A} mice [58]. Ngn1 is a transcription factor able to induce neuronal differentiation in MSCs [58]. Two weeks after transplantation, injected cells were found within the brain, spinal cord and liver, and some cells had migrated into the spinal cord parenchyma [58]. The neural induction of hMSCs with neurogenin1 seemed to potentiate the migration

Table 1 Summary of BM-MSC injections in ALS rodent model

ALS model	Delivery Method	Cell numbers	Age	Sacrifice to evaluate graft	Outcomes	Cell graft	Reference
SOD1^{G93A}mice — hBM-MSC after 5 passages in culture	Intravenous	3×10^6in 0.3 ml of L-DMEM	Pre-symptomatic (8 w)	14 days post-injection	Increased lifespan of 18 days, delayed disease onset of 14 days and reduced motor neuron loss	Very few cells in grey and white matter of lumbar spinal cord. Considerable number of cells in kidney, lung and spleen.	[61]
SOD1^{G93A}mice — hBM-MSC expressing Ngn1 after 5 passages in culture	Intravenous	1×10^6in 0.1 ml of PBS	Pre-symptomatic (8 w) or symptom onset (14–16 w)	14 days post-injection	Increased lifespan of 3 days, delayed disease onset of 5 days and reduced motor neuron loss.	Very few cells in brainstem and spinal cord. Cells mostly found in kidney.	[58]
SOD1^{G93A}mice — mBM-MSCs expressing Luciferase expanded for 8–15 passages	Intravenous	1×10^6in 0.2 ml of PBS	Symptom onset	24 h, 3 weeks and 4 weeks post-injection	Increased lifespan of 17 days, delayed decline in motor performance and weight loss.	Cells detected in spinal cord and hypothalamus after 24 h and 48 h. Very few cells after 20 days. No cells after 35 days	[58, 62]
SOD1^{G93A}mice — hBM-MSC-derived neural-like cells from neurosphere	Cisterna Magna	1×10^5in 10 µl of PBS	Pre-symptomatic	10 days post-injection	No benefits	Subarachnoid space near cisterna magna and within cerebellum.	[63]
SOD1^{G93A}mice — ALS-hBM-MSC after 3 passages in culture	Cisterna Magna	1×10^6in 10 µl of ALS-CSF	Pre-symptomatic	7 weeks post-injection	Increased lifespan of 8 days, slowed decline in rotarod test and increased motor neuron survival	Ventricular system and subarachnoid space. Some cells into brain and spinal cord.	[64]
SOD1^{G93A}mice — hBM-MSC after 3–4 passages in culture	Cisterna Magna	5×10^5in 5 µl of PBS	Pre-symptomatic	3 weeks post-injection	Increased lifespan of 14 days, delayed disease onset of 6 days and reduced astrogliosis	Not shown	[67]
SOD1^{G93A}rats — GFP-hBM-MSCs	Cisterna Magna	5×10^5in 10 µl of PBS	Symptom onset	14 days post-injection	Increased lifespan of 14 days and reduced motor neuron loss. Preservation of PNN.	No graft	[66]
SOD1^{G93A}rats — BrdU-labelled mBM-MSC after 15 passages in culture	Cisterna Magna	2×10^6in 15 µl of Opti-MEM	Symptom onset	35 days post-injection	Increased lifespan of 16 days, slowed disease progression, reduced motor neuron loss and inflammation.	White and grey matter of spinal cord. Substantial differentiation into astrocyte phenotype	[54]
SOD1^{G93A}mice — Bisbenzimide -hBM-MSC after 3–8 passages in culture	Cisterna lumbaris (L5-L6)	3×10^6in 5 µl of PBS	Symptom onset	14 days post-injection	Reduced astrogliosis and microglial activation.	Lumbar, cervical and thoracic meninges. Migration into spinal cord parenchyma.	[68]
SOD1^{G93A}mice — Bisbenzimide -hBM-MSC after 3–5 passages in culture	Intraspinal (L1-L2)	1×10^6in 2 µl of PBS	Pre-symptomatic (28 w)	10 weeks post-injection (38 w)	Reduced astrogliosis and microglial activation. Improved motor function and delayed neuron death	Close to injection site. Migration up to 2 mm toward ventral horn.	[70]
SOD1^{G93A}rats — GFP-hBM-MSC engineered to secrete GDNF	Intramuscular after focal injuries	1.3×10^5in	Pre-symptomatic (80 days)	Disease end-point	Prolonged survival, reduction in denervated motor endplates and reduced motor neuron loss	Between basal lamina and muscle fibres	[72]

hBM-MSC human bone marrow-derived mesenchymal stem cells, DMEM Dulbecco's modified eagle medium, Ngn1 neurogenin-1, PBS phosphate buffered saline, mBM-MSC mouse bone marrow-derived mesenchymal stem cells, ALS-hBM-MSC human bone marrow-derived mesenchymal stem cells derived from ALS patient, ALS-CSF cerebrospinal fluid derived from ALS patient, GFP-hBM-MSC green fluorescent protein labelled hBM-MSC, PNN perineural net, BrdU bromodeoxyuridine, GDNF glial derived neural factor capacity and survival of engrafted cells into the central nervous system (CNS) of SOD1^{G93A} mice, resulting in enhanced and prolonged benefits [58]. The migration capacity might be explained by high expression of chemokine receptors such as CCR2 and CXCR4, which were significantly more expressed after neurogenin1 induction. [58]. Interestingly, when MSCs were injected at a pre-symptomatic stage, disease onset in the treated group was delayed by 5 days with an increase in life span of only 3 days. Conversely, when injected close to disease onset, Ng1-MSCs were able to increase survival by about 7 days, suggesting the importance of the time of intervention for stem cell therapy in ALS [58].

Furthermore, the Uccelli group demonstrated that mouse BM-MSCs isolated from non-transgenic mice, were therapeutically effective when transplanted during the symptomatic stage of the disease in the SOD1^{G93A} mice [62]. In this study, mBM-MSCs expanded ex-vivo for 8–15 passages, were transfected with the Luciferase gene reporter vector pL-Luc-HI for in vivo tracking and injected into the tail vein of SOD1^{G93A} mice. The mice that received the MSC transplantation showed an extended survival of 17 days, delayed decline in motor performance and decreased weight loss when compared to the control PBS-injected mice [62]. In addition, the transplantation of MSCs alleviated the pathology of the disease in the ALS spinal cord, by reducing astrogliosis and microglial activation, and by restoring antioxidant components such as glutathione-S-transferase and metallothioneins to their baseline level of expression and activity. However, the engraftment efficiency of intravenous delivered cells within the CNS was very low, with luciferase-positive cells almost completely absent twenty days post- injection. This suggested that MSCs delivered by the intravenous route, can exert clinically positive effects during the disease course that do not correlate with the efficiency of long-term engraftment in the host [62].

Intrathecal delivery

Using a different approach, several authors have injected a variable number of BM-MSCs directly into the cisterna magna of pre-symptomatic SOD1^{G93A} mice [63–66]. Direct injection into the CSF allows the obstacle of the brain blood barrier (BBB) to be bypassed. Moreover, the injected cells may migrate along the spinal cord possibly reaching segments specifically affected by motor neuron degeneration.

Indeed, it has been demonstrated that the injected BM-MSCs were able to delay disease onset, improve motor performance, ameliorate motor neuron death and prolong survival in transplanted SOD1^{G93A} mice [64–67]. These beneficial effects were enhanced by multiple intrathecal injections or by using a considerable number of

MSCs (1×10^6) [64, 65]. However, injected cells rarely migrated into the parenchyma, suggesting a neuroprotective effect of MSCs from the CSF [64, 65, 67]. In fact, it was shown that injection of MSCS into the CSF of SOD1^{G93A} mice consistently inhibited microglial activation and the release of inflammatory molecules, possibly by diffusion of soluble factors where direct contact between cells is not a requirement [67].

In 2009, Boucherie and colleagues, investigated the therapeutic potential of rat wild-type (WT) bromodeoxyuridine-labelled BM-MSCs (BrdU-MSC) by intrathecal injection in SOD1^{G93A} transgenic rats, at disease onset [54]. Stem cell transplantation in SOD1^{G93A} rats resulted in a reduction in the rate of disease progression, as the first signs of paralysis were detected 2 weeks later in in comparison to control mice. Moreover, treated mice showed reduced local inflammatory response and an increase in life span of 16 days [54]. Interestingly, this is the only study to show a significant trans-differentiation of MSCs into astrocyte-like cells in vivo. Indeed, transplanted BrdU-MSCs were found to penetrate into the grey matter of the ventral horns, and stained positively for the astrocyte marker GFAP [54]. Remarkably, around 40% of the BrdU-MSCs that successfully migrated in proximity to motor neurons, co-localized with the astrocyte marker, and about 30% of the GFAP-positive cells were actually positive for the BrdU. This study demonstrated a considerable local chimerization of the astroglial population near the site of motor neuron injury in the lumbar spinal cord of SOD1^{G93A} rats [54]. However, cell fusion events with resident astrocytes cannot be excluded. Surprisingly, the overall level of astrogliosis was not changed upon MSCs treatment, and the loss of expression of the astrocyte glutamate reuptake transporter (GLT-1), typically observed in SOD1^{G93A} rats, was not rescued [54].

The perineural net (PNN) is a specialized matrix structure present at a high density around motor neurons and is fundamental in axon development as well as neuronal plasticity [66]. Modification and deterioration of the PNN has been observed in the spinal cord of SOD1^{G93A} rats during neurodegeneration [66]. Interestingly, intrathecal delivery of hBM-MSCs into early post-symptomatic SOD1^{G93A} rats, resulted in partial rescue of PNN structures suggesting a role of MSCs in reactivating CNS plasticity [66]. In this study, stem cell injection increased survival of 14 days in comparison to the placebo group.

Boido et al. (2014) injected a total of 300,000 bisbenzimide pre-labelled hMSCs into the cisterna lumbaris (L5-L6 level) of early symptomatic SOD1^{G93A} mice [68]. Although the treated mice showed only a slight delay in motor neuron loss and slowing of motor performance decline, astgliosis and microgliosis were consistently attenuated in recipient mice in comparison to the controls [68]. Two weeks post-transplantation, transplanted cells were found mostly concentrated on lumbar, thoracic and cervical meninges, but considerable numbers of bisbenzimide positive cells were found in proximity to motor neurons within the spinal cord [68]. It is noteworthy that the use of bisbenzimide as a marker for cell transplantation has been questioned since the dye may transfer from labelled cells to host cells [69].

Intraparenchymal delivery

Other authors have attempted to inject human or mouse MSCs directly into the dorsal horn of spinal cord of SOD1^{G93A} mice [70, 71]. In the Vercelli group experiments, hMSCs were found to engraft, migrate to the ventral horn close to α-motor neurons and survive more than 10 weeks after surgery, although without signs of differentiation into neurons or astrocytes [70]. Also, male but not female recipient mice showed a consistent (38%) increased motor neuron survival as well as reduced gliosis and attenuated astrocyte activation in comparison to control mice [70]. Though the authors claimed an extended lifespan in male treated mice, not all of the experimental groups were followed until the disease end-point, and a Kaplan-Meier survival curve was not shown.

Intramuscular delivery

Since early pathologic mechanisms of disease involve destruction of neuromuscular junctions before motor neuron death, intramuscular injection of MSCs at early stages of disease has also been proposed. hBM-MSCs, genetically engineered to express green fluorescent protein (GFP) and to constitutively secrete GDNF, were injected into the forelimb triceps brachii muscles of pre-symptomatic SOD1^{G93A} rats [72].

The intramuscular transplantation of MSCs did not delay disease onset, however, survival was prolonged by 18 days. Furthermore, a reduction of endplate denervation in SOD1^{G93A} rats was observed, when compared to the control vehicle group [72]. However, MSCs were not able to regenerate motor end-plates, nor to reduce neuroinflammation [72]. Moreover, to obtain significant survival and integration of MSCs in the host, the induction of focal muscle injuries was necessary.

MSCs in ALS: Clinical trials
Mazzini trials: Intraparenchymal delivery of autologous BM-MSC

Despite the absence of any preclinical data, in 2001 Mazzini et al. embarked upon the first clinical trial in order to evaluate the safety and feasibility of MSC injection into the spinal cord of sporadic ALS patients [73]. The study comprised the recruitment of 7 SALS patients with spinal onset and severe lower limb impairment without respiratory complications [73]. Autologous

mesenchymal bone marrow-derived stem cells were expanded for 3–4 weeks under good manufacturing practice (GMP) conditions and cytogenetic analysis, viability and cytofluorimetric analysis for characterization of antigens were carried out before infusion [73]. However, no detailed data was provided.

In this study, following three hours in serum-free medium, a variable number of cells ranging from 7 to 152 million were suspended in 1–2 ml of autologous CSF and transplanted directly into the parenchyma of spinal cord at thoracic level (T7-T9) [73, 74].

The patient follow-up was performed every 3 months for six years. After surgery, no signs of increased neurological defects or toxicity were observed, indicating that implantation into the spinal cord of ex vivo expanded MSCs was safe and well tolerated by patients [73, 74].

To further validate the safety of the therapy, in 2010 a second Phase I clinical trial was conducted in another 10 patients following the same protocol as described above, with slight modifications [75]. Cells (11–122 million) were transplanted in the anterior horn at the thoracic level (T4-T6) with different numbers of injection sites (2 to 5) [75]. Two years post-surgery, no tumour formation, side effects or toxicity had been detected [75].

A long-term (9 years) safety study, concluded in 2012, was carried out by the same authors on the basis of 19 ALS patients who underwent autologous MSCs implantation in two separate phase I studies from 2001 to 2003 [76]. Importantly, magnetic resonance imaging (MRI) analysis demonstrated no tumour formation or abnormal cell growth, indicating that ex vivo expansion of ALS patient-derived MSCs does not affect karyotype or cellular senescence, making their use safe in the clinic [76]. No data describing stem cell characterization were shown and evidence of engraftment in post-mortem tissues have not yet been described.

Blanquer trial: Intraparenchymal delivery of autologous BMNC

Based on promising results in a mouse model of MND [77], Blanquer et al. tested the safety and tolerability of intraspinal transplantation of mononuclear cells derived from autologous bone marrow (BMNC) in ALS patients in an open label phase I clinical trial [78]. The study was performed on 11 sporadic ALS patients with spinal onset and no evidence of significant respiratory dysfunction [78].

Briefly, patients received two infusions of BMNC diluted in 1 ml of saline solution into two different sites along the posterior column of spinal cord at thoracic level after laminectomy, with the help of a specially designed micromanipulator [79]. A variable number (138,000 to 60,287 × 10^6) of BMNC cells, including an average of 2.77 × 10^6 CD34+, 2.31 × 10^6 CD117+ and 1.30 × 10^6 CD133+ cells, were injected [78].

After 1 year of follow up, no severe adverse effects or acceleration of the disease progression related to the treatment were observed, demonstrating the safety and feasibly of the described procedure in ALS patients [78]. Moreover, spinal cord pathology on post mortem material showed preservation of motor neurons at the injection sites [78]. Interestingly, preserved motor neurons were surrounded by spherical CD90+ cells negative for neuronal markers, CD45 (hematopoietic stem cells) and CD68 (monocytes/macrophages) markers [78]. These motor neurons did not show any sign of degeneration [77, 78].

Karussis trial: Intrathecal and intravenous delivery of autologous MSCs

In 2010, a phase 1/2 clinical trial was conducted in Israel in 15 patients with multiple sclerosis (MS) and 19 ALS patients [80]. In order to enhance the potential benefits of MSC transplantation, after 40–60 days in culture, a median of 60 million autologous MSCs were transplanted intrathecally in combination with a mean of 20 million MSCs delivered intravenously [80]. Also, in 9 patients MSCs were pre-labelled with ferumoxides in order to track their fate in vivo by MRI [80].

At the end of 25 months of follow-up, no severe adverse effects were registered in any of the patients, with signs of disease stabilization in some patients during the first 6 months after the intervention [80]. Furthermore, MRI screening 24 h, 48 h, 1 and 3 months after the infusion of cells, showed the presence of ferumoxides in nerve roots, meninges and the parenchyma of the spinal cord. However, these results are not conclusive of the presence of MSCs in the CNS, since the contrast agent can be ingested by phagocytes which have migrated to inflammatory lesions [80]. Also, flow cytometry analysis and subsequent proliferative response assay of peripheral blood monocytes obtained from ALS patients 4 h and 24 h after infusion of MSCs, showed a dramatic increase in CD4+ CD25+ regulatory T cells, coupled with a reduction in activated dendritic cells and lymphocyte proliferation, demonstrating the immediate immunomodulatory properties of MSCs following transplantation [80].

Oh trial: Repeated intrathecal infusion of autologous BM-MSCs

Very recently, a single open-label clinical trial was performed in order to evaluate the clinical feasibility and safety of two repeated infusions of autologous MSCs into the CSF by lumbar puncture in 8 ALS patients [81]. At intervals of 26 days, 1×10^6 MSC cells per kg were injected diluted in autologous CSF [81].

After 1 year, no deaths were recorded and the procedure was considered safe, without long-term adverse effects [81]. In addition, CSF samples of two patients were collected before both the first and the second injection in order to evaluate cytokine levels. Il-10, TGF-β (I, II and III) and IL-6 levels were increased after MSC transplantation, while the level of the monocyte chemoattractant protein 1 (MCP-1) was decreased [81]. A phase II clinical trial in 64 ALS patients is on-going, with a placebo control group allowing proper evaluation of efficacy and safety (NCT01363401).

The same group performed repeated intrathecal MSC injections in another 37 patients between 2007 and 2010, with the aim of identifying MSC markers capable of predicting the response in ALS patients [82]. First, they measured the level of various trophic factors in MSC cultures from each patient by ELISA assay. They then transplanted MSCs from different patients in the SOD1^{G93A} mouse model and analysed differences in onset, MN loss and immunoreactivity [82]. The authors concluded that the beneficial effects (symptom improvement and slowing of decline) observed in a proportion of patients, were positively correlated with the increased capacity of MSC cells to secrete VEGF, ANG and TGF-β in vitro [82]. Moreover, the clinical efficacy observed in some patients was confirmed also in SOD1^{G93A} mice which exhibited prolonged survival and lower levels of neuroinflammation [82].

Adipose tissue: A fat tissue source for mesenchymal stem cells

Mesenchymal stem cells represent an ideal source of adult stem cells for cell therapy given their immunosuppressive nature, low potential for immunogenicity and trans-differentiation capacity. However, the collection of MSC from bone marrow is an invasive procedure which can be painful and anaesthesia is often required [83]. Moreover, the proportion of stem cells within the total cell population in bone marrow aspirate is usually about 0.001–0.002% which leads to extended culture times and increased expense in order to obtain sufficient GMP cells for clinical application [83].

Subcutaneous (buttocks and abdomen) and visceral (omentum) white adipose tissue (WAT) may represent an alternative source of stromal adult stem cells since they can be obtained by minimally invasive, simple procedures such as liposuction or lipectomy and they are relatively abundant, representing 1% of WAT cells after processing [83–85]. Several names and abbreviations have been used to refer to adipose-derived mesenchymal stem cells. Here, the abbreviation ADSC will be used.

In the literature, the method for isolation of ADSCs from human fat is performed following almost always the same protocol described by Zuk and colleagues [83]. An illustration of the ADSC isolation method is showed in Fig. 2.

Briefly, fresh lipoaspirate is washed extensively to eliminate red blood cells and contaminant debris, followed

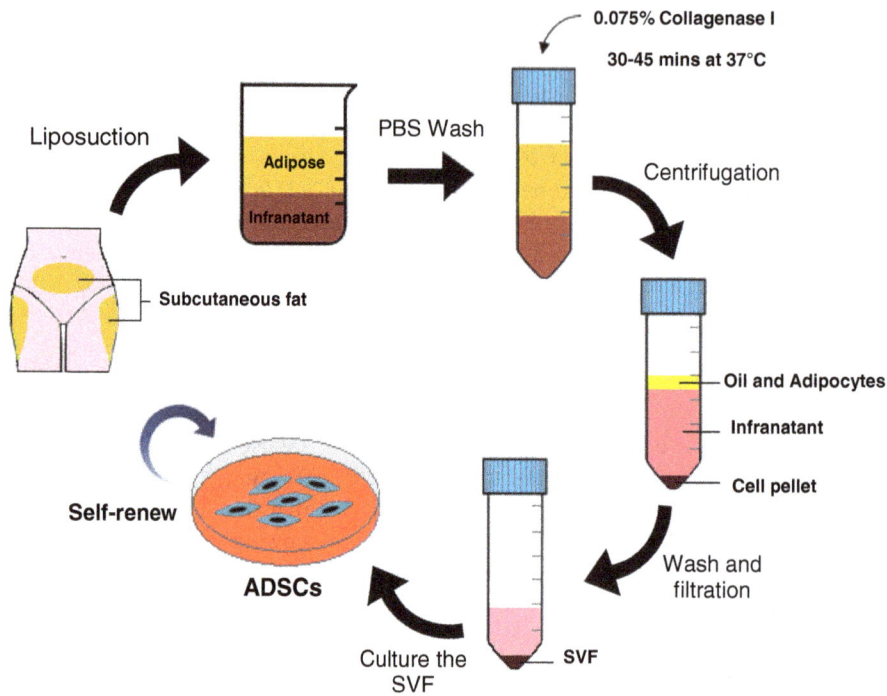

Fig. 2 Isolation process to obtain ADSCs from human lipoaspirate. Fresh lipoaspirate is extensively washed in PBS to remove blood and contaminants. The adipose tissue is then enzymatically digested and the stromal vascular fraction (SVF) is obtained by filtration and centrifugation. Culture of the SVF in standard plastic tissue culture flasks results in the selection and expansion of the adipose stem cell population

by extracellular matrix digestion with collagenase. After enzymatic neutralization, the homogenate is centrifuged to obtain the stromal-vascular fraction (SVF) pellet. The pellet is then suspended in culture medium and left overnight in a flask in the incubator at 37 °C with 5% CO_2. After incubation, cells are washed with phosphate buffered saline (PBS) to remove residual non-adherent cells. The culture medium usually consists of Dulbecco's modified eagle medium (DMEM) supplemented with foetal bovine serum (FBS), penicillin and streptomycin.

In spite of some differences in the expression of cluster of differentiation (CD) markers such as CD49d and CD106, ADSC cells are phenotypically similar to BM-MSC cells, showing fibroblast-like morphology, characteristic expression of mesenchymal stem cell markers (CD44+, CD105+, CD73+, CD90+, CD29+, CD45−, CD34−, CD14− CD19−), lack of major histocompatibility complex class II (MHC-II) and the capacity to differentiate into osteoblasts, chondrocytes and adipocytes in specific culture conditions [83]. Thus, hADSCs comply with all the minimum criteria for the characterization of hMSCs, established in 2005, by the International Society for Cellular Therapy (ISCT) [86].

Like MSCs obtained from bone marrow aspirates, hADSCs secrete several soluble factors such as BDNF, NGF, hepatocyte growth factor (HGF), vascular endothelial growth factor (VEGF), insulin-like growth factor-1 (IGF-1) and basic fibroblast growth factor (bFGF) that may contribute to neurotropism, neuroprotection and tissue regeneration by paracrine mechanisms [87].

Even though the literature appears controversial, there is evidence supporting the potential of ADSCs to trans-differentiate into progenitors or mature cells of ectodermal origin, therefore opening the way to a future investigation of the feasibility of cell replacement in neurodegenerative disorders (Safford et al., 2002; Krampera et al., 2007; Ahmadi et al., 2012; Feng et al., 2014).

In vitro neuronal differentiation capacity of ADSC

The capacity of ADSCs to differentiate in vitro into mature, stable and functional neurons is an open field of debate among researchers. Table 2 summarises the protocols for neuronal differentiation of ADSCs published in literature. Usually, the differentiation protocol consists of expanding ADSCs as adherent cells for several passages, followed by induction with media containing different cocktails of chemical agents, cytokines and growth factors [88–92].

A different method to obtain neuron-like cells from ADSCs is based on neurosphere formation capacity, generally achieved by culturing cells in EGF and bFGF conditioned serum-free media [93, 94]. A neurosphere

Table 2 Summary of protocols to obtain neural trans-differentiation of hADSCs

Culture method	Differentiation protocol	Neuronal/glial marker expressed	Comments	Reference
Adherent method	24 h pre-incubation in DMEM/FCS 20% followed by 24 h incubation in DMEM containing BHA, valproic acid, forskolin, hydrocortisone and insulin.	Nestin (developing nervous system cells) NeuN (neuronal nuclei) GFAP (mature astrocytes) I-NFM (Neurons)	Cells started to lose their neuronal morphology after 4–5 days and all died in 14 days.	[88]
Adherent method	14 days incubation in DMEM containing insulin, indomethacin and IBMX	Vimentin (Schwann cells) Trk-A (central nervous system) NSE (early neuronal progenitors)	Low neuronal marker expression also in undifferentiated ADSCs. 25% differentiation rate obtained. Cells not able to generate action potentials.	[90]
Adherent method with or without human Schwann cells	24 h pre-incubation in DMEM/FBS 20% and β-mercaptoethanol followed by 8–16 h incubation in DMEM containing DMSO, β-mercaptoethanol and BHA	GFPA S-100 (Astrocytes and Schwann cells) NeuN Nestin Gal-C (Oligodendrocyte)	Cell morphology turned back to fibroblast shape after 72 h in normal basal medium. Co-culture with human irradiated Schwann cells enhanced survival (12 days) and expression of myelin proteins.	[91]
Adherent method	7 days incubation in DMEM containing bFGF followed by 7 days incubation in DMEM containing forskolin	GFPA I-NFM Tuj –1 (neuron specific β-III tubulin) Nestin SNAP-25 (synaptic marker) CNPase (Oligodendrocyte)	Inward and outward ion current in patch-clamp experiment. High mRNA expression of ion channels. Low differentiation marker expression also in undifferentiated ADSCs.	[92]
Neurosphere method followed by maturation on poly-D-lysine	8 days pre-incubation in DMEM containing β-mercaptoethanol and b-FGF followed by 7 days incubation in neural basal medium (N2B27) and further 7 days in N2B27 medium containing EGF and bGFG. Final maturation achieved from neurosphere dissociated progenitors after 14 day culture in N2B27 media containing retinoic acid and BDNF	MAP2 (mature neurons) Nestin Sox1(neural tube development) Pax6 (human neuroepithelium) Vimentin	Inward and outward ion currents in patch-clamp experiment. High mRNA expression of ion channels	[95]

DMEM Dulbecco's modified eagle medium, *FCS* foetal calf serum, *BHA* butylated hydroxyanisole, *GFAP* glial fibrillary acid protein, *I-NFM* intermediate neurofilament, *IBMX* isobutylmethylxantine, *Trk-A* tropomyosin receptor kinase A, *NSE* neuron specific enolase, *DMSO* dimethyl sulfoxide, *S-100* S protein 100, *Gal-C* galactosylceramidase, *CNPase* 2,3-Cyclic-nucleotide 3′-phosphodiesterase, *EGF* epidermal growth factor, *BDNF* brain derived neurotrophic factor, *MAP2* microtubule-associated protein 2 is a cluster of cells containing neural precursors able to proliferate and survive as floating and non-adherent structures. The neurosphere can be dissociated, seeded onto a poly-L-lysine feeder layer and differentiated by adding neuronal induction components [93–95]. Alternatively, ADSCs are cultured in the presence of ESCs or Schwann cells either in the presence or absence of induction factors [91, 96]. In particular, when co-cultured with Schwann cells, ADSCs showed long-lasting (12 days) Schwann-like cell morphology and expression of myelin protein [91]. Pre-irradiation of Schwann cells excluded eventual cellular fusion artefacts [91]. Since the addition of supernatant from Schwann cell cultures failed to differentiate ADSCs, the authors speculated that the addition of specific chemical components or growth factors to the ADSC cultures, may promote the initial steps toward differentiation in vitro, which can be completed in the appropriate microenvironment and by required cell-to-cell interaction with mature cells in vivo.

The trans-differentiation of ADSCs towards motor neuron-like cells has also been reported. In 2012, Abdanipour and Tirahini [97] induced rat ADSCs to trans-differentiate into motor neuron-like cells by a two-step protocol. ADSCs were committed to neural progenitors expressing nestin, neurofilament 68 and neuro D by pre-induction for 24 h with selegiline. Selegiline is an inhibitor of monoamine oxidase B (MAO-B) which was used to trans-differentiate BM-MSCs into dopaminergic neural-like cells and proved to be a safer pre-inducer in comparison to the toxic β-mercaptoethanol and butylated hydroxyanisole compounds, widely used for ectodermal differentiation of MSC [97]. The maturation of the pre-induced ADSCs into a motor-neuron phenotype was then achieved by incubation with Shh and RA, resulting in a differentiation efficiency of around 70%. The resultant motor neuron-like cells (MNLCs) were characterized by an initial and transient high expression of oligo-2 and islet-1 (markers for early motor neuron commitment during in vitro differentiation), followed by a decrease in these two markers accompanied by an increase in the expression of the motor neuron marker HLBX9 [97]. Mature MNLCs, but not high HLBX9 expressing cells, were functionally tested for the capacity to release pre-synaptic vesicles by staining and destaining with the fluorescent probe FM1–43. Quantitative analysis of vesicle release after stimulation, showed a 4-fold increase in comparison to pre-induced ADSCs. MNLCs, also formed innervation-like contacts with myotubes in a co-culture in vitro system [97].

Very recently, the same authors proposed a different method to obtain MNLCs from rat ADSCs [98]. ADSCs were first converted into neurospheres by induction with NM medium consisting of DMEM, B27, EGF and bFGF for 7 days. Next, neural stem cells (NSC) were obtained by neurosphere dissociation into single cells, and incubation for 10 days with NM supplemented with 10% FBS. Maturation into motor neurons was achieved by incubation with Shh and RA for 5 days, followed by addition in culture media of BDNF, GDNF, CTNF and NT-3 for another 7 days [98]. During the maturation process of ADSC-NSCs into motor neurons, an increase in the expression of islet-1, HB9 and ChAT was observed, with MN-like cells positive for the neural marker MAP2 at day 14 of maturation. These findings were documented by both immunocytochemistry and RT-PCR. The functional activity of mature MNLCs was investigated by quantification of the release of synaptic vesicles by FM1–43 loading and release experiments upon ion stimulation. The synaptic vesicle activity correlated with changes in intracellular calcium concentration and membrane depolarization, as demonstrated by further investigations utilizing calcium and voltage-sensitive dyes [98].

Is the trans-differentiation of ADSCs into neurons real?

The differentiation into neurons is commonly described as morphological changes such as body retraction, bi- or multi-polar shape and branching extension, and by the expression of neuronal markers revealed by immunohistochemistry (IHC), western blotting (WB) and quantitative RT-PCR analysis. However, several studies showed that the neural-like phenotype obtained by chemical induction was a very fast but transient event which may be a result of cytoskeletal rearrangement due to the toxicity of compounds added into the induction media [99, 100]. Furthermore, several neuronal markers considered to confirm neuron maturation such as Nestin, NSE, trk-A and vimentin are already present at low levels in undifferentiated ADSCs [89, 90, 92, 95, 101].

Thus, morphological changes and expression of neuronal markers on the cell surface should not be considered as a definitive proof of neuronal differentiation, and functional characterization (i.e. electrophysiology) is necessary. However, very few studies confirmed electrical activity of ADSC-derived neurons by patch-clamp experiments [92, 95].

In addition, the efficiency and reproducibility of differentiation protocols described in the literature is low, and neuronal induction of ADSCs gives rise to a heterogeneous population of undifferentiated cells, neuron-like cells and astroglial-like cells with different degrees of maturation [91, 92]. Together with the fact that untreated ADSCs often show slight expression of neuronal progenitor markers, these results suggest the presence of specific cell subtypes with different neuronal differentiation potential [102]. This is supported by the existence of variability in the secretome of hADSCs obtained from different donors and maintained in separated cultures [103].

In vivo studies with ADSCs

For the first time in 2013, the therapeutic potential of ADSCs was investigated in the SOD1^{G93A} mouse model [104]. ADSCs were isolated from C57BL/6 GFP-expressing mice, and a total of two million cells were injected into the tail vein of B6SJL-SOD1^{G93A} mice after the first clinical signs of disease. The control group received injection of PBS only as vehicle. mADSCs delayed the motor performance decline and transiently attenuated motor neuron death, in comparison to the controls. However, no differences in the degree of astrogliosis, nor in survival were observed between the two groups [104]. The authors claimed that GFP-positive cells were found to migrate into damaged CNS areas, such as the grey matter in the spinal cord, however, low magnification images showing the entire spinal cord section or co-staining with neuronal specific markers were not shown and histology on PBS-treated control spinal cord sections was not performed. Finally, increased levels of trophic factors such as GDNF and bFGF were found in spinal cord homogenates of ADSC injected mice. This was despite the fact that mADSC used in this study were not capable of producing GDNF in vitro. It is likely that, in addition to trophic factor production and secretion, ADSCs could have an indirect biological effect by stimulating the secretome of surrounding astrocytes, which are known to produce GDNF [104].

Recently, another group tested the therapeutic potential of human ADSCs isolated from three healthy donors aged 64, 69 and 84 [105]. Female transgenic SOD1^{G93A} mice before clinical evidence of disease received 1×10^6 hADSCs by intravenous (IV) or 2×10^5 hADSCs by intracerebroventricular (ICV) injections. As a control, the sham group received PBS only.

Rotarod test and paw grip endurance were monitored and a reduction of 15% was considered as disease onset. The endpoint (survival) was defined by the lack of a righting reflex within 30 s after being placed on their side [105]. The authors found that disease onset in mice that received ICV injections was significantly delayed by 26 days, while in mice infused IV there was only an 11 day delay in disease onset. Remarkably, survival was prolonged by 24 days and 9 days respectively in ICV and IV mice when compared to the controls [105].

IHC evaluation of the spinal cord of ICV transplanted mice revealed that 6.8% of transplanted cells survived up to 4 weeks post-injection. However, only 0.7% migrated to the grey matter of the lumbar spinal cord and very few cells were positive for neuronal markers (MAP2 or I-NFM). In contrast, after IV infusion very few undifferentiated cells were found to engraft in the meninges of the spinal cord [105]. In addition, when the TUNEL assay was performed on spinal cord from ICV mice, reduced levels of apoptosis were seen in the anterior grey

matter compared to IV and control recipients. Also, RT-PCR and ELISA assays on spinal cord homogenates showed a significantly higher concentration of neurotrophic factors in the ICV group in comparison to controls [105]. ELISA assay on the supernatant from hADSC cultures showed high levels of neurotrophic factors that are relevant in neuroprotection such as IGF-1 and VEGF [105]. The anti-apoptotic effect was further confirmed in vitro by culturing primary neural cells from normal mice with hADSC conditioned media [105].

To date, these are the only two published studies using ADSCs in an experimental model of ALS. However, the therapeutic potential of ADSCs has been tested in other experimental models of neurodegeneration. In particular, the use of ADSCs showed encouraging results in animal models of chronic stroke, Parkinson's disease, Alzheimer's disease and traumatic brain injury and ageing [106–109]. The use of ADSCs in ALS patients has not been tested so far. However, currently two different clinical trials are recruiting participants.

A clinical trial sponsored by The Royan Institute in Iran will test the safety of intravenous injections of ADSCs derived from healthy donors (2 million cells/kg) in 8 ALS patients (ClinicalTrial.gov identifier: NCT02492516). The Andalusian Initiative for Advanced Therapies is recruiting 40 ALS patients for a phase I/II, multicentre, randomized, placebo controlled clinical trial to evaluate the safety and efficacy of intravenous infusion of different concentrations of autologous ADSCs (ClinicalTrials.gov identifier: NCT02290886).

MSCs for ALS therapy: Proposed mechanisms of action

The in vitro differentiation of mesenchymal stem cells into neuron-like cells brought great enthusiasm into the idea of cellular replacement as a therapeutic strategy in ALS. However, there are many practical issues to be solved. The real trans-differentiation of MSCs into neurons has been questioned and further investigation in order to study molecular pathways and optimized protocols enhancing the efficiency, stability and degree of maturation are needed. Also, only a few studies have reported MSCs or MSC-derived NSCs showing signs of in vivo maturation when transplanted into mice (detailed in the next section).

More importantly, for therapeutic efficacy, the transplanted cells should engraft, migrate to affected areas of degeneration, survive, mature and integrate into the pre-existing neuronal circuits forming synapses, extending long axon projections to reach muscles and regenerating neuromuscular junctions. All this must occur within a hostile microenvironment where other motor neurons are dying and activated microglia and astrocytes are sustaining an inflammatory milieu [30, 31].

Moreover, different pathological mechanisms described in ALS such as glutamate excitotoxicity [22], oxidative stress [26] and loss of metabolic support [110] may affect the viability of transplanted cells and inhibit maturation. Finally, stem cell maturation and integration into the host neuronal circuits could last a relatively long time, which may not be compatible with the fast progression rate of the disease.

Besides the challenge of cell replacement in ALS, in recent years increased attention has been paid to the "bystander effect" mechanism through which MSCs could exert their therapeutic effect. Different mechanisms have been proposed to explain the role of MSCs in neuroprotection. Although the precise mechanisms are still unknown, the secretion of anti-inflammatory cytokines and growth factors by MSCs may influence the progression of ALS in multiple ways, including endogenous regenerative processes such as neuronal plasticity, angiogenesis and axonal re-myelination [66, 111].

The delivery of growth factors such as BDNF, insulin-like growth factor-1 (IGF-I), vascular endothelial growth factor (VEGF) and glial derived neurotrophic factor (GDNF) into ALS experimental models has been very promising since these factors were shown to be neuroprotective, improved motor function and prolonged motor neuron survival [112]. However, translation into the clinic failed to provide any beneficial effect in ALS patients [112]. This is thought to be related to the small amount of growth factor that effectively reached the central nervous system (CNS) either because of an inability to cross the blood brain barrier or because of the short half-life after intravenous injection [112]. Moreover, intrathecal injections of growth factors did not result in relevant benefits for ALS patient [112].

The use of MSCs as "carriers" for the uninterrupted supply of growth factors has been proposed, having shown positive results in an ALS rodent model [113, 114]. Indeed, MSCs transduced to overexpress specific growth factors (GDNF, VEGF) or neuroprotective agents (e.g. glucagon-like peptide 1) transplanted into SOD1^{G93A} rodent models, significantly preserved neuromuscular junctions, attenuated motor neuron death, improved motor function, delayed symptom onset and prolonged survival [113, 114]. Recently, the Karussis group and Brainstorm-Cell therapeutics completed an open lab phase 1/2 clinical trial evaluating the safety and feasibility of intrathecal injections of MSCs induced to secrete neurotrophic factors (BDNF, GDNF) (NurOwn™) in 12 ALS patients (NCT01051882). Although, no results have been published so far, the details of another two separate active clinical trials can be found at ClinicalTrials.gov. An open label phase 2a escalating-dose trial (NCT01777646) and a phase 2 randomized, double-blind trial (NCT02017912) in order to evaluate safety and efficacy of multiple intramuscular and intrathecal combined injection of NurOwn™ cells into ALS patients are reported as in progress.

Through paracrine activity and cell-to-cell contacts, MSCs were able to induce astrocytes and glial cells to secrete enhanced levels of GDNF, VEGF and CNTF (ciliary neurotrophic factor) both in vitro and in the SOD1^{G93A} mice, resulting in anti-apoptotic effects and motor neuron protection [104, 115].

Another potential mechanism by which MSC could participate in tissue repair, is in the secretion of exosomes [116]. Exosomes are membrane vesicles originating from the inner cell membrane, which contain proteins, mRNAs and microRNAs. The content of exosomes, after their secretion from stem cells, could be transferred to neighbouring cells and mediate a plethora of biological pathways from free radical scavenging to the activation of self-regenerative programmes [117]. Interestingly, exosomes derived from murine adipose derived stem cells (ADSCs), were able to protect both naïve and SOD1^{G93A} transfected (overexpression of the human SOD1 gene with the G93A mutation) NSC34 motor neuron-like cells from oxidative stress in an in vitro culture system, with a significant reduction of apoptosis events and an increase in cell viability [118].

MSCs may act by modulating astrocyte dysfunction since they showed the ability to induce expression of glutamate re-uptake transporter 1 (GLT1) and inhibit caspase-3 cleavage in SOD1^{G93A} mutated astrocytes, thus limiting excitotoxicity [119].

Several studies on experimental models of ALS demonstrated the capacity of MSCs to attenuate astrogliosis [67, 68, 70]. When transplanted into SOD1^{G93A} mice, MSCs may exert immunomodulatory effects indirectly by stimulating host cells to secrete anti-inflammatory interleukins (IL) such as IL-10, IL-3 and IL-13 [68].

Intrathecal delivery of hMSCs into SOD1^{G93A} mice slowed disease progression, but increased lymphocyte infiltration into the spinal cord [120]. However, hMSCs cultured with peripheral blood mononuclear cells (PBMC) derived from ALS patients increased the proportion of regulatory T cells accompanied by enhanced production of anti-inflammatory cytokines such as IL-4, IL-10 and transforming growth factor-beta (TGFβ) [120]. Thus, when injected into the cerebrospinal fluid (CSF) of ALS mice, MSCs could exert their beneficial immunomodulation by stimulating regulatory T cell proliferation, activation and migration to areas of CNS inflammation [120]. MSCs were shown to inhibit maturation and activation of dendritic cells in vitro, and prevent lymphocyte migration into the spinal cord of experimental autoimmune encephalomyelitis mice [121, 122]. MSCs were also able to suppress proliferation, maturation and activation of pro-inflammatory Th1 and Th17 cells, with a concomitant switch toward active CD4$^+$ CD25 Foxp3 regulatory T cells in vitro [123].

T regulatory cells are reduced in patients with aggressive ALS and reduced levels of these cells in early disease correlates with rapid progression of neurodegeneration [124]. Interestingly, peripheral blood monocytes obtained from ALS patients 4 h and 24 h after an intravenous infusion of MSCs, showed a dramatic increase in CD4+ CD25+ regulatory T cells, coupled with a reduction in activated dendritic cells and lymphocyte proliferation [80].

The establishment of a sustained pro-inflammatory milieu in ALS spinal cord has been demonstrated which is probably accompanied by the shift of microglia cells from an anti-inflammatory state (often referred to as M2 in the literature) to an active neurotoxic state (often referred to as M1 in the literature) [125].

Of interest, MSC-conditioned media significantly inhibited the production and secretion of pro-inflammatory cytokines in microglia activated by lipopolysaccharide (LPS) [126] [127]. This, has been attributed to the capacity of MSCs to secrete TGF-β, which in turn inhibited the NFκB pathway and restored a protective microglial phenotype [127]. Thus, through paracrine effects, MSCs could modulate the functional properties of microglia by switching the detrimental M1 activated microglial state to the beneficial M2 activated microglial state after LPS induction [127].

Therefore, the immunomodulatory properties of MSCs may play an important role in attenuating neuroinflammatory processes during the progression of ALS and further work is needed in order to explore this specific mechanism.

An overview of the potential beneficial effects that MSCs could exert in modulating pathophysiology in neurodegenerative conditions is summarized in Fig. 3.

Delivery route for MSCs in ALS

One of the major technical issues in ALS cellular therapy is to effectively deliver stem cells into the CNS. Several studies demonstrated that injecting human stem cells directly into the spinal cord of ALS rodents is feasible, safe and efficient [40, 70, 71, 128]. The surgical procedure for intraspinal infusion of hMSCs into the spinal cord of ALS patients by specifically designed microinjection manipulators have also been shown to be safe in open-label clinical trials [75, 76, 78, 79, 129]. However, direct CNS injection remains an invasive procedure which could cause serious clinical complications and permanent damage to CNS areas already affected by the disease. Thus, it might be a considerable ethical issue in clinical trials when investigating the efficacy of the therapy, especially where placebo controls are required.

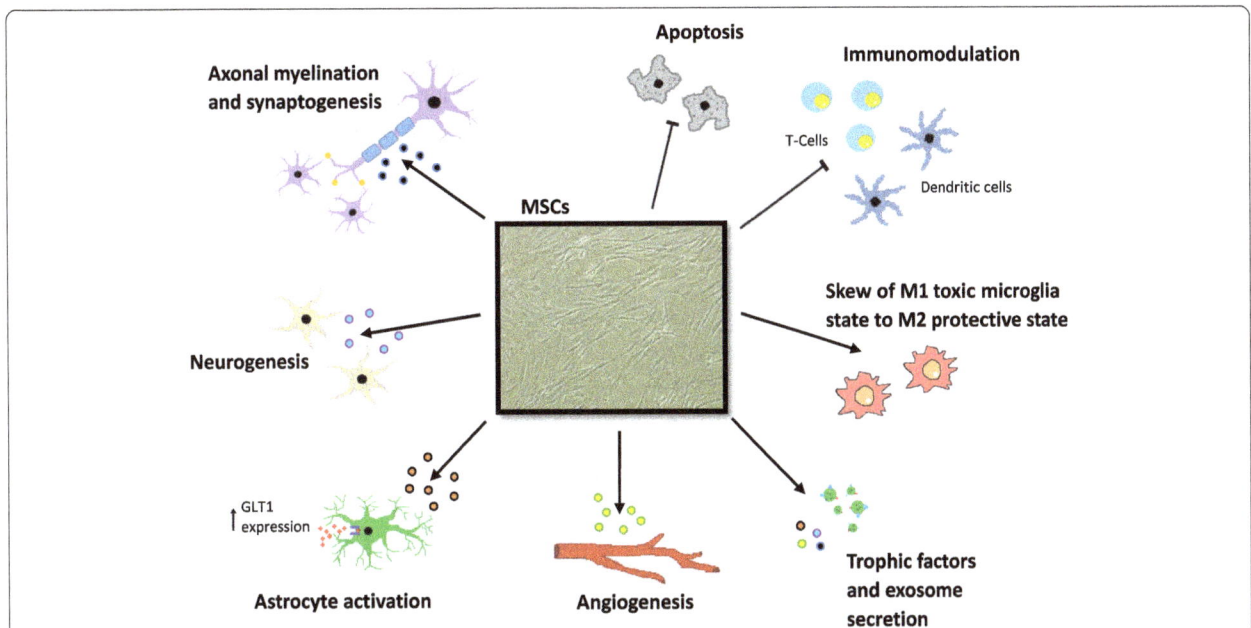

Fig. 3 Potential mechanisms of mesenchymal stem cell efficacy in neurodegeneration. Transplanted MSCs may provide therapeutic responses through paracrine effects and cell-to-cell contacts with resident neural cells. The capacity of MSCs to secrete cytokines, growth factors and exosomes could potentially induce and support regeneration processes, including angiogenesis, synaptogenesis, axonal re-myelination and neurogenesis. Because of their immunomodulatory properties, MSCs could attenuate inflammatory responses in the central nervous system by inhibiting maturation and migration of dendritic cells, suppression of lymphocyte activation and proliferation, and by reducing gliosis. Moreover, MSCs possess anti-apoptotic properties, and may limit excitotoxicity by modulating astrocyte functions

Since early pathologic mechanisms of disease involve destruction of neuromuscular junctions before motor neuron death, intramuscular injection of MSCs at an early stage of disease has also been proposed. Intramuscular injections of hMSCs engineered to overexpress GDNF into SOD1^{G93A} rats resulted in delayed disease onset and prolonged survival, but MSCs were not able to regenerate motor end-plates, nor to ameliorate motor neuron loss [72].

Given the immunomodulatory properties, together with the homing capacity in response to inflammatory signals, hMSCs showed beneficial effects when infused intravenously in ALS animal models [58, 61]. However, even though intravenous infusion could be the easiest and safest way for stem cell delivery, very few cells appear to be able to migrate, penetrate and engraft into the spinal cord parenchyma. Thus, a large number of cells may need to be transplanted in order to obtain effective results in human subjects.

The delivery of stem cells into the CSF surrounding the spinal cord by intrathecal injection may be a useful compromise, since stem cells would be placed in proximity to damaged areas without direct delivery into the spinal cord parenchyma. Furthermore, it would be possible to perform multiple injections both at the cervical and lumbar levels, allowing stem cells to migrate towards more affected areas of neurodegeneration/inflammation [67]. In some preclinical studies, stem cells were able to migrate from the CSF into the parenchyma, however, the mechanisms of migration remains unknown [64, 68]. Figure 4 is a representation of different proposed strategies to deliver MSCs into ALS patients with the relative advantages and disadvantages.

Strategies to enhance tissue penetration

The study of CNS inflammation models allowed the discovery of chemokines, receptors, adhesion molecules, and inhibitors that govern and regulate lymphocyte migration, extravasation and penetration into the CNS parenchyma. Even though the migration of lymphocytes from the blood to the CSF has been extensively studied, very little is known about the transmigration of lymphocytes from the perivascular space to the CNS parenchyma, where astrocytes and the basal membrane constitute a second impermeable barrier [130].

Curiously, important chemokines released during inflammation which stimulate lymphocyte migration through the BBB such as CXCL12 and CXCL10, were shown to inhibit infiltration into the parenchyma, inducing lymphocytes to persist in the perivascular space [131, 132]. Conversely, production of metalloproteases such as MP-2 and MP-9 seems to be necessary in order to break the dystroglycan basal membrane required for penetration into the CNS [130, 133].

MSCs express several chemokine receptors and homing properties similar to that of lymphocytes which allow them to migrate into damaged or inflamed tissues. However, donor age and the number of passages in culture were shown to negatively influence the stem cell's expression of homing factors [134].

Interestingly, Corti and colleagues have performed intrathecal and intravenous injection in SOD1^{G93A} mice of hiPSC-derived neural cells after being sorted for expression of the integrin VLA4 (CD49d) by FACS [49]. A considerable number of transplanted cells were able to migrate into the grey and white matter of spinal cord [49].

Engineering MSCs in order to induce overexpression of chemokine receptors or factors involved in homing and migration to sites of inflammation, may enhance the delivery into the spinal cord parenchyma. The characterization of chemokines and relative concentration in spinal cord and CSF of ALS models during different stages of disease would be of interest to identify the best candidate and also the peak of inflammatory chemokine production in order to define the ideal time of intervention for stem cell injection.

Future directions in clinical trials

During the past two decades, several clinical trials investigated the use of stem cells in patients with ALS, mostly focusing on the safety and feasibility of the intervention. Nonetheless, as reported by Appel and Armon, stem cells have often been transplanted into ALS patients with limited preclinical data, without providing details on adverse effects and using small numbers of participants [135]. Moreover, the long-term safety of stem cell transplantation (e.g. non acceleration of disease progression associated with the cell implantation) has been evaluated by comparison with historical control groups. This is an important limitation since heterogeneity in the patient population and differences in clinical care between the treated group and historical controls may affect the readouts [135].

Although single-armed, small phase I/II clinical trials found that cell-based therapy for ALS is relatively safe and feasible, it is uncertain whether stem cell transplantation may be clinically beneficial leading to functional improvements and of the slowing of disease progression. The majority of the clinical trials were principally focused on the safety and feasibility of the surgical procedure related to the stem cell implantation. Secondly, these clinical trials were not powered to demonstrate any clinical benefit [136].

In 2016, Abdul et al. published a systematic review aiming to assess the effectiveness of stem cell therapy in people with ALS, compared with a placebo or no additional treatment [136]. However, the authors could not identify any randomized controlled trial (RCT), quasi-

Fig. 4 Delivery strategies for the transplantation of MSCs in ALS. **a** Intrathecal delivery of MSCs into the spinal cord CSF; **b** Systemic delivery of MSCs; **c** Local delivery of MSCs directly into the spinal cord parenchyma. For each delivery route, advantages and disadvantages are summarized

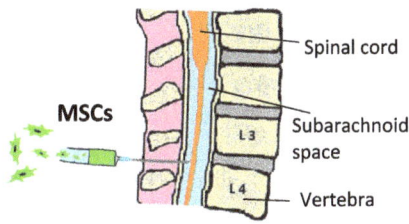

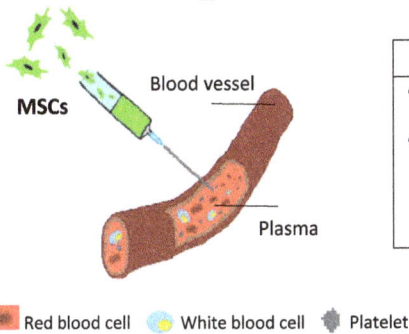

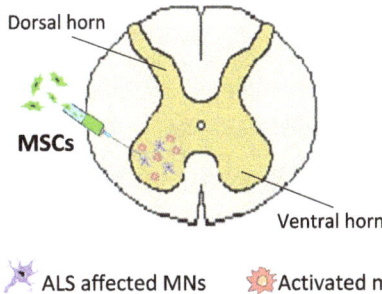

RCT or cluster RCT involving the use of stem cells in ALS/MND patients. Thus, there is an absence of high-quality published evidence to assess the safety and efficacy of stem cell transplantation in ALS [136]. Moreover, when analyzing the single arm phase I/II clinical studies available in the literature, the authors found substantial variability between clinical trials in terms of selection criteria, intervention methods and objective outcomes, with the involvement of small number of participants and a short-term follow-up period [136].

To investigate the long-term safety and efficacy of cellular therapy for ALS, well-designed prospective randomized-controlled trials with larger sample size,

long-term-follow up and standardization of cell products, are urgently needed [136].

Recently, the ALS Clinical Trials Workshop (Airlie Conference, Virginia, 2016), driven by the ALS community, clinicians, researches, industry representatives, government representatives, ALS patients and family members, released and submitted to the FDA the draft version of the "Guidance for Industry on Drug Development for Amyotrophic Lateral Sclerosis". The manuscript has been drafted with the intention of improving and accelerating the drug development process, including guidelines for a more effective clinical trial design in ALS [137]. In particular, the guideline highlighted the importance of reducing clinical and genetic heterogeneity when establishing the patient selection criteria. With regards to clinical heterogeneity, inclusion and exclusion criteria for patient enrolment must be well justified for each study, which could vary depending on the phase of development [137].

Selection criteria should also depend on the specific trial goals, since some therapies may be more effective in early stage of disease or in specific sub-group of patients. Thus, investigators should endeavor to incorporate reliable predictive and prognostic biomarkers for clinical trial eligibility or stratification criteria [137].

Because of the multifactorial nature of ALS, post-hoc analysis of reliable biological markers and neurophysiological data is extremely important, since in specific sub-groups of patients a beneficial effect could be missed during the analysis. However, responder analyses must only be used as hypothesis generating, which will need to be confirmed and further investigated in future trials [137].

Importantly, although early phase trials are not meant to investigate efficacy, for cell-based therapies which embrace potentially invasive delivery methods and lifelong biological effects, evaluation of efficacy should be included in the design of phase I trials. Furthermore, a long-term monitoring plan to evaluate tumorigenesis, stem cell engraftment and long-term efficacy should be included [137].

Finally, RCTs with placebo controls is considered as the gold standard for clinical investigation. However, in rare, rapidly progressive and untreatable diseases such as ALS, the requirement for a placebo could be revisited, especially if the intervention involves invasive methods. While in phase III clinical trials a randomized placebo group is indispensable, in earlier phase studies, the use of historical controls and predictive algorithms could be accepted. However, the development of target-specific biomarkers, standardization of outcome measures and validation of surrogate end-points is essential, especially in cell-based studies in which the mechanisms mediating the therapeutic effect are not well established.

Conclusions

During the last decade, the great advances achieved in regenerative medicine have created an unprecedented enthusiasm and new hope for amelioration of the devastating and until now incurable disease that is ALS. The initial exciting idea of replacing lost of motor neurons, with MSCs is unlikely to be achieved, although other strategies may provide some promise for stem cell derived motor neuron replacement [138]. Indeed, transplanted cells should differentiate and integrate with the host spinal motor circuits within the toxic and non-permissive environment that characterizes ALS. However, the neuroprotective and immunomodulatory potential of MSCSs

could match perfectly with the multifactorial nature of ALS.

Among different types of stem cells, MSCs represent a promising candidate for clinical application. However, several technical issues need to be addressed including: route of administration, optimal dose, and differentiation state and neuroprotective mechanisms of transplanted cells. In addition, in the majority of pre-clinical experiments stem cell injection was performed before disease onset. This is an important limitation for translation into the clinic where the diagnosis takes several months and early markers of disease are lacking [139]. Another limitation is the exclusive use of the SOD1^{G93A} model, which may reflect the pathological features of only a very small proportion of patients. Although these mice represent a robust model of ALS, only a small proportion of ALS cases are caused by SOD1 mutations [140]. Thus, the use of other ALS models such those driven by mutant TDP-43 and C9ORF72 expansions would be of interest [141].

Also, despite the excellent utility of the SOD1^{G93A} mice in revealing pathological ALS features, translation of promising therapies from this model has failed in human clinical trials [142]. Apart from considerable differences between rodents and humans, the answer to this problem could be attributed to the existence of a high rate of intra- and inter-laboratory variability [142]. Such variability could be improved by a more meticulous preclinical design, use of defined inbred mouse strains, transgene copy number analysis and trying to standardize preclinical investigation methods [142, 143].

In general, the presence of injected stem cells within the host nervous system of treated rodents was evaluated only a few days or weeks post-transplantation. Thus, the design of experiments looking at the long-term survival and integration of cells is necessary.

Evaluation of the presence of injected cells in the host has been carried out by the exclusive use of immunohistochemistry. Adopting advanced microscopy techniques such as confocal and two-photon microscopy would be of great interest to confirm stem cell engraftment, which could also allow tracking in vivo the fate of transplanted cells [144, 145].

In addition, rate of proliferation, stemness properties, longevity and differentiation capacity of MSCs declines considerably with time when culturing cells as monolayers [146]. The advent of 3D culture systems, along with enormous progress in the fabrication of biomaterials must be considered. When maintained in 3D culture systems such as hanging drops, low-adhesion plates, porous scaffolds or hydrogels, hMSCs showed increased proliferation and migration capacity, enhanced colony-forming efficiency, higher expression of stem cell markers, greater neuronal differentiation ability and greater cellular engraftment after transplantation in animals [146–148].

Thus, the regenerative potential of stem cells could be considerably improved by adopting 3D culture methods. Transplantation of bio-scaffolds or encapsulating MSCs to sustain favorable conditions for stem cell survival, growth, migration and maturation is showing promising results in experimental models of spinal cord injury, traumatic brain injury and nerve regeneration, and must be considered in ALS models where the presence of a hostile microenvironment is one of the main factors that negatively affects stem cell engraftment and therefore therapeutic potential [147, 149, 150].

The optimal maturation level for the transplantation of stem cells to obtain the greatest therapeutic benefit is also unclear. If undifferentiated cells may represent the best way to obtain immunomodulation and trophic factor production, induced neural progenitors may overcome the possibility of tumour formation, along with the possibility of in vivo maturation and integration into existing neuronal circuits.

A combination strategy could be interesting, where intravenous infusion of immature cells may generate permissive environmental conditions for the successive implantation of neuronal committed cells within the CSF. This would require an in-depth study of the maturation process of MSCs into neurons, trying to understand, optimize and standardize differentiation protocols that promote the generation of stable precursors.

Last but not least, although autologous transplantation can reduce the probability of immune rejection, it has been reported that patient-derived MSCs may have impaired or reduced therapeutic effects [151, 152]. Other evidence indicates no functional alteration or accelerated cellular senescence in BM-MSCs derived from sporadic cases of ALS [153]. Moreover, it was shown that there was the possibility to functionally restore defective ALS-derived MSCs by correcting alterations in DNA methylation [153, 154]. However, the identification of MSC biological markers predictive of a positive/negative therapeutic response in ALS patients would be of great value [82]. In relation to the use of autologous MSCs in patients carrying ALS causative genetic mutations, stem cells could be genetically corrected by adopting CRISPR-Cas9-mediated gene editing technology [155].

In conclusion, several strategies have been tested in the SOD1^{G93A} mouse model, but with different hurdles. All the discussed parameters should be reconsidered and optimized before the translation of stem cell therapy from mice to humans in order to avoid undesirable de-lays or therapy failure as has happened for most of the promising results derived from SOD1^{G93A} transgenic mouse models, with failure of translation into clinical benefits for ALS patients.

Abbreviations
ADSC: Adipose derived stem cells; ALS: Amyotrophic lateral sclerosis; BBB: Blood brain barrier; BDNF: Brain derived neurotrophicfFactor; bFGF: basic fibroblast growth factor; BM: Bone marrow; BMNC: Bone marrow mononuclear cells; CD: Cluster of differentiation; CNS: Central nervous system; CNTF: Ciliary neurotrophic factor; CSF: Cerebrospinal fluid; DCX: Doublecortin; DMEM: Dulbecco's modified eagle medium; FALS: Familial amyotrophic lateral sclerosis; FBS: Foetal bovine serum; FUS: Fused in sarcoma protein; GDNF: Glial derived neurotrophic factor; GFAP: Glial fibrillary acidic protein; GFP: Green fluorescent protein; GLT1: Glutamate re-uptake transporter 1; GMP: Good manufacturing practice; hESC: human embryonic stem cells; HGF: Hepatocyte growth factor; ICV: Intracerebroventricular; IGF-I: Insulin-like growth factor-1; IHC: Immunohistochemistry; IL: Interleukin; iPSC: induced pluripotent stem cells; ISCT: International Society for Cellular Therapy; IV: Intravenous; MAO-B: Monoamine oxidase B; MCP-1: Monocyte chemoattractant protein 1; MHC-II: Major histocompatibility complex class II; MND: Motor neuron disease; MNLCs: Motor neuron-like cells; MNPs: Motor neuron progenitors; MNs: Motor neurons; MS: Multiple sclerosis; MSCs: Mesenchymal stem cells; NGF: Nerve growth factor; Ngn1: Neurogenin1; NPs: Neural progenitors; NSC: Neural stem cells; NT-3: Neurotrophin 3; OPTN: Optineurin; PBMC: Peripheral blood mononuclear cell; PBS: Phosphate buffered saline; PNN: Perineural net; RA: Retinoic acid; RCT: Randomized controlled trial; SALS: Sporadic amyotrophic lateral sclerosis; SCI: Spinal cord injury; Shh: Sonic hedgehog; SMA: Spinal muscular atrophy; SOD1: Superoxide dismutase 1; SVF: Stromal vascular fraction; TARDBP: TAR DNA-binding protein 43; TGFα: Transforming growth factor-alpha; TGFβ: Transforming growth factor-beta; VCP: Valosin containing protein; VEGF: Vascular endothelial growth factor; WAT: White adipose tissue; WB: Western blotting; WT: Wild-type

Acknowledgements
University of Sheffield-Tongji University Joint Doctoral Researcher Programme (YC, PJS, RM), the NIHR Sheffield Biomedical Research Centre for Translational Neuroscience (PJS). Medical Research Council (MRC) Award Number: MR/M010864/1 (KN). Medical Research Council (MRC) award Number: MR/M010864/1 (PJS). MND Association Award Number: 983-797 (RJM).

Funding
This work was funded by a University of Sheffield-Tongji University collaborative PhD scholarship awarded to YC. PJS is an NIHR Senior Investigator and this work was also supported by the NIHR Sheffield Biomedical Research Centre for Translational Neuroscience.

Authors' contributions
All authors assisted in the planning and conception of the review article, YC drafted the manuscript and figures, RJM, PJS, KN and XJ edited the manuscript. All authors read and approved the final manuscript.

Competing interests
The authors declare that they have no competing interests.

Author details
[1]Sheffield Institute for Translational Neuroscience (SITraN), Department of Neuroscience, Faculty of Medicine, Dentistry and Health, University of Sheffield, 385a Glossop Rd S10 2HQ, Sheffield, UK. [2]Tongji University School of Medicine, 1239 Siping Rd, Yangpu Qu, Shanghai, China.

References

1. Walling AD. Amyotrophic lateral sclerosis: Lou Gehrig's disease. Am Fam Physician. 1999;59(6):1489–96.
2. Andersen PM, Al-Chalabi A. Clinical genetics of amyotrophic lateral sclerosis: what do we really know? Nat Rev Neurol. 2011;7(11):603–15.
3. Rosen DR, Siddique T, Patterson D, Figlewicz DA, Sapp P, Hentati A, et al. Mutations in cu/Zn superoxide dismutase gene are associated with familial amyotrophic lateral sclerosis. Nature. 1993;362(6415):59–62.
4. Kabashi E, Valdmanis PN, Dion P, Spiegelman D, McConkey BJ, Vande Velde C, et al. TARDBP mutations in individuals with sporadic and familial amyotrophic lateral sclerosis. Nat Genet. 2008;40(5):572–4.
5. Rutherford NJ, Zhang YJ, Baker M, Gass JM, Finch NA, YF X, et al. Novel mutations in TARDBP (TDP-43) in patients with familial amyotrophic lateral sclerosis. PLoS Genet. 2008;4(9):e1000193.
6. Kwiatkowski TJ Jr, Bosco DA, Leclerc AL, Tamrazian E, Vanderburg CR, Russ C, et al. Mutations in the FUS/TLS gene on chromosome 16 cause familial amyotrophic lateral sclerosis. Science. 2009;323(5918):1205–8.
7. Vance C, Rogelj B, Hortobagyi T, De Vos KJ, Nishimura AL, Sreedharan J, et al. Mutations in FUS, an RNA processing protein, cause familial amyotrophic lateral sclerosis type 6. Science. 2009;323(5918):1208–11.
8. Maruyama H, Morino H, Ito H, Izumi Y, Kato H, Watanabe Y, et al. Mutations of optineurin in amyotrophic lateral sclerosis. Nature. 2010;465(7295):223–6.
9. Johnson JO, Mandrioli J, Benatar M, Abramzon Y, Van Deerlin VM, Trojanowski JQ, et al. Exome sequencing reveals VCP mutations as a cause of familial ALS. Neuron. 2010;68(5):857–64.
10. Shaw CE, Capturing VCP. Another molecular piece in the ALS jigsaw puzzle. Neuron. 2010;68(5):812–4.
11. Deng HX, Chen W, Hong ST, Boycott KM, Gorrie GH, Siddique N, et al. Mutations in UBQLN2 cause dominant X-linked juvenile and adult-onset ALS and ALS/dementia. Nature. 2011;477(7363):211–5.
12. Renton AE, Majounie E, Waite A, Simon-Sanchez J, Rollinson S, Gibbs JR, et al. A hexanucleotide repeat expansion in C9ORF72 is the cause of chromosome 9p21-linked ALS-FTD. Neuron. 2011;72(2):257–68.
13. DeJesus-Hernandez M, Mackenzie IR, Boeve BF, Boxer AL, Baker M, Rutherford NJ, et al. Expanded GGGGCC hexanucleotide repeat in noncoding region of C9ORF72 causes chromosome 9p-linked FTD and ALS. Neuron. 2011;72(2):245–56.
14. Cirulli ET, Lasseigne BN, Petrovski S, Sapp PC, Dion PA, Leblond CS, et al. Exome sequencing in amyotrophic lateral sclerosis identifies risk genes and pathways. Science. 2015;347(6229):1436–41.
15. Freischmidt A, Wieland T, Richter B, Ruf W, Schaeffer V, Muller K, et al. Haploinsufficiency of TBK1 causes familial ALS and fronto-temporal dementia. Nat Neurosci. 2015;18(5):631–6.
16. Poppe L, Rue L, Robberecht W, Van Den Bosch L. Translating biological findings into new treatment strategies for amyotrophic lateral sclerosis (ALS). Exp Neurol. 2014;262 Pt B:138–151.
17. Gurney ME, Pu H, Chiu AY, Dal Canto MC, Polchow CY, Alexander DD, et al. Motor neuron degeneration in mice that express a human cu,Zn superoxide dismutase mutation. Science. 1994;264(5166):1772–5.
18. Cleveland DW, Bruijn LI, Wong PC, Marszalek JR, Vechio JD, Lee MK, et al. Mechanisms of selective motor neuron death in transgenic mouse models of motor neuron disease. Neurology. 1996;47(4 Suppl 2):S54–S61; discussion S-2.
19. Lagier-Tourenne C, Polymenidou M, Hutt KR, AQ V, Baughn M, Huelga SC, et al. Divergent roles of ALS-linked proteins FUS/TLS and TDP-43 intersect in processing long pre-mRNAs. Nat Neurosci. 2012;15(11):1488–97.
20. Kitamura A, Inada N, Kubota H, Matsumoto G, Kinjo M, Morimoto RI, et al. Dysregulation of the proteasome increases the toxicity of ALS-linked mutant SOD1. Genes Cells. 2014;19(3):209–24.
21. Highley JR, Kirby J, Jansweijer JA, Webb PS, Hewamadduma CA, Heath PR, et al. Loss of nuclear TDP-43 in amyotrophic lateral sclerosis (ALS) causes altered expression of splicing machinery and widespread dysregulation of RNA splicing in motor neurones. Neuropathol Appl Neurobiol. 2014;40(6):670–85.
22. Alexander GM, Deitch JS, Seeburger JL, Del Valle L, Heiman-Patterson TD. Elevated cortical extracellular fluid glutamate in transgenic mice expressing human mutant (G93A) cu/Zn superoxide dismutase. J Neurochem. 2000;74(4):1666–73.
23. Shi P, Gal J, Kwinter DM, Liu X, Zhu H. Mitochondrial dysfunction in amyotrophic lateral sclerosis. Biochim Biophys Acta. 2010;1802(1):45–51.
24. Saxena S, Cabuy E, Caroni PA. Role for motoneuron subtype-selective ER stress in disease manifestations of FALS mice. Nat Neurosci. 2009;12(5):627–36.

25. Zhang B, Tu P, Abtahian F, Trojanowski JQ, Lee VM. Neurofilaments and orthograde transport are reduced in ventral root axons of transgenic mice that express human SOD1 with a G93A mutation. J Cell Biol. 1997;139(5):1307–15.
26. Barber SC, Shaw PJ. Oxidative stress in ALS: key role in motor neuron injury and therapeutic target. Free Radic Biol Med. 2010;48(5):629–41.
27. Clement AM, Nguyen MD, Roberts EA, Garcia ML, Boillee S, Rule M, et al. Wild-type nonneuronal cells extend survival of SOD1 mutant motor neurons in ALS mice. Science. 2003;302(5642):113–7.
28. Pramatarova A, Laganiere J, Roussel J, Brisebois K, Rouleau GA. Neuron-specific expression of mutant superoxide dismutase 1 in transgenic mice does not lead to motor impairment. J Neurosci. 2001;21(10):3369–74.
29. Kang SH, Li Y, Fukaya M, Lorenzini I, Cleveland DW, Ostrow LW, et al. Degeneration and impaired regeneration of gray matter oligodendrocytes in amyotrophic lateral sclerosis. Nat Neurosci. 2013;16(5):571–9.
30. Alexianu ME, Kozovska M, Appel SH. Immune reactivity in a mouse model of familial ALS correlates with disease progression. Neurology. 2001;57(7):1282–9.
31. Feeney SJ, McKelvie PA, Austin L, Jean-Francois MJ, Kapsa R, Tombs SM, et al. Presymptomatic motor neuron loss and reactive astrocytosis in the SOD1 mouse model of amyotrophic lateral sclerosis. Muscle Nerve. 2001;24(11):1510–9.
32. Ferraiuolo L. The non-cell-autonomous component of ALS: new in vitro models and future challenges. Biochem Soc Trans. 2014;42(5):1270–4.
33. Thomson JA, Itskovitz-Eldor J, Shapiro SS, Waknitz MA, Swiergiel JJ, Marshall VS, et al. Embryonic stem cell lines derived from human blastocysts. Science. 1998;282(5391):1145–7.
34. Shin S, Dalton S, Stice SL. Human motor neuron differentiation from human embryonic stem cells. Stem Cells Dev. 2005;14(3):266–9.
35. Rossi SL, Nistor G, Wyatt T, Yin HZ, Poole AJ, Weiss JH, et al. Histological and functional benefit following transplantation of motor neuron progenitors to the injured rat spinal cord. PLoS One. 2010;5(7):e11852.
36. Wyatt TJ, Rossi SL, Siegenthaler MM, Frame J, Robles R, Nistor G, et al. Human motor neuron progenitor transplantation leads to endogenous neuronal sparing in 3 models of motor neuron loss. Stem Cells Int. 2011;2011:207230.
37. Toma JS, Shettar BC, Chipman PH, Pinto DM, Borowska JP, Ichida JK, et al. Motoneurons derived from induced pluripotent stem cells develop mature phenotypes typical of endogenous spinal Motoneurons. J Neurosci. 2015;35(3):1291–306.
38. Mothe A, Tator CH. Isolation of neural stem/progenitor cells from the periventricular region of the adult rat and human spinal cord. J Vis Exp. 2015;99:e52732.
39. Xu L, Ryugo DK, Pongstaporn T, Johe K, Koliatsos VE. Human neural stem cell grafts in the spinal cord of SOD1 transgenic rats: differentiation and structural integration into the segmental motor circuitry. J Comp Neurol. 2009;514(4):297–309.
40. Xu L, Shen P, Hazel T, Johe K, Koliatsos VE. Dual transplantation of human neural stem cells into cervical and lumbar cord ameliorates motor neuron disease in SOD1 transgenic rats. Neurosci Lett. 2011;494(3):222–6.
41. Yan J, Xu L, Welsh AM, Hatfield G, Hazel T, Johe K, et al. Extensive neuronal differentiation of human neural stem cell grafts in adult rat spinal cord. PLoS Med. 2007;4(2):e39.
42. Yan J, Xu L, Welsh AM, Chen D, Hazel T, Johe K, et al. Combined immunosuppressive agents or CD4 antibodies prolong survival of human neural stem cell grafts and improve disease outcomes in amyotrophic lateral sclerosis transgenic mice. Stem Cells. 2006;24(8):1976–85.
43. Xu L, Yan J, Chen D, Welsh AM, Hazel T, Johe K, et al. Human neural stem cell grafts ameliorate motor neuron disease in SOD-1 transgenic rats. Transplantation. 2006;82(7):865–75.
44. Takahashi K, Yamanaka S. Induction of pluripotent stem cells from mouse embryonic and adult fibroblast cultures by defined factors. Cell. 2006;126(4):663–76.
45. Takahashi K, Tanabe K, Ohnuki M, Narita M, Ichisaka T, Tomoda K, et al. Induction of pluripotent stem cells from adult human fibroblasts by defined factors. Cell. 2007;131(5):861–72.
46. Dimos JT, Rodolfa KT, Niakan KK, Weisenthal LM, Mitsumoto H, Chung W, et al. Induced pluripotent stem cells generated from patients with ALS can be differentiated into motor neurons. Science. 2008;321(5893):1218–21.
47. Karumbayaram S, Novitch BG, Patterson M, Umbach JA, Richter L, Lindgren A, et al. Directed differentiation of human-induced pluripotent stem cells generates active motor neurons. Stem Cells. 2009;27(4):806–11.

48. Popescu IR, Nicaise C, Liu S, Bisch G, Knippenberg S, Daubie V, et al. Neural progenitors derived from human induced pluripotent stem cells survive and differentiate upon transplantation into a rat model of amyotrophic lateral sclerosis. Stem Cells Transl Med. 2013;2(3):167–74.

49. Nizzardo M, Simone C, Rizzo F, Ruggieri M, Salani S, Riboldi G, et al. Minimally invasive transplantation of iPSC-derived ALDHhiSSCloVLA4+ neural stem cells effectively improves the phenotype of an amyotrophic lateral sclerosis model. Hum Mol Genet. 2014;23(2):342–54.

50. Pittenger MF, Mackay AM, Beck SC, Jaiswal RK, Douglas R, Mosca JD, et al. Multilineage potential of adult human mesenchymal stem cells. Science. 1999;284(5411):143–7.

51. Woodbury D, Schwarz EJ, Prockop DJ, Black IB. Adult rat and human bone marrow stromal cells differentiate into neurons. J Neurosci Res. 2000;61(4):364–70.

52. Hermann A, Gastl R, Liebau S, Popa MO, Fiedler J, Boehm BO, et al. Efficient generation of neural stem cell-like cells from adult human bone marrow stromal cells. J Cell Sci. 2004;117(Pt 19):4411–22.

53. Rivera FJ, Couillard-Despres S, Pedre X, Ploetz S, Caioni M, Lois C, et al. Mesenchymal stem cells instruct oligodendrogenic fate decision on adult neural stem cells. Stem Cells. 2006;24(10):2209–19.

54. Boucherie C, Schafer S, Lavand'homme P, Maloteaux JM, Hermans E. Chimerization of astroglial population in the lumbar spinal cord after mesenchymal stem cell transplantation prolongs survival in a rat model of amyotrophic lateral sclerosis. J Neurosci Res. 2009;87(9):2034–46.

55. Sanchez-Ramos J, Song S, Cardozo-Pelaez F, Hazzi C, Stedeford T, Willing A, et al. Adult bone marrow stromal cells differentiate into neural cells in vitro. Exp Neurol. 2000;164(2):247–56.

56. Wislet-Gendebien S, Hans G, Leprince P, Rigo JM, Moonen G, Rogister B. Plasticity of cultured mesenchymal stem cells: switch from nestin-positive to excitable neuron-like phenotype. Stem Cells. 2005;23(3):392–402.

57. Joe IS, Jeong S-G, Cho G-W. Resveratrol-induced SIRT1 activation promotes neuronal differentiation of human bone marrow mesenchymal stem cells. Neurosci Lett 2014;584:97–102.

58. Chan-Il C, Young-Don L, Heejaung K, Kim SH, Suh-Kim H, Kim SS. Neural induction with neurogenin 1 enhances the therapeutic potential of mesenchymal stem cells in an amyotrophic lateral sclerosis mouse model. Cell Transplant. 2013;22(5):855–70.

59. Choi YK, Lee DH, Seo YK, Jung H, Park JK, Cho H. Stimulation of neural differentiation in human bone marrow mesenchymal stem cells by extremely low-frequency electromagnetic fields incorporated with MNPs. Appl Biochem Biotechnol. 2014;174(4):1233–45.

60. Lewis CM, Suzuki M. Therapeutic applications of mesenchymal stem cells for amyotrophic lateral sclerosis. Stem Cell Res Ther. 2014;5(2):32.

61. Zhao CP, Zhang C, Zhou SN, Xie YM, Wang YH, Huang H, et al. Human mesenchymal stromal cells ameliorate the phenotype of SOD1-G93A ALS mice. Cytotherapy. 2007;9(5):414–26.

62. Uccelli A, Milanese M, Principato MC, Morando S, Bonifacino T, Vergani L, et al. Intravenous mesenchymal stem cells improve survival and motor function in experimental amyotrophic lateral sclerosis. Mol Med. 2012;18: 794–804.

63. Habisch HJ, Janowski M, Binder D, Kuzma-Kozakiewicz M, Widmann A, Habich A, et al. Intrathecal application of neuroectodermally converted stem cells into a mouse model of ALS: limited intraparenchymal migration and survival narrows therapeutic effects. J Neural Transm (Vienna). 2007; 114(11):1395–406.

64. Kim H, Kim HY, Choi MR, Hwang S, Nam KH, Kim HC, et al. Dose-dependent efficacy of ALS-human mesenchymal stem cells transplantation into cisterna magna in SOD1-G93A ALS mice. Neurosci Lett. 2010;468(3):190–4.

65. Zhang C, Zhou C, Teng JJ, Zhao RL, Song YQ. Multiple administrations of human marrow stromal cells through cerebrospinal fluid prolong survival in a transgenic mouse model of amyotrophic lateral sclerosis. Cytotherapy. 2009;11(3):299–306.

66. Forostyak S, Homola A, Turnovcova K, Svitil P, Jendelova P, Sykova E. Intrathecal delivery of mesenchymal stromal cells protects the structure of altered perineuronal nets in SOD1 rats and amends the course of ALS. Stem Cells. 2014;32(12):3163–72.

67. Zhou C, Zhang C, Zhao R, Chi S, Ge P. Human marrow stromal cells reduce microglial activation to protect motor neurons in a transgenic mouse model of amyotrophic lateral sclerosis. J Neuroinflammation. 2013;10:52.

68. Boido M, Piras A, Valsecchi V, Spigolon G, Mareschi K, Ferrero I, et al. Human mesenchymal stromal cell transplantation modulates neuroinflammatory

milieu in a mouse model of amyotrophic lateral sclerosis. Cytotherapy. 2014; 16(8):1059–72.

69. Iwashita Y, Crang AJ, Blakemore WF. Redistribution of bisbenzimide Hoechst 33342 from transplanted cells to host cells. Neuroreport. 2000;11(5):1013–6. Epub 2000/05/03

70. Vercelli A, Mereuta OM, Garbossa D, Muraca G, Mareschi K, Rustichelli D, et al. Human mesenchymal stem cell transplantation extends survival, improves motor performance and decreases neuroinflammation in mouse model of amyotrophic lateral sclerosis. Neurobiol Dis. 2008;31(3):395–405.

71. Knippenberg S, Thau N, Schwabe K, Dengler R, Schambach A, Hass R, et al. Intraspinal injection of human umbilical cord blood-derived cells is neuroprotective in a transgenic mouse model of amyotrophic lateral sclerosis. Neurodegener Dis. 2012;9(3):107–20.

72. Suzuki M, McHugh J, Tork C, Shelley B, Hayes A, Bellantuono I, et al. Direct muscle delivery of GDNF with human mesenchymal stem cells improves motor neuron survival and function in a rat model of familial ALS. Mol Ther. 2008;16(12):2002–10.

73. Mazzini L, Fagioli F, Boccaletti R, Mareschi K, Oliveri G, Olivieri C, et al. Stem cell therapy in amyotrophic lateral sclerosis: a methodological approach in humans. Amyotroph Lateral Scler Other Motor Neuron Disord. 2003;4(3):158–61.

74. Mazzini L, Mareschi K, Ferrero I, Vassallo E, Oliveri G, Nasuelli N, et al. Stem cell treatment in amyotrophic lateral sclerosis. J Neurol Sci. 2008;265(1–2):78–83.

75. Mazzini L, Ferrero I, Luparello V, Rustichelli D, Gunetti M, Mareschi K, et al. Mesenchymal stem cell transplantation in amyotrophic lateral sclerosis: a phase I clinical trial. Exp Neurol. 2010;223(1):229–37.

76. Mazzini L, Mareschi K, Ferrero I, Miglioretti M, Stecco A, Servo S, et al. Mesenchymal stromal cell transplantation in amyotrophic lateral sclerosis: a long-term safety study. Cytotherapy. 2012;14(1):56–60.

77. Cabanes C, Bonilla S, Tabares L, Martinez S. Neuroprotective effect of adult hematopoietic stem cells in a mouse model of motoneuron degeneration. Neurobiol Dis. 2007;26(2):408–18.

78. Blanquer M, Moraleda JM, Iniesta F, Gomez-Espuch J, Meca-Lallana J, Villaverde R, et al. Neurotrophic bone marrow cellular nests prevent spinal motoneuron degeneration in amyotrophic lateral sclerosis patients: a pilot safety study. Stem Cells. 2012;30(6):1277–85.

79. Blanquer M, Perez-Espejo MA, Martinez-Lage JF, Iniesta F, Martinez S, Moraleda JMA. Surgical technique of spinal cord cell transplantation in amyotrophic lateral sclerosis. J Neurosci Methods. 2010;191(2):255–7.

80. Karussis D, Karageorgiou C, Vaknin-Dembinsky A, Gowda-Kurkalli B, Gomori JM, Kassis I, et al. Safety and immunological effects of mesenchymal stem cell transplantation in patients with multiple sclerosis and amyotrophic lateral sclerosis. Arch Neurol. 2010;67(10):1187–94.

81. KW O, Moon C, Kim HY, SI O, Park J, Lee JH, et al. Phase I trial of repeated intrathecal autologous bone marrow-derived mesenchymal stromal cells in amyotrophic lateral sclerosis. Stem Cells Transl Med. 2015;4(6):590–7.

82. Kim HY, Kim H, KW O, SI O, Koh SH, Baik W, et al. Biological markers of mesenchymal stromal cells as predictors of response to autologous stem cell transplantation in patients with amyotrophic lateral sclerosis: an investigator-initiated trial and in vivo study. Stem Cells. 2014;32(10):2724–31.

83. Zuk PA, Zhu M, Mizuno H, Huang J, Futrell JW, Katz AJ, et al. Multilineage cells from human adipose tissue: implications for cell-based therapies. Tissue Eng. 2001;7(2):211–28.

84. Meyer J, Salamon A, Herzmann N, Adam S, Kleine HD, Matthiesen I, et al. Isolation and differentiation potential of human Mesenchymal stem cells from adipose tissue harvested by water jet-assisted liposuction. Aesthet Surg J. 2015;35(8):1030–9.

85. Baglioni S, Francalanci M, Squecco R, Lombardi A, Cantini G, Angeli R, et al. Characterization of human adult stem-cell populations isolated from visceral and subcutaneous adipose tissue. FASEB J. 2009;23(10):3494–505.

86. Dominici M, Le Blanc K, Mueller I, Slaper-Cortenbach I, Marini F, Krause D, et al. Minimal criteria for defining multipotent mesenchymal stromal cells. The International Society for Cellular Therapy position statement. Cytotherapy. 2006;8(4):315–7.

87. Han C, Zhang L, Song L, Liu Y, Zou W, Piao H, et al. Human adipose-derived mesenchymal stem cells: a better cell source for nervous system regeneration. Chin Med J. 2014;127(2):329–37.

88. Safford KM, Hicok KC, Safford SD, Halvorsen YD, Wilkison WO, Gimble JM, et al. Neurogenic differentiation of murine and human adipose-derived stromal cells. Biochem Biophys Res Commun. 2002;294(2):371–9.

89. Zuk PA, Zhu M, Ashjian P, De Ugarte DA, Huang JI, Mizuno H, et al. Human

adipose tissue is a source of multipotent stem cells. Mol Biol Cell. 2002; 13(12):4279–95.

90. Ashjian PH, Elbarbary AS, Edmonds B, DeUgarte D, Zhu M, Zuk PA, et al. Vitro differentiation of human processed lipoaspirate cells into early neural progenitors. Plast Reconstr Surg. 2003;111(6):1922–31.

91. Krampera M, Marconi S, Pasini A, Galie M, Rigotti G, Mosna F, et al. Induction of neural-like differentiation in human mesenchymal stem cells derived from bone marrow, fat, spleen and thymus. Bone. 2007;40(2):382–90.

92. Jang S, Cho HH, Cho YB, Park JS, Jeong HS. Functional neural differentiation of human adipose tissue-derived stem cells using bFGF and forskolin. BMC Cell Biol. 2010;11:25.

93. Qian DX, Zhang HT, Ma X, Jiang XD, Comparison XRX. Of the efficiencies of three neural induction protocols in human adipose stromal cells. Neurochem Res. 2010;35(4):572–9.

94. Ahmadi N, Razavi S, Kazemi M, Oryan S. Stability of neural differentiation in human adipose derived stem cells by two induction protocols. Tissue Cell. 2012;44(2):87–94.

95. Feng N, Han Q, Li J, Wang S, Li H, Yao X, et al. Generation of highly purified neural stem cells from human adipose-derived mesenchymal stem cells by Sox1 activation. Stem Cells Dev. 2014;23(5):515–29.

96. Bahmani L, Taha MF, Javeri A. Coculture with embryonic stem cells improves neural differentiation of adipose tissue stem cells. Neuroscience. 2014;272:229–39.

97. Abdanipour A, Tiraihi T. Induction of adipose-derived stem cell into motoneuron-like cells using selegiline as preinducer. Brain Res. 2012;1440:23–33.

98. Darvishi M, Tiraihi T, Mesbah-Namin SA, Delshad A, Taheri T. Motor neuron Transdifferentiation of neural stem cell from adipose-derived stem cell characterized by differential gene expression. Cell Mol Neurobiol. 2016;

99. Neuhuber B, Gallo G, Howard L, Kostura L, Mackay A, Fischer I. Reevaluation of in vitro differentiation protocols for bone marrow stromal cells: disruption of actin cytoskeleton induces rapid morphological changes and mimics neuronal phenotype. J Neurosci Res. 2004;77(2):192–204.

100. Lu P, Blesch A, Tuszynski MH. Induction of bone marrow stromal cells to neurons: differentiation, transdifferentiation, or artifact? J Neurosci Res. 2004; 77(2):174–91.

101. Woodbury D, Reynolds K, Black IB. Adult bone marrow stromal stem cells express germline, ectodermal, endodermal, and mesodermal genes prior to neurogenesis. J Neurosci Res. 2002;69(6):908–17.

102. Fu L, Zhu L, Huang Y, Lee TD, Forman SJ, Shih CC. Derivation of neural stem cells from mesenchymal stem cells: evidence for a bipotential stem cell population. Stem Cells Dev. 2008;17(6):1109–21.

103. Kalinina N, Kharlampieva D, Loguinova M, Butenko I, Pobeguts O, Efimenko A, et al. Characterization of secretomes provides evidence for adipose-derived mesenchymal stromal cells subtypes. Stem Cell Res Ther. 2015;6:221.

104. Marconi S, Bonaconsa M, Scambi I, Squintani GM, Rui W, Turano E, et al. Systemic treatment with adipose-derived mesenchymal stem cells ameliorates clinical and pathological features in the amyotrophic lateral sclerosis murine model. Neuroscience. 2013;248:333–43.

105. Kim KS, Lee HJ, An J, Kim YB, Ra JC, Lim I, et al. Transplantation of human adipose tissue-derived stem cells delays clinical onset and prolongs life span in ALS mouse model. Cell Transplant. 2014;23(12):1585–97.

106. Kim JM, Lee ST, Chu K, Jung KH, Song EC, Kim SJ, et al. Systemic transplantation of human adipose stem cells attenuated cerebral inflammation and degeneration in a hemorrhagic stroke model. Brain Res. 2007;1183:43–50.

107. Park D, Yang G, Bae DK, Lee SH, Yang YH, Kyung J, et al. Human adipose tissue-derived mesenchymal stem cells improve cognitive function and physical activity in ageing mice. J Neurosci Res. 2013;91(5):660–70.

108. Yan Y, Ma T, Gong K, Ao Q, Zhang X, Gong Y. Adipose-derived mesenchymal stem cell transplantation promotes adult neurogenesis in the brains of Alzheimer's disease mice. Neural Regen Res. 2014;9(8):798–805.

109. Schwerk A, Altschuler J, Roch M, Gossen M, Winter C, Berg J, et al. Adipose-derived human mesenchymal stem cells induce long-term neurogenic and anti-inflammatory effects and improve cognitive but not motor performance in a rat model of Parkinson's disease. Regen Med. 2015;10(4):431–46.

110. Ilieva H, Polymenidou M, Cleveland DW. Non-cell autonomous toxicity in neurodegenerative disorders: ALS and beyond. J Cell Biol. 2009;187(6):761–72.

111. Kingham PJ, Kolar MK, Novikova LN, Novikov LN, Wiberg M. Stimulating the neurotrophic and angiogenic properties of human adipose-derived stem cells enhances nerve repair. Stem Cells Dev. 2014;23(7):741–54.

112. Henriques A, Pitzer C, Schneider A. Neurotrophic growth factors for the treatment of amyotrophic lateral sclerosis: where do we stand? Front Neurosci. 2010;4:32.

113. Krakora D, Mulcrone P, Meyer M, Lewis C, Bernau K, Gowing G, et al. Synergistic effects of GDNF and VEGF on lifespan and disease progression in a familial ALS rat model. Mol Ther. 2013;21(8):1602–10.

114. Knippenberg S, Thau N, Dengler R, Brinker T, Petri S. Intracerebroventricular injection of encapsulated human mesenchymal cells producing glucagon-like peptide 1 prolongs survival in a mouse model of ALS. PLoS One. 2012; 7(6):e36857.

115. Sun H, Benardais K, Stanslowsky N, Thau-Habermann N, Hensel N, Huang D, et al. Therapeutic potential of mesenchymal stromal cells and MSC conditioned medium in amyotrophic lateral sclerosis (ALS)–in vitro evidence from primary motor neuron cultures, NSC-34 cells, astrocytes and microglia. PLoS One. 2013;8(9):e72926.

116. Han C, Sun X, Liu L, Jiang H, Shen Y, Xu X, et al. Exosomes and their therapeutic potentials of stem cells. Stem Cells Int. 2016;2016:7653489.

117. Bonafede R, Scambi I, Peroni D, Potrich V, Boschi F, Benati D, et al. Exosome derived from murine adipose-derived stromal cells: Neuroprotective effect on in vitro model of amyotrophic lateral sclerosis. Exp Cell Res. 2015;340(1): 150–8.

118. Bonafede R, Scambi I, Peroni D, Potrich V, Boschi F, Benati D, et al. Exosome derived from murine adipose-derived stromal cells: Neuroprotective effect on in vitro model of amyotrophic lateral sclerosis. Exp Cell Res. 2016;340(1): 150–8.

119. Gu R, Hou X, Pang R, Li L, Chen F, Geng J, et al. Human adipose-derived stem cells enhance the glutamate uptake function of GLT1 in SOD1(G93A)-bearing astrocytes. Biochem Biophys Res Commun. 2010;393(3):481–6.

120. Kwon MS, Noh MY, KW O, Cho KA, Kang BY, Kim KS, et al. The immunomodulatory effects of human mesenchymal stem cells on peripheral blood mononuclear cells in ALS patients. J Neurochem. 2014;131(2):206–18.

121. Zappia E, Casazza S, Pedemonte E, Benvenuto F, Bonanni I, Gerdoni E, et al. Mesenchymal stem cells ameliorate experimental autoimmune encephalomyelitis inducing T-cell anergy. Blood. 2005;106(5):1755–61.

122. Ramasamy R, Fazekasova H, Lam EW, Soeiro I, Lombardi G, Dazzi F. Mesenchymal stem cells inhibit dendritic cell differentiation and function by preventing entry into the cell cycle. Transplantation. 2007;83(1):71–6.

123. Luz-Crawford P, Kurte M, Bravo-Alegría J, Contreras R, Nova-Lamperti E, Tejedor G, et al. Mesenchymal stem cells generate a CD4+CD25+Foxp3+ regulatory T cell population during the differentiation process of Th1 and Th17 cells. Stem Cell Res Ther. 2013;4(3):65.

124. Henkel JS, Beers DR, Wen S, Rivera AL, Toennis KM, Appel JE, et al. Regulatory T-lymphocytes mediate amyotrophic lateral sclerosis progression and survival. EMBO Mol Med. 2013;5(1):64–79.

125. Brites D, Vaz AR. Microglia centered pathogenesis in ALS: insights in cell interconnectivity. Front Cell Neurosci. 2014;8:117.

126. Ooi YY, Dheen ST, Tay SS. Paracrine effects of mesenchymal stem cells-conditioned medium on microglial cytokines expression and nitric oxide production. Neuroimmunomodulation. 2015;22(4):233–42.

127. Noh MY, Lim SM, KW O, Cho KA, Park J, Kim KS, et al. Mesenchymal stem cells modulate the functional properties of microglia via TGF-beta secretion. Stem Cells Transl Med. 2016;5(11):1538–49.

128. Knippenberg S, Rath KJ, Boselt S, Thau-Habermann N, Schwarz SC, Dengler R, et al. Intraspinal administration of human spinal cord-derived neural progenitor cells in the G93A–SOD1 mouse model of ALS delays symptom progression, prolongs survival and increases expression of endogenous neurotrophic factors. J Tissue Eng Regen Med. 2015;11(3):751–64.

129. Riley J, Glass J, Feldman EL, Polak M, Bordeau J, Federici T, et al. Intraspinal stem cell transplantation in amyotrophic lateral sclerosis: a phase I trial, cervical microinjection, and final surgical safety outcomes. Neurosurgery. 2014;74(1):77–87.

130. Wilson EH, Weninger W, Hunter CA. Trafficking of immune cells in the central nervous system. J Clin Invest. 2010;120(5):1368–79.

131. McCandless EE, Wang Q, Woerner BM, Harper JM, Klein RS. CXCL12 limits inflammation by localizing mononuclear infiltrates to the perivascular space during experimental autoimmune encephalomyelitis. J Immunol. 2006; 177(11):8053–64.

132. Muller M, Carter SL, Hofer MJ, Manders P, Getts DR, Getts MT, et al. CXCR3 signaling reduces the severity of experimental autoimmune encephalomyelitis by controlling the parenchymal distribution of effector and regulatory T cells in the central nervous system. J Immunol. 2007;179(5):2774–86.

133. Agrawal S, Anderson P, Durbeej M, van Rooijen N, Ivars F, Opdenakker G, et

al. Dystroglycan is selectively cleaved at the parenchymal basement membrane at sites of leukocyte extravasation in experimental autoimmune encephalomyelitis. J Exp Med. 2006;203(4):1007–19.

134. Corti S, Locatelli F, Papadimitriou D, Donadoni C, Del Bo R, Fortunato F, et al. Multipotentiality, homing properties, and pyramidal neurogenesis of CNS-derived LeX(ssea-1)+/CXCR4+ stem cells. FASEB J. 2005;19(13):1860–2.

135. Appel SH, Armon C. Stem cells in amyotrophic lateral sclerosis: Ready for prime time? Neurology. 2016;87:348–9. United States.

136. Abdul Wahid SF, Law ZK, Ismail NA, Azman Ali R, Lai NM. Cell-based therapies for amyotrophic lateral sclerosis/motor neuron disease. Cochrane Database Syst Rev. 2016;11:Cd011742.

137. Guidance for Industry Drug Development for Amyotrophic Lateral Sclerosis. 2016. [Internet] http://www.alsa.org/advocacy/fda/assets/als-drug-development-guidance-for-public-comment-5-2-16.pdf. Accessed 23 Aug 2017.

138. Bryson JB, Machado CB, Crossley M, Stevenson D, Bros-Facer V, Burrone J, et al. Optical control of muscle function by transplantation of stem cell-derived motor neurons in mice. Science. 2014;344(6179):94–7.

139. Robberecht W, Philips T. The changing scene of amyotrophic lateral sclerosis. Nat Rev Neurosci. 2013;14(4):248–64.

140. Abel O, Powell JF, Andersen PM, Al-Chalabi A. ALSoD: a user-friendly online bioinformatics tool for amyotrophic lateral sclerosis genetics. Hum Mutat. 2012;3(9):1345–51.

141. Arnold ES, Ling SC, Huelga SC, Lagier-Tourenne C, Polymenidou M, Ditsworth D, et al. ALS-linked TDP-43 mutations produce aberrant RNA splicing and adult-onset motor neuron disease without aggregation or loss of nuclear TDP-43. Proc Natl Acad Sci U S A. 2013;110(8):E736–45.

142. Mead RJ, Bennett EJ, Kennerley AJ, Sharp P, Sunyach C, Kasher P, et al. Optimised and rapid pre-clinical screening in the SOD1(G93A) transgenic mouse model of amyotrophic lateral sclerosis (ALS). PLoS One. 2011;6(8): e23244.

143. Bennett EJ, Mead RJ, Azzouz M, Shaw PJ, Grierson AJ. Early detection of motor dysfunction in the SOD1G93A mouse model of amyotrophic lateral sclerosis (ALS) using home cage running wheels. PLoS One. 2014;9(9): e107918.

144. Scott MK, Akinduro O, Lo CC. In vivo 4-dimensional tracking of hematopoietic stem and progenitor cells in adult mouse calvarial bone marrow. J Vis Exp. 2014;91:e51683.

145. Malide D, Metais JY, Dunbar CE. In vivo clonal tracking of hematopoietic stem and progenitor cells marked by five fluorescent proteins using confocal and multiphoton microscopy. J Vis Exp. 2014;90:e51669.

146. Cheng NC, Wang S, Young TH. The influence of spheroid formation of human adipose-derived stem cells on chitosan films on stemness and differentiation capabilities. Biomaterials. 2012;33(6):1748–58.

147. Gao S, Zhao P, Lin C, Sun Y, Wang Y, Zhou Z, et al. Differentiation of human adipose-derived stem cells into neuron-like cells which are compatible with photocurable three-dimensional scaffolds. Tissue Eng Part A. 2014;20(7–8): 1271–84.

148. Cheng NC, Chen SY, Li JR, Young TH. Short-term spheroid formation enhances the regenerative capacity of adipose-derived stem cells by promoting stemness, angiogenesis, and chemotaxis. Stem Cells Transl Med. 2013;2(8):584–94.

149. Shen CC, Yang YC, Liu BS. Peripheral nerve repair of transplanted undifferentiated adipose tissue-derived stem cells in a biodegradable reinforced nerve conduit. J Biomed Mater Res A. 2012;100(1):48–63.

150. Shrestha B, Coykendall K, Li Y, Moon A, Priyadarshani P, Yao L. Repair of injured spinal cord using biomaterial scaffolds and stem cells. Stem Cell Res Ther. 2014;5(4):91.

151. Koh SH, Baik W, Noh MY, Cho GW, Kim HY, Kim KS, et al. The functional deficiency of bone marrow mesenchymal stromal cells in ALS patients is proportional to disease progression rate. Exp Neurol. 2012;233(1):472–80.

152. Cho GW, Noh MY, Kim HY, Koh SH, Kim KS, Kim SH. Bone marrow-derived stromal cells from amyotrophic lateral sclerosis patients have diminished stem cell capacity. Stem Cells Dev. 2010;19(7):1035–42.

153. Ferrero I, Mazzini L, Rustichelli D, Gunetti M, Mareschi K, Testa L, et al. Bone marrow mesenchymal stem cells from healthy donors and sporadic amyotrophic lateral sclerosis patients. Cell Transplant. 2008;17(3):255–66.

154. YS O, Kim SH, Cho GW. Functional restoration of amyotrophic lateral sclerosis patient-derived Mesenchymal stromal cells through inhibition of DNA Methyltransferase. Cell Mol Neurobiol. 2016;36(4):613–20.

155. Wu Y, Zhou H, Fan X, Zhang Y, Zhang M, Wang Y, et al. Correction of a genetic disease by CRISPR-Cas9-mediated gene editing in mouse spermatogonial stem cells. Cell Res. 2015;25(1):67–79.

10

SOD1 protein aggregates stimulate macropinocytosis in neurons to facilitate their propagation

Rafaa Zeineddine[1,2], Jay F. Pundavela[1,2], Lisa Corcoran[1,2], Elise M. Stewart[3], Dzung Do-Ha[1,2], Monique Bax[1,2], Gilles Guillemin[4], Kara L. Vine[1,2], Danny M. Hatters[5], Heath Ecroyd[1,2], Christopher M. Dobson[6], Bradley J. Turner[7], Lezanne Ooi[1,2], Mark R. Wilson[1,2], Neil R. Cashman[8] and Justin J. Yerbury[1,2*]

Abstract

Background: Amyotrophic Lateral Sclerosis is characterized by a focal onset of symptoms followed by a progressive spread of pathology that has been likened to transmission of infectious prions. Cell-to-cell transmission of SOD1 protein aggregates is dependent on fluid-phase endocytosis pathways, although the precise molecular mechanisms remain to be elucidated.

Results: We demonstrate in this paper that SOD1 aggregates interact with the cell surface triggering activation of Rac1 and subsequent membrane ruffling permitting aggregate uptake via stimulated macropinocytosis. In addition, other protein aggregates, including those associated with neurodegenerative diseases (TDP-43, Htt$_{ex1}$46Q, a-synuclein) also trigger membrane ruffling to gain entry into the cell. Aggregates are able to rupture unstructured macropinosomes to enter the cytosol allowing propagation of aggregation to proceed.

Conclusion: Thus, we conclude that in addition to basic proteostasis mechanisms, pathways involved in the activation of macropinocytosis are key determinants in the spread of pathology in these misfolding diseases.

Keywords: Protein aggregation, Transmission, Macropinocytosis

Background

The hallmark of Amyotrophic Lateral Sclerosis (ALS) is the selective death of upper and lower motor neurons in the motor cortex, brainstem and spinal cord, leading to loss of voluntary muscle control, muscle atrophy and invariably death. The specific causes of most cases of ALS are undefined, although approximately 10 % are inherited. The best-studied familial ALS (fALS) cases are from families possessing mutations in the gene encoding copper/zinc superoxide dismutase (Cu/Zn SOD, *SOD1*) [1]. There is, however, a rapidly growing list of other genes in which mutations have been implicated in fALS. These include *ALS2, SETX, FUS, VAPB, ANG, TARDBP, OPTN, VCP, UBQLN2, PFN1, SQSTM1*, and a hexanucleotide repeat in a non-coding region of *C9ORF72* [2]. Current

clinical practices are such that by the time that a diagnosis is confirmed disease progression is well under way and as many as 50 % of motor units may already have been affected [3]. There is now very strong evidence in humans that neurodegeneration in ALS begins focally and then spreads amongst adjacent motor neurons or through axonal pathways throughout the three dimensional anatomy of the central nervous system [4–6]. More detailed knowledge of the action of this spreading is crucial, as is identifying a means of early detection of the disease if we are to therapeutically slow disease progression.

In common with other neurodegenerative diseases, such as Alzheimer's Disease and Parkinson's Disease [7, 8], there is growing evidence that disruptions to proteostasis, protein misfolding and aggregation are the underlying mechanisms driving neurodegeneration in ALS [9]. Of particular interest is the fact that, although nucleation of protein aggregation appears to

* Correspondence: jyerbury@uow.edu.au
[1]Illawarra Health and Medical Research Institute, Wollongong, Australia2522
[2]School of Biological Sciences, Faculty of Science, Medicine and Health, University of Wollongong, Wollongong, Australia2522
Full list of author information is available at the end of the article

be a stochastic process [10], suggesting that protein aggregation should cause a random pattern of cell death, cell death in ALS occurs in an ordered and progressive manner. One way to explain such ordered progression is the prion-like propagation of protein misfolding and aggregation between adjacent cells. In addition, recent work has indicated that secondary processes, notably nucleation [11–13], takes place on the surface of aggregates, and along with other diffusional or active transport of protein aggregates between cells can give rise to cell-to-cell propagation of the type that is often defined as prion-like behaviour.

In the specific context of ALS, previous work has shown that exogenously applied mutant SOD1 aggregates induce protein aggregation in cells overexpressing mutant SOD1 [14]. Importantly, recent work shows that injection of spinal cord homogenates from symptomatic G93A SOD1 mice into the sciatic nerve of mice expressing G85R SOD1-YFP, below the threshold for triggering disease, has been shown to kindle protein aggregation and subsequent ALS-like phenotype [15]. In addition, we have recently shown, using cell lines and primary neurons, that propagation of SOD1 misfolding is dependent upon the passage of misfolded SOD1 (either mutant or wt) from cell-to-cell, a process that can be neutralized by antibodies reactive with misfolded SOD1 epitopes [16]. We have also shown that soluble and aggregated SOD1 can be taken up by neuroblastoma cells (mouse NSC-34 and human SHSY5Y), after which it accumulates in cytosolic inclusions [17]. Clues to understanding the entry of aggregates into cells comes from studies that show uptake of aggregates of SOD1 can be blocked with EIPA, wortmannin, IPA-3 [14] and rottlerin [16, 17], which inhibit Na^+/H^+ exchangers, phosphoinositide 3-kinases (PI3K), P21 protein (Cdc42/Rac)-activated kinase 1 (PAK-1) and protein kinase C (PKC), respectively (suppressing signalling events that promote actin rearrangement and pinosome closure). These findings suggest the involvement of fluid phase pinocytosis, possibly macropinocytosis, in the aggregate uptake process. Similarly, we have shown that cellular uptake of soluble SOD1 can be blocked by co-treatment with EIPA or rottlerin also suggesting that a form of pinocytosis plays a role in this process [17].

Macropinocytosis is a form of non-selective endocytosis used by cells to engulf large amounts of solute macromolecules (fluid phase) or particles too large for other forms of endocytosis. Macropinocytosis is typically defined as a transient, externally induced, actin-dependent endocytic process associated with vigorous perturbations, such as ruffles and blebs, in the plasma membrane [18]. The activation of this process results in a transient increase in receptor-independent fluid phase endocytosis in large vesicles or vacuoles (0.5–10 μm) termed macropinosomes [18, 19]. Macropinosomes do not have a coat to guide their formation and are heterogeneous in size and shape. Macropinocytosis provides non-phagocytic cells with the ability to take up large particles, but the process must be triggered by an external stimulus. Bacteria, viruses, apoptotic bodies and necrotic cells have all been shown to induce the ruffling behaviour typical of macropinocytosis resulting in their uptake along with fluid [18].

There are a number of viruses, including the vaccinia virus and adenovirus [20], that have been shown to hijack macropinocytosis pathways to enter cells, including the Japanese encephalitis virus that triggers macropinocytosis in neurons [21]. A lack of physical structure is thought to result in the loss of integrity of the macropinosome membrane and may explain why particles (e.g. bacteria and virions) can escape the macropinosomes and reach the cytosol [22]. There is emerging evidence that prions and prion-like proteins may also enter cells via macropinocytosis allowing the propagation of their aggregation [14, 16, 17, 23, 24]. However, the small molecule inhibitors utilized to define macropinocytosis, such as EIPA, are not specific to a single cellular event and depending on the cell type can prevent various forms of endocytosis [25].

We show here however, that aggregates of SOD1 trigger activation of the Rho GTPase Rac1, leading to membrane ruffling and fluid phase uptake in neurons that defines macropinocytosis and that this facilitates aggregate entry into cells. In addition, we show that these aggregates can escape macropinosomes to be deposited in the cytosol. We further show that this process is not specific for SOD1 but rather can be triggered by a variety of protein aggregates, including model protein aggregates (α-lactalbumin) and those associated with neurodegenerative diseases (TDP-43, $Htt_{ex1}46Q$ and α-synuclein). We conclude that the infectious prion-like spread of protein aggregation in a range of neurodegenerative diseases is dependent on cells activating ruffling and subsequent macropinocytosis in a manner analogous to viral entry and propagation through activation of macropinocytosis.

Results

SOD1 aggregates are taken up by cells and promote wtSOD1 inclusion formation

We, and others, have previously shown that aggregated human SOD1 can be taken up by neuronal cells [14, 16, 17]. Here we confirm these results using recombinantly produced properly folded and dimeric human SOD1 that was aggregated in vitro to form fibrillar structures, as previously described [26] (Additional file 1A-B). The preformed SOD1 aggregates were then added to the media of the motor neuron like cell line NSC-34.

Following incubation of the cells with the SOD1 aggregates for 60 min, the aggregates could be detected in association with the cells by flow cytometry (Fig. 1a). In addition, human SOD1, including SDS resistant high molecular weight (HMW) species, was detected in lysates from trypsin treated cells (Fig. 1a). Furthermore, to eliminate the possibility that SOD1 aggregates were bound primarily to the cell surface we treated cells with trypsin and observed no difference in SOD1 signal consistent with SOD1 being inside cells (Additional file 2). Putative uptake of SOD1 was quantified by flow cytometry and it was found that soluble (properly folded)

wtSOD1 and non-aggregated ALS associated mutant G93A SOD1 are taken up by cells to a similar extent to that of aggregated wtSOD1 (Fig. 1b). This is consistent with previous work showing uptake of soluble wt and mutant SOD1 [17] and may reflect the proposed role of non-classically secreted SOD1 in signal transduction [27, 28]. In contrast, there was no statistically significant increase in immunofluorescence after incubation with an unrelated control protein GST, suggesting that the uptake of both soluble and aggregated forms of SOD1 is relatively specific (Fig. 1b). The uptake of aggregates is dependent upon cell surface proteins, since

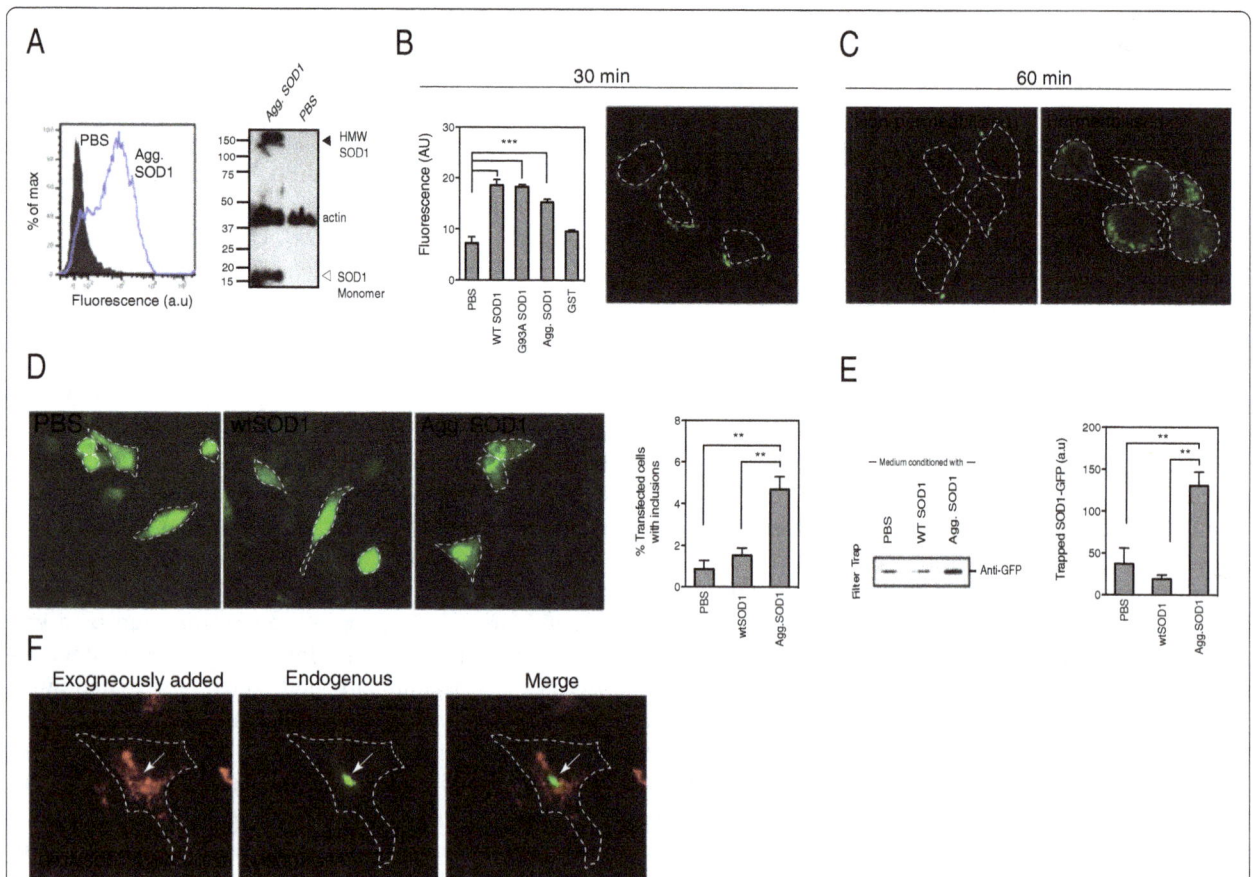

Fig. 1 Exogenously applied SOD1 aggregates enter cells and induce endogenous SOD1 aggregation. a Left panel Quantitative analysis of SOD1 association with NSC-34 cells using flow cytometry. Cells were either incubated with PBS (grey) or aggregated wtSOD1 (60 min incubation; blue line). Right panel Western blot of cell lysates detecting human SOD1 (and actin as a loading control). (b) Left panel Association with cells was quantified using flow cytometry. NSC-34 cells were treated with aggregated human SOD1 protein for 30 min and subsequently detected using immunofluorescence. Results shown are means ± SE, n = 3, ** p < 0.01. Right panel Confocal laser scanning micrograph of aggregated wtSOD1 interacting with NSC34 cells after 30 min on ice to slow endocytosis. White dotted line represents cell membrane. (c) Confocal laser scanning micrographs of biotinylated wtSOD1 aggregates incubated with NSC34 cells for 60 min then either permeabilized with Triton x-100 or not, and subsequent detection using SA-Alexa488. (d) NSC-34 cells were transfected with wtSOD1-GFP and then incubated with either PBS, wtSOD1 (non-aggregated) or aggregated SOD1 and the number of cells with inclusions counted at 72 h. Results shown are means ± SE, n = 3, * p < 0.05. A minimum of 150 cells were counted per treatment and the average % of transfected cells with inclusions calculated across a minimum of 5 fields of view per treatment. (e) Cell lysates were further analyzed by filter trap assay. Any trapped SOD1-GFP material was measured using an anti-GFP antibody to avoid measuring aggregated material added to cells. Quantification of filter trap assays using a densitometer. Values are the mean intensity of trapped aggregated material averaged over 3 experiments. Results shown are means ± SE, n = 3, ** p < 0.01. (f) Exogenously added and endogenously produced SOD1 aggregates do not substantively colocalise. G93A SOD1 aggregates were labelled with Alexa-633 and added to NSC-34 cells expressing wtSOD1-GFP. After 48 h the cells were imaged using laser scanning confocal microscopy. Little colocalisation of Alexa633 and GFP signal was observed

trypsinization of cell surface proteins prior to treatment with aggregates significantly inhibited aggregate association with cells (Additional file 1C). In addition, uptake occurs relatively rapidly; SOD1 aggregates were associated with the surface of NSC-34 cells after 30 min incubation (Fig. 1b), and after 60 min are no longer detected on the surface but instead are only detected following permeabilisation of cells with Triton X-100 (Fig. 1c).

Previous work has shown that exogenously added preformed aggregates of mutant SOD1 containing fibrils can induce aggregation of intracellular SOD1 in cells overexpressing mutant SOD1 [14], but not in those expressing wtSOD1. Recently we have shown that wtSOD1 can indeed participate in the propagation of misfolded SOD1 within and between cells [16, 29]. To further examine the induced aggregation of intracellular wtSOD1, we transfected NSC-34 cells with wtSOD1-GFP and added soluble or aggregated recombinant SOD1 to the media. After 48 h of incubation there were more cells that contained wtSOD1-GFP inclusions when treated with aggregated SOD1 than when treated with soluble SOD1 (Fig. 1d). As the exogenously added aggregates were not labelled with GFP these cellular inclusions could not be attributed to the uptake of aggregates but must have formed from intracellular wtSOD1-GFP. The number of cells expressing wtSOD1-GFP that spontaneously developed inclusions was low (< 1 % for cells treated only with PBS) and occurred only in cells expressing very high levels of wtSOD1-GFP [29, 30]. As we did not observe substantive colocalisation of the exogenously applied SOD1 aggregates and SOD1-GFP, our results suggest accumulation of SOD1-GFP occurs alongside aggregates taken up from the media (Fig. 1f). Exogenous application of aggregated SOD1 resulted in a highly significant ($p < 0.0001$) increase (from 0.85 +/− 0.42 % to 4.7 +/− 0.62 %) in the proportion of cells containing inclusions (Fig. 1d). We confirmed these data with a filter trap assay using cell lysates (Fig. 1e). Increased levels of SOD1-GFP were trapped on the cellulose membrane when cells were treated with aggregated wtSOD1 than those treated with soluble wtSOD1 or PBS alone (Fig. 1e; $p < 0.001$). Similar results were also seen when aggregates made from several mutant SOD1 variants that cause ALS were aggregated in vitro and added to cells expressing wtSOD1-GFP (Additional file 3).

SOD1 aggregates escape endolysosomal system to access the cytosol

The mechanism by which exogenously applied SOD1 aggregates induce the formation of cytoplasmic inclusions containing intracellular SOD1 likely involves the escape of SOD1 from membrane bound endolysosomes. To test whether SOD1 leaks from endo-lysosomal compartments following its uptake, NSC-34 cells were incubated with

SOD1 aggregates at 37 °C and following incubation at incremental time intervals co-stained for SOD1 aggregates and lysosomes. Exogenous SOD1 aggregates co-localised with Lysotracker (fluorescent in mildly acidic compartments) until 30 min, after which low levels of SOD1 could be observed outside the acidic endo-lysosomal system (Fig. 2a). To determine if SOD1 aggregates had entered the cytosol we first performed sub-cellular fractionation of cells. Immunoblotting of cytosolic, membrane (ER/Golgi), nuclear and cytoskeletal fractions demonstrated that aggregated SOD1 predominantly fractionated with the cytoskeleton fraction (Fig. 2b). We observe upon boiling in SDS that the aggregates no longer appear as high molecular weight species stuck in the loading gel (see Fig. 1a), but are reduced to apparent cross-linked species as previously observed [31]. These results are consistent with SOD1 aggregates having a density comparable to cytoskeleton elements and, in addition, suggests cytosolic exposure of SOD1 aggregates. There was also a very small amount of high molecular weight SOD1 observed in the nuclear fraction, again consistent with cytosolic exposure (outside of the endo-lysosome system). However, in confocal microscopy experiments aggregates were not observed within the nucleus (Fig. 2d) suggesting aggregated material either bound the nuclear membrane or pelleted at a similar density to the nuclear fraction.

To confirm that aggregates were present outside any membrane enclosed compartments we used selective permeabilization; Triton- X-100 disrupts all cellular membranes, while digitonin permeabilizes only the plasma membrane [32] (see also control membrane enclosed [Lysosomal associated membrane protein 1; LAMP1, Binding immunoglobulin protein; BiP, Early endosome antigen 1; EEA1] and cytosolic proteins shown in Fig. 2c). After 60 min incubation, human SOD1 aggregates were detected only after Triton X-100 permeabilization (Fig. 2d). However, after 120 min, SOD1 aggregates could also be detected after permeabilization by digitonin, consistent with aggregate presence in the cytosol. Soluble human SOD1 was also able to escape the endosome system, such that it was detected in the cytosol after digitonin permeabilization (Additional file 4). In contrast, when the control protein RAP-GST (known to be internalized by receptor mediated endocytosis) was added to cells for 120 min it was not detected after digitonin permeablization (Additional file 4), consistent with its retention in an endosomal-lysosomal compartment.

Macropinosomes are thought to be 'leaky' due to their lack of physical structure [22]. In order to test the possibility that SOD1 aggregates are rupturing macropinosomes we specifically permeabilized only the plasma membrane with digitonin and then stained for galectin-3 after 2 h of incubation with SOD1 aggregates. Galectin-3 is a non-classically secreted β-galactoside binding lectin

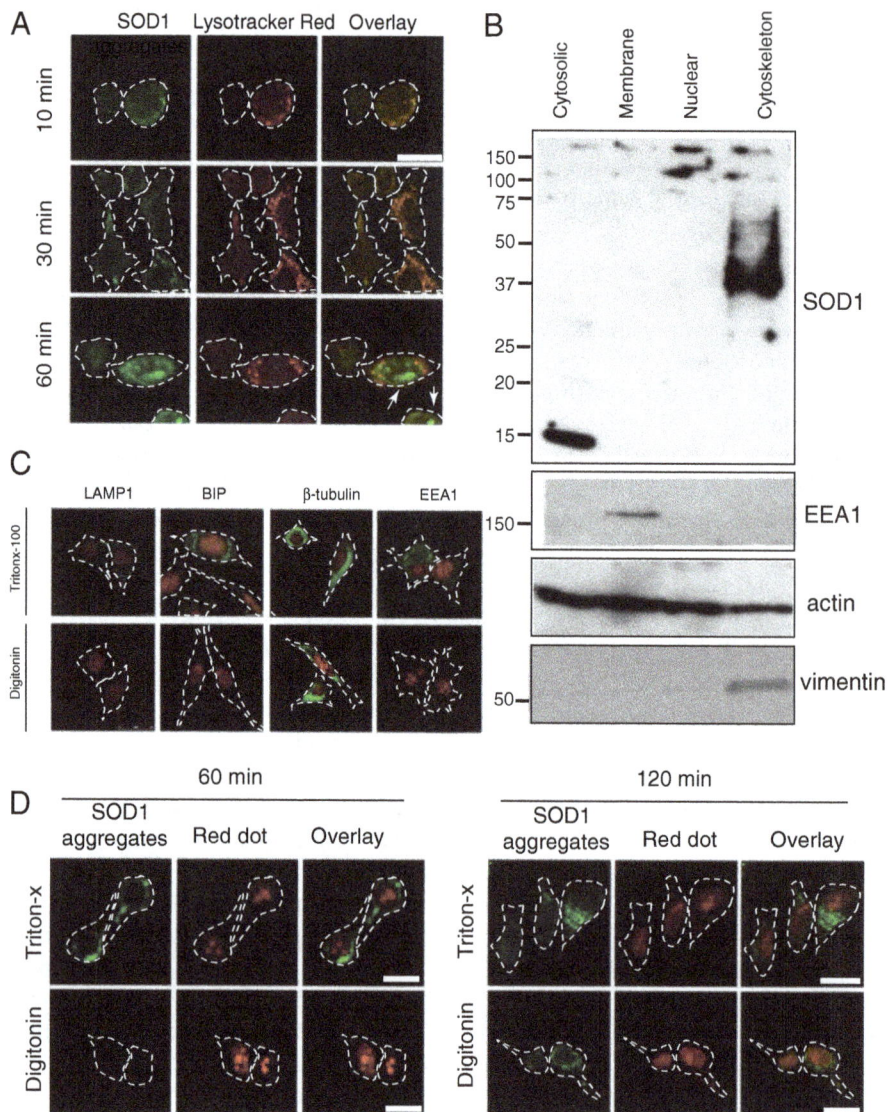

Fig. 2 Internalized aggregates entering via the endocytic pathway escape from the endosomes to the cytosol. **a** Confocal microscopy of the co-staining of wtSOD1 aggregates (20 μg/mL) taken up by NSC-34 cells after 10, 30 and 60 min at 37 °C, with Lysotracker Red. Fixed and permeabilized cells were immunostained with an anti-human specific SOD1 antibody. Bars represent 25 μm. Arrowheads indicate areas of localisation of SOD1 outside the acidic compartment. (**b**) Western blotting of cytosolic, membrane (ER/Golgi), nuclear and cytoskeleton fractions (10 μg) collected from NSC-34 cells treated with wtSOD1 aggregates (20 μg/mL) for 2 h at 37 °C. Western blots were stained for the presence of human SOD1, EEA1, actin and vimentin. (**c**) Digitonin selectively permeabilizes plasma membrane of NSC-34 cells. NSC-34 Cells were treated with either digitonin (10 μM) or Triton-x100 (0.5 %) and then immunostained for membrane bounded markers LAMP1, BIP and EEA and the cytosolic β-tubulin. Membrane bounded markers were not detected when permeabilized with digitonin indicating the specificity of digitonin for plasma membrane. Cells were counterstained with Red Dot 2. (**d**) Laser scanning confocal micrographs of NSC-34 cells were treated with aggregated human SOD1 protein for 60 or 120 min then fixed and permeabilized with either Triton-x100 (0.5 %) or digitonin (10 μM). SOD1 aggregates were detected using Alexa488 conjugated to streptavidin and counter stained with the nuclear dye Red Dot 2. SOD1 aggregates are only detected upon digitonin permeabilization after 120 min SOD1 incubation. White dotted line represents cell membrane

that has been shown to be enriched in Rab positive endosomes [33] and also redistributes from the cytosol to endosome fragments upon endosome rupture [34, 35]. We utilized our selective permeabilization method (see Fig. 2c) to examine increased cytosolic exposure of galectin-3 indicating rupture of endosomal compartments. Cells permeabilized by digitonin and treated with PBS alone showed very little galectin-3 staining compared to cells permeabilized with Triton x-100 (Fig. 3), consistent with a large fraction of galectin-3 being located on the inside endosomal compartments [33] in NSC-34 cells. Compared to controls, the cultures treated with misfolded G93A SOD1 or aggregated SOD1 contained an increase in staining for galectin-3 indicative of endosome rupture

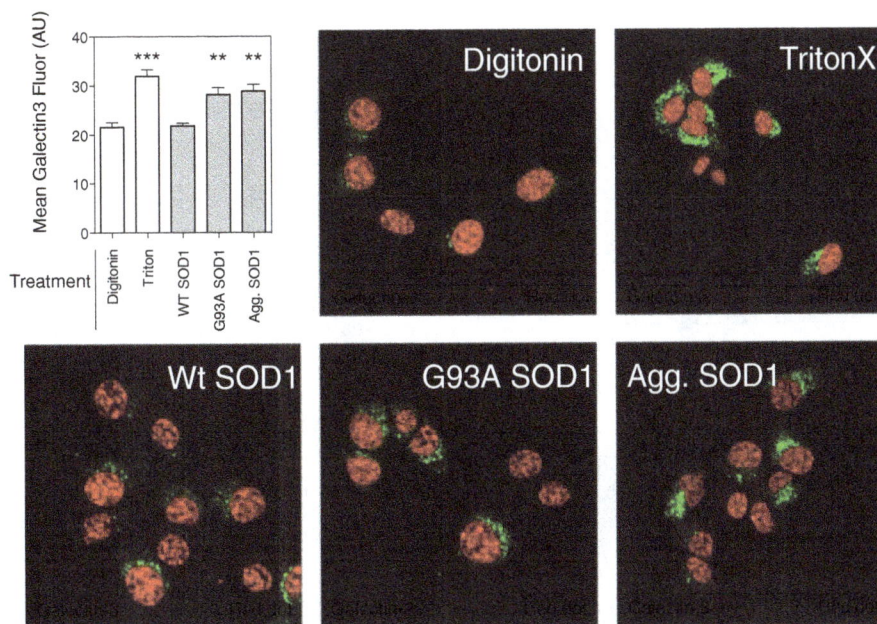

Fig. 3 Endosome rupture by SOD1 aggregates. NSC-34 cells were incubated with either PBS (digitonin and Triton X-100 treatments), non-aggregated wt or G93A SOD1 or aggregated G93A SOD1 for 2 h before permeabilizatin (digitonin for the SOD1 treatments), fixation, immunostaining of galectin-3 and the mean fluorescence per cell quantified. A minimum of 150 cells were counted per treatment across a minimum of 5 fields of view per treatment and the mean galectin-3 fluorescence per cell calculated. Results shown are means ± SE, ** $p < 0.01$, *** $p < 0.001$. Confocal microscopy of the immunostaining of galectin-3 after treatment with PBS and the SOD1 preparations, counterstained with RedDot

and exposure of galectin-3 (Fig. 3). In addition, we treated human red blood cells with the SOD1 samples and the amount of membrane disruption was measured by free hemoglobin (Additional file 5A). Soluble mutant G93A SOD1, and aggregated SOD1 increased the amount of free hemoglobin consistent with an ability to damage biological membranes (Additional file 5A). Lastly, we generated unilamellar vesicles and examined for interaction of SOD1 aggregates. Similar to previous findings for fibrillar aggregates [36], aggregates of SOD1 interacted with liposomes and deformed their structure (Additional file 5B). Together, these data are consistent with SOD1 aggregates disrupting biological membranes and escaping in to the cytosol.

Aggregated SOD1 triggers ruffling and subsequent macropinocytosis in neurons

Previous studies have shown that small molecules that inhibit actin rearrangement, or Na$^+$/H$^+$ exchangers, Pak-1, PI3K, and PKC suppress aggregate uptake [14, 16, 17], consistent with macropinocytosis. However, it has not been shown whether macropinocytosis is triggered through an interaction of SOD1 with cells or whether aggregates are taken up by some other constitutive process. Initially, we used EIPA (an inhibitor of the Na$^+$/H$^+$ exchanger and subsequent endocytosis) and rottlerin (an inhibitor of PKC), as reported previously [14, 16, 17], to confirm the involvement of macropinocytosis-like pathways in the uptake of SOD1

aggregates into NSC-34 cells. Aggregate uptake was inhibited by both EIPA and rottlerin ($p < 0.001$; Fig. 4a-b), however inhibitors of clathrin (chlorpromazine) or caveolin (genistein) dependent endocytosis had no significant effect on this process (Fig. 4a-b). Macropinocytosis is a form of fluid phase endocytosis that engulfs solutes at whatever concentrations they are found in the extracellular medium, rather than concentrating ligands at the cell surface. EIPA, cytochalasin D (an inhibitor of actin rearrangement) and rottlerin inhibited fluid phase uptake (quantified as dextran-Alexa647 uptake) stimulated by phorbol 12-myristate 13-acetate (PMA) treatment of NSC-34 cells, but genistein and chlorpromazine did not, demonstrating the specificity of the inhibitors to PKC-dependent fluid phase uptake (Additional file 6A). Similar results were found regardless of whether or not the aggregates were wt or mutant G93A SOD1 (Additional file 6B). While a similar pattern of SOD1 uptake inhibition was found when soluble non-aggregated wtSOD1 was applied to cells (largest decreases in fluorescence when co-incubated with EIPA and rottlerin; Additional file 6C), non-aggregated G93A SOD1 uptake was inhibited by similar levels regardless of the inhibitor used (Additional file 6D).

We next investigated whether there were any perturbations to the cell surface membrane caused by incubation with SOD1. Field emission scanning electron microscopy (FESEM) imaging of cells treated with PMA showed increased membrane perturbations, including

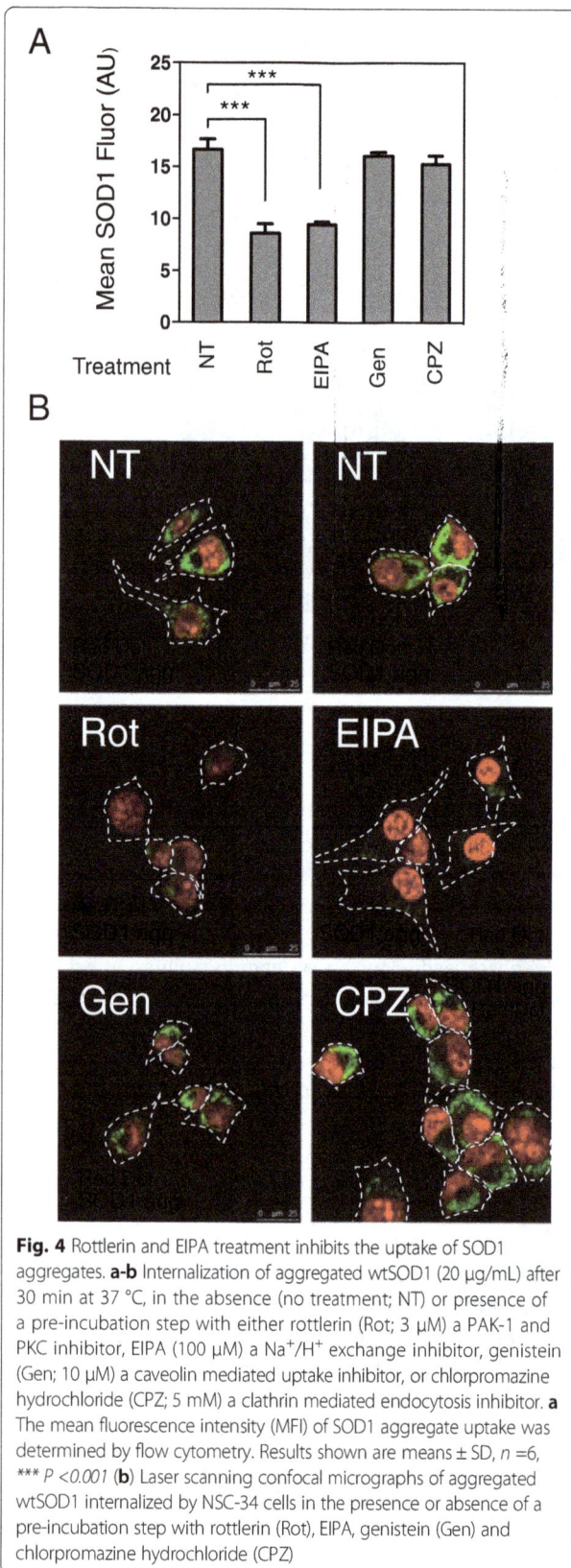

Fig. 4 Rottlerin and EIPA treatment inhibits the uptake of SOD1 aggregates. **a-b** Internalization of aggregated wtSOD1 (20 μg/mL) after 30 min at 37 °C, in the absence (no treatment; NT) or presence of a pre-incubation step with either rottlerin (Rot; 3 μM) a PAK-1 and PKC inhibitor, EIPA (100 μM) a Na^+/H^+ exchange inhibitor, genistein (Gen; 10 μM) a caveolin mediated uptake inhibitor, or chlorpromazine hydrochloride (CPZ; 5 mM) a clathrin mediated endocytosis inhibitor. **a** The mean fluorescence intensity (MFI) of SOD1 aggregate uptake was determined by flow cytometry. Results shown are means ± SD, $n = 6$, *** $P < 0.001$ (**b**) Laser scanning confocal micrographs of aggregated wtSOD1 internalized by NSC-34 cells in the presence or absence of a pre-incubation step with rottlerin (Rot), EIPA, genistein (Gen) and chlorpromazine hydrochloride (CPZ)

ruffles and blebs (Fig. 5a), consistent with an activation of macropinocytosis. Incubation with soluble G93A SOD1 did not induce such perturbations, although incubation with aggregated G93A SOD1 induced pronounced membrane ruffling and blebbing consistent with macropinosome formation (Fig. 5a). To exclude the possibility that cells were blebbing due to apoptosis, we examined the cells for active caspase 3, however there was no caspase 3 activation in cells treated with aggregates above basal (PBS treated) levels (Additional file 7). To visualize and quantify the extent of membrane perturbation we used the membrane dye FM® 1-43FX, as used previously for studies of membrane perturbation during growth cone ruffling [37]. Fluorescence from FM 1-43FX was significantly increased ($p < 0.001$) upon treatment of cells with SOD1 aggregates, consistent with an increase in membrane perturbation (Fig. 5b). In contrast, there was no increase in fluorescence following incubation with soluble SOD1 (Fig. 5b).

Next, to explore whether the interaction of SOD1 aggregates with cells triggers fluid phase uptake, we incubated NSC-34 cells in the presence of both SOD1 and dextran-Alexa647 and quantified uptake of the latter using flow cytometry. Aggregated SOD1 triggered a significant increase ($p < 0.001$) in dextran uptake compared to that in the absence of treatment or following incubation with soluble SOD1 (Fig. 5c). Whilst there was a small increase in dextran uptake in cells treated with soluble SOD1 compared to those not treated (Fig. 5c) this was thus not attributable to stimulated macropinocytosis as it occurred in the absence of membrane ruffling (Fig. 5a). Finally, we examined the role of the Rho GTPase, Rac1, in the uptake of SOD1 aggregates. Initially we probed for the presence of activated Rac1 using an ELISA based assay. Incubation of cells with aggregated but not with soluble SOD1 resulted in a significant increase ($p < 0.05$) in the amount of activated Rac1 (Rac1-GTP; Fig. 5d) in NSC-34 cells. In addition, the uptake of SOD1 aggregates was significantly suppressed ($p < 0.001$) by pre-treatment and subsequent co-incubation of aggregates with the Rac1 inhibitor W56 (Fig. 5e). To confirm that Rac1 was downstream of membrane ruffling we treated cells with PMA or SOD1 aggregates in the presence or absence of W56 and then examined for membrane perturbations using FM1-43FX. We observed that in the case of both PMA and aggregate treated cells W56 suppressed membrane perturbation (Additional file 8).

We also used human iPSC-derived motor neuron cultures to determine whether or not these effects are also observed in human neurons (differentiation characterized in Additional file 9). The motor neuron cultures contained 90.5 ± 1.4 % SMI32-positive cells and 88.8 ± 1.4 % Islet 1-positive cells, with large cell bodies, consistent with a large proportion of the cells having a motor

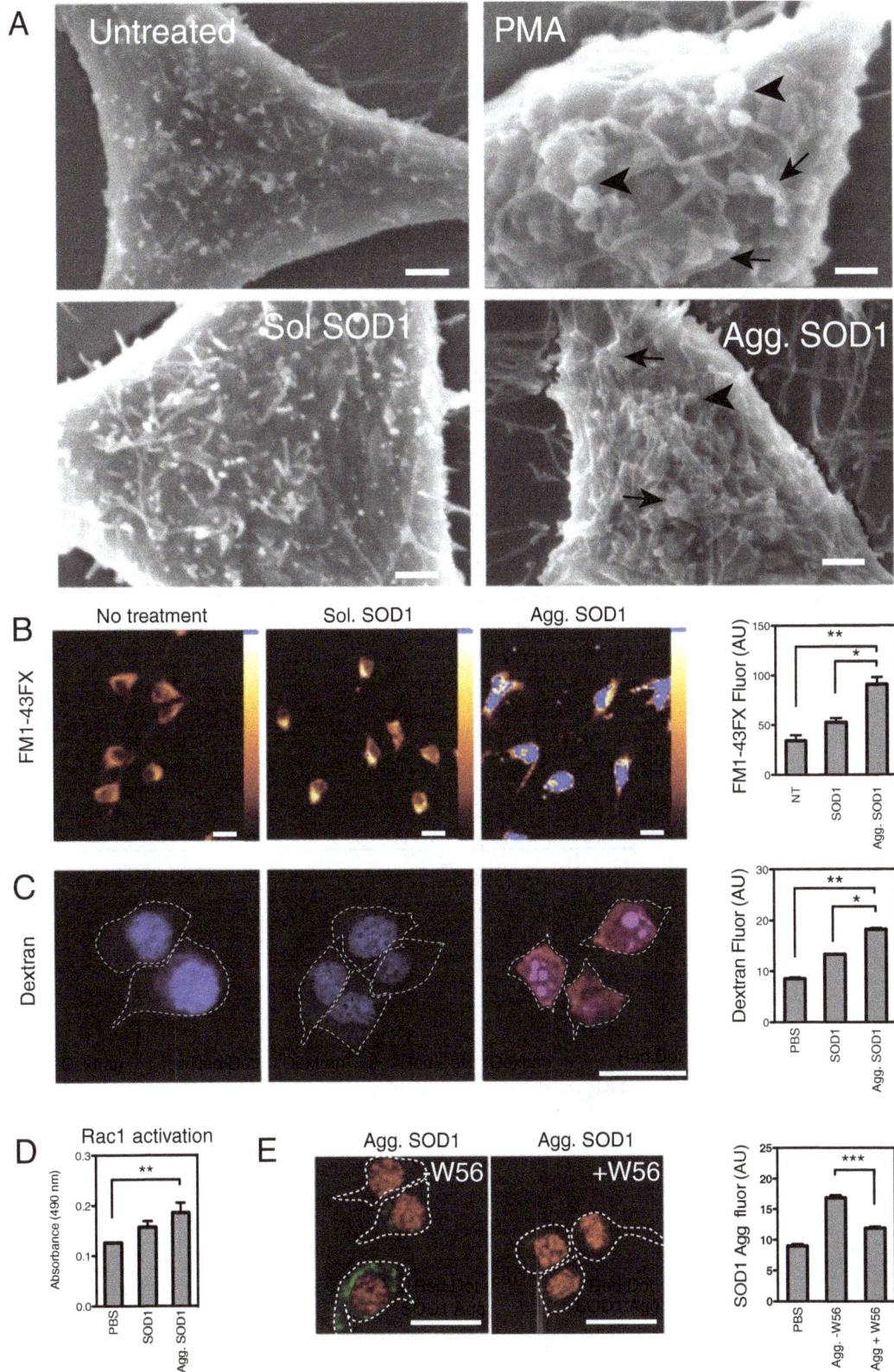

Fig. 5 (See legend on next page.)

Fig. 5 Aggregated SOD1 induces ruffles and blebs, dextran uptake and activation of RAC1. **a** Field emission SEM of cells treated with SOD1 aggregates or controls, non-aggregated SOD1 (sol SOD1), PMA or PBS (untreated). Increases in membrane perturbations can be observed, such as ruffles (black arrow) and blebs (black arrow head). Bars represent 2 μm. (**b**) Laser scanning confocal micrographs of treated cells stained with the membrane dye FM1-43FX to measure membrane perturbation and fluorescence intensity per cell was quantified using ImageJ. Scale bars represent 20 μm. A minimum of 200 cells were scored per treatment. Results shown are means ± SD of three experiments, * $p < 0.05$ ** $p < 0.01$. (**c**) The induction of fluid phase uptake was measured using fluorescently labelled dextran. Laser scanning confocal micrographs of dextran-Alexa647 uptake in treated NSC-34 cells. Outline of cells are indicated with white dashed lines. Scale bars represent 20 μm. (**e**) Flow cytometry quantification of dextran uptake in the treated NSC-34 cells. Results shown as means ± SD of 6 experiments * $p < 0.05$ ** $p < 0.01$. (**d**) Rac1 activation in treated NSC-34 cell lysates was measured using a Rac1 activation ELISA assay that probes for Rac1-GDP. Results are mean ± SD of 6 experiments, ** $p < 0.01$. (**e**) Addition of a Rac1 inhibitor reduces SOD1 uptake. Laser scanning confocal micrographs of SOD1 aggregate uptake in the presence of absence of W56, mean fluorescence per cell was calculated using ImageJ. Data are mean fluorescence intensity per cell of a minimum of 100 cells ± SD, $p < 0.001$

neuron morphology (Additional file 10). Treatment of human motor neuron cultures with aggregated SOD1 promoted membrane perturbations, such as ruffling and blebbing (Fig. 6 arrowheads). This membrane perturbation, quantified with the membrane dye FM1-43, was significantly increased compared to cells treated with PBS alone and similar to that induced by PMA (Fig. 7a-b, Additional file 11B). Furthermore, human neurons treated with SOD1 aggregates exhibited an increase in fluid phase uptake (Fig. 7c-d, Additional file 11A). Lastly, as observed for NSC-34 cells, the uptake of SOD1 aggregates into neurons was suppressed by the Na$^+$/H$^+$ exchanger inhibitor, EIPA (Fig. 7e, Additional file 11C), the inhibitor of PKC, rottlerin (Fig. 7f, Additional file 11C) and the Rac1 inhibitor, W56 (Fig. 7g, Additional file 11C).

Activation of membrane ruffling is not restricted to SOD1 aggregates

Given that SOD1 aggregates were found to trigger the activation of membrane ruffling and entry via macropinocytosis, we sought to determine if triggering of membrane ruffling was responsible for a generic cellular response to aggregates. We therefore examined the uptake of disease-associated fibrillar aggregates formed by TDP-43, Htt$_{ex1}$-46Q, α-synuclein, and also of amorphous and fibrillar aggregates formed from the model protein α-lactalbumin [38] into NSC-34 cells (Fig. 8, Additional file 12). Using laser scanning confocal microscopy we confirmed the uptake of aggregates in each case (Fig. 8a) and, with the exception of α-synuclein, the levels of uptake were significantly suppressed by EIPA (Fig. 8a-b).

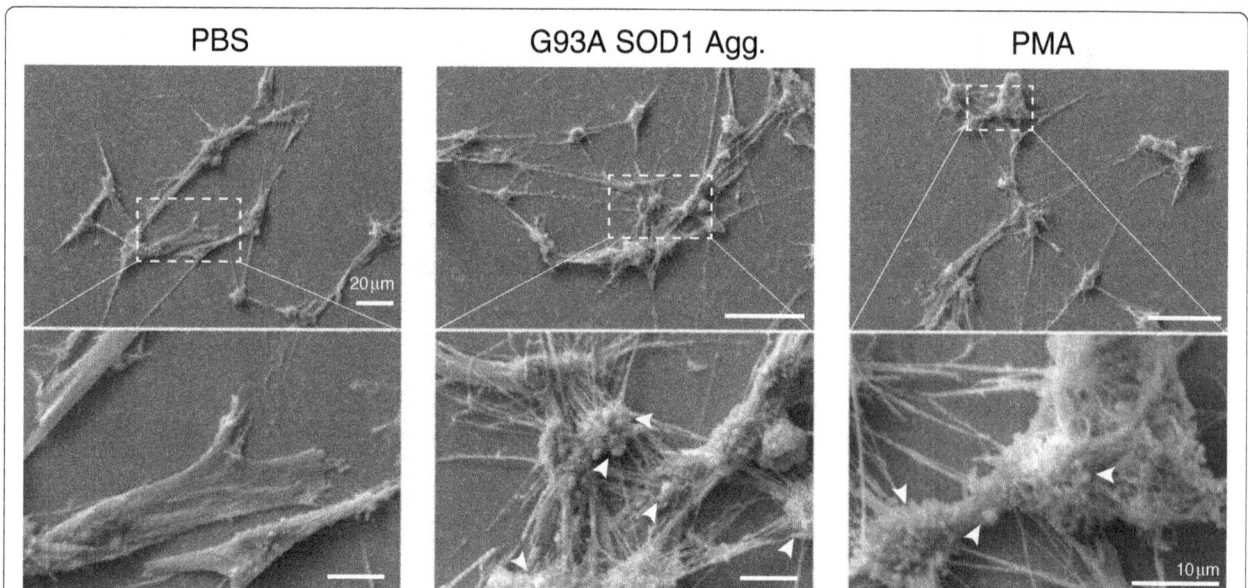

Fig. 6 Aggregated SOD1 induces membrane ruffling in iPSC derived human motor neurons. Field emission SEM of motor neurons treated with SOD1 aggregates, and PBS or PMA controls. The area in the dashed box is enlarged in the bottom panels. Increases in membrane perturbations can be observed, such as ruffles and blebs (white arrow heads). Bars represent 20 μm in top row and 10 μm in the bottom row. Data shown is from experiments performed on cells derived from one fibroblast line and represents experiments performed on cells from 2 individuals

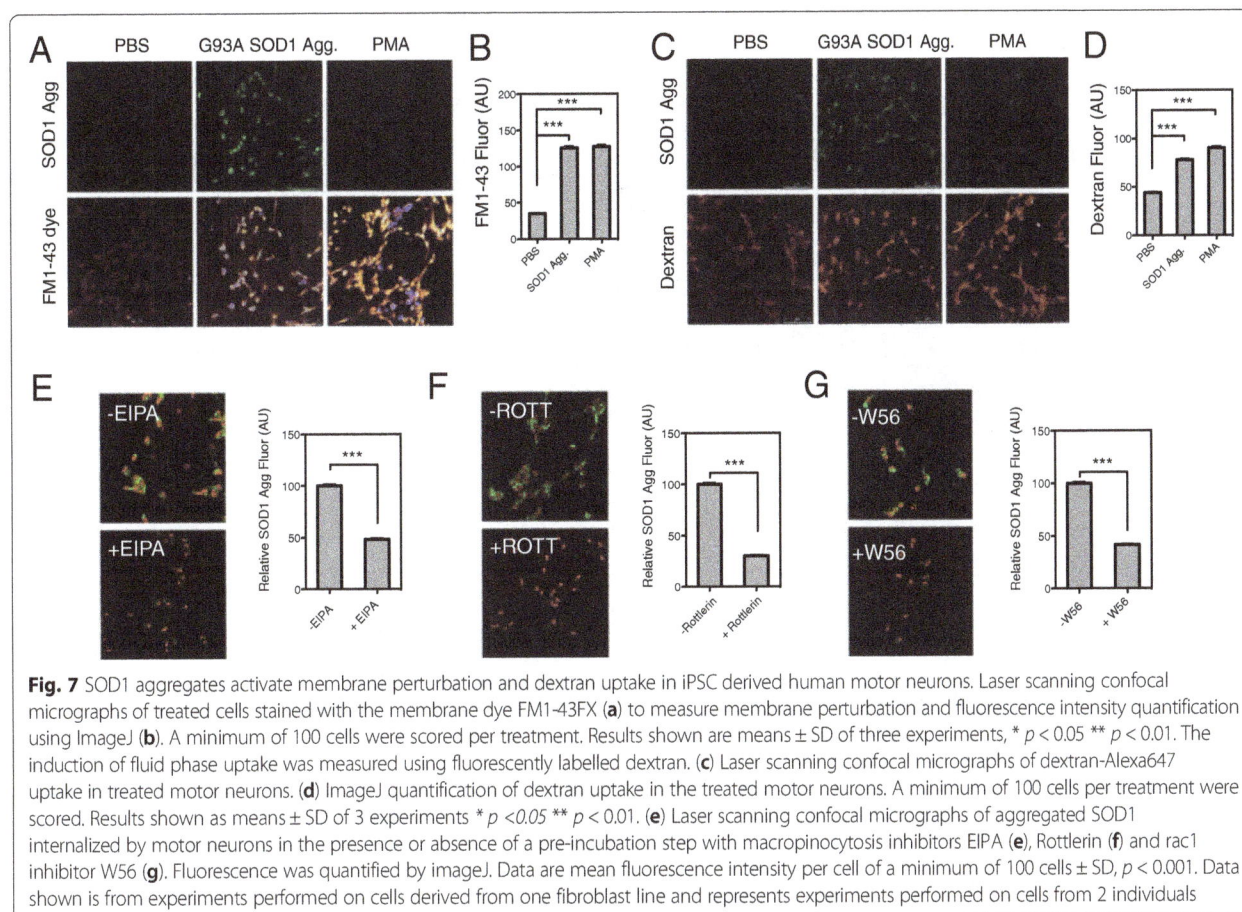

Fig. 7 SOD1 aggregates activate membrane perturbation and dextran uptake in iPSC derived human motor neurons. Laser scanning confocal micrographs of treated cells stained with the membrane dye FM1-43FX (**a**) to measure membrane perturbation and fluorescence intensity quantification using ImageJ (**b**). A minimum of 100 cells were scored per treatment. Results shown are means ± SD of three experiments, * $p < 0.05$ ** $p < 0.01$. The induction of fluid phase uptake was measured using fluorescently labelled dextran. (**c**) Laser scanning confocal micrographs of dextran-Alexa647 uptake in treated motor neurons. (**d**) ImageJ quantification of dextran uptake in the treated motor neurons. A minimum of 100 cells per treatment were scored. Results shown as means ± SD of 3 experiments * $p < 0.05$ ** $p < 0.01$. (**e**) Laser scanning confocal micrographs of aggregated SOD1 internalized by motor neurons in the presence or absence of a pre-incubation step with macropinocytosis inhibitors EIPA (**e**), Rottlerin (**f**) and rac1 inhibitor W56 (**g**). Fluorescence was quantified by imageJ. Data are mean fluorescence intensity per cell of a minimum of 100 cells ± SD, $p < 0.001$. Data shown is from experiments performed on cells derived from one fibroblast line and represents experiments performed on cells from 2 individuals

Moreover, all aggregates induced a significant ($p < 0.01$) increase in the uptake of the fluid phase marker dextran-Alexa647 (Fig. 8c) and an increase in membrane perturbations, as illustrated in FESEM images (Fig. 8d). Thus, a broad range of aggregated proteins, both amorphous and amyloid-like, are able to induce membrane perturbations that facilitate their cellular uptake in a similar manner to that of SOD1 (Fig. 8).

Discussion

The work presented here reveals that both soluble and aggregated SOD1 are taken up by neuronal cells via fluid phase endocytosis pathways. In addition we show that aggregated but not soluble SOD1 triggers activation of Rac1 and subsequent membrane ruffling, and thus itself stimulates macropinocytosis, not only in cell lines but also in human iPSC derived motor neurons. This process differs from that responsible for the uptake of soluble SOD1, which is independent of membrane ruffling and occurs presumably via a constitutive form of pinocytosis in the case of the wtSOD1 and potentially via a range of mechanisms in the case of soluble G93A SOD1. SOD1 aggregates are not permanently maintained in a membrane bound compartment once inside the cells, but rupture macropinosomes and escape into the cytosol where they can induce further aggregation. In addition, the data presented here shows that other protein aggregates, including those of TDP-43, Htt$_{ex1}$-46Q, α-synuclein, and α-lactalbumin, can also trigger significant perturbations in the plasma membrane of neurons allowing the uptake of large fibrillar or amorphous protein aggregates.

Various viruses, such as the vaccinia virus, adenovirus 3, herpes simplex virus 1 and HIV, utilize macropinocytosis to gain entry to cells. This phenomenon is likely to be due to the fact that macropinosomes are not restricted in size, enabling even large virions to be internalized, and that many cell types, not just professional phagocytes (such as macrophages), have the ability to activate the macropinocytosis pathways [18]. Indeed, macropinocytosis can be activated in neurons by interactions with large viral particles [21]. In the specific context of ALS we show that aggregates formed by SOD1 can activate the same macropinocytosis pathways as those utilized by virions and that this can result in the propagation of aggregation. In addition, we show that aggregates formed from TDP-43, which are also associated with ALS, stimulate ruffling and mediates their

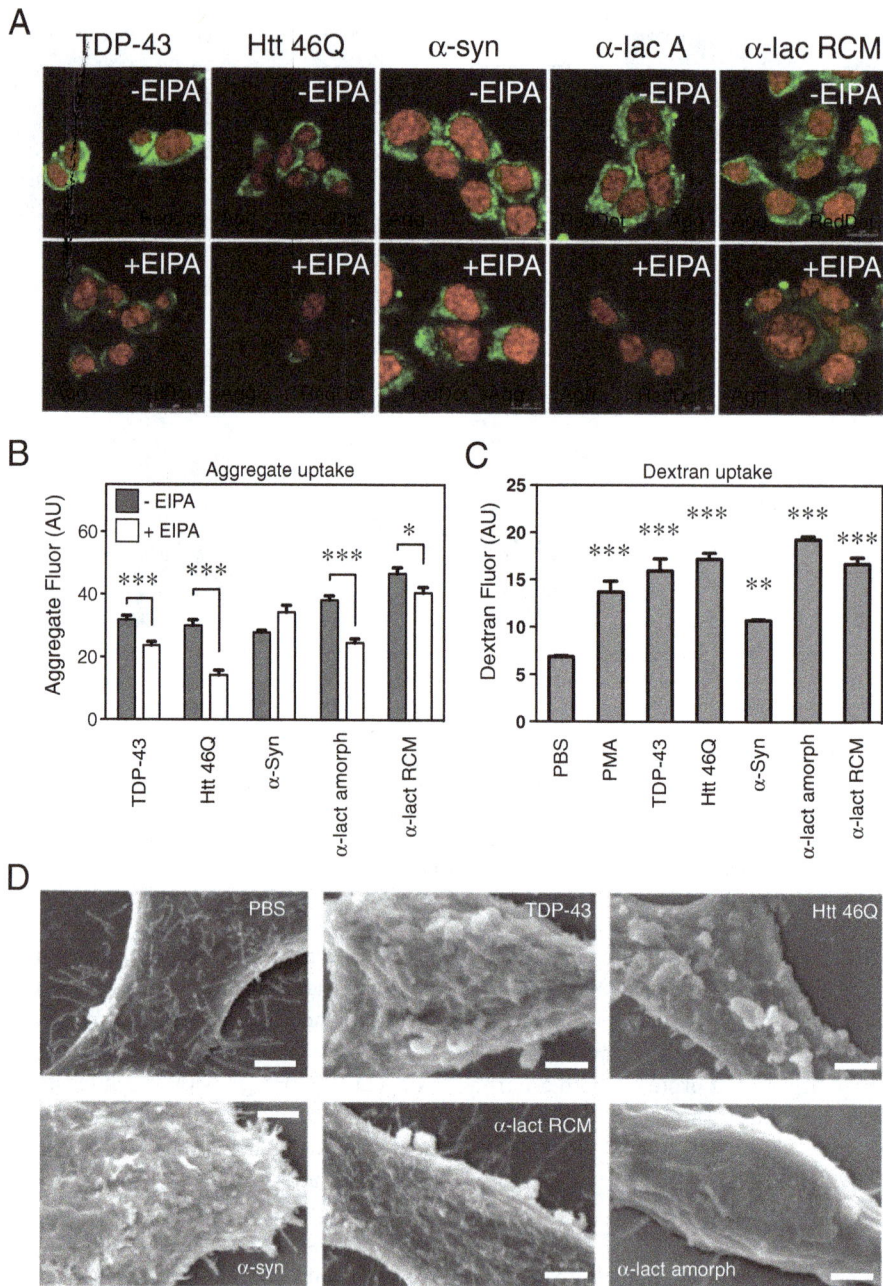

Fig. 8 Other aggregated proteins are capable of stimulating plasma membrane ruffling (**a**) Laser scanning confocal micrographs of uptake of TDP-43, Htt$_{ex1}$46Q, α-synuclein, and α-lactalbumin aggregates into NSC-34 cells. Cells were incubated with the aggregated proteins (20 μg/mL) in the presence or absence of EIPA. Fixed and permealized cells were labelled with an ALEXA-488 conjugated to SA (green) and RedDot 2 (red). (**b**) ImageJ quantification of SOD1 uptake in to treated NSC-34 cells. Results shown as mean fluorescence intensity per cell, minimum 50 cells, ± SD, ** $p < 0.01$. (**c**) Flow cytometry of NSC-34 cells co-treated with protein aggregates and dextran-Alexa647. Results shown as means ± SD, $n = 3$, *** $P < 0.001$. (**d**) Field emission SEM of cells treated with protein aggregates

subsequent cellular uptake. Previous work has shown that amyloid fibrils can enhance HIV viral infection [39], it is interesting to speculate that this behaviour could be due to the potent ability of such aggregates to stimulate macropinocytosis.

Our data are consistent with the notion that protein aggregates could be an active part of ALS disease progression, possibly through secondary nucleation [40], or another prion-like aggregate propagation process. Recent work provides striking evidence that this may indeed drive disease progression as focal injection of spinal cord homogenates from symptomatic G93A SOD1 triggers progressive motor neuron disease in mice expressing G85R SOD1-YFP below the threshold for disease [15]. Our data however, does not directly demonstrate seeding of aggregation and as such we cannot rule out the possibility that the stress of aggregate uptake induces further aggregation in the absence of seeding. We have also shown that Rac1 and protein kinase C (PKC) pathways are actively involved in aggregate uptake. Interestingly, intracellular mutant SOD1 has been found to interact with and activate Rac1 [41]. Rac1, a Rho GTPase, has been identified as an important and central player in triggering membrane ruffles associated with virus entry into cells and has been found to do so by activating downstream effectors of actin polymerisation [42]. In addition, while the precise role of PKC in virus entry is still unclear, its activation with PMA (as used in this study) can induce ruffling and fluid uptake in the absence of ligands that bind the cell surface [43].

There is a growing wave of evidence that is consistent with the hypothesis that protein aggregates propagate between cells and that this is responsible for the orderly progression of disease pathology seen in some neurological disorders [44–49]. The most startling evidence shows that healthy cells grafted into the brains of people with Parkinson's disease acquires intracellular inclusions of α-synuclein, known as Lewy bodies [47]. Evidence suggests that large fibrillar aggregates of a range of proteins (tau, α-synuclein, and expanded polyglutamine repeats) are able to gain access to the cytoplasmic compartment via an incompletely understood mechanism and induce protein aggregation [44, 45, 48, 49]. We show here that aggregates of proteins associated with ALS, Parkinson's and Huntington's disease all trigger both membrane ruffling and fluid uptake; findings indicating the stimulation of macropinocytosis.

While much of the focus on toxic aggregate species has been placed on oligomers, our data adds to work already published that demonstrates large insoluble aggregates can be taken up by cells and subsequently promote propagation of aggregation [16, 23, 44–49]. It has previously been shown that aggregation of α-synuclein can be triggered in an acidic environment and that this, through secondary nucleation, may produce a range of aggregates including toxic oligomers [40]. Taken together, these data suggest that the propagation of large insoluble aggregates through cellular uptake may be responsible for the perpetual propagation and generation of toxic oligomeric species. This conclusion, together with the knowledge of intracellular pathways that result in macropinosome formation and closure, provide possible therapeutic targets for halting the propagation of aggregation in these disorders. For example, we have previously shown that microglia recognize protein aggregates through CD14, scavenger and toll-like receptors, and hence may use receptor-mediated endocytosis, rather than macropinocytosis, to facilitate the uptake of aggregates and to promote their degradation [50, 51]. This distinction between microglia and neurons provides a possible approach to specifically block the uptake of aggregates by neurons.

Materials and methods
Cell culture
The mouse neuroblastoma x spinal cord hybrid cell line (NSC-34 cells [52]) were routinely cultured in DMEM/F12 supplemented with 10 % (v/v) FBS and 2 mM GlutaMAX. Cells were maintained in an incubator at 37 °C under a humidified atmosphere containing 5 % (v/v) CO_2. Human fibroblasts were sourced from non-ALS individuals (female aged 62 and male aged 59 at the time of collection) and reprogrammed into induced pluripotent stem cells using mRNA (Miltenyi). Pluripotency was confirmed by PluriTest and differentiation of the cells [53]. Karyotyping was carried out in iPSCs, to ensure chromosomal abnormalities were not introduced during reprogramming and culture. Immunocytochemistry confirmed the expression of the pluripotency marker Oct4 (Additional file 9A).

Differentiation of pluripotent stem cells into motor neurons was carried out as in [54] and one clone from each line was used in experiments. Motor neurons (150,000 cells) were plated onto laminin (20 μg/mL) and fibronectin (10 μg/mL) coated 13 mm coverslips. The timeline summarizes the differentiation stages and the growth factor conditions used during differentiation (Additional file 9B). The morphological changes of each cell line were examined at each stage of the differentiation process (Additional file 9B).

Confirmation of motor neuron phenotype was carried out, including expression analysis by quantitative reverse transcription PCR and immunocytochemistry. The differentiated neurons expressed the motor neuron specific markers SMI32 and islet 1 (Additional file 9C). Immunocytochemistry identified the presence of extended dendrites ~100 μm in length. Quantitative reverse transcription PCR analysis identified the expression of the motor neuron specific gene *MNX1* (that encodes the transcription factor homeobox 9, HB9) [55]. *MNX1* was specifically expressed in motor neurons and *MNX1* was silent in pluripotent stem cells. The cholinergic specific marker acetylcholine esterase (*ACHE* that encodes the enzyme responsible for the degradation of the neurotransmitter acetylcholine) was specifically expressed in cholinergic motor neurons. The expression levels for both *MNX1* and *ACHE*, were normalized to the housekeeper gene *GAPDH* (Additional file 8D).

Application of aggregates to cells

Wt and G93A SOD1 were expressed and purified from *E.coli* as previously outlined [50, 56]. SOD1 aggregation was performed in vitro as previously described [50]. Briefly, solutions of purified wt or G93A mutant SOD1 protein (1 mg/mL) in PBS were co-incubated with 20 mM dithiothreitol (DTT) and 5 mM ethylenediaminetetraacetic acid (EDTA) for 72 h at 37 °C with shaking; aggregated SOD1 was washed several times to remove DTT and EDTA. NSC-34 cells were cultured in 12 well plates and were transfected with wt or mutant SOD1-GFP using lipofectamine 2000 (following the manufacturer's instructions). Lipofectamine was removed after 5 h and replaced with 10 % FCS in DMEM. After 24 h the aggregates, or soluble (non-aggregated) wtSOD1 as a control, were added in fresh media to transfected or naïve NSC-34 cells. Cells were incubated for a further 48 h and then imaged. In other experiments, aggregates were added to untransfected NSC-34 cells and incubated for various time periods in the presence or absence of pathway inhibitors before fixation and detection of aggregates (see online methods for details). In some experiments, NSC34 cells were incubated with 20 µg/mL of human wt and mutant SOD1 aggregates for 1 h at 37 °C. Post incubation, cells were washed three times in PBS and incubated with trypsin (0.25 %, Invitrogen) for 5 min to remove surface-bound aggregates. The resulting detached cells were centrifuged at $1100 \times g$ for 5 min, re-plated in media, and allowed to recover for 6 h at 37 °C before fixation for immunocytochemistry.

Aggregation and biotinylation of wt and G93A SOD1 aggregates

SOD1 aggregation was performed in vitro as previously described 50. Aggregated SOD1 was labelled with biotinamidohexanoic acid 3-sulfo-N-hydroxysuccinimide ester sodium salt in DMSO for 2 h at RT. The unconjugated biotin was then separated by centrifugation ($21\,000 \times g$ for 30 min) and washed three times with PBS. The purified aggregates were then resuspended in PBS (pH 7.4). A bicinchoninic acid protein assay was performed to determine the amount of protein in solution. Aggregated forms of other proteins were obtained by incubation under conditions previously described, Httex146Q [57] , TDP-43 [58], α-synuclein [59], and α-lactalbumin [38].

Cell surface binding and internalization of aggregated SOD1

NSC-34 cells were initially incubated with 20 µg/mL of aggregated SOD1 for 30 min at 4 °C. Cells were then fixed with 4 % (w/v) paraformaldehyde (PFA) in PBS (pH 7.4) before immunodetection. In separate experiments, cells were incubated with 20 µg/mL of aggregated wtSOD1 for 60 min at 4 °C, fixed with 4 % (w/v)

PFA in PBS (pH 7.4) and permeabilized, or not, with Triton x-100. SOD1 was then detected using anti-SOD1 antibodies. Cells were imaged using a Leica TCS SPII laser scanning confocal microscope (Heidelberg, Germany). In addition, quantitative analysis of SOD1 internalisation into NSC-34 cells was performed using flow cytometry using a BD LSRII (California, USA). Cells were incubated with 20 µg/mL of aggregated SOD1 for 60 min at 4 °C. Cells incubated with PBS (pH 7.4) alone acted as the control. Similar experiments were performed in the presence of the dye, Lysotracker Red as per the manufacturer's instructions. In addition, some cells were treated with trypsin and washed extensively before being lysed after incubation with aggregated wtSOD1 for 60 min. The cell lysates were analysed by Western blotting.

Internalisation of aggregated SOD1 was measured in the presence or absence of a range of compounds that inhibit various internalisation mechanisms. NSC34 cells were pre-treated with various endocytic inhibitors including 100 µM 5-N-ethyl-N-isopropyl-amiloride (EIPA), 5 µM chlorpromazine hydrochloride (CPZ), 10 µM genistein (Gen) or 3 µM rottlerin (Rot) diluted in 1 % BSA/PBS for 30 min at 37 °C, followed by 20 µg/mL aggregated wtSOD1 for 30 min at 37 °C. Cells were then fixed and permeabilized before detection of biotinylated aggregates with SA- Alexa 488. Cells were washed once with PBS medium and analysed using a LSR II flow cytometer (BD Biosciences, San Diego, CA) (excitation 488 nm, emission collected with 515 ± 20 band-pass filters). The mean fluorescence intensity (MFI) of relative SOD1 uptake was determined using FlowJo software (Tree Star, Ashland, OR). For confocal microscopy, cells remained on glass coverslips and incubated in wells as outlined for flow cytometry. Sytox Red (5 nM) was used as a counter stain. Results are the average of at least five independent experiments.

Field emission scanning electron microscopy (FESEM)

NSC-34 cells in phenol-red serum free culture medium were plated into 12-well plates with 19 mm glass coverslips (7×10^4 cells/ ml/well) and starved of serum for 24 h, and treated with 20 µg/mL soluble or aggregated proteins in PBS or PBS containing 200 nM PMA for 2 h at 37 °C. Post incubation, cells were washed three times in PBS then fixed in 2.5 % glutaraldehyde/ 4 % PFA in 0.1 M phosphate buffer (pH 7.4) for 3 h at 4 °C. The cells were then washed three times in phosphate buffer and postfixed in 2 % OsO4/ water at RT for 1 h. After washing with water, the cells were dehydrated using a gradient of ethanol at 30, 50, 70, 80, 90 and 100 % (30 min per incubation) at RT. The cells were then critical point dried for 2 h using a LEICA CPD030 (Vienna, Austria) and coated with graphite-gold in a sputter coater. The samples were analysed with a JEOL 6490LV

SEM (Tokyo, Japan) operated at 10 kV at a 10 mm working distance and a spot size setting of 35.

Rac1 activation assays

NSC-34 cells were treated with 20 µg/mL of soluble and aggregated G93A SOD1 for 30 min at 37 °C. The cells were washed twice with cold PBS and harvested by treatment with 0.05 % trypsin for 10 min at 37 °C. Rac1 activation was measured using a G-LISA activation kit (Kit #BK128 Cytoskeleton, Inc. (Denver, USA) as per the manufacturer's recommendations.

Transmission electron microscopy

Negative staining was performed using substrate carbon-coated nickel grids (Proscitech Kirwan, Australia). Protein was loaded onto the grid and washed three times with milli-Q water. Subsequently, 2 % (w/v) uranyl acetate (ProsciTech Kirwan, Australia) in 0.22 µm sterile filtered milli Q water was added for 2 min to stain the proteins negatively. The grids were analysed using a JEOL 2011 TEM (Tokyo, Japan) operated at 200 kV and Images taken using a Gatan Orius digital camera (California, USA).

Pharmacological inhibitors and antibodies

Pharmacological inhibitors were prepared in either DMSO or 20 % acetonitrile/water according to the manufacturer's recommendations and used at the indicated concentrations. EIPA, CPZ, Gen, and Rot were purchased from Sigma Aldrich. The Rac1 inhibitor W56 was purchased from Tocris Bioscience.

Specific antibodies including mouse anti-beta actin (ab8226), rabbit anti-EEA1 antibody (ab2900), Anti-LAMP1 [H4A3], anti-beta actin antibody [AC-15], anti-beta tubulin antibody, anti-neuron specific beta III tubulin were purchased from Abcam. Alexa Fluor 488 goat anti-mouse, Alexa Fluor 488 goat anti-rabbit, streptavidin Alexa Fluor 633 conjugate, streptavidin Alexa Fluor 488 conjugate, Alexa Fluor 488 donkey anti-sheep, Alexa Fluor 488 donkey anti-rabbit, SYTOX Red dead cell stain, FM® 1-43FX fixable analogue of FM® 1–43 membrane stain were purchased from Invitrogen Life Technologies. Donkey anti-sheep/goat IgG HRP conjugate and goat anti-mouse IgM + IgG + IgA (H + L) HRP conjugates were purchased from Millipore.

Sheep anti-SOD1 was purchased from Thermo Fisher Scientific. Mouse monoclonal anti-human TARDBP antibody (clone k1B8) was purchased from Abnova. Anti-BiP/GRP78 was purchased from BD Transduction Laboratories. FITC-conjugated sheep anti-mouse was purchased from Silenus. RedDot 2 was obtained from Biotium. Goat Anti-Rabbit IgG (H + L)-HRP Conjugate was obtained from Bio-Rad.

Selective permeability of cells

NSC-34 cells were incubated with 20 µg/mL of biotinylated aggregated wt and G93A SOD1 in PBS for either 60 or 120 min at 37 °C. Post incubation, cells were fixed and permeabilized with either 10 µM digitonin or 0.5 % Triton-x100 (v/v) for either 10 or 30 min at 4 °C respectively. The cells were washed three times in PBS, blocked in 5 % BSA/PBS, for subsequent detection using SA-Alexa 633. Cells were visualised using a TCS SP laser scanning confocal microscopy (Leica Microsystems, Wetzlar, Germany) using a 60x objective. The He Ne laser (633 nm) was used and emission was collected at 645 +/− 20 nm using a standard PMT. Data were acquired in Leica Application Suite (Leica Microsystems).

Cellular subfractionation

NSC-34 cells were incubated with 20 µg/mL of aggregated SOD1 in PBS for 120 min at 37 °C. Post incubation the cytosolic (CEB), membrane (MEB), nuclear (NEB) and cytoskeletal proteins (PEB) were extracted from NSC-34 cells using a Subcellular Protein Fractionation Kit for Cultured Cells (Thermo Fisher Scientific) according to the manufacturer's instructions. Aliquots of cell extract (20 µg protein/lane) were separated under reducing conditions (5 % β-mercaptoethanol) using discontinuous TGX Stain-Free™ Precast Gels separating gels (BioRad). Proteins were then transferred to nitrocellulose membranes (Bio-Rad, Hercules, CA) then blocked with heat denatured casein (HDC) in PBS (pH 7.4) for 1 h at 37 °C. To detect exogenously applied SOD1, sheep polyclonal anti-human SOD1 was used. To test the quality of the fractionation, rabbit anti-EEA1, anti- vimentin and mouse anti- actin antibody diluted in HDC/PBS for 1 h at 37 °C were used to probe the MEB and PEB fractions. Membranes were visualised using chemiluminescent substrate and Amersham Hyperfilm ECL (GE Healthcare, Little Chalfont, Bukinghamshire, UK). Images of films were collected using a GS-800 Calibrated Densitometer (Bio-Rad).

Membrane dye uptake

NSC-34 cells were treated with 20 µg/mL of soluble or aggregated wt or G93A SOD1, PBS alone, or a positive control containing 200 nM PMA in PBS for 2 h at 37 °C. The cells were then washed twice in PBS and incubated with 10 µM of FM® 1-43FX membrane stain in PBS for 7 min at 37 °C. Excess dye was removed by several washes in PBS and cells were returned to the incubator for 4 min. This procedure was repeated to give a total of 8 min of incubation in PBS. Post incubation, ice-cold PBS was added to stop endocytosis and prepare cells for fixation in 4 % (w/v) PFA/PBS (pH 7.4) for 20 min at 4 °C. Post fixation, cells were washed twice in PBS and incubated with 1x RedDot 2 for 10 min at RT.

Fluid phase uptake assays

Pinocytosis involves uptake of solutes from the extracellular medium. One well established solute is dextran. To quantify the amount of fluid phase solute uptake, NSC34 cells were treated with either 20 µg/mL of soluble and biotinylated aggregated wt and G93A SOD1, Htt$_{ex1}$46Q, α-synuclein, TDP-43, and α-lactalbumin in PBS alone or containing 200 nM PMA for 30 min at 37 °C. Prior to harvesting or fixation, cells were incubated for 15 min with 0.5 mg/ml 10 kDa 647-dextran (Invitrogen) at 37 °C. The cells were then placed on ice to stop dextran uptake and cells were washed three times with ice cold PBS and once with low pH buffer (0.1 M sodium acetate, 0.05 M NaCl, pH 5.5) for 10 min. The cells were then prepared for either flow cytometry or confocal laser scanning microscopy as described above. For flow cytometry, dextran uptake was displayed as fluorescence mean of three or more independent experiments.

Fixed cell antibody staining of iPSCs

The iPSCs were plated on matrigel-coated 8 mm coverslips at a density of 25,000 cells and cultured for 3 days before staining. Cells were fixed with 4 % (v/v) PFA at room temperature for 10 min, permeabilized with 0.5 % (v/v) TritonX-100 in phosphate buffered saline (PBS) and blocked with 5 % (w/v) bovine serum albumin (BSA) in PBS.

The iPSC colonies were stained with Oct3/4 (mouse 1:500) (Stem Cell Technologies) primary antibody overnight at 4C and anti-mouse Alexa Fluor 488 (1:1000) (Life Technologies) secondary antibody for 1 h at room temperature.

Fixed cell antibody staining of motor neurons

Cells were plated on coverslips coated with laminin (20 µg/mL) and fibronectin (10 µg/mL) at a density of 42,000 cells/cm^2. Cells were fixed using 4 % (v/v) PFA at room temperature for 10 min. The cells were permeabilized with 0.5 % (v/v) Triton X-100 in PBS at room temperature for 15 min. Cells were blocked with 5 % (w/v) bovine serum albumin (BSA) in PBS at room temperature for 1 h. SMI32 primary antibody (Abcam) was diluted 1:800 in PBS 5 % BSA and incubated at 4 °C overnight. Secondary antibodies, Alexa Fluor 488 anti-sheep IgG antibody (1:1000 in PBS 5 % BSA) was incubated with the cells for 1 h at room temperature. Images of stained cells were taken on a Leica DMI6000B confocal microscope and acquired using the LAS AF 2.3.5 software.

Quantitative RT-PCR

RNA was extracted and purified from differentiated cell using the ISOLATE II RNA Mini Kit (Bioline, USA), as per manufacturer's instructions. The purified RNA was quantified using a Nanodrop 2000C (Thermo Fisher Scientific, USA).

RNA was reverse transcribed into complementary DNA (cDNA) for subsequent analysis. Reagents for cDNA preparation were obtained from Promega (USA). Five µg of purified RNA was annealed to random primers (0.75 µg) and oligo dT primers (0.75 µg) by incubating at 65 °C for 4 min, followed by 1 min incubation on ice. For reverse transcription, Moloney-murine leukaemia virus reverse transcriptase (M-MLV RTase) (150 U), 96 nmol dNTPs, RNasin (60 U) and 1x MMLV RTase Buffer were added to the reaction mixture and then incubated at 37 °C for 100 min.

The primers for qRT-PCR were obtained from Sigma Aldrich (USA) (unless stated otherwise) and had the following sequences:

acetylcholinesterase (AChE)
forward: 5'-GGAACCGCTTCCTCCCCAAATTG-3',
reverse: 5'-TGCTGTAGTGGTCGAACTGGTTCTTC-3';
Homeobox 9 (MNX1)
forward: 5'-GTTCAAGCTCAACAAGTACC-3',
reverse: 5'-GGTTCTGGAACCAAATCTTC-3'; GFAP
forward: 5'-CTGGATCTGGAGAGGAAGATTGA
GTCG-3',
reverse: 5'-CTCATACTGCGTGCGGATCTCTTTCA-3';
glyceraldehyde 3-phosphate dehydrogenase (GAPDH)
forward: 5'-GAGCACAAGAGGAAGAGAGAGACCC-3',
reverse: 5'-GTTGAGCACAGGGTACTTTATTGATGG
TACATG-3'. The final qRT-PCR reaction consisted of 10 µL of SYBR Select Master Mix, 800 nM of each forward and reverse primer, 2 µL of cDNA in a final reaction volume of 20 µL. Each reaction was run in duplicate and a negative control (water) and no reverse transcription (RNA) control was included as well as a positive control using cDNA of human putamen. The amplification consisted of 40 cycles, of 95 °C for 15 s (activation step), 58 °C for 15 s (annealing step) and 72 °C for 1 min. A melting curve analysis was conducted to confirm the presence of the appropriate amplified target. The acquired data was normalized against quantitative expression levels of the housekeeping gene GAPDH and analyzed using the comparative threshold cycle method.

Preparation of giant unilamellar vesicles

The rapid evaporation method was used to prepare giant unilamellar vesicles for confocal microscopy as described in [36]. Briefly, soy L-α-phosphatidylcholine (Avanti Polar Lipids Inc) was dissolved in CHCl$_3$:MeOH (2:1) to give a phospholipid concentration of 5 mM. Liposome buffer (50 mM HEPES, 107 mM NaCl, 1 mM EDTA, 0.1 M sucrose, pH 7.4, 2.5 mL) was then added to the lipid/solvent solution in a 50 mL round bottom flask and the two phases mixed by vigorous pipetting. The organic solvent was removed by rotary evaporator under reduced pressure (final pressure 44 mbar) for 5 min at 35 °C. The resulting liposome suspension was stored overnight at 4 °C prior to confocal microscopy studies.

Additional files

Additional file 1: SOD1 aggregates in to fibril like structures that associate with cells via membrane proteins.

Additional file 2: SOD1 aggregates are internalized in NSC-34 cells.

Additional file 3: Aggregates made from a variety of SOD1 mutants induce formation of wtSOD1-GFP aggregates.

Additional file 4: Aggregated and soluble SOD1 enter the cytosol of NSC-34 cells.

Additional file 5: Disruption of membrane structure by SOD1 aggregates.

Additional file 6: Small molecule inhibitors block macropinocytosis.

Additional file 7: Addition of SOD1 does not induce rapid apoptosis.

Additional file 8: Rac1 activation is downstream of membrane ruffling.

Additional file 9: Characterization of iPSC derived motor neurons.

Additional file 10: Characterization of iPSC derived motor neurons.

Additional file 11: wtSOD1 aggregates activate membrane perturbation and dextran uptake in iPSC derived human motor neurons.

Additional file 12: Morphology of protein aggregates using TEM.

Competing interests
N.R.C. is the founder, Chief Scientific Officer, and Chairman of Amorfix Life Sciences.

Authors' contributions
JJY conceptualized, designed and supervised the experiments, analyzed the data and wrote the paper. RZ designed and performed experiments, analyzed data and wrote the paper. ES, JP, LC, DD, MB performed experiments and analyzed data. GG, DMH, HE, CMD, LO contributed resources and to writing/editing the manuscript. MRW and NRC contributed to experimental design and writing of the manuscript. All authors read and approved the final manuscript.

Acknowledgments
RZ is supported by an Australian Postgraduate Award. NRC is supported by donations from the Allen T. Lambert Neural Research Fund and the Temerty Family Foundation, and also by grants from PrioNet Canada, the Canadian Institutes of Health Research (CIHR), and Biogen-Idec Corp. JJY is supported by an ARC Discovery Early Career Award, and by NHMRC project grant 1003032. BJT is supported by NHMRC Project Grant 1008910, MND Research Institute of Australia and Victorian Government's Operational Infrastructure Support Grant. DMH is supported by an ARC Future Fellowship and NHMRC project grants. CMD is supported by the Wellcome Trust. LO is supported by an NHMRC project grant and the Motor Neurone Disease Research Institute of Australia. NRC declares that he is Founder, Chief Scientific Officer and Chairman of Amorfix Life Sciences. HE is supported by an ARC Future Fellowship (FT110100586).

Author details
[1]Illawarra Health and Medical Research Institute, Wollongong, Australia2522. [2]School of Biological Sciences, Faculty of Science, Medicine and Health, University of Wollongong, Wollongong, Australia2522. [3]Intelligent Polymer Research Institute, University of Wollongong, Wollongong, Australia2522. [4]Australian School for Advanced Medicine, Macquarie University, Sydney, Australia2109. [5]Department of Biochemistry and Molecular Biology and Bio21 Molecular Science and Biotechnology Institute, University of Melbourne, Parkville, Australia3010. [6]Department of Chemistry, University of Cambridge, Cambridge CB2 1EW, UK. [7]Florey Institute of Neuroscience and Mental Health, University of Melbourne, Parkville, Australia3010. [8]Department of Medicine (Neurology), University of British Columbia and Vancouver Coastal Health Research Institute, Brain Research Centre, University of British Columbia, Vancouver, CanadaV6T 2B5.

References
1. Rosen DR, Siddique T, Patterson D, Figlewicz DA, Sapp P, Hentati D, et al. Mutations in Cu/Zn superoxide dismutase gene are associated with familial amyotrophic lateral sclerosis. Nature. 1993;362(6415):59–62.
2. Renton AE, Chio A, Traynor BJ. State of play in amyotrophic lateral sclerosis genetics. Nat Neurosci. 2014;17(1):17–23.
3. Aggarwal A, Nicholson G. Detection of preclinical motor neurone loss in SOD1 mutation carriers using motor unit number estimation. J Neurol Neurosurg Psychiatry. 2002;73(2):199–201.
4. Shaw PJ. Toxicity of CSF in motor neurone disease: a potential route to neuroprotection. Brain. 2002;125(Pt 4):693–4.
5. Brettschneider J, Del Tredici K, Irwin DJ, Grossman M, Robinson JL, Toledo L, et al. Sequential distribution of pTDP-43 pathology in behavioral variant frontotemporal dementia (bvFTD). Acta Neuropathol. 2014;127(3):423–39.
6. Ravits JM, La Spada AR. ALS motor phenotype heterogeneity, focality, and spread: deconstructing motor neuron degeneration. Neurology. 2009;73(10):805–11.
7. Chiti F, Dobson CM. Protein misfolding, functional amyloid, and human disease. Annu Rev Biochem. 2006;75:333–66.
8. Knowles TP, Vendruscolo M, Dobson CM. The amyloid state and its association with protein misfolding diseases. Nat Rev Mol Cell Biol. 2014;15(6):384–96.
9. Pasinelli P, Brown RH. Molecular biology of amyotrophic lateral sclerosis: insights from genetics. Nat Rev Neurosci. 2006;7(9):710–23.
10. Hortschansky P, Schroeckh V, Christopeit T, Zandomeneghi G, Fandrich M. The aggregation kinetics of Alzheimer's beta-amyloid peptide is controlled by stochastic nucleation. Protein Sci. 2005;14(7):1753–9.
11. Knowles TP, Waudby CA, Devlin GL, Cohen SI, Aguzzi A, Vendruscolo M, et al. An analytical solution to the kinetics of breakable filament assembly. Science. 2009;326(5959):1533–7.
12. Knowles TP, White DA, Abate AR, Agresti JJ, Cohen SI, Sperling RA, et al. Observation of spatial propagation of amyloid assembly from single nuclei. Proc Natl Acad Sci U S A. 2011;108(36):14746–51.
13. Cohen SI, Linse S, Luheshi LM, Hellstrand E, White DA, Rajah L, et al. Proliferation of amyloid-beta42 aggregates occurs through a secondary nucleation mechanism. Proc Natl Acad Sci U S A. 2013;110(24):9758–63.
14. Munch C, O'Brien J, Bertolotti A. Prion-like propagation of mutant superoxide dismutase-1 misfolding in neuronal cells. Proc Natl Acad Sci U S A. 2011;108(9):3548–53.
15. Ayers JI, Fromholt S, Koch M, DeBosier A, McMahon B, Xu G,et al. Experimental transmissibility of mutant SOD1 motor neuron disease. Acta Neuropathol. 2014;128(6):791–803.
16. Grad LI, Yerbury JJ, Turner BJ, Guest WC, Pokrishevsky E, O'Neill MA, et al. Intercellular propagated misfolding of wild-type Cu/Zn superoxide dismutase occurs via exosome-dependent and -independent mechanisms. Proc Natl Acad Sci U S A. 2014;111(9):3620–5.
17. Sundaramoorthy V, Walker AK, Yerbury J, Soo KY, Farg MA, Hoang V, et al. Extracellular wildtype and mutant SOD1 induces ER-Golgi pathology characteristic of amyotrophic lateral sclerosis in neuronal cells. Cell Mol Life Sci. 2013;70(21):4181–95.
18. Swanson JA, Watts C. Macropinocytosis. Trends Cell Biol. 1995;5(11):424–8.
19. Mercer J, Helenius A. Virus entry by macropinocytosis. Nat Cell Biol. 2009;11(5):510–20.

20. Mercer J, Helenius A. Gulping rather than sipping: macropinocytosis as a way of virus entry. Curr Opin Microbiol. 2012;15(4):490–9.

21. Kalia M, Khasa R, Sharma M, Nain M, Vrati S. Japanese encephalitis virus infects neuronal cells through a clathrin-independent endocytic mechanism. J Virol. 2013;87(1):148–62.

22. Conner SD, Schmid SL. Regulated portals of entry into the cell. Nature. 2003;422(6927):37–44.

23. Holmes BB, DeVos SL, Kfoury N, Li M, Jacks R, Yanamandra K, et al. Heparan sulfate proteoglycans mediate internalization and propagation of specific proteopathic seeds. Proc Natl Acad Sci U S A. 2013;110(33):E3138–47.

24. Wadia JS, Schaller M, Williamson RA, Dowdy SF. Pathologic prion protein infects cells by lipid-raft dependent macropinocytosis. PLoS One. 2008;3(10), e3314.

25. Ivanov AI. Pharmacological inhibition of endocytic pathways: is it specific enough to be useful? Methods Mol Biol. 2008;440:15–33.

26. Yerbury JJ, Gower D, Vanags L, Roberts K, Lee JA, Ecroyd H. The small heat shock proteins alphaB-crystallin and Hsp27 suppress SOD1 aggregation in vitro. Cell Stress Chaperones. 2013;18(2):251–7.

27. Damiano S, Petrozziello T, Ucci V, Amente S, Santillo M, Mondola P. Cu-Zn superoxide dismutase activates muscarinic acetylcholine M1 receptor pathway in neuroblastoma cells. Mol Cell Neurosci. 2013;52:31–7.

28. Turner BJ, Atkin JD, Farg MA, Zang DW, Rembach A, Lopes EC, et al. Impaired extracellular secretion of mutant superoxide dismutase 1 associates with neurotoxicity in familial amyotrophic lateral sclerosis. J Neurosci. 2005;25(1):108–17.

29. Grad LI, Guest WC, Yanai A, Pokrishevsky E, O'Neill MA, Gibbs E, et al. Intermolecular transmission of superoxide dismutase 1 misfolding in living cells. Proc Natl Acad Sci U S A. 2011;108(39):16398–403.

30. Graffmo KS, Forsberg K, Bergh J, Birve A, Zetterstrom P, Andersen PM, et al. Expression of wild-type human superoxide dismutase-1 in mice causes amyotrophic lateral sclerosis. Hum Mol Genet. 2013;22(1):51–60.

31. Deng HX, Shi Y, Furukawa Y, Zhai H, Fu R, Liu E, et al. Conversion to the amyotrophic lateral sclerosis phenotype is associated with intermolecular linked insoluble aggregates of SOD1 in mitochondria. Proc Natl Acad Sci U S A. 2006;103(18):7142–7.

32. Nizard P, Tetley S, Le Drean Y, Watrin T, Le Goff P, Wilson MR, et al. Stress-induced retrotranslocation of clusterin/ApoJ into the cytosol. Traffic. 2007;8(5):554–65.

33. Schneider D, Greb C, Koch A, Straube T, Elli A, Delacour D, et al. Trafficking of galectin-3 through endosomal organelles of polarized and non-polarized cells. Eur J Cell Biol. 2010;89(11):788–98.

34. Freeman D, Cedillos R, Choyke S, Lukic Z, McGuire K, Marvin S, et al. Alpha-synuclein induces lysosomal rupture and cathepsin dependent reactive oxygen species following endocytosis. PLoS One. 2013;8(4), e62143.

35. Maier O, Marvin SA, Wodrich H, Campbell EM, Wiethoff CM. Spatiotemporal dynamics of adenovirus membrane rupture and endosomal escape. J Virol. 2012;86(19):10821–8.

36. Milanesi L, Sheynis T, Xue WF, Orlova EV, Hellewell AL, Jelinek R, et al. Direct three-dimensional visualization of membrane disruption by amyloid fibrils. Proc Natl Acad Sci U S A. 2012;109(50):20455–60.

37. Kolpak AL, Jiang J, Guo D, Standley C, Bellve K, Fogarty K, et al. Negative guidance factor-induced macropinocytosis in the growth cone plays a critical role in repulsive axon turning. J Neurosci. 2009;29(34):10488–98.

38. Kulig M, Ecroyd H. The small heat-shock protein alphaB-crystallin uses different mechanisms of chaperone action to prevent the amorphous versus fibrillar aggregation of alpha-lactalbumin. Biochem J. 2012;448(3):343–52.

39. Munch J, Rucker E, Standker L, Adermann K, Goffinet C, Schindler M, et al. Semen-derived amyloid fibrils drastically enhance HIV infection. Cell. 2007;131(6):1059–71.

40. Buell AK, Galvagnion C, Gaspar R, Sparr E, Vendruscolo M, Knowles TP, et al. Solution conditions determine the relative importance of nucleation and growth processes in alpha-synuclein aggregation. Proc Natl Acad Sci U S A. 2014;111(21):7671–6.

41. Harraz MM, Marden JJ, Zhou W, Zhang Y, Williams A, Sharov VS, et al. SOD1 mutations disrupt redox-sensitive Rac regulation of NADPH oxidase in a familial ALS model. J Clin Invest. 2008;118(2):659–70.

42. Sanchez EG, Quintas A, Perez-Nunez D, Nogal M, Barroso S, Carrascosa AL, et al. African swine fever virus uses macropinocytosis to enter host cells. PLoS Pathog. 2012;8(6), e1002754.

43. Swanson JA. Phorbol esters stimulate macropinocytosis and solute flow through macrophages. J Cell Sci. 1989;94(Pt 1):135–42.

44. Clavaguera F, Bolmont T, Crowther RA, Abramowski D, Frank S, Probst A, et al. Transmission and spreading of tauopathy in transgenic mouse brain. Nat Cell Biol. 2009;11(7):909–13.

45. Desplats P, Lee HJ, Bae EJ, Patrick C, Rockenstein E, Crews L, et al. Inclusion formation and neuronal cell death through neuron-to-neuron transmission of alpha-synuclein. Proc Natl Acad Sci U S A. 2009;106(31):13010–5.

46. Jucker M, Walker LC. Self-propagation of pathogenic protein aggregates in neurodegenerative diseases. Nature. 2013;501(7465):45–51.

47. Li JY, Englund E, Holton JL, Soulet D, Hagell P, Lees AJ, et al. Lewy bodies in grafted neurons in subjects with Parkinson's disease suggest host-to-graft disease propagation. Nat Med. 2008;14(5):501–3.

48. Ren PH, Lauckner JE, Kachirskaia I, Heuser JE, Melki R, Kopito RR. Cytoplasmic penetration and persistent infection of mammalian cells by polyglutamine aggregates. Nat Cell Biol. 2009;11(2):219–25.

49. Volpicelli-Daley LA, Luk KC, Patel TP, Tanik SA, Riddle DM, Stieber A, et al. Exogenous alpha-synuclein fibrils induce Lewy body pathology leading to synaptic dysfunction and neuron death. Neuron. 2011;72(1):57–71.

50. Roberts K, Zeineddine R, Corcoran L, Li W, Campbell IL, Yerbury JJ. Extracellular aggregated Cu/Zn superoxide dismutase activates microglia to give a cytotoxic phenotype. Glia. 2013;61(3):409–19.

51. Medeiros LA, Khan T, El Khoury JB, Pham CL, Hatters DM, Howlett GJ, et al. Fibrillar amyloid protein present in atheroma activates CD36 signal transduction. J Biol Chem. 2004;279(11):10643–8.

52. Cashman NR, Durham HD, Blusztajn JK, Oda K, Tabira T, Shaw IT. Neuroblastoma x Spinal Cord (NSC) Hybrid Cell Lines Resemble Developing Motor Neurons. Dev Dynam. 1992;194:209–21.

53. Muller FJ, Schuldt BM, Williams R, Mason D, Altun G, Papapetrou EP, et al. A bioinformatic assay for pluripotency in human cells. Nat Methods. 2011;8(4):315–7.

54. Bilican B, Livesey MR, Haghi G, Qiu J, Burr K, Siller R, et al. Physiological normoxia and absence of EGF is required for the long-term propagation of anterior neural precursors from human pluripotent cells. PLoS One. 2014;9(1), e85932.

55. Arber S, Han B, Mendelsohn M, Smith M, Jessell TM, Sockanathan S. Requirement for the homeobox gene Hb9 in the consolidation of motor neuron identity. Neuron. 1999;23(4):659–74.

56. Lindberg MJ, Tibell L, Oliveberg M. Common denominator of Cu/Zn superoxide dismutase mutants associated with amyotrophic lateral sclerosis: Decreased stability of the apo state. Proc Natl Acad Sci U S A. 2002;99(26):16607–12.

57. Olshina MA, Angley LM, Ramdzan YM, Tang J, Bailey MF, Hill AF, et al. Tracking mutant huntingtin aggregation kinetics in cells reveals three major populations that include an invariant oligomer pool. J Biol Chem. 2010;285(28):21807–16.

58. Johnson BS, Snead D, Lee JJ, McCaffery JM, Shorter J, Gitler AD. TDP-43 is intrinsically aggregation-prone, and amyotrophic lateral sclerosis-linked mutations accelerate aggregation and increase toxicity. J Biol Chem. 2009;284(30):20329–39.

59. Aquilina JA, Shrestha S, Morris AM, Ecroyd H. Structural and functional aspects of hetero-oligomers formed by the small heat shock proteins alphaB-crystallin and HSP27. J Biol Chem. 2013;288(19):13602–9.

11

Viral expression of ALS-linked ubiquilin-2 mutants causes inclusion pathology and behavioral deficits in mice

Carolina Ceballos-Diaz[1], Awilda M. Rosario[1], Hyo-Jin Park[1,2], Paramita Chakrabarty[1], Amanda Sacino[1], Pedro E. Cruz[1], Zoe Siemienski[1], Nicolas Lara[1], Corey Moran[1], Natalia Ravelo[1,2], Todd E. Golde[1] and Nikolaus R. McFarland[1,2]*

Abstract

Background: *UBQLN2* mutations have recently been associated with familial forms of amyotrophic lateral sclerosis (ALS) and ALS-dementia. *UBQLN2* encodes for ubiquilin-2, a member of the ubiquitin-like protein family which facilitates delivery of ubiquitinated proteins to the proteasome for degradation. To study the potential role of ubiquilin-2 in ALS, we used recombinant adeno-associated viral (rAAV) vectors to express UBQLN2 and three of the identified ALS-linked mutants (P497H, P497S, and P506T) in primary neuroglial cultures and in developing neonatal mouse brains.

Results: In primary cultures rAAV2/8-mediated expression of UBQLN2 mutants resulted in inclusion bodies and insoluble aggregates. Intracerebroventricular injection of FVB mice at post-natal day 0 with rAAV2/8 expressing wild type or mutant UBQLN2 resulted in widespread, sustained expression of ubiquilin-2 in brain. In contrast to wild type, mutant UBQLN2 expression induced significant pathology with large neuronal, cytoplasmic inclusions and ubiquilin-2-positive aggregates in surrounding neuropil. Ubiquilin-2 inclusions co-localized with ubiquitin, p62/SQSTM, optineurin, and occasionally TDP-43, but were negative for α-synuclein, neurofilament, tau, and FUS. Mutant UBLQN2 expression also resulted in Thioflavin-S-positive inclusions/aggregates. Mice expressing mutant forms of UBQLN2 variably developed a motor phenotype at 3–4 months, including nonspecific clasping and rotarod deficits.

Conclusions: These findings demonstrate that UBQLN2 mutants (P497H, P497S, and P506T) induce proteinopathy and cause behavioral deficits, supporting a "toxic" gain-of-function, which may contribute to ALS pathology. These data establish also that our rAAV model can be used to rapidly assess the pathological consequences of various *UBQLN2* mutations and provides an agile system to further interrogate the molecular mechanisms of ubiquilins in neurodegeneration.

Keywords: Ubiquilin-2, Amyotrophic lateral sclerosis (ALS), Proteinopathy, Somatic brain transgenesis, Mouse model

* Correspondence: nikolaus.mcfarland@neurology.ufl.edu
[1]Center for Translational Research in Neurodegenerative Disease, Department of Neuroscience, University of Florida, 1275 Center Dr, PO Box 100159, Gainesville, FL 32610, USA
[2]Department of Neurology, College of Medicine, University of Florida, 1149 S Newell Dr, L3-100, PO Box 100236, Gainesville, FL 32610, USA

Background

Several mutations in the *UBQLN2* gene have recently been identified and associated with X-linked familial ALS and ALS-dementia [1–3]. *UBQLN2* encodes ubiquilin-2, a member of the ubiquitin-like family of proteins that facilitate delivery of polyubiquitinated proteins to the proteasome for degradation [1]. In humans there are at least 4 ubiquilins. Each is widely expressed, except for ubiquilin-3 which is testes specific [4]. Ubiquilins are characterized by an N-terminal ubiquitin-biding domain (UBA), a variable number of Sti1-like repeats, and a C-terminal ubiquitin-like domain (UBL) that associates with the proteasome. Identified ALS-linked mutations (P497S/H, P506TS/T, and P525S) are primarily located in a C-terminal proline-rich domain that contains 12 PXX repeats [1]; however, 3 have been identified outside this region [2]. Recently, another mutation was identified within the proline-rich region in *UBQLN2* and linked to familial ALS (c.1490C > T, p.P497L) [3]. Mutations in ubiquilin-2 have been proposed to alter proteasome mediated protein clearance, suggesting a loss-of-function and possible cause for abnormal protein accumulation and deposition [1]. However, ubiquilins have also been implicated in ER-associated protein degradation and autophagy [5–7]. Examination of protein inclusions in pathological tissue from both sporadic ALS and ALS-dementia demonstrate the presence of ubiquilin-2 in inclusions and co-localization with other proteins such as ubiquitin and p62/SQSTM1, further suggesting a role for ubiquilin-2 in proteinopathy and in ALS pathology [1, 8, 9]. Few studies to date, however, have examined the role of ubiquilin-2 and consequence of identified mutations—so far limited to P497H mutant—on the development of ALS pathology [10, 11].

To determine the pathological consequences of *UBQLN2* mutants, we developed rAAV 2/8 vectors to compare the effects of overexpression of wild type (WT) and three of the recently identified ALS-mutant ubiquilins in primary neuroglial cultures and in the developing mouse brain. In mice we utilized "somatic brain transgenesis" (SBT) to rapidly introduce and express *UBQLN2* mutants in throughout the brain. Although having more limited and variable expression compared to traditional transgenic models, SBT still allows for rapid, widespread expression and screening of genes of interest before expending the time and expense developing traditional transgenic models [12, 13]. Our findings demonstrate that overexpression of pathological forms of mutant ubiquilin-2 compared to WT all develop widespread inclusion pathology, including amyloid-like aggregates, that persists over 6 months and which is associated with mild, early motor deficits. These studies provide further insight into the *in vivo* effects of expression of ALS-linked mutant forms of ubiquilin-2 in mice. Furthermore, our SBT mouse models demonstrate a powerful and complementary approach to traditional transgenics that will allow further dissection of pathological mechanisms of ubiquilin-2 mutants and their role in development of ALS and ALS-dementia.

Results

To study the effects of recently described ALS-linked *UBQLN2* mutants on pathology we cloned wild-type (WT) and three mutant forms of ubiquilin-2 (P497S, P497H and P506T) into rAAV vectors for expression in developing mouse brain. Viral expression was first tested in primary neuroglial cultures before moving to mice.

Viral expression of ubiquilin-2 mutants in mixed neuroglia cultures results in large punctate intracellular accumulations

Recombinant AAV2/8 expressing ubiquilin-2 WT or ALS-linked mutants (P497S, P497H and P506T) was used to transduce primary neuroglial cultures at DIV + 6. Four days post-transduction cells were analyzed by immunofluorescence and biochemistry. Neurons were identified by MAP2 and astrocytes by GFAP co-immunostaining. Ubiquilin-2 expression was primarily observed in neurons in E16 cultures, but also seen in some astrocytes. In cells expressing ubiquilin-2 WT or pathologic mutants, there was low level of diffuse ubiquilin-2 immunoreactivity throughout the neuronal perikarya. Most notably, large accumulations of ubiquilin-2 were seen in both the neuronal cytoplasm and processes. Intracellular ubiquilin-2-postive accumulations, although present in cultures transduced with AAV-*UBQLN2*(WT), were larger and more prevalent in cultures transduced with mutant *UBQLN2* (Fig. 1a). Also, neurons transduced with either P497S, P497H or P506T mutant ubiquilin-2 displayed frequent ubiquilin-2-postive punctate accumulations in neuronal processes with a "bead on a string"-like appearance, suggesting an altered subcellular distribution. These puncta were more apparent in cultures transduced with the P497H and P506T *UBQLN2* mutants and associated with apparent dystrophic changes in neurites. Some ubiquilin-2-postive accumulations were located outside neurons and colocalized with the astrocytic marker GFAP, but not the microglial marker Iba-1 (Fig. 1b). Preliminary screen to identify subcellular localization of intracellular ubiquilin-2 accumulations revealed no colocalization with early endosomal markers such as EEA1 or Rab5; late endosomes, Rab7; autophagosomes, LC3; or lysosomes, LAMP1 (data not shown).

To further assess viral expression of WT and mutant ubiquilin-2 in primary cultures, we performed Western blots on fractionated cell lysates. Notably, mutant forms of ubiquilin-2, but not WT, accumulated in the SDS soluble fraction suggesting that ALS-linked mutant

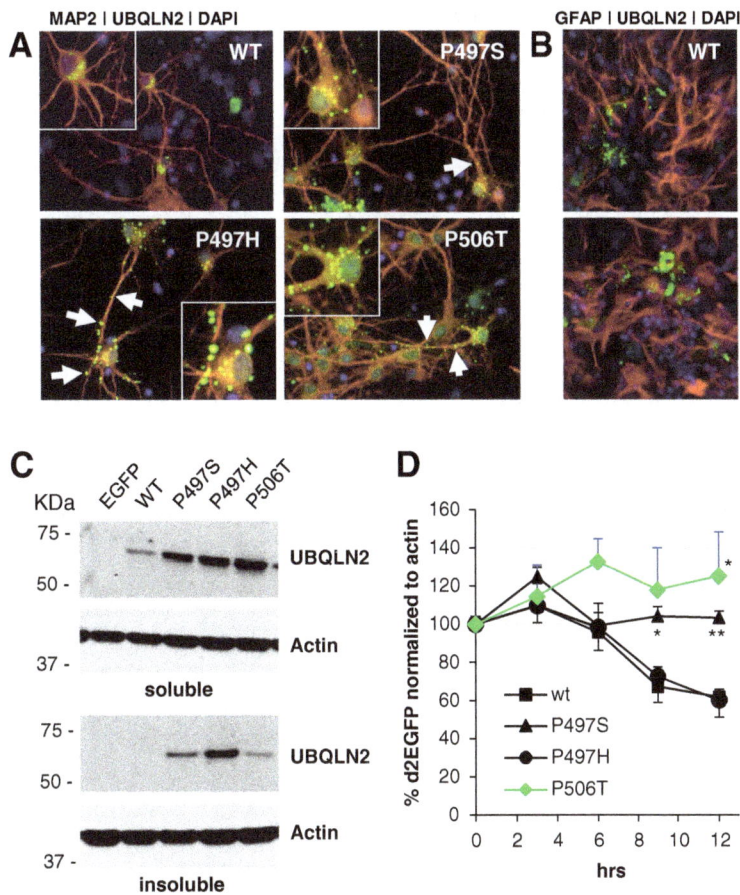

Fig. 1 Mutant Ubiquilin-2 overexpression results in punctate intracellular accumulations in primary mixed neuroglia cultures. **a**. Cells transduced with AAV-*UBQLN2*(WT) show ubiquilin-2 immunoreactivity (*green*) diffusely present in the cytoplasm and cell processes with few small punctate accumulations. In contrast, *UBQLN2* mutants (P497S, P497H, and P506T) result in large intracellular ubiquilin-2 accumulations both in neuronal soma and processes (red, labelled with MAP2). Ubiquilin-2 accumulations in processes have a "bead on a string"-like appearance particularly for P497H and P506T mutants. **b**. Some ubiquilin-2 accumulations (*green*) are outside of neurons and colocalized with astrocytes in culture, labeled with GFAP-imunoreactivity (*red*). **c**. Western blot of TX-soluble and insoluble fractions show that all *UBQLN2* mutants and not WT accumulate in the TX-insoluble/SDS fraction, suggesting formation insoluble aggregates. **d**. Graph of d2EGFP signal normalized to actin in HEK293 cells transfected with WT and mutant ubiquilin-2. Both P497S and P506T mutants show impaired proteasomal degradation of the d2EGFP reporter compared to the P497H mutant and WT ubiquilin-2. $*p < 0.05$, $**p < 0.01$

ubiquilins form Triton X-100 (TX) insoluble aggregates (Fig. 1c). As mutations in ubiquilin-2 have been suggested to reduce proteasomal degradation [1], we investigated the effect of expression of different ALS-linked mutant ubiquilin-2 on UPS function in HEK293 cells using the reporter d2EGFP. Twenty-four hours post transfection cells were treated with cyclohexamide and then harvested at 3 h intervals and assessed for d2EGFP levels which were normalized to β-actin. Expression of both the P497S and P506T mutants significantly reduced the rate of d2EGFP proteasomal degradation relative to WT ubiquilin-2 (Fig. 1d). Interestingly, the P497H mutant showed no change in d2EGFP degradation compared to WT in contrast to that previously reported [1].

SBT expression of ubiquilin-2 mutants results in widespread inclusion pathology

To investigate the role of *UBLQN2* and ALS-liked mutations in pathology, we used somatic brain transgenesis with rAAV serotype 2/8 to express either EGFP-control, WT or one of three different mutant forms of ubiquilin-2 (P497S, P497H, and P506T) in the developing mouse brain. Non-transgenic FVB mice all received bilateral i.c.v. injections of virus at P0. Mice injected with rAAV2/8-*UBQLN2* wild type and ALS-linked mutants all demonstrated widespread neuronal (specific) expression of ubiquilin-2 in the olfactory bulb, cortex, hippocampus, thalamus, striatum, brainstem, and cerebellum as early as 1 month post-injection, and maintained at both 3 and 6 month time points (Fig. 2). In sites near to

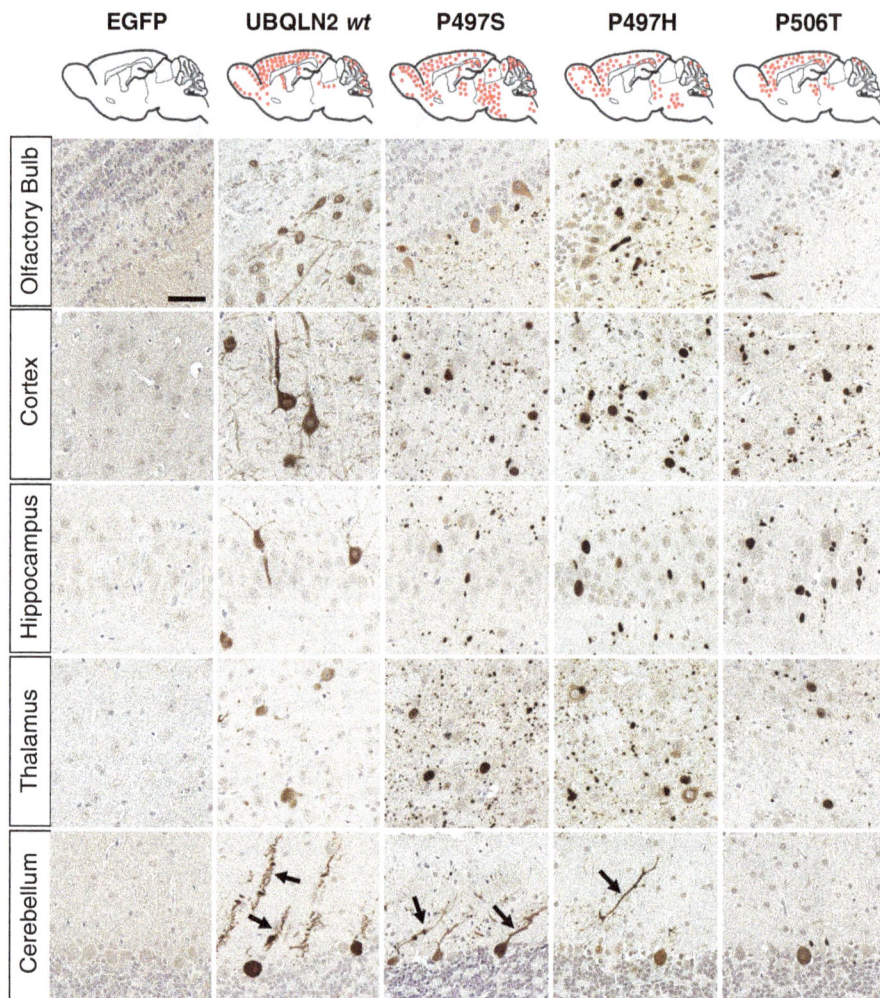

Fig. 2 Viral expression of ubiquilin-2 at 6 months. Representative schema of sagittal section shows the overall distribution of AAV-UBQLN2 expression in mouse brain after ICV injection (SBT model). Photos show ubiquilin-2 immunostaining in representative sections animals injected with AAV expressing either EGFP control or WT vs P497S, P497H, or P506T mutant ubiquilin-2. WT ubiquilin-2 expression is homogeneous throughout the neuronal perykaria, including processes. Mutant ubiquilin-2 shows altered subcellular expression, often concentrating in the nucleus, but also resulting cytoplasmic inclusions. Ubiquilin-2-positive "aggregates" are seen also in adjacent neuropil. Arrows point out alteration in purkinje cell dendritic arbors for mutant vs WT ubiquilin-2. (Scale same for all photomicrographs, bar = 50 μm)

the injection such as cortex, hippocampus, thalamus and striatum, nearly 30–40 % neurons were transduced. Western blots of whole brain tissue lysates similarly indicated sustained ubiquilin-2 expression through the 6 month time point with levels reaching 10–40 % that of endogenous mouse ubiquilin-2 (Fig. 3). Transduced neurons expressing human ubiquilin-2, however, were easily identified by immunohistochemistry relative to background endogenous mouse ubiquilin-2, suggesting several-fold overexpression. Expression of WT ubiquilin-2 in neurons was diffuse, involving the soma and proximal dendrites, and included few small punctate cytoplasmic accumulations (see Fig. 4, confocal images). In contrast, expression of each of the mutant forms of ubiquilin-2 resulted in large intracellular neuronal

inclusions and extensive neuropil aggregates in the surrounding gray matter, similar to that recently described by Gorrie et al. in transgenic mice with the P497H mutant ubiquilin-2 [10]. Whereas WT ubiquilin-2 was mainly cytoplasmic and diffuse, mutant ubiquilin-2 expression also appeared to have more prominent nuclear localization. As early as 1 month dystrophic changes were also seen in the dendritic arbors of purkinje cells expressing mutant ubiquilin-2, which appeared to have reduced branching architecture (Fig. 2). Glial markers showed only a rare ubiquilin-2-positive astrocyte in areas of abundant viral expression (Fig. 4). Despite the presence of abundant large inclusion seen in mice expressing mutant forms of ubiquilin-2, there was no apparent neurodegeneration or cell loss even in 6 month

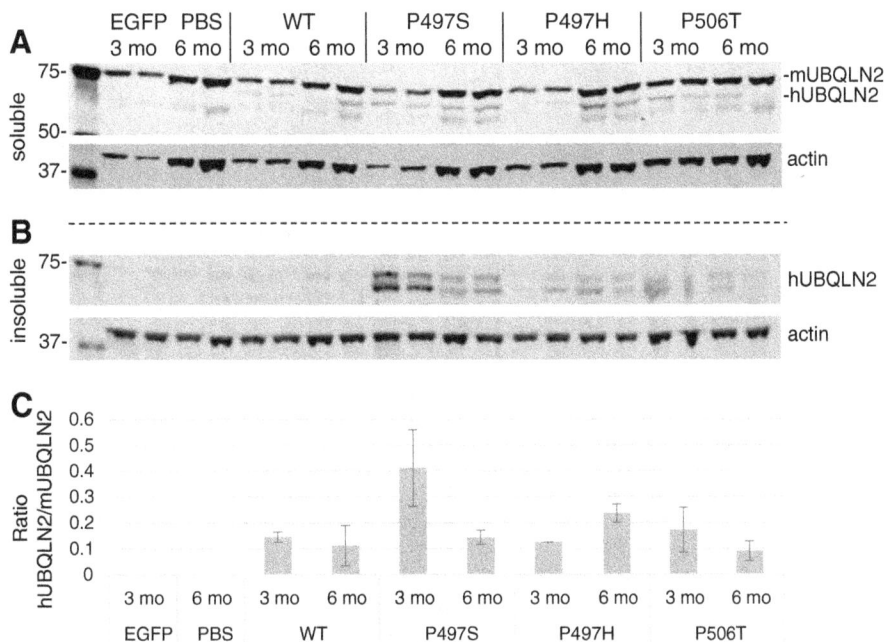

Fig. 3 Viral expression of human ubiquilin-2 in whole brain lysates. Western blots of brain lysates from 3 and 6 month animals demonstrate sustained expression of WT ubiquilin-2 and mutants. In the Trition-X100 soluble fraction (**a**) three bands are seen for ubiquilin-2: top is mouse UBQLN2 whereas middle and lower (truncated?) bands represent human UBQLN2. **b**) Only mutant forms of human UBQLN2 are seen in the Triton insoluble fractions. **c**) Graph of human vs endogenous mouse UBQLN2 expression in whole brain (Triton soluble) lysates. $N = 2$–3 sample each with mean ± SD ratio shown

mice. Tissues were immunostained for apoptotic cell markers including caspase-3/7 and tunnel stain, and both negative (data not shown). Examination of hematoxylin & eosin stained sections also showed no evident cell loss or degeneration of brain regions overexpressing ubiquilin-2.

Mutant ubiquilin-2 inclusions colocalize with TDP-43 and are ThioS-positive

As ubiquilin-2 has been found colocalized with other proteins in ALS inclusions, such as ubiquitin, p62, and FUS [1, 14], we examined brain tissue from mice for colocalization of these and several other neuropathological proteins including pSer129-synuclein, tau, phospho-tau, and TDP-43, which is found both in frontotemporal dementia (FTLD-U) and ALS brains. Minimal differences were noted in expression patterns between 1, 3, and 6 month mice. As expected, ubiquilin-2-positive inclusions and aggregates co-stained for ubiquitin, p62, and optineurin (Fig. 5). However, ubiquilin-2 inclusions did not colocalize with FUS (except for that within nuclei) or phosphorylated α-synuclein using the pSer129/81A antibody, which has recently shown also to bind phosphorylated neurofilament subunit L, or NFL [15] (data not shown). Inclusions also did not colocalize with tau, consistent with published data that indicate no correlation of ubiquilin-2 with tau pathology [16].

However, in mice expressing the mutant ubuiqilin-2(P506T) cytoplasmic TDP-43 aggregates, immunostained with antibodies to either phospho-TDP-43 (403–404) or (409–410) epitopes, were associated with ubiquilin-2-positive inclusions (Fig. 6). These findings suggest that ubiquilin-2(P506T) may be more prone than the P497S/H mutants to cause proteinopathy involving TDP-43 pathology that is seen in frontotemporal dementia (FTD). Interestingly, expression of mutant forms and not WT, of ubiquilin-2 also resulted in inclusions or aggregates that stained positive for ThioflavinS suggesting induction of amyloid pathology (Fig. 7) further supporting the notion that ALS-linked ubiquilin-2 mutants induce proteinopathy via misfolding and aggregation of proteins.

Viral SBT of ALS-linked *UBQLN2* mutants results in an early motor deficits

So far in mice aged to 6 months we have not observed significant cell loss or neurodegeneration as determined by tunnel, caspase-3/7 or hematoxylin and eosin staining. However, at 3–4 months several mice expressing mutant ubiquilin-2 (P497S: 7 of 9, P497H: 2 of 9, and P506T: 4 of 9 mice) developed a nonspecific clasping phenotype (Fig. 8a). On rotarod testing mice expressing mutant ubiquilin-2 also showed significant impairment compared to mice expressing WT ubiquilin-2 (Fig. 8b).

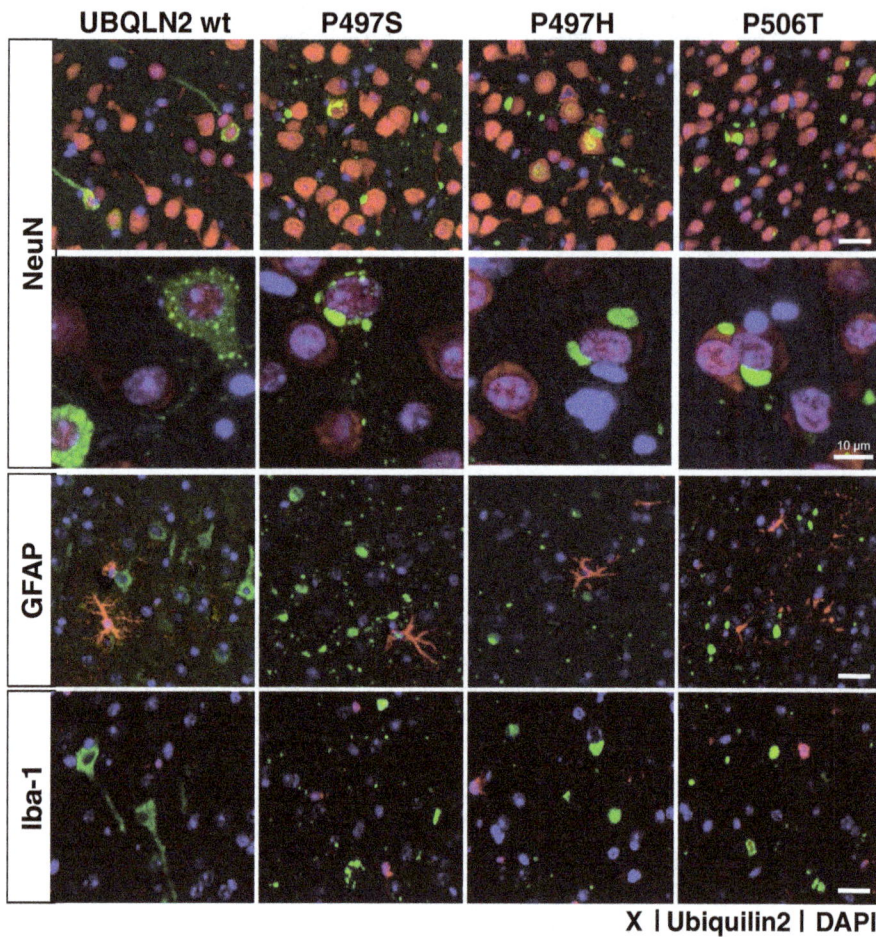

Fig. 4 AAV expression of *UBQLN2* WT and mutants is specific to neurons. Images are merged photos of representative cortical areas from 6 month mice stained with immunofluorescence for NeuN/GFAP/Iba-1 (*red*), ubiquilin-2 (*green*), and DAPI (*blue*). The top 2 rows show colocalization of ubiquilin-2 accumulations with NeuN-positive neurons. Row 2 includes high-power confocal images that demonstrate differences in the distribution of ubiquilin-2-containing inclusions in NeuN labeled neurons; large inclusions are seen for all mutant forms in contrast to WT ubiquilin-2. Glial markers GFAP (row 3) and Iba-1 (row 4) rarely colocalize with ubiquilin-2. (Scale bar = 50 μm unless otherwise noted)

Despite the appearance of relative stable pathological features, these findings suggest progression of pathology and that more prolonged expression of ALS-linked ubiquilin-2 using our novel rAAV model system may result in a more disease-relevant motor phenotype.

Discussion

UBQLN2 mutations have recently been added to the list of potential genes that cause familial ALS and ALS-FTD [1, 2]. *UBQLN2* encodes for ubiquilin-2, a member of the ubiquitin-like family of proteins that facilitate transport of ubiquitinated proteins to the proteasome for degradation. Although evidence to date suggests that ALS-linked ubiquilin-2 mutants have reduced proteasomal function and cause a potential loss-of-function [1], the role of ubiquilin-2 in ALS pathology remains unclear. To determine the functional consequences of ALS-linked *UBQLN2* mutations, we developed rAAV

vectors to express WT and three of the identified ubiquilin-2 mutants (P497, P497H, and P506T) in primary neuronal cells and in the developing mouse brain. In primary cultures we found that viral overexpression of ubiquilin-2 resulted in large intracellular accumulations that were more prominent and distributed along neuronal processes for mutant forms than for WT ubiquilin-2. Fractionated lysates from these cultures demonstrated also that mutant ubiquilin-2, but not WT, were present in TX-insoluble (SDS soluble) fractions, suggesting tendency for mutant forms of ubiquilin-2 to form insoluble aggregates. To determine whether viral expression ALS-linked mutant ubiquilin-2 could induce pathological and behavioral abnormalities in mice, we developed a model system using somatic brain transgenesis, or SBT, to widely and rapidly overexpress ubiquilin-2 in the developing mouse nervous system. We demonstrate herein that mice injected i.c.v. with rAAV-ubiquilin-2

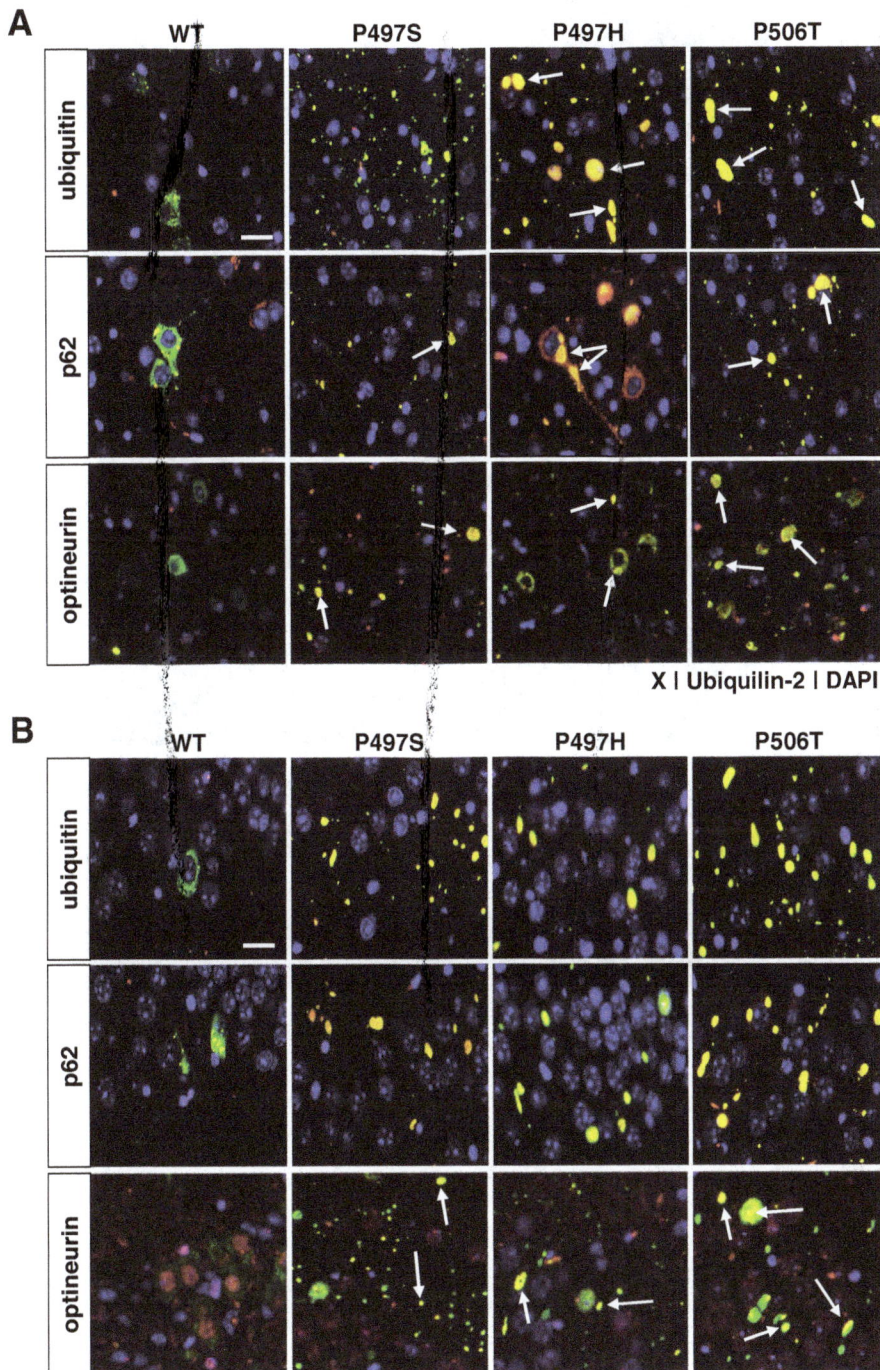

Fig. 5 Ubiquilin-2 inclusions colocalize with ubiquitin, p62, and optineurin. Merged immunofluorescent images are from **a**) cortex and **b**) hippocampus from 6 month mice and show staining for ubiquitin/p62/optineurin (*red*), ubiquilin-2 (*green*), and DAPI (*blue*). In contrast to WT, pathological (mutant) ubiquilin-2 form large intracellular and neuropil inclusions that frequently colocalize (indicated as yellow, representing overlap *red* and *green* signal) with ubiquitin, p62, and optineurin. (bar = 25 μm)

mutants and aged up to 6 months develop early, widespread neuronal inclusion pathology, dystrophic neurite changes, and motor deficits.

To date few studies have examined the *in vivo* consequences of ALS-linked ubquilin-2 in brain and spinal cord. Recently, Gorrie et al. [10] published the first findings from transgenic mice that express one of the ALS-linked mutant ubquilin-2 (P497H) under the direction of the *UBQLN2* promoter. Progressive ubiquilin-2 pathology was observed in these mice and particularly

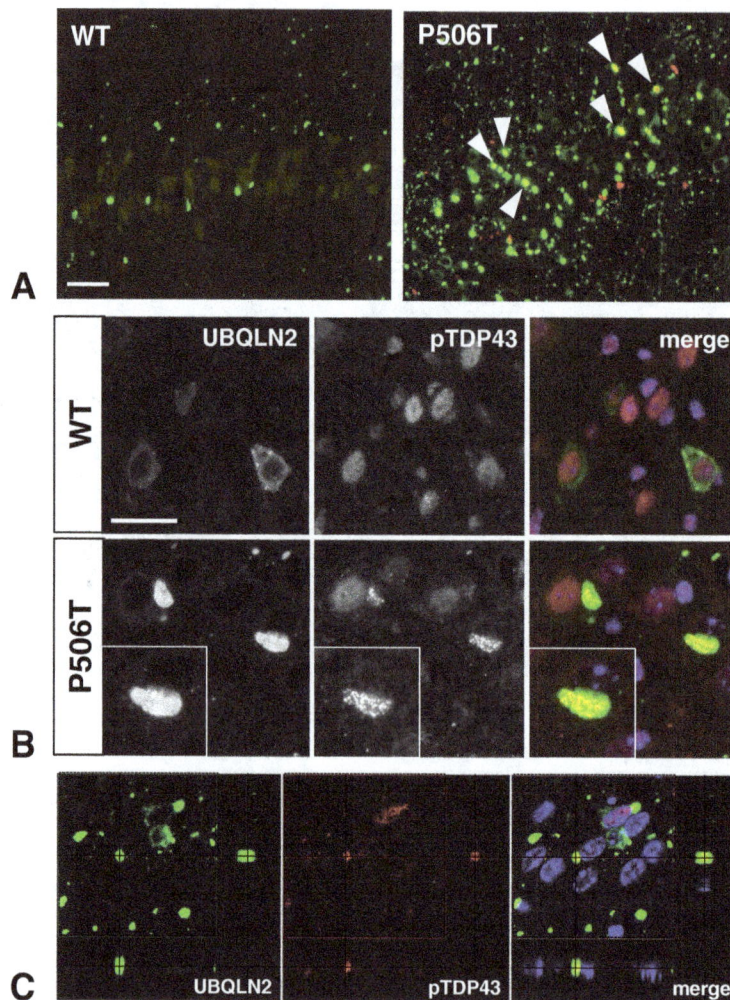

Fig. 6 TDP43 colocalizes with ubiquilin-2 in mice expressing mutant UBQLN2 (P506T). **a**) Low power merged immunofluorescent images of CA3 hippocampus from mice injected with rAAV expressing WT or P506T mutant ubiquilin-2 and aged 6 months. TDP43 (*red*) colocalizes (*arrowheads*) with several ubiquilin-2-positive (*green*) inclusions in mutant P506T expressing mice. (bar = 25 μm) **b**) Higher power photomicrographs show cytoplasmic TDP43 puncta stained with the phospho-TDP43 antibody (403–404) within a large cytoplasmic ubiquilin-2-positive inclusion. (bar = 25 μm) **c**) Confocal Z-slice section analysis of ubiquilin-2 inclusions (*green*) similarly demonstrates colocalization of phosphorylated TDP43 (*red*) in brain tissue from mice expressing mutant UBQLN2 (P506T)

prominent in the hippocampal gyrus, but also in the frontal and temporal lobes with increasing age, similar to that seen in human ALS tissues [1]. Abundant ubiquilin-2-positve neuropil aggregates in gray matter, but not in white matter, were noted [10] and similar to that observed in our mouse brains transduced with rAAV-UBQLN2 mutants. These findings suggest that ubiquilin-2 aggregates are localized to dendrites rather than axons. Indeed, electron microscopy studies indicate primary somatodendritic aggregates which are prominent in dendritic spines in hippocampal and cortical tissues and which may contribute to altered spine density and plasticity [10]. The findings from our mouse models are complimentary and together these models indicate that expression of ALS-linked ubiquilin-2 mutants cause

progressive ubiquilin-2 pathology involving aggregate formation and proteinopathy. However, the link between these findings, neurodegeneration, and development of ALS remains unclear. In both our mouse SBT model and the $UBQLN2^{P497H}$ transgenic mice, neuronal loss and neurodegeneration have not been observed. However, more recently, Wu et al. in a similar transgenic model in rats did show neuronal loss proceeded by formation of ubiquilin-2 aggregates and evidence of impaired autophagy and endosomal function [11]. Lack of evidence for neurodegeneration in our model may possibly be explained by relative low viral transduction of neurons (estimated at 30–40 %, greatest in regions near the ventricles); however, detailed analyses with both tunnel and caspase 3/7 were unrevealing. Nevertheless, in

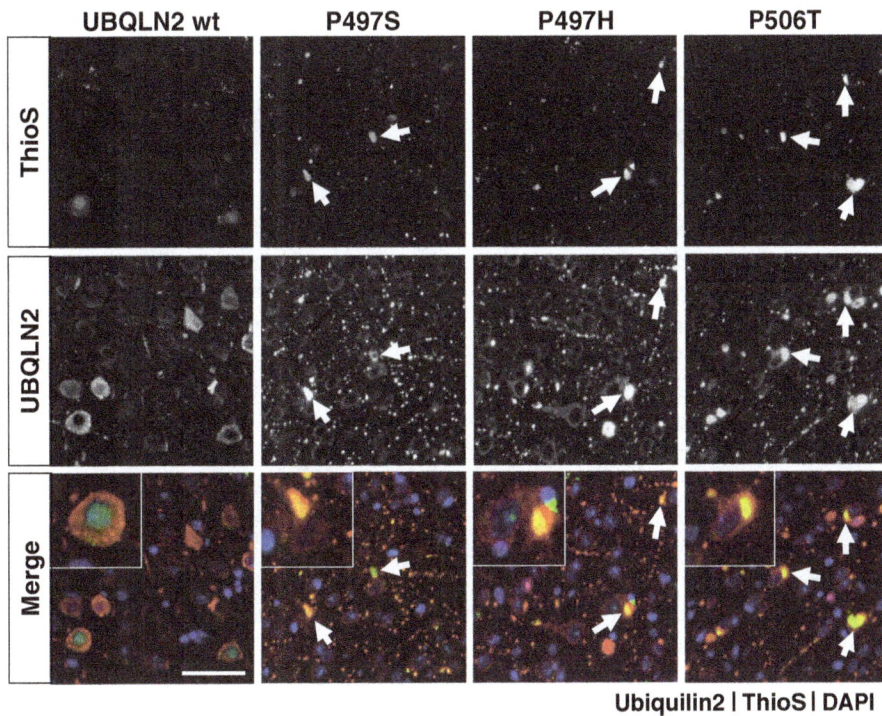

Fig. 7 Mutant ubiquilin-2 expression induces ThioS-positive inclusions. Photos show Thioflavin-S staining that colocalizes (arrows; yellow in merged images) with intracellular ubiquilin-2-positive inclusions seen in mice injected with rAAV expressing mutant but not WT ubiquilin-2. Images shown are from mice aged 6 months, but similar findings were seen also in younger mice. (bar = 50 μm)

our study SBT mice expressing mutant UBQLN2 variably developed clasping and rotarod deficits as early as 3–4 months, which although nonspecific may indicate progressive pathology and possible later development of a more disease-relevant motor phenotype. This finding is in contrast to recent transgenic P497H models that report evidence for cognitive rather than motor deficits [10, 11], which may have relevance to ALS-FTD and other neurodegenerative dementias. To fully determine the utility of our novel rAAV model system, we will need

to further establish the effects of mutant ubiquilin-2 expression in mouse brain and spinal cord beyond 6 months to determine whether we can induce pathological and phenotypic changes, such as paresis, expected for ALS/ALS-FTD.

Evidence to date indicates that ubiquilins play important roles in multiple protein recycling and degradation pathways, including the UPS, ERAD, and autophagy [17]. Although the function of ubiquilin-2 remains unclear, its homology to ubiquilin-1 suggests a similar

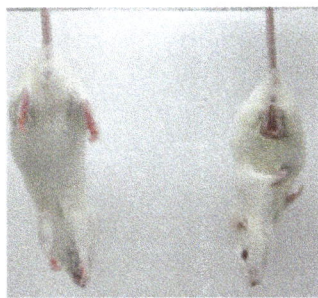

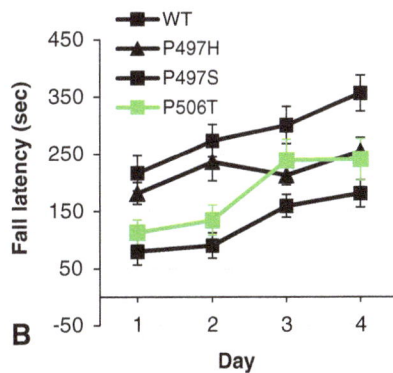

Fig. 8 Behavioral deficits in mice. **a)** Mice expressing ALS-mutant ubiquilin-2 develop a clasping phenotype at 3–4 months. **b)** Rotarod performance for mice at 3 months expressing mutant ubiquilin-2 P497S ($p < 0.0001$) and P506T ($p < 0.01$) was significantly impaired compared to those expressing WT ubiquilin-2. Data shown as mean ± SEM; $N = 9$ for each group

function and role in the UPS and degradation of proteins. Identified ALS-linked mutations in ubiquilin-2 all localize to a proline-rich (PXX repeat) region that is distinct from either the N-terminal UBL (ubiquitin-like) domain that interacts with the proteasome or the C-terminal UBA (ubiquitin-associated) domain that associates with ubiquitinated proteins, suggesting that ALS mutants may leave these functional domains intact. ALS-linked mutations in ubiquilin-2 have been shown *in vitro* to impair proteasomal degradation and these findings appear consistent with its primary function in the UPS [1]. Recently *in vivo* data from bigenic mice expressing both $UBQLN2^{P497H}$ and the ubiquitinated protein substrate, Ub^{G67V}-GFP, appears to support these findings. Ub^{G67V}-GFP accumulated in the brain of bigenic mice expressing $UBQLN2^{P497H}$ suggesting impaired UPS function [10]. Furthermore, ubiquilin-2 deposits in brain sections from these mice colocalized with antibodies to proteasome subunits. These findings appear to indicate that mutant ubiquilin-2(P497H) may still function to bring ubiquitinated proteins to the proteasome, but somehow interferes with proteasomal degradation, leading to accumulation and abnormal deposition proteins. Our data indicate that ALS-linked ubiquilin-2 variants may have differential effects on UPS function. Indeed the P497H mutant had little effect on d2EGFP levels and was similar to WT, whereas expression of both the P497S and P506T mutants impaired d2EGFP metabolism (Fig. 7). These data suggest that alternative protein degradation mechanisms may be involved such as the autophagy-lysosomal system to explain the effects of these ubiquilin-2 mutants on proteinopathy seen in our models.

Recent studies also implicate ubiquilin-2 in macroautophagy. Early studies demonstrated that ubiquilin-1 binds the target of rapamycin (mTOR) kinase in mammalian cells, a critical regulator of macroautophagy [18]. Both ubiquilin-1 and 2 have also been shown to colocalize with the microtubule-associated protein 1 light chain 3 (LC3), a membrane component of autophagosomes, and have been implicated in the maturation of autophagic vesicles [5]. Notably, knockdown of ubiquilin-2 (and 1) rendered cells expressing either a Alzheimer's-related presenilin mutant or a huntingtin polyglutamine expansion more susceptible to starvation-induced death, whereas overexpression is protective, further supporting a role in autophagy and neurodegenerative disease [5]. The effects of ALS-linked mutations on ubiquilin-2 function in macroautophagy have not been explored and remain unclear. We hypothesize that expression of ubiquilin-2 mutants may impair macroautophagy, as well as UPS function, disrupting proteostasis and contributing to protein accumulation, aggregate formation, cell stress and cytotoxicity.

To date, few studies have identified protein interactors with ubiquilin-2 or ALS-linked mutants. UBA and UBL domains in ubiquilins are known to interact with polyubiquitinated proteins and the proteasome, respectively, consistent with their function in the UPS [4]. In addition, ubiquilins have been shown to interact with components of the ERAD including Erasin and p97/VCP (valosin-containing protein) that form a complex at the ER membrane to direct degradation of misfolded protein as part of the unfolded protein response [6]. More recently, ubiquilin-2 was shown to interact with the ubiquitin regulatory X domain-containing protein 8 (UBXD8), which mediates translocation of ERAD substrates such as p97/VCP, and this interaction was impaired by the ubiquilin-2 mutant (P497) [19]. Although ubiquilin-2 has been colocalized with several other proteins *in vitro* and *in vivo* including LC3 [5], p62/SQSTM1, ubiquitin [1], and optineurin [10], direct interactions have not been demonstrated. Our data indicate colocalization of ubiquilin-2 inclusions with cytoplasmic, phospho-TDP-43 in mice expressing the P506T mutant ubiquilin-2. Recent evidence suggests that ubiquilin-2 binds to C-terminal fragments of TDP-43 [1, 20]. TDP-43 and in particular mislocalization and aggregation of C-terminal fragments of TDP-43 have been implicated in both ALS and FTD pathology. Together, these data provide an incomplete picture of proteins that may interact with ubiquilin-2 or ALS-linked mutants that may be critical to understanding both the normal function of ubiquilin-2 as well as how identified mutations alter its function and may influence development of ALS/ALS-FTD pathology.

Conclusions

We demonstrate using rAAV techniques that overexpression of ALS-linked mutant *UBQLN2* induce pathological accumulations of ubiquilin-2 in neurons, insoluble aggregates, and early behavioral deficits in our SBT mouse model. Our findings lend support to the notion that mutant ubiquilin-2 expression result in a (toxic) gain of function, disrupting proteostasis. Although traditional transgenic approaches are being used to investigate the pathological consequences of ubiquilin-2 mutant expression in mice [21], we report here the first use of a novel somatic brain transgenic approach using rAAV serotype 8 that shows a similar pattern of widespread neuronal inclusion pathology in brain. This approach has several advantages in that we are able to relatively rapidly test several of the recently reported ubiquilin-2 variants and highlight potential differences in their pathological effects, as well as noted a potential relevant motor phenotype not previously reported. Clearly there are several limitations to SBT including variability among injections and limited viral expression. However, the use of rAAV provides agility to easily modify future constructs to test specific portions of the ubiquilin-2 that may differentially affect aggregation and pathology or to express in select cell types to address possible non-cell autonomous effects suggested in ALS [22].

Methods
Cloning and rAAV preparation
Both WT and mutant *UBQLN2* (P497S, P497H and P50T) constructs were generated using PCR and were subcloned into recombinant adeno-associated viral (rAAV) vectors, serotype 2, with expression cassette containing a cytomegalovirus enhancer/chicken beta actin (CBA) promoter, bovine growth hormone polyA, and woodchuck hepatitis virus post-transcriptional regulatory element (WPRE). AAV control vector expressing EGFP was prepared as previously described by Chakrabarty et al. [13]. Recombinant AAV constructs were packaged into AAV with serotype 2/8 capsid using methods derived from Zolotukhin et al. [23]. Briefly, we co-transfected rAAV into HEK293T cells with linear polyethylenimines (PEI, Polysciences) along with AAV helper plasmid 8 (Plasmid Factory, Germany). Cells were harvested, lysed, and virus isolated with an iodixanol gradient, and then buffer exchanged to sterile PBS, pH 7.2. Viral titers (genome copies per mL) were determined by quantitative PCR (Bio-Rad, CFX384) as previously described and [13]. AAV titers were as follows: *UBQLN2* WT 2.30×10^{13} gc/mL, P497S 1.38×10^{13} gc/mL, P497H 1.30×10^{13} gc/mL, P506T 1.26×10^{13} gc/mL, and EGFP 2×10^{13} gc/mL. All freshly prepared AAVs were aliquoted and stored at -80 °C until use. *Neuroglial cultures.* Primary mixed neuronal-glial cultures were prepared as previously described by Sacino et al. [24]. Briefly, mouse cortices from B6C3HF1 mice were isolated at E16. The tissue was dissociated by digestion with papain solution (Worthington Biochemical Corp, NJ) and 50ug/ml DNase I (Sigma, MO) at 37 for 20 min. After digestion cortices were washed three times with Hank's Balanced Salt Solution (HBSS, Life Technologies) to remove the papain and place in media consisting of Neurobasal (Life Technologies) supplemented with 0.02 % NeuroCult™ SM1 (STEMCELL Technologies Inc., Vancouver), 0.5 mM GlutaMax (GIBCO, Life Technologies), 5 % Fetal Bovine Serum (Hyclone, GE Life Sciences) and 0.01 % Pen-strep (GIBCO, Life Technologies). The tissue was triturated in the same media and dissociated cells were plated in CC2-coated cell Lab-Tek II 8-chamber slides (Fisher Scientific) at a density of 20,000 cells per well for imaging and in poly-D-lysine (Sigma, MO) coated 6-well plates for biochemical analysis. Cells were maintained at 37 °C in a humidified incubator with 5 % CO_2.

Double Immunofluorescence analysis of mixed neuroglia cultures
Cells were transduced at DIV-6 (days *in vitro*) with rAAV2/8 *UBQLN2* WT and mutants to a final concentration of 10^{11} gc/ml. At DIV-10 cells were fixed with 4 % paraformaldehyde in PBS (0.01 M phosphate buffered saline, pH 7.4), then washed with PBS and blocked in 5 % goat serum with 0.1 % triton X-100 in PBS for 1 h, and then incubated overnight in primary antibodies: UBQLN2 (1:500; Abcam) and MAP2 (1: 1000; Abcam). Cells were washed in PBS and then incubated in secondary antibody goat-anti mouse conjugated to Alexa-488 and goat anti-rabbit conjugated to Alexa-594 (1:1000; Life technologies). Nuclei were counterstained with mounting media containing 4′,6-diamidino-2-phenylindole (DAPI). Images were captured using Olympus BX-60 epi-fluorescence microscope with DP71 digital camera.

Biochemical fractionation followed by western blot analysis
Cells for Western blot were extracted using TBS (tris-buffered saline) and 1 % triton X-100 supplemented with proteinase and phosphate inhibitors (TBS-T buffer), vortexed, and incubated on ice for 5 min. Tissue samples from adult mouse brain were weighed (wet weight), then digested mechanically in 4× volume of same lysis buffer (ice-cool), and similarly incubated on ice for 5 min. Lysates were centrifuge at 100,000 g for 20 min at 4 °C, the supernatant saved (soluble fraction), and the pellets re-washed with TBS-T buffer and re-centrifuged with the same buffers to remove any trace of the soluble fraction. The insoluble fractions were the extracted from the remaining pellets using 2 % SDS (sodium dodecyl sulfate) and sonication. Equal amounts of Soluble and Insoluble fractions were visualized by SDS protein electrophoresis and detected by mouse monoclonal UBQLN2 antibody (1:1000; Abcam). Ubiquilin-2 was normalized to actin (AC15, Sigma) in blots.

Proteasomal assay
HEK293 cells were transfected with a UPS reporter vector encoding d2EGFP. 24 h post transfection, cells were re-plated into 12-well plates and transfected with either wild type or mutant ubiquilin-2. 24 h after second transfection, cells were treated with 30 µg/ml of cyclohexamide (Sigma) for 0, 3, 6, 9, or 12 h. At each time point, cells were harvested, washed in ice-cold PBS and lysed in RIPA buffer including protease inhibitors. Equal amounts of protein were loaded for Odyssey blotting, and the d2EGFP levels were normalized to β-actin. Data were collected from three independent experiments.

Mice, neonatal injections, and behavioral assessment
All animal husbandry and procedures were approved by the University of Florida Institutional Animal Care and

Use Committee and conformed to the NIH guidelines for animal research. B5C3HF1 and FVB mice were obtained from Harlan labs (Tampa, FL) for use in these studies. Neonatal mice were kept with parent mother until weaned. Mice were otherwise housed three to five per cage, given food and water *ad libitum*, and kept on a 12 h light/dark cycle.

AAV were injected in newborn mice P0 (0–24 h old) as described in Chakrabarty et al. [13]. Briefly, rAAV-UBQLN2 were delivered to non-transgenic FVB mice via bilateral intracerebroventricular (i.c.v.) injections. Each injection included 2 μL rAAV ($1-3x10^{13}$ gc/mL) expressing UBQLN2 WT or P497S, P497H, P506T mutant or EFGP (control) into both cerebral ventricles. For each virus, approximately 12–18 mice were injected (2–3 litters). Mice were observed and underwent periodic SHIRPA primary screen testing [25]. At 3 months a subset of mice ($n = 9$ per group) performed rotarod testing. Mice were sacrificed at set timepoints: 1 month ($n = 2-3$ per group), 3 months ($n = 6-8$) and 6 months ($n = 6-8$) post-injection. Animals were euthanized by CO_2 inhalation, briefly perfused transcardially with PBS, and brains harvested immediately. Half of the brain was fixed in 10 % formalin, washed and embedded in paraffin for sections; the other half was flash-frozen for later biochemical analysis.

Rotarod testing

Mice were trained in groups of 3–5 on a Rotamex-5 apparatus (Columbus Inst., OH). Mice were given a series of pre-training trials the day before testing, including 3, 5 min runs on the rotarod at constant speed (5 rpm). During the following 4 consecutive days, mice were tested with 4, 5 min trials (40–60 min inter-trial interval) with gradual acceleration of the rod from 4 to 40 rpm. The speed and latency to fall were recorded for each trial. Best performances from each of the 4 test trials on each consecutive day were analyzed and groups compared using repeated measures ANOVA.

Immunohistochemistry and immunofluorescence analysis of brain sections

Paraffin embedded brains were cut into 8 μm sagittal sections. Sections were deparaffinized and dehydrated in xylenes and serial alcohol concentrations (70–100 %) followed by water antigen retrieval, steam, or retrieval solution (Dako) for 30 min followed by hydrogen-peroxide incubation. Sections were immunostained with primary antibody to UBQLN2 (Sigma; 1:500) and other specific antibodies (as listed below) overnight, and then developed using Immpress polymer detection reagents (Vector Labs). Sections were counterstained using hematoxylin solution. Separate sections also underwent hematoxylin and eosin staining. Brain images were

scanned using ScanscopeXT image scanner (Aperio/Leica USA). For double immunofluorescence sections were immunostained with primary antibody to UBQLN2 (5 F5, Novus Biologicals; or HPA006431, Sigma-Aldrich) in combination with other antibodies including: ubiquitin (Ab7780, Abcam, Cambridge, MA), p62 (SQSTM1, Proteintech, Chicago, IL), GFAP (Dako, Carpinteria, CA), Iba-1 (Abcam), MAP2 (Abcam), caspase 3, α-synuclein (Syn1, BD Biosciences, San Jose, CA), pSer129-synclein [26], NFL (neurofilament, C28E10, Cell Signaling Technologies; or monoclonal NR4, Sigma-Aldrich), PHF1 (provided by Dr. Peter Davis), TDP-43 (Cosmo Bio, Carlsbad, CA), phospho-TDP43 (403/404 and 409/410 antibodies, Cosmo Bio), FUS (Bethyl, Montgomery, TX), Matrin-3 (2539C3a, Abcam), Optineurin (Abcam), and VCP/p97 (Abcam). For visualization fluorescent conjugated antibodies, Alexa 594-goat anti-mouse or anti-rabbit and Alexa 488-goat anti mouse at 1:500, were used. Fluorescent images were captured using either Olympus BX60 microscope with epifluorescence, confocal spinning disc (Olympus DSU-IX81) or laser confocal microscope (Leica TCS SP2 AOBS spectral) for analysis.

Abbreviations
ALS: Amyotrophic lateral sclerosis; ERAD: Endoplasmic reticulum associated degradation; FTD: Frontotemporal lobar dementia; FUS: Fused in sarcoma; icv: Intracerbroventricular; NFL: Neurofilament light chain; rAAV: Recombinant adeno-associated virus; SBT: Somatic brain transgenesis; TDP-43: Transactive response DNA binding protein 43; UBA: Ubiquitin binding domain; UBQLN2: Ubiquilin-2; UBL: Ubiquitin-like domain; UPS: Ubiquitin-proteasome system.

Competing interests
The authors declare that they have no competing interest.

Authors' contributions
CCD carried out the molecular studies, immunoassays, animal procedures, behavioral testing, histology, analysis and drafting of the manuscript. AMR generated the virus, performed histochemistry, and participated in animal procedures and testing. HJP performed the proteasomal assays. PC participated in the study design and animal procedures. AS assisted with animal procedures. PEC cloned the molecular and viral constructs. ZS performed the histopathology. NL assisted with animal procedures and histology. CM contributed to the histopathology. NR participated in the histology. TEG participated in overall design and conception of the study, and manuscript preparation and editing. NRM participated in the experimental design, coordination, interpretation, drafting and editing of the manuscript. All authors read and approved the final manuscript.

Acknowledgements
We would like to thank Dr. Benoit Giasson for providing us anti-pSer129 α-synuclein antibody (81A). This work was supported by NIH grant NS067024 to NRM, the Ellison Medical Foundation to TEG, and the Florida Practice Associates.

References
1. Deng HX, Chen W, Hong ST, Boycott KM, Gorrie GH, Siddique N, et al. Mutations in UBQLN2 cause dominant X-linked juvenile and adult-onset ALS and ALS/dementia. Nature. 2011;477:211–5.

2. Synofzik M, Maetzler W, Grehl T, Prudlo J, Vom Hagen JM, Haack T, et al. Screening in ALS and FTD patients reveals 3 novel UBQLN2 mutations outside the PXX domain and a pure FTD phenotype. Neurobiol Aging. 2012;33:2949 e2913–2947.

3. Fahed AC, McDonough B, Gouvion CM, Newell KL, Dure LS, Bebin M, Bick AG, Seidman JG, Harter DH, Seidman CE: UBQLN2 mutation causing heterogeneous X-linked dominant neurodegeneration. Annals of neurology 2014, 75(5):793-798.

4. Marin I. The ubiquilin gene family: evolutionary patterns and functional insights. BMC Evol Biol. 2014;14:63.

5. Rothenberg C, Srinivasan D, Mah L, Kaushik S, Peterhoff CM, Ugolino J, et al. Ubiquilin functions in autophagy and is degraded by chaperone-mediated autophagy. Hum Mol Genet. 2010;19:3219–32.

6. Lim PJ, Danner R, Liang J, Doong H, Harman C, Srinivasan D, et al. Ubiquilin and p97/VCP bind erasin, forming a complex involved in ERAD. J Cell Biol. 2009;187:201–17.

7. Kim TY, Kim E, Yoon SK, Yoon JB. Herp enhances ER-associated protein degradation by recruiting ubiquilins. Biochem Biophys Res Commun. 2008;369:741–6.

8. Mizusawa H, Nakamura H, Wakayama I, Yen SH, Hirano A. Skein-like inclusions in the anterior horn cells in motor neuron disease. J Neurol Sci. 1991;105:14–21.

9. Kiernan MC, Vucic S, Cheah BC, Turner MR, Eisen A, Hardiman O, et al. Amyotrophic lateral sclerosis. Lancet. 2011;377:942–55.

10. Gorrie GH, Fecto F, Radzicki D, Weiss C, Shi Y, Dong H, Zhai H, Fu R, Liu E, Li S, et al: Dendritic spinopathy in transgenic mice expressing ALS/dementia-linked mutant UBQLN2. Proceedings of the National Academy of Sciences of the United States of America 2014, 111(40):14524-14529.

11. Wu Q, Liu M, Huang C, Liu X, Huang B, Li N, Zhou H, Xia XG: Pathogenic Ubqln2 gains toxic properties to induce neuron death. Acta neuropathologica 2014, 129(3):417-428.

12. Kim J, Miller VM, Levites Y, West KJ, Zwizinski CW, Moore BD, et al. BRI2 (ITM2b) inhibits Abeta deposition in vivo. J Neurosci. 2008;28:6030–6.

13. Chakrabarty P, Rosario A, Cruz P, Siemienski Z, Ceballos-Diaz C, Crosby K, et al. Capsid Serotype and Timing of Injection Determines AAV Transduction in the Neonatal Mice Brain. PLoS One. 2013;8:e67680.

14. Fecto F, Yan J, Vemula SP, Liu E, Yang Y, Chen W, et al. SQSTM1 mutations in familial and sporadic amyotrophic lateral sclerosis. Arch Neurol. 2011;68:1440–6.

15. Sacino AN, Brooks M, Thomas MA, McKinney AB, McGarvey NH, Rutherford NJ, et al. Amyloidogenic alpha-synuclein seeds do not invariably induce rapid, widespread pathology in mice. Acta Neuropathol. 2014;127:645–65.

16. Nolle A, van Haastert ES, Zwart R, Hoozemans JJ, Scheper W. Ubiquilin 2 is not associated with tau pathology. PLoS One. 2013;8:e76598.

17. Fecto F, Siddique T. Making connections: pathology and genetics link amyotrophic lateral sclerosis with frontotemporal lobe dementia. J Mol Neurosci. 2011;45:663–75.

18. Wu S, Mikhailov A, Kallo-Hosein H, Hara K, Yonezawa K, Avruch J. Characterization of ubiquilin 1, an mTOR-interacting protein. Biochim Biophys Acta. 2002;1542:41–56.

19. Xia Y, Yan LH, Huang B, Liu M, Liu X, Huang C. Pathogenic mutation of UBQLN2 impairs its interaction with UBXD8 and disrupts endoplasmic reticulum-associated protein degradation. J Neurochem. 2014;129:99–106.

20. Cassel JA, Reitz AB. Ubiquilin-2 (UBQLN2) binds with high affinity to the C-terminal region of TDP-43 and modulates TDP-43 levels in H4 cells: characterization of inhibition by nucleic acids and 4-aminoquinolines. Biochim Biophys Acta. 1834;2013:964–71.

21. DATATOP. a multicenter controlled clinical trial in early Parkinson's disease. Parkinson Study Group. Arch Neurol. 1989;46:1052–60.

22. Ilieva H, Polymenidou M, Cleveland DW. Non-cell autonomous toxicity in neurodegenerative disorders: ALS and beyond. J Cell Biol. 2009;187:761–72.

23. Zolotukhin S, Potter M, Zolotukhin I, Sakai Y, Loiler S, Fraites Jr TJ, et al. Production and purification of serotype 1, 2, and 5 recombinant adeno-associated viral vectors. Methods. 2002;28:158–67.

24. Sacino AN, Thomas MA, Ceballos-Diaz C, Cruz PE, Rosario AM, Lewis J, et al. Conformational templating of alpha-synuclein aggregates in neuronal-glial cultures. Mol Neurodegener. 2013;8:17.

25. Lalonde R, Eyer J, Wunderle V, Strazielle C. Characterization of NFH-LacZ transgenic mice with the SHIRPA primary screening battery and tests of motor coordination, exploratory activity, and spatial learning. Behav Processes. 2003;63:9–19.

26. Waxman EA, Duda JE, Giasson BI. Characterization of antibodies that selectively detect alpha-synuclein in pathological inclusions. Acta Neuropathol. 2008;116:37–46.

12

Brca1 is expressed in human microglia and is dysregulated in human and animal model of ALS

Harun Najib Noristani[1†], Jean Charles Sabourin[2†], Yannick Nicolas Gerber[1,2], Marisa Teigell[1], Andreas Sommacal[3], Maria dM Vivanco[4], Markus Weber[3] and Florence Evelyne Perrin[1,2,5*]

Abstract

Background: There is growing evidence that microglia are key players in the pathological process of amyotrophic lateral sclerosis (ALS). It is suggested that microglia have a dual role in motoneurone degeneration through the release of both neuroprotective and neurotoxic factors.

Results: To identify candidate genes that may be involved in ALS pathology we have analysed at early symptomatic age (P90), the molecular signature of microglia from the lumbar region of the spinal cord of hSOD1[G93A] mice, the most widely used animal model of ALS. We first identified unique hSOD1[G93A] microglia transcriptomic profile that, in addition to more classical processes such as chemotaxis and immune response, pointed toward the potential involvement of the tumour suppressor gene breast cancer susceptibility gene 1 (Brca1). Secondly, comparison with our previous data on hSOD1[G93A] motoneurone gene profile substantiated the putative contribution of Brca1 in ALS. Finally, we established that Brca1 protein is specifically expressed in human spinal microglia and is up-regulated in ALS patients.

Conclusions: Overall, our data provide new insights into the pathogenic concept of a non-cell-autonomous disease and the involvement of microglia in ALS. Importantly, the identification of Brca1 as a novel microglial marker and as possible contributor in both human and animal model of ALS may represent a valid therapeutic target. Moreover, our data points toward novel research strategies such as investigating the role of oncogenic proteins in neurodegenerative diseases.

Keywords: Microglia, Transcriptomics, hSOD1[G93A] mice, ALS patients, Brca1

Background

Amyotrophic lateral sclerosis (ALS) is characterised by selective motoneurones degeneration in the spinal cord, brainstem and motor cortex leading to progressive muscle weakness, atrophy and paralysis. Approximately 90 % of ALS patients are sporadic whilst 10 % are familial cases with genetic mutations in SOD1 (Cu/Zn superoxide dismutase 1), FUS (fused in sarcoma), TARDBP (also known as TDP-43) and C9ORF72, among others [1]. Transgenic mice over-expressing the human mutated gene for SOD1 develop an adult-onset paralysis that closely recapitulates human ALS [2]. Recent studies have established that ALS is a complex multi-factorial disease that involves several cellular partners including glial cells [3].

Microglia, the resident immune cells of the central nervous system (CNS), when activated, release pro- and anti-inflammatory cytokines and chemokines that are generally associated with M1 and M2 phenotypes [4, 5]. Microglia have a dual role in ALS with an early protective effect on motoneurones but also a detrimental effect due to the secretion of neurotoxic factors [6]. It is hypothesised that progressive motoneurone death results from the combination of intrinsic motoneurones vulnerability and toxicity from neighbouring cells such as microglia [6]. In ALS patients and animal models, there is a clear microglia activation [3], in particular we have shown an early involvement of microglia in hSOD1[G93A] mice [7]. Understanding the contribution of microglia to motoneurone degeneration is of high priority. One means of analysing the role of a cell population in a process network is to study gene expression alterations in this given population. In

* Correspondence: florence.perrin@inserm.fr

†Equal contributors

[1]Institute for Neurosciences of Montpellier (INM), INSERM U1051, 80, rue Augustin Fliche, 34091 Montpellier, Cedex 5, France

[2]"Integrative Biology of Neurodegeneration", IKERBASQUE Basque Foundation for Science and Neuroscience Department, University of the Basque Country, Bilbao, Spain

Full list of author information is available at the end of the article

addition, an integrative comparison of the specific molecular signatures of several cellular partners is necessary to decipher the crosstalk between these cells. We have previously identified gene dysregulation in pure motoneurones from the lumbar spinal cord of hSOD1^{G93A} mice [8] and two other mouse models of motoneurone disease [9]. We revealed a unique motoneurone gene expression profile characterised by an absence of dysregulation of genes associated with cell death and a massive up-regulation of genes involved in cell growth [8].

Growing evidence points toward mitochondrial dysfunction and oxidative DNA damage in ALS [10]. Defence mechanisms, including SOD, counteract excessive accumulation of reactive oxygen species, however in ALS, cellular antioxidant defences are insufficient leading to damage of nucleic acids, proteins and lipids [11]. Inherited mutations in breast cancer susceptibility gene 1 (Brca1), a well-known tumour suppressor implicated in familial breast and ovarian cancers, is one of the best defined risk factor for development of breast and ovarian cancer. Brca1 plays important roles in a broad spectrum of functions including transcription regulation, cell cycle checkpoint activation, apoptosis, chromosomal remodelling, ubiquitination and DNA repair [12]. The role of Brca1 in each of these processes remains to be fully understood but it is hypothesized that it act as a scaffold for the formation of complexes with a wide range of proteins [13]. This ability of Brca1 to interact with different proteins may underlie its involvement in a variety of cellular processes [13]. Brca1 also exerts a protective role against oxidative stress via up-regulation of antioxidant genes and maintenance of the redox balance through up-regulating the expression of heat shock protein HSP27 [14, 15].

In breast cancer, Brca1 cellular localisation as well as the significance of its altered localisation, is still a matter of debate. It had been recently shown that in normal breast, Brca1 nuclear expression is strong and uniform in parenchymal cells whereas in malignant cells its expression is reduced if not absent from the nucleus and is, in some cases, observed in the cytoplasm [16]. Interestingly, altered expression of Brca1 was associated with poor prognosis and shortened survival. In the adult rodent CNS, the presence of Brca1 is detected only in neurons [17] whereas a high Brca1 expression is observed in embryonic [17, 18] and adult neural stem cells and is involved in cell proliferation [18].

Here we identify putative Brca1 involvement in ALS via hSOD1^{G93A} microglia gene profiling and comparisons to our previous transcriptomic findings in hSOD1^{G93A} motoneurones. We then demonstrated that Brca1 is a novel marker of human microglia and is up-regulated in ALS patients.

Results

Transcriptomic analysis of FACS isolated microglia from control and hSOD1^{G93A} lumber spinal cord

We have previously described early microglial disturbances in hSOD1^{G93A} male mice reflected at P90 by a heterogeneous Iba1$^+$ microglial distribution with higher density within the grey matter in hSOD1^{G93A} mice as compared to control [7, 19]. Since activated microglia/macrophages exhibit increased CD11b expression, we carried out CD11b immunostaining (Fig. 1a & b). CD11b-positive microglia displayed enlarged somata with short and thick processes that are typical of a reactive phenotype and were predominantly found in hSOD1^{G93A} mice (Fig. 1b). To further analyse transcriptomic modification specifically in microglia, we isolated microglia of hSOD1^{G93A} and control littermate males at early symptomatic age (P90) from the lumbar spinal cord (L1-L5) that corresponds to the onset of degeneration. Microglia were isolated by fluorescence-activated cell sorting (FACS) using CD11b (Fig. 1c–e). We observed a 1.65-fold increase in the total number of CD11b$^+$ microglia in hSOD1^{G93A} versus controls (26 350; $n = 15$ in hSOD1^{G93A} and 15 900; $n = 26$ in control; Fig. 1c & d). RNA extracted from FACS purified microglia was of high quality (Fig. 1f) and microarrays analysis revealed 630 dysregulated genes (260 down-regulated and 370 up-regulated, Additional file 1: Table S1).

Cross-talk between microglia and motoneurones

We had previously identified dysregulated genes in hSOD1^{G93A} motoneuronse during disease progression [8, 9]. To unravel potential molecular cross-talk between microglia and motoneurones, we performed a comparative analysis of gene dysregulation in both cell populations. Comparison of dysregulated genes at P90 between motoneurones (102 genes) and microglia (668 genes) revealed 19 common genes (Additional file 2: Figure S1A). Process network rankings were clearly different in the commonly dysregulated genes (in motoneurones and microglia) and uniquely dysregulated genes. Antigen presentation was classified first in the common group, whilst cytoskeleton and cytoplasmic microtubules genes were top ranked in motoneurones only set (Additional file 3: Table S2A). Similarly, cellular processes analysis ranked first immune response and antigen presentation in the common group whereas response to stress, regulation of immune response, system development and wounding response were the top 4 ranked processes in motoneurones only group (Additional file 3: Table S2B). Signalling and metabolic pathway analysis revealed immune response and cytoskeleton remodelling as first ranked in the commonly and motoneurone

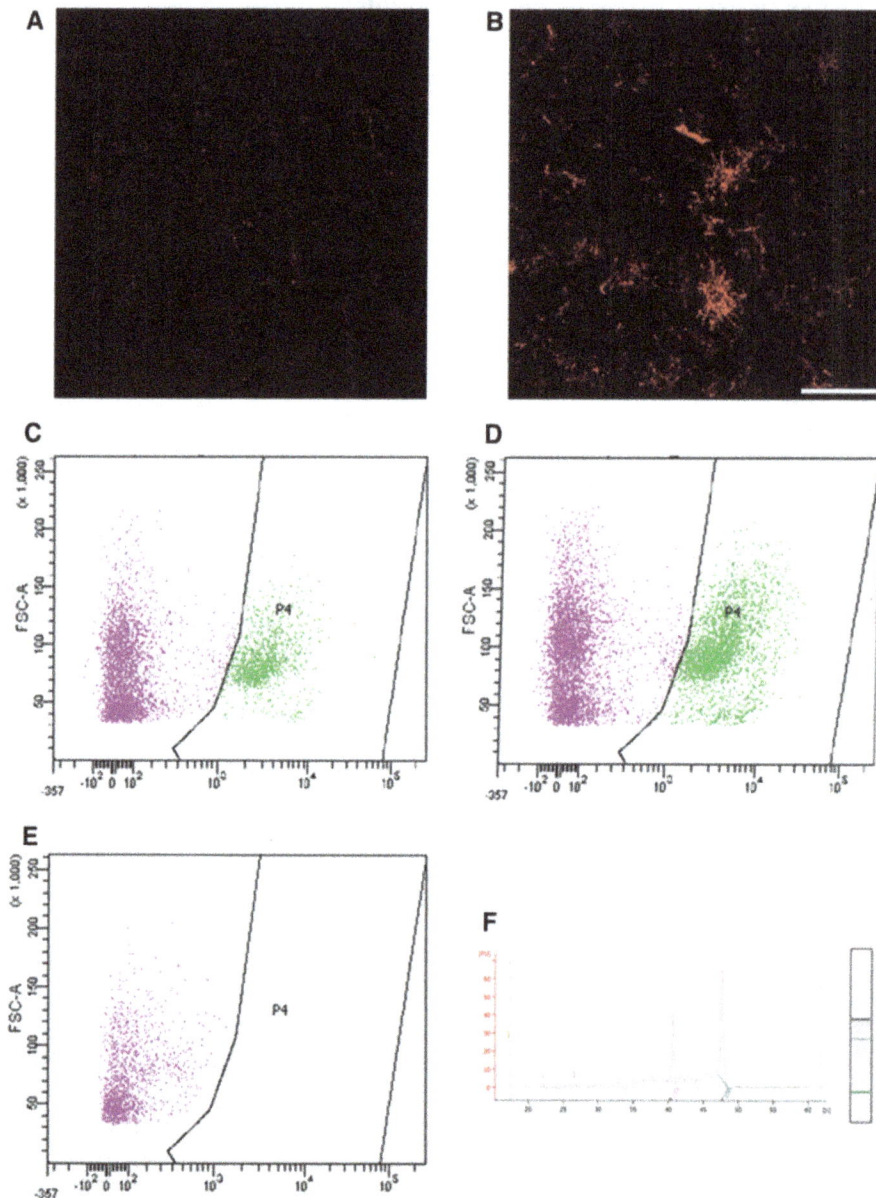

Fig. 1 FACS analysis of CD11b+ microglia in control and hSOD1^{G93A} mice from the lumbar segment of the spinal cords at 90 days of age. Microglia were sorted by flow cytometry using the microglia marker CD11b. **a** Confocal images of CD11b expression in spinal cord microglia from control at 90 day of age and (**b**) from transgenic hSOD1^{G93A} mice at early symptomatic age. *Scale bars* (**a & b**): 50 μm. **c–d** Representative flow cytometry analysis dot plot displaying microglia profiles. **c** Control and (**d**) hSOD1^{G93A} spinal microglia at P90. In both (**c**) control and (**d**) hSOD1^{G93A} surrounded areas, designed as *"P4"*, correspond to the labelled cells. **e** Negative control (without CD11b labelling). The X-axis represents the intensity of fluorescence and the Y axis the size of the cells. **f** RNA quality isolated from FACSed microglia

only dysregulated genes, respectively (Additional file 3: Table S2C).

We have previously shown that microglial reactivity precedes neuronal death in hSOD1^{G93A} mice [7]; to seek for potential modifications in microglia that could trigger motoneurone death, we compared dysregulated genes at P90 in microglia and P120 in motoneurones. Our previous microarrays analysis of microdissected motoneurones at the end stage of the disease (P120)

showed no dysregulation of genes associated with cell death [8], this most likely reflects that dissected motoneurones were at an early demise stage. Indeed, we selected motoneurones that had an identifiable nucleus and a diameter of at least 25 μm, picking a subpopulation of neurones that may resist degeneration. Three hundred twenty genes were uniquely dysregulated in hSOD1^{G93A} motoneurones; 603 uniquely dysregulated in hSOD1^{G93A} microglia; 65 genes were common (Additional file 2: Figure S1B). Clear differences were highlighted not only between the genes that were commonly and uniquely dysregulated but also in the ranking as compared to the previous analysis (microglia and motoneurones at P90, Additional file 4: Table S3). Particularly, inflammation and immune response were ranked top in motoneurones (Additional file 4: Table S3A). Interestingly, signalling and metabolic pathway analysis revealed the involvement of heme metabolism and DNA damage in both motoneurones and microglia (Additional file 4: Table S3C).

Unique transcriptomic profiles of hSOD1^{G93A} microglia

To identify processes and pathways modified in hSOD1^{G93A} microglia, we carried out gene ontology enrichment and network analysis (Additional file 5: Table S4A–C; Fig. 2). Process network analysis ranked as first chemotaxis (Additional file 5: Table S4A, Fig. 2a) with 23 dysregulated transcripts out of 137 annotated genes in this process (17 %, $p = 2.1$E-08) (Additional file 5: Table S4A). Out of the 18 most significantly dysregulated genes, 4 were down-regulated with a maximum of 2-fold whereas 14 were up-regulated (Fig. 2a). The gene coding for osteopontin (SPP1) presents a 16.8-fold increase (Additional file 1: Table S1). Regulation of angiogenesis (ranked 8th, Additional file 5: Table S4A, Fig. 2e) displayed 22 dysregulated genes (223 genes in this process, 9.8 %, $p = 7.3$E-04), with 16 being up-regulated. Inflammation network was also dysregulated in hSOD1^{G93A} microglia (ranked 9th, 9 % of the annotated genes in this process, $p = 1.4$E-04, Additional file 5: Table S4A, Fig. 2d) with 14 up-regulated genes (including a 12.6 fold increase for IGF-1, Fig. 2d). GO cellular processes analysis ranked immune response as first (61/1505 genes, 4 %, $p = 1.3$E-18, Additional file 5: Table S4B, Fig. 2b). Out of the 38 most significantly dysregulated genes 5 were down-regulated with a maximum of 2.97-fold decrease for the gene coding for alpha-synuclein, whereas 33 were up-regulated. Genes coding for CCL5 (5.1-fold change (FC)) and CXCL13 (5.7-FC) were the most up-regulated (Additional file 1: Table S1). Regulation of blood coagulation was ranked 3rd (50/665 genes, 7.5 %, $p = 1.8$E-09, Additional file 5: Table S4B, Fig. 2f). Amongst the 29 most significantly dysregulated genes 8 were down-regulated and 21 were up-regulated. Hypoxia was the 4th dysregulated cellular processes (31/416 genes, 7.45 %, $p = 8.3$E-09, Additional file 5: Table S4B). Out of the 20 most significantly dysregulated genes 4 were down-regulated and 16 were up-regulated (Fig. 2c).

Breast cancer 1 (Brca1) pathway is dysregulated in hSOD1^{G93A} mice

Pathways map analysis ranked as the third position DNA damage and specifically the involvement of Brca1

as a transcription regulator (Additional file 5: Table S4C, Figs. 2g and 3). Indeed, in hSOD1^{G93A} microglia (7/30 genes, 23 %; $p = 1.6$E-05, Additional file 5: Table S4C) were dysregulated in the canonical Brca1 pathway. GADD45α and SP3 transcription factor were downregulated with FC of 2.6 and 1.9, respectively. Genes coding for p21 (2.18-FC), PCNA (1.85-FC), STAT1 (1.9-FC), c-Myc (1.8-FC) and Brca1 (1.76-FC) were up-regulated (Additional file 1: Table S1 and Fig. 2g). Concomitant dysregulation of these genes clearly pointed toward a potential involvement of Brca1 as a transcription regulator (Fig. 2g and red and blue thermometers labelled in Fig. 3). Interestingly, even if Brca1 transcript itself was not dysregulated in motoneurones, 4 genes that are involved in Brca1 pathway were also up-regulated in hSOD1^{G93A} motoneurones namely p21: 7.88-FC; GADD45α: 5.19-FC; Rb protein: 2.44-FC and ATF-1: 2.38-FC, (Fig. 2h and red thermometers labelled 2 in Fig. 3). To confirm microarray findings, we carried out quantitative real-time polymerase chain reaction (qPCR) in pure populations of hSOD1^{G93A} and wild type microglia and assessed the expression profiles of all candidate genes involved in Brca1 pathway (Additional file 6: Figure S2). In addition, we have also included microglial samples at 60 days of age to assess the potential involvement of microglial Brca1 at the initial stages of the disease progression in hSOD1^{G93A} mice (Additional file 6: Figure S2A). Our qPCR results showed no significant dysregulation of the genes involved in Brca1 pathway at 60 days of age (Additional file 6: Figure S2A). However, at 90 days of age, and similarly to our microarrays results, we found up-regulation of Brca1, Cdkn1a, Myc, Pcna and Stat1 as well as down-regulation of Gadd45a and Sp3 in hSOD1^{G93A} microglia (Additional file 6: Figure S2B). It is important to note that dysregulation in Cdkn1a, Myc, Pcna, Stat1, Gadd45a and Sp3 transcripts may also be involved in other signalling pathways. These findings confirm Brca1 involvement in hSOD1^{G93A} microglia is specifically triggered at 90 days of age when the pronounced microgliosis becomes evident.

Brca1 protein is expressed in human microglia and is up-regulated in ALS patients

To investigate Brca1 protein expression in human microglia, we performed dual immunofluorescence labelling using Brca1 and CD11b antibodies (Fig. 4). Brca1 staining in human control samples revealed ramified microglial population throughout the spinal cord displaying small cell bodies with long and thin processes (Fig. 4a & d) that co-localised with CD11b-positive microglia (Fig. 4b & e, c & f). Similarly, single immunoperoxidase detection of Brca1 revealed microglial profile that were identical to Iba1 (the most commonly used

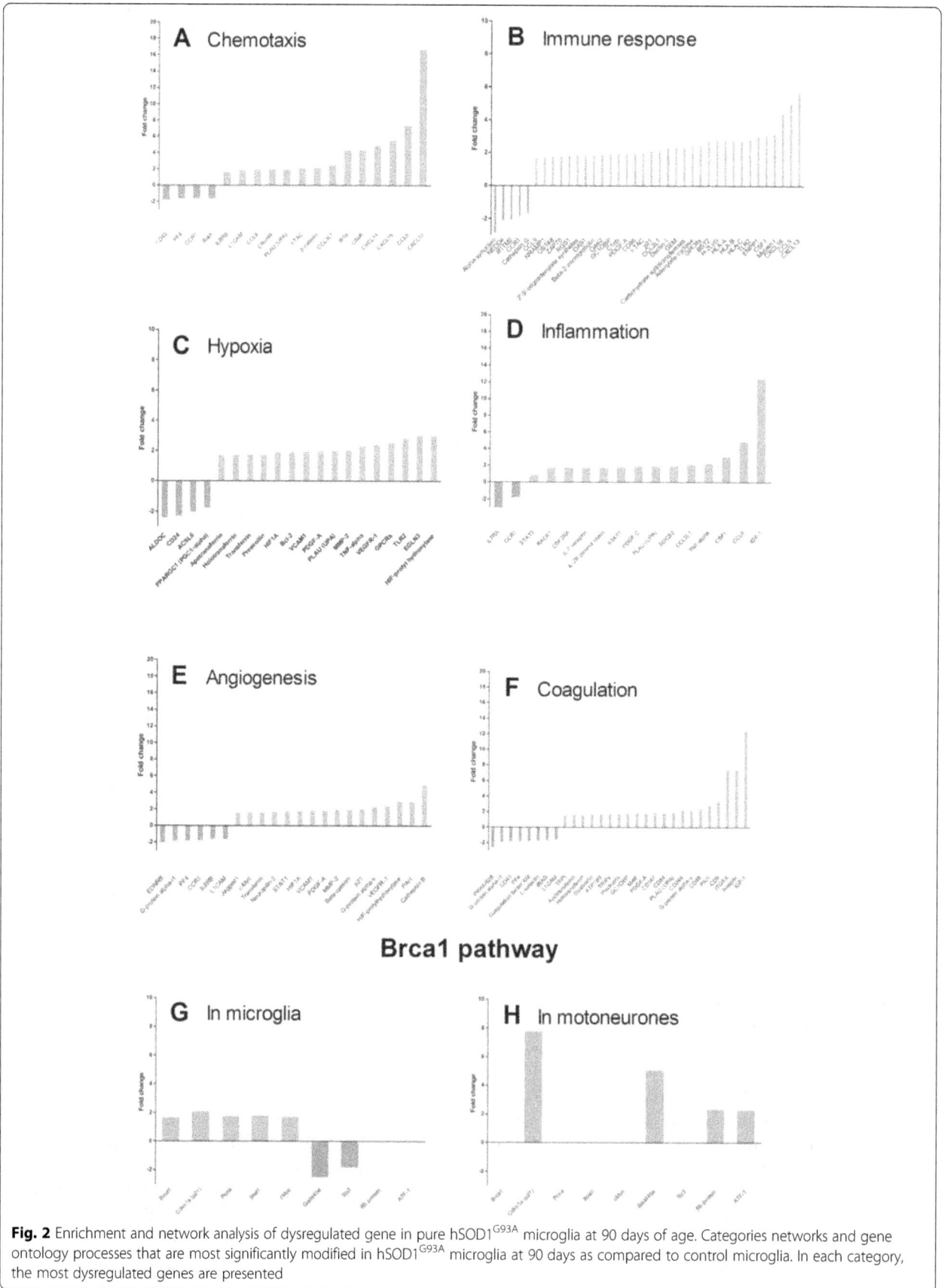

Brca1 pathway

Fig. 2 Enrichment and network analysis of dysregulated gene in pure hSOD1^{G93A} microglia at 90 days of age. Categories networks and gene ontology processes that are most significantly modified in hSOD1^{G93A} microglia at 90 days as compared to control microglia. In each category, the most dysregulated genes are presented

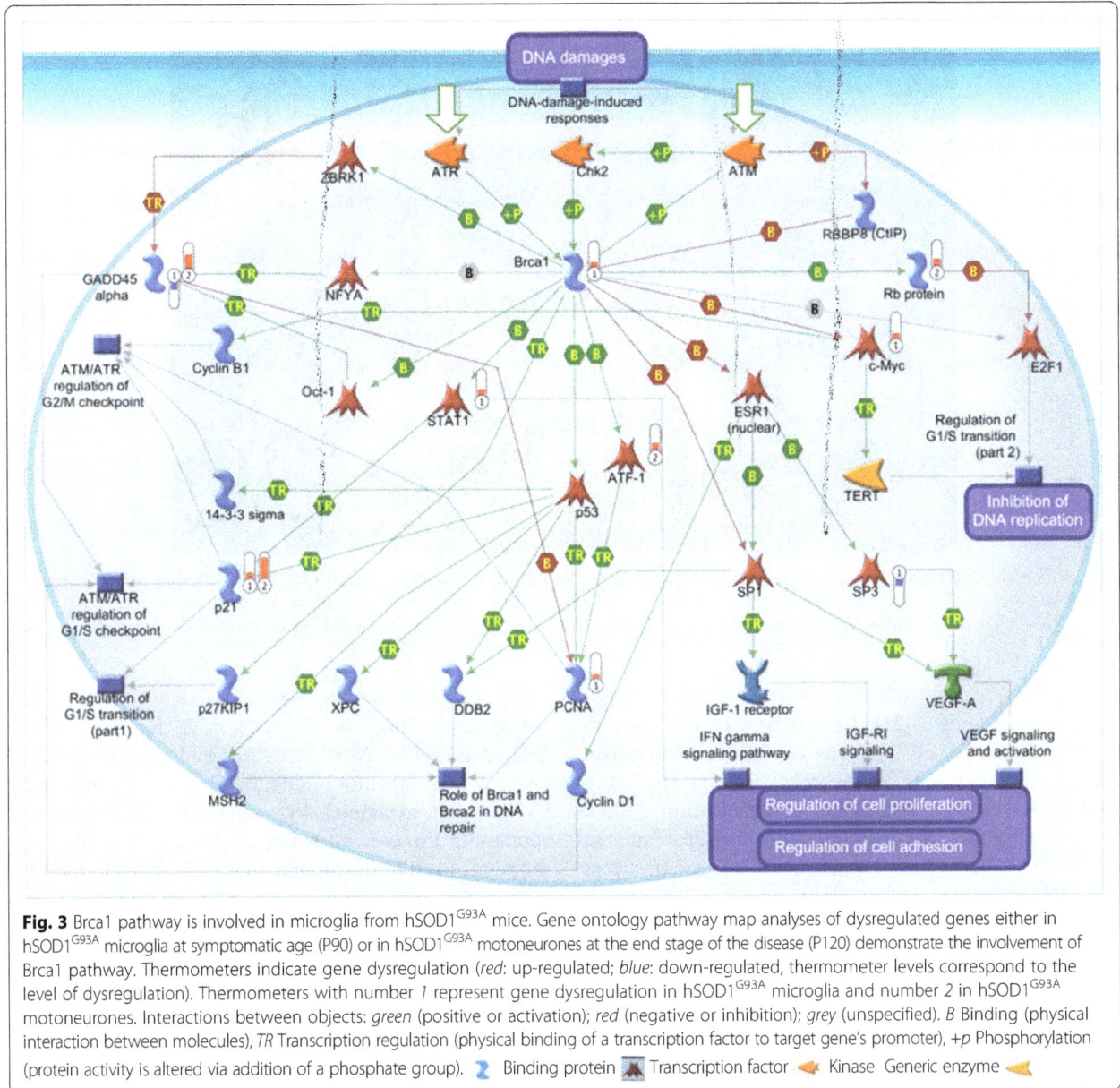

Fig. 3 Brca1 pathway is involved in microglia from hSOD1^{G93A} mice. Gene ontology pathway map analyses of dysregulated genes either in hSOD1^{G93A} microglia at symptomatic age (P90) or in hSOD1^{G93A} motoneurones at the end stage of the disease (P120) demonstrate the involvement of Brca1 pathway. Thermometers indicate gene dysregulation (*red*: up-regulated; *blue*: down-regulated, thermometer levels correspond to the level of dysregulation). Thermometers with number *1* represent gene dysregulation in hSOD1^{G93A} microglia and number *2* in hSOD1^{G93A} motoneurones. Interactions between objects: *green* (positive or activation); *red* (negative or inhibition); *grey* (unspecified). *B* Binding (physical interaction between molecules), *TR* Transcription regulation (physical binding of a transcription factor to target gene's promoter), *+p* Phosphorylation (protein activity is altered via addition of a phosphate group). Binding protein Transcription factor Kinase Generic enzyme

microglia marker) using adjacent human spinal cord sections (Fig. 5). Ramified microglia were evident in control cases following both Brca1 and Iba1 immunoperoxidase labelling (Fig. 5a–d). On the other hand, Brca1-positive microglia displayed enlarged cell bodies with short/thick processes in ALS cases similar to Iba1 immunostaining (Fig. 5e–h).

Finally, to determine Brca1 dysregulation in ALS, we quantified Brca1 immunoreactivity between the control and ALS spinal cords (Fig. 6). Brca1 expression was more evident in ALS compared to control cases (Fig. 6a & b, c & d). Quantitative analysis revealed a significant 78.2 % increase in Brca1 intensity within the white matter in ALS samples compared to controls (26.4 vs 47.1,

$p = 0.015$; Fig. 6e). Within the grey matter, we observed a 32.8 % increase in Brca1 intensity in ALS samples compared to controls, however data variations in control samples kept them from attaining statistical significance (49.7 vs 66, $p = 0.0545$; Fig. 6f).

Discussion

Non-cell autonomous toxicity plays a major role in ALS [20] but microglia participation is dual and complex. Microglia reactivity over the course of the disease may be characterised by a continuum of activation states from a M2 neuroprotective state to a deleterious M1 state. In culture, microglia have, at disease onset, a M2 phenotype whereas they are typified by a M1 phenotype

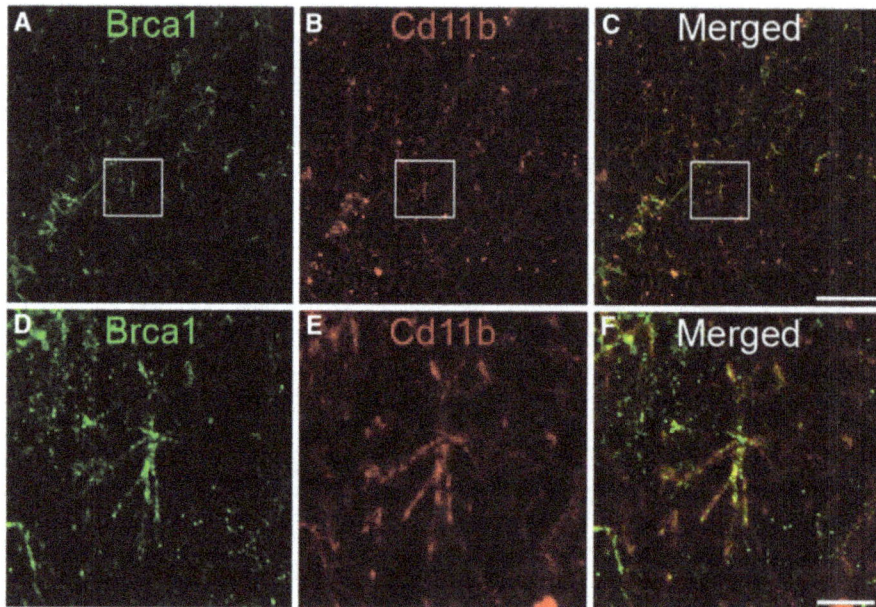

Fig. 4 Microglial expression of Brca1 in human spinal cords. Confocal micrographs displaying Brca1 (**a**, **d**), CD11b (**b**, **e**) and dual Brca1/CD11b expression (**c**, **f**) expression by microglia within the human spinal cord. Brca1 labelled microglia displayed typical ramified morphology with small cell bodies and large and thin processes that completely colocalised with CD11b-positive microglia (**c** & **f**). *Scale bars* (**a**–**c**): 50 μm; (**d**–**f**): 10 μm

at disease end-stage [21]. Comparison of our data to previous studies [21, 22] reveals an up-regulation of five M2 priming genes (*Clec7a*, *Igf1*, *Mmp12*, *Spp1* and *Lgals3*) and a down-regulation of *Retnla* and *F13a1*. Interestingly, four M1 priming genes are up-regulated *CD86*, *Tnfα*, *Bcl2a1*a and *Cxcl10*, whilst growth arrest and DNA-damage-inducible alpha gene (*Gadd45gip1*) is down-regulated. A previous study has reported the gene-expression profile of isolated microglia in hSOD1^{G93A} mice and shown that potentially neuroprotective and neurotoxic factors are induced concurrently during disease progression [23]. The authors have analysed microglia from the entire spinal cord whereas we have restricted our investigations to the lumbar segment where onset of degeneration occurs. We report that hSOD1^{G93A} microglia from the lumbar region of the spinal cord over-express *progranulin*, *Igf1* and *osteopontin*, all potential neurotrophic factors, and thus confirmed findings from a previous study [23]. Interestingly, we had previously identified in pure motoneurones of two mouse models of motoneurone disease (hSOD1^{G93A} and *pmn*) an increase in *IGFBP*. Also, an *IGFBP* that binds to *IGF-1* and *IGF-2* (nephroblastoma over-expressed gene) was up-regulated at all disease stages in hSOD1^{G93A} mice [8] and *IGFBP4* mRNA was induced at pre-symptomatic age in *pmn* mice [9]. We also confirmed the up-regulation of potential neurotoxic factors (including *Mmp12*, *tnf-α* and interferon-induced protein with tetratricopeptide repeats) [23]. However, we did not confirm the dysregulation of

the genes coding for *IL-1β*, *IL-α*, *IL-10*, *Ifnar 1* and *Ifnar 2* as well as *Nox2* at P90. It had been shown that delayed forelimb motor impairment in ALS mice may be partially explained by augmented protective responses in the cervical spinal cords [24], thus gene expression profile of lumbar hSOD1^{G93A} microglia is potentially more homogenous and is more likely to reflect a pathological gene profile than microglia taken from the entire spinal cord. Together, these data confirm that microglia activation states are best characterised as a continuum of M2 and M1 states [21] with a M2 phenotype at early stage of the disease that evolves into a M1 phenotype at disease end-stage.

An unexpected finding was the up-regulation in hSOD1^{G93A} microglia of *Brca1* with a 1.76 fold. Using *in silico* comparison with data from Chiu et al. [23], we found that *Brca1* was also deregulated in their study and presented a steady increased with 2.78 and 3.08 fold changes at P100 and P130, respectively. In our study, *Brca1* involvement was substantiated by the concomitant dysregulation of a number of other genes. As previously stated, *Igf1* was robustly up-regulated in hSOD1^{G93A} microglia; a complex interplay between *Brca1* and *IGF* signalling pathways had been reported in familial cancer, in particular through the convergence of Brca1-mediated tumour protective pathways and IGF1 receptors-mediated cell survival [25, 26]. This simultaneous up-regulation may represent a potential neuroprotective phenotype of microglia in ALS

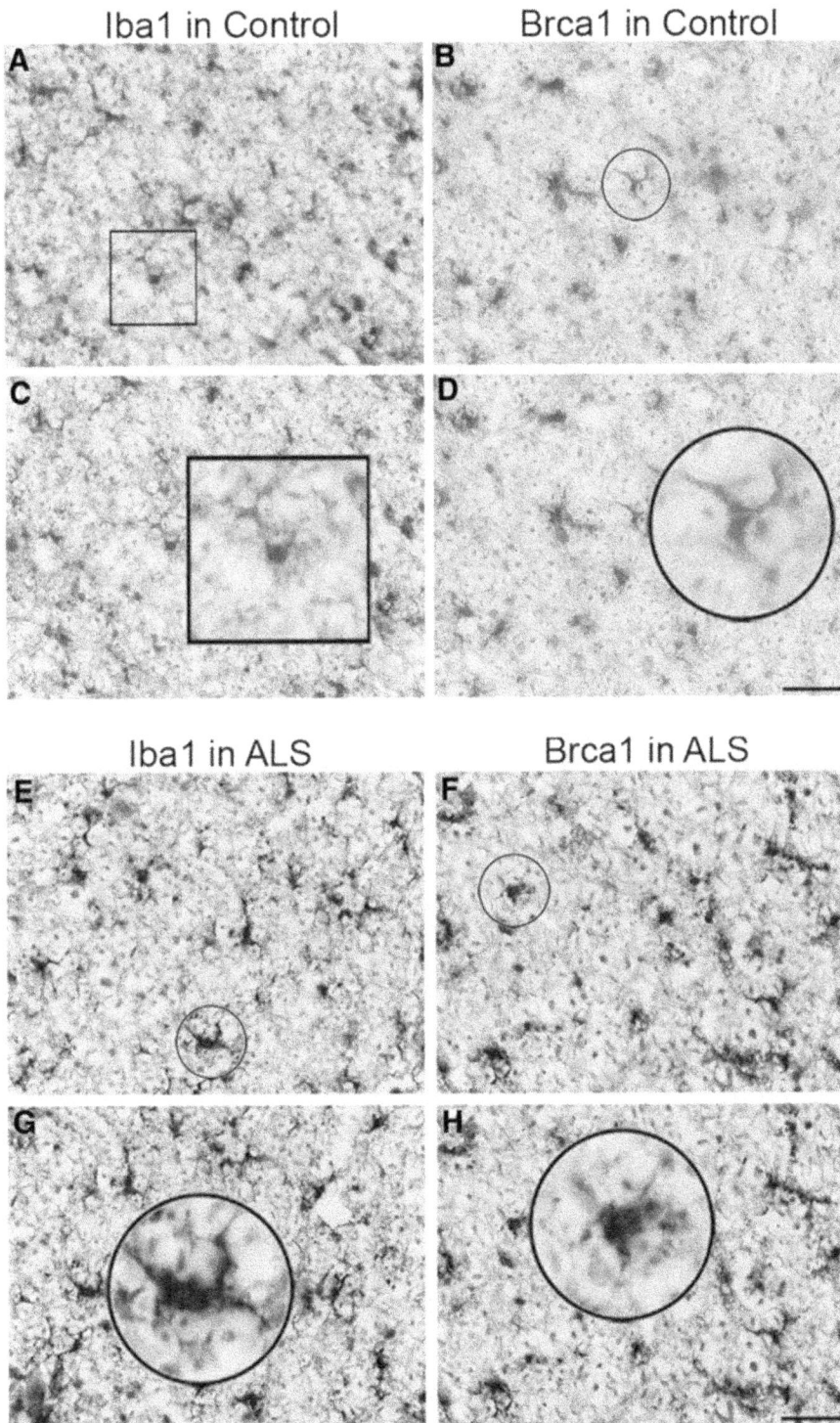

Fig. 5 Microglial Iba1 and Brca1 expression within adjacent human control and ALS spinal cord. Brightfield micrographs indicating Iba1 and Brca1 expression within adjacent sections of control (**a–d**) and ALS (**e–h**) spinal cords. Both Ibal and Brca1-labelled microglia displayed typical ramified morphology in the control spinal cords with small cell bodies and large and thin processes (**c & d**). Microglial morphology displayed similar features following Iba1 (**a & c**) and Brca1 (**b & d**) immuno staining. In ALS spinal cords, Ibal and Brca1-labelled microglia displayed both ramified and activated microglia with enlarged cell bodies and short and thick processes (**g & h**). Microglial morphology were similar using Iba1 (**e & g**) or Brca1 (**f & h**) immuno staining. *Scale bars* (**a–h**): 50 μm

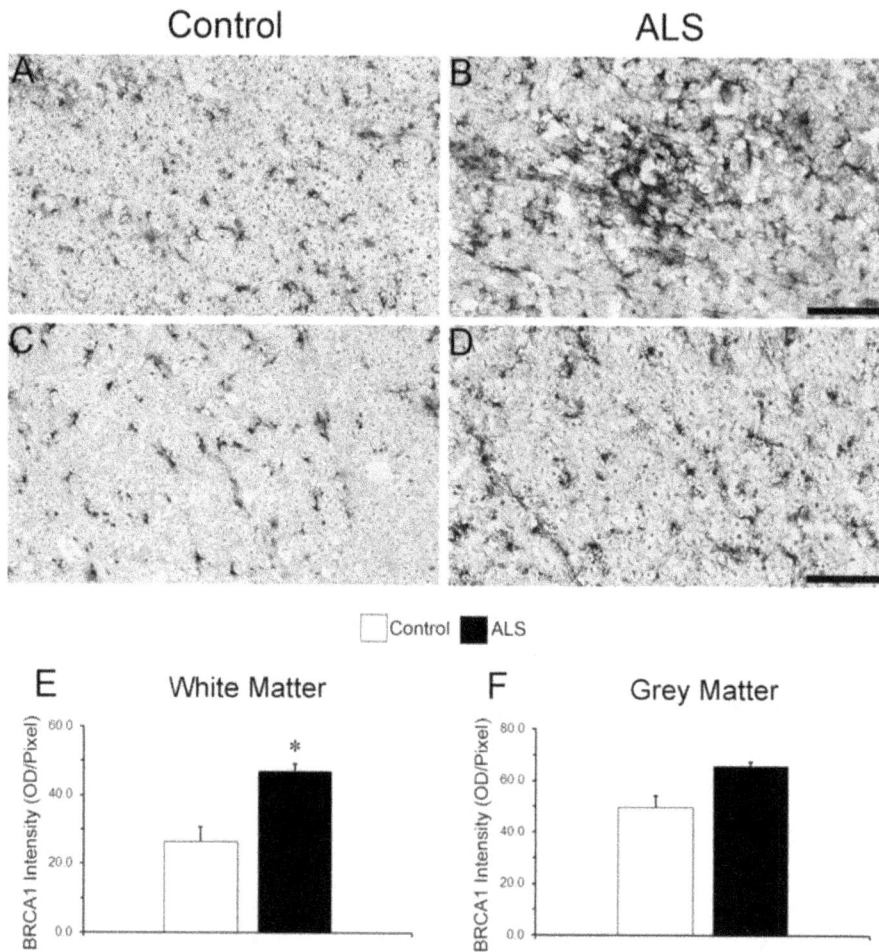

Fig. 6 Up-regulation of microglial Brca1 expression in human ALS spinal cords. Brightfield micrographs displaying Brca1 expression within the spinal cords of control (**a & c**) and ALS cases (**b & d**). *Bar graphs* showing the increase in Brca1 intensity within the white (**e**) and grey (**f**) matters of the spinal cord in ALS compared to control cases. *Bars* represent mean ± SEM ($n = 5$ for ALS and 14 for controls). *$p < 0.05$. *Scale bar* (**a–d**): 100 μm

at early stage. Converging elements toward the involvement of Brca1 was also pointed through the dysregulation of genes linked to *Brca1* and belonging to the DNA damage pathway (Fig. 3). Indeed, *GADD45* was down-regulated in hSOD1^{G93A} microglia (P90) and up-regulated in motoneurones (P120) and it had been demonstrated that *Brca1* can modulate *GADD45* that in turn mediates DNA repair mechanisms and regulates growth arrest [15]. Importantly, we found that the gene coding for cyclin-dependent kinase inhibitor 1A (*p21*) was up-regulated both in hSOD1^{G93A} microglia (P90) and motoneurones (P120). Indeed, *p21* is a downstream target of *p53* and regulates several processes such as DNA repair, cell cycle arrest, cell differentiation and apoptosis. Through its antioxidant effects, *p21* also protects cells from oxidative damage *in vitro* and *in vivo* [15]. Activation of microglial cells and acquisition of deleterious M1 state is associated with an increased

generation of reactive oxygen species (ROS) [27] that is likely to participate in motoneurone demise. Polarisation of microglia/macrophages to pro- and anti-inflammatory states is driven by cytokines and other factors such as ROS within the tissue microenvironment [28]. While the functional role of deregulated *Brca1* pathway in microglia remains to be determined, one hypothesis is that it may represent an attempt to counteract the detrimental effects of ROS and reflect an antioxidative defence mechanism through modulation of microglia polarisation.

Brca1 is implicated in a broad spectrum of functions; it regulates transcription and cell cycle progression, it is also involved in function that preserve genomic stability such as DNA repair pathways [29] and protection against oxidative damage to DNA. Many of these functions have been associated with CNS development but also with neurodegenerative diseases and in particular with ALS. Brca1 is required for normal cerebral cortex size development [30] by preventing apoptosis [31]. Using a neural progenitor-specific driver to delete *Brca1*, Pao et al. demonstrated an important role of *Brca1* in apoptotic and centrosomal functions in neuronal progenitors that may underlie DNA damage and brain size during development [31]. *Brca1* is also associated with lack of spinal cord neural tube closure in *spina bifida* meningomyelocele [32, 33]. Moreover, *Brca1*-deficient embryos presented disorganised neuroepithelium associated with rapid proliferation and enhanced cell death [32].

De-regulation in *Brca1* expression had been reported in Alzheimer's [34, 35] and Huntington's diseases [36]. Even though motor neuron diseases are not typical paraneoplastic syndromes, association with breast cancer had been regularly reported [37–41]. Moreover, there are occasional reports on improvement of motor neuron syndrome after cancer treatment [42–44].

Conclusion

Here we identify putative *Brca1* involvement in ALS via hSOD1^{G93A} microglia gene profiling and comparisons to our previous transcriptomic findings in hSOD1^{G93A} motoneurones. Nevertheless, mRNA up-regulation of *Brca1* in hSOD1^{G93A} microglia could be simply anecdotal if it were restricted to a mouse model of ALS. This is not the case since we demonstrated that Brca1 protein is specifically expressed by human microglia and is significantly up-regulated in ALS patients.

These results substantiate that microglia are key non-cell autonomous players in the disease. Thus, the identification of the putative Brca1 involvement in a mouse model and human ALS provides new insights into the pathogenesis of ALS and points towards novel therapeutic targets.

Methods
Animals
Transgenic mice carrying the G93A human SOD1 mutation, B6SJL-Tg (SOD1-G93A)1Gur/J (ALS mice, high copy number) were purchased from The Jackson Laboratory (Bar Harbor, ME, USA) and bred on a B6SJL background. Transgenic mice were housed in controlled conditions (hygrometry, temperature and 12 h light/dark cycle). Ninety days old (P90, symptomatic) males were used for transcriptomic analysis and immunohistochemistry. Litter-matching between groups were done. We carried out all animal experiments in accordance with the guidelines approved by the French Ministry of Agriculture and following the European Council directive (2010/63/UE). We minimised the number and suffering of animals.

Flow cytometry sorting of spinal cord microglia from SOD^{G93A} and control littermate mice
Mice were deeply anesthetised with tribromoethanol (500 mg/kg) and intracardially perfused with cold RNAse-free 0.1 M phosphate base saline (PBS, Invitrogen, Carlsbad, USA); spinal cords were dissected. Only the lumbar (L1 - L5) segment was used and dissociated in 750 µl PBS, 100 µl trypsin 13 mg/ml, 100 µl hyaluronidase 7 mg/ml, 50 µl kinurenic acid 4 mg/ml (Sigma Aldrich, Saint Louis, USA) and 20 µl DNAseI 10 mg/ml (Roche, Rotkreuz, Switzerland) for 30 min at 37 °C. Finally, gentle mechanic dissociation was carried out by pipetting. Cell suspension was sieved on a 40 µm cell strainer (BD Biosciences, Franklin Lakes, USA). To eliminate myelin, cells were re-suspended in PBS-25 % sucrose and centrifuged for 20 min at 750 g. Cells were incubated for 20 min on ice in the primary antibody CD11b-APC 1/100 in PBS (BD biosciences, Franklin Lakes, USA) that specifically labels microglia. Cells were washed with cold PBS and re-suspended in PBS 7-AAD 2 µg/ml (Sigma Aldrich). Cells were sorted with a FACS ARIA (BD Biosciences, Franklin Lakes, USA), equipped with a 488 nm Laser Sapphire 488–20. Size threshold, morphology and 7-AAD were used to eliminate cellular debris and dead cells.

Microarray analysis of gene transcripts
Our data comply with the "Minimal Information About Microarray Experiment (MIAME)" guidelines. Total RNA was isolated using RNeasy Mini Kit, (Qiagen, Maryland, USA) including DNAse treatment to remove potential genomic DNA contamination. We tested the quality of the starting RNA and of the amplified cRNA (Agilent 2100 bioanalyzer, RNA 6000 Pico LabChip, Palo Alto, USA) and proceeded only if the RNA quality was satisfactory. A criterion was a cut point for RNA integrity number (RIN) at 7 [45]. Fifty nanograms of RNA per chip were hybridized (three chips per condition) following a T7-based double amplification procedure.

Hybridization targets were obtained following a double amplification procedure according to the protocol developed by Affymetrix (GeneChip® Eukaryotic Small Sample Target Labeling Assay Version II, Affymetrix, Santa Clara, USA) and previously used [8, 9]. A hybridization mixture containing 5.5 µg of biotinylated cRNA was generated. The biotinylated cRNA was hybridized to Affymetrix GeneChip® MOE 430 2.0. Three chips per group (wild type and hSOD1^{G93A}) were hybridized, each corresponding to microglia from at least six pooled mice. Chips were visualised on a 3000 gene scanner (Affymetrix, Santa Clara, USA). We selected the differentially expressed transcripts using the Affymetrix software MAS 5.0 and carried out pair-wise comparison analyses where each of the mutant samples was compared to each of their respective control samples. This analysis is based on the Mann–Whitney pair-wise comparison test and allows the ranking of the results by concordance as well as the calculation of significance (p value) of each identified gene expression [46, 47]. A gene must exhibit 50 % or more of the "present" calls in all samples to be considered "expressed" and has two or more "present" calls among the three sets of samples. Fold differences were calculated as the ratio between the average values within each condition. Signal values and detection calls (present or absent) for all samples were determined using Affymetrix MAS5.0. Based on power analysis, we had selected a cut off threshold of 1.75 (p (α) 0.05, β 0.80) to identify transcripts that are differentially expressed between the controls and hSOD1^{G93A} mutant mice. Statistics: t-test with un-equal variance. Pathway analysis was done with MetaCore (Thomson Reuters).

Quantitative real-time polymerase chain reaction

Candidate genes involved in Brca1 pathway were validated using qPCR. Similar to microarray, total RNA was extracted as described above from CD11-positive microglia isolated using FACS and used as a template in real time PCR. At least two animals were used for each analysis. To assess the involvement of microglia *Brca1* at initial stages of the disease progression, we carried out qPCR at 60 and 90 days of age in hSOD1^{G93A} and wild type mice. One round of amplification was done following the first cycle (first cDNA and cRNA synthesis) of the Affymetrix double amplification procedure before undertaking reverse transcription with random hexamers (Superscript II, Invitrogen, Carlsbad, CA). Real time PCR using Syber Green PCR Master Mix and Abi Prism SDS 7900 HT (Applied Biosystems, Foster City, CA) was done according to the manufacturer's protocol. All amplicons were designed within the 3′ end of the cDNA using Primer Express Software 2.0 (Applied Biosystems, Foster City, CA) and when possible, overlapped exon-exon junctions. For the sequences of the primers, see Additional file 7: Table S5. All samples were analysed in triplicate and the values were normalised to four reference genes mitochondrial ribosomal protein S9 (*RPS9*), TATA box binding protein (*TBP*), actin β and eukaryotic translation elongation factor 1 (*EEF1*).

Human spinal cord samples

Human low thoracic and lumbar (T11-L5) spinal cords were obtained from 14 controls (males and females; 23 to 74 years of age; mean age: 52.4 years) and five ALS patients (males and females; 66 to 79 years of age; mean age: 71 years) from the Kantonsspital St. Gallen Fachbereichsleiter Muskelzentrum/ALS clinic under the approval of the Swiss legislation and from

the New York Brain Bank–Taub Institute, Columbia University (NYBB), New York, USA. All donors had given their written consent for the autopsy and we followed the Declaration of Helsinki.

Immunohistochemistry

Mice were anesthetised with tribromoethanol (500 mg/kg) and perfused intracardially with cold PBS followed by cold 4 % paraformaldehyde (PFA, Sigma Aldrich). Spinal cords were removed and post fixed for 2 h in 4 % PFA. Samples were cryoprotected in sucrose 30 %, included in Tissue Teck (Sakura, Alphen aan den Rijn, The Netherlands), frozen and kept at −80 °C until processing.

For mice, free floating spinal cord transverse sections (20 μm) were washed twice in PBS (5 min), treated for 30 min in PBS containing lysine (20 mM, pH 7.2) and for 15 min in 1 % H$_2$O$_2$. Sections were blocked for 1 h with PBS containing bovine serum albumin (BSA, 1 %, Sigma Aldrich) and Triton X-100 (0.1 %, Fisher Scientific, Illkirch, France) and then incubated 48 h at 4 °C with CD11b (1/200, Developmental Studies Hybridoma Bank, Iowa, USA) primary antibody. Alexa-conjugated 594 secondary antibody was used (1/1000; Molecular Probes, Eugene, OR, USA).

For human spinal cord 22 μm-thick cryosections of lumbar and lower thoracic segments were collected on super frost plus slides and were processed as described above. For dual fluorescence labelling, sections were placed in a cocktail of rat anti CD11b (1/100, Hybridoma Bank, University of Iowa, USA) and rabbit anti-Brca1 (1/100, Santa Cruz Biotechnology, Dallas, USA) primary antibodies for 48 h at 4 °C. Sections were washed in 0.1 M PBS followed by incubation in corresponding secondary antibodies conjugated to Alexa 488 and 594 (1/1000; Molecular Probes, Eugene, OR, USA). For peroxidase labelling, sections were placed for 48 h at 4 °C in either rabbit anti Iba1 (macrophage/microglia-specific calcium-binding protein) (1/1000, Wako Pure Chemical Industries, Osaka, Japan) or rabbit anti-Brca1 (1/100, Santa Cruz Biotechnology, Dallas, USA) primary antibodies. Spinal cord sections were then incubated in donkey anti-rabbit (1/500, Jackson Immunoresearch, Carlsbad, USA) antibody for 2 h at 4 °C. Sections were then washed in TRIS buffer and enzymatic revelation was done with nickel enhanced DAB and H$_2$O$_2$ 0.1 % as a substrate. Sections were then dehydrated in ascending concentration of ethanol and finally xylene. Coverslips were applied using Entellan (Merck KGaA, Darmstadt, Germany).

Morphometric bright field photographs had been obtained and analysed using NanoZoomer RS slide scanner (NanoZoomer Digital Pathology System and NDP view software, Hamamatsu, Japan). For immunofluorescence images, we used laser scanning inverted confocal microscopy (Leica SP5, Mannheim, Germany). Laser intensity and detector sensitivity settings were kept constant for all image acquisitions within a given experiment. Brca1 staining intensity measurement was done by measuring their optical density (OD) using ImageJ (National Institutes of Health, USA), as described previously [48]. For each given sample we analysed at least three 22-μm-thick section with 330 μm distance from each other. Statistics: un-paired t-test done with GraphPad Prism version 5.03 (GraphPad software, CA, USA). Significance was accepted at $p \le 0.05$. Results are expressed as mean ± S.E.M.

Additional files

Additional file 1: Table S1. Database of differential expression comparison of hSOD1^{G93A} microglia microarray data relative to control microglia at 90 days of age. We list information for each dysregulated genes in hSOD1^{G93A} microglia as compared to control microglia. With both the p-value and the step-up p-value that is the false discovery rate (FDR) analogue of the p-value. Three chips were used per condition (wild type and SOD1^{G93A}) with microglia from lumbar spinal cord of at least six pooled mice.

Additional file 2: Figure S1. Comparison of gene dysregulation in microglia and motoneurones. (A) Venn diagrams showing that 19 genes are commonly dysregulated in microglia and motoneurones at symptomatic age (P90). (B) Comparison of dysregulated genes in microglia at P90 and motoneurones at disease end stage shows that 65 genes are commonly dysregulated, 603 genes are uniquely dysregulated in hSOD1^{G93A} microglia and 320 uniquely in hSOD1^{G93A} motoneurones. Three chips were used per condition (wild type and SOD1^{G93A}) with microglia from lumbar spinal cord of at least six pooled mice.

Additional file 3: Table S2. Comparison of gene dysregulation in both microglia and motoneurones at symptomatic age (P90) and in motoneurone only (P90) using gene ontology enrichment and network analysis. In all tables the top scored categories have the lowest p-value. Table S2A: Process networks ranking. Table S2B: Gene ontology processes ranking and Table S2C: Pathway maps ranking.

Additional file 4: Table S3. Comparison of gene dysregulation in microglia at symptomatic age (P90) and in motoneurone at the end stage of the disease (P120) using gene ontology enrichment and network analysis. In all tables the top scored categories have the lowest p-value. Table S3A: Process networks ranking. Table S3B: Gene ontology processes ranking and Table S3C: Pathway maps ranking.

Additional file 5: Table S4. Gene ontology enrichment and network analysis of gene dysregulation in microglia at symptomatic age (P90). In all tables the top scored categories have the lowest p-value. Table S4A: Process networks. Table S4B: Gene ontology processes and Table S4C: Pathway maps. Percentage of dysregulated genes corresponds to the ratio of dysregulated genes in our data out of annotated genes in the given category (Gene Ontology).

Additional file 6: Figure S2. Quantitative real-time polymerase chain reaction (qPCR) validation of microarray findings related to candidate genes involved in Brca1 pathway. To confirm the microarray results, the seven identified genes involved in Brca1 pathway were analysed by real time qPCR. Bar graphs showing up-regulation of Brca1, Cdkn1a, Myc, Pcna and Stat1 as well as down-regulation of Gadd45a and Sp3 in hSOD1^{G93A} microglia at 90 (B) but not 60 days (A) as compared to control microglia. For each sample, real time PCR was done in triplicate.

Additional file 7: Table S5. Candidate genes involved in Brca1 pathway selected for qPCR to validate the microarray data.

Abbreviations

ALS: Amyotrophic lateral sclerosis; CNS: Central nervous system; DAB: Diaminobenzidine; ER: Endoplasmic reticulum; FACS: Fluorescence-activated cell sorting; FALS: Familial amyotrophic lateral sclerosis; FC: Fold change; GO: Gene ontology; OD: Optical density; PBS: Phosphate base saline; PFA: Paraformaldehyde; pmn: Progressive motor neuronopathy; RIN: RNA integrity number; ROS: Reactive oxygen species; SOD: Super oxide dismutase.

Competing interests

The authors declare that they have no competing interests.

Authors' contributions

HNN: participated in the design of the study, performed immunohistology, participated to the analysis and interpretation of data and helped to draft the manuscript. JCS: participated in the design of the study, carried out FACS and participated to immunohistology. YNG: participated to acquisition of FACS data. MT: participated to immunohistology. AS: performed autopsy. MdmV: participated to acquisition of FACS data. MW: performed patient selection and obtained patients consent. FEP: conception, design of the work; analysis and interpretation of data, drafting the work and final approval. All authors read and approved the final manuscript.

Acknowledgments

We are grateful to ALS patients and their relatives that donate their tissues. We acknowledge the New York Brain Bank–The Taub Institute, Columbia University (NYBB). The hybridoma CD11b antibody developed by Timothy A. Springer was obtained from the Developmental Studies Hybridoma Bank developed under the auspices of the NICHD and maintained by the University of Iowa, Department of Biology, Iowa city, IA 52242. We thank the iGE3Genomics Platform, University of Geneva Switzerland for their assistance in transcriptomic and qPCR analysis.
This work was supported by the Spanish Government, Plan Nacional de I+D+I 2008–2011 and ISCIII-Subdirección General de Evaluación y Fomento de la investigación (PI10/00709) [to FEP], the Government of the Basque Country grant (Proyectos de Investigacion Sanitaria and Fondo Comun de Cooperacion Aquitania-Euskadi) [to FEP], the "Fondation pour la Recherche Médicale" [to FEP] and the French Government, ANR-FNS grant, GliALS (N° ANR-14-CE36-0009-01) [to FEP], the patient organisations "Demain Debout Aquitaine" [to YNG and HNN] and "Verticale" [to FEP and HNN].

Author details

¹Institute for Neurosciences of Montpellier (INM), INSERM U1051, 80, rue Augustin Fliche, 34091 Montpellier, Cedex 5, France. ²"Integrative Biology of Neurodegeneration", IKERBASQUE Basque Foundation for Science and Neuroscience Department, University of the Basque Country, Bilbao, Spain. ³Kantonspital St. Gallen. FachMuskelzentrum/ALS clinic, St. Gallen, Switzerland. ⁴CIC bioGUNE, Cell Biology & Stem Cells Unit, Technological Park of Bizkaia, Derio, Spain. ⁵Department "Biologie-Mécanismes du Vivant" Faculty of Science, University of Montpellier, Montpellier, France.

References

1. Leblond CS, Kaneb HM, Dion PA, Rouleau GA. Dissection of genetic factors associated with amyotrophic lateral sclerosis. Exp Neurol. 2014;262 Pt B:91–101.
2. Gurney ME, Pu H, Chiu AY, Dal Canto MC, Polchow CY, Alexander DD, et al. Motor neuron degeneration in mice that express a human Cu, Zn superoxide dismutase mutation. Science. 1994;264:1772–5.
3. Philips T, Rothstein JD. Glial cells in amyotrophic lateral sclerosis. Exp Neurol. 2014;262 Pt B:111–20.
4. Crain JM, Nikodemova M, Watters JJ. Microglia express distinct M1 and M2 phenotypic markers in the postnatal and adult central nervous system in male and female mice. J Neurosci Res. 2013;91:1143–51.
5. Michelucci A, Heurtaux T, Grandbarbe L, Morga E, Heuschling P. Characterization of the microglial phenotype under specific pro-inflammatory and anti-inflammatory conditions: effects of oligomeric and fibrillar amyloid-beta. J Neuroimmunol. 2009;210:3–12.
6. Brites D, Vaz AR. Microglia centered pathogenesis in ALS: insights in cell interconnectivity. Front Cell Neurosci. 2014;8:117.

7. Gerber YN, Sabourin JC, Rabano M, Vivanco M, Perrin FE. Early functional deficit and microglial disturbances in a mouse model of amyotrophic lateral sclerosis. PLoS One. 2012;7, e36000.

8. Perrin FE, Boisset G, Docquier M, Schaad O, Descombes P, Kato AC. No widespread induction of cell death genes occurs in pure motoneurons in an amyotrophic lateral sclerosis mouse model. Hum Mol Genet. 2005;14:3309–20.

9. Perrin FE, Boisset G, Lathuiliere A, Kato AC. Cell death pathways differ in several mouse models with motoneurone disease: analysis of pure motoneurone populations at a presymptomatic age. J Neurochem. 2006;98:1959–72.

10. Coppede F. An overview of DNA repair in amyotrophic lateral sclerosis. ScientificWorldJournal. 2011;11:1679–91.

11. Caestecker KW, Van de Walle GR. The role of BRCA1 in DNA double-strand repair: past and present. Exp Cell Res. 2013;319:575–87.

12. Somasundaram K. Breast cancer gene 1 (BRCA1): role in cell cycle regulation and DNA repair–perhaps through transcription. J Cell Biochem. 2003;88:1084–91.

13. Savage KI, Harkin DP. BRCA1, a 'complex' protein involved in the maintenance of genomic stability. FEBS J. 2015;282:630–46.

14. Bae I, Fan S, Meng Q, Rih JK, Kim HJ, Kang HJ, et al. BRCA1 induces antioxidant gene expression and resistance to oxidative stress. Cancer Res. 2004;64:7893–909.

15. Vurusaner B, Poli G, Basaga H. Tumor suppressor genes and ROS: complex networks of interactions. Free Radic Biol Med. 2012;52:7–18.

16. Rakha EA, El-Sheikh SE, Kandil MA, El-Sayed ME, Green AR, Ellis IO. Expression of BRCA1 protein in breast cancer and its prognostic significance. Hum Pathol. 2008;39:857–65.

17. Bernard-Gallon DJ, De Latour MP, Sylvain V, Vissac C, Aunoble B, Chassagne J, et al. Brca1 and Brca2 protein expression patterns in different tissues of murine origin. Int J Oncol. 2001;18:271–80.

18. Korhonen L, Brannvall K, Skoglosa Y, Lindholm D. Tumor suppressor gene BRCA-1 is expressed by embryonic and adult neural stem cells and involved in cell proliferation. J Neurosci Res. 2003;71:769–76.

19. Gerber YN, Sabourin JC, Hugnot JP, Perrin FE. Unlike physical exercise, modified environment increases the lifespan of SOD1G93A mice however both conditions induce cellular changes. PLoS One. 2012;7, e45503.

20. Ilieva H, Polymenidou M, Cleveland DW. Non-cell autonomous toxicity in neurodegenerative disorders: ALS and beyond. J Cell Biol. 2009;187:761–72.

21. Liao B, Zhao W, Beers DR, Henkel JS, Appel SH. Transformation from a neuroprotective to a neurotoxic microglial phenotype in a mouse model of ALS. Exp Neurol. 2012;237:147–52.

22. Hickman SE, Kingery ND, Ohsumi TK, Borowsky ML, Wang LC, Means TK, et al. The microglial sensome revealed by direct RNA sequencing. Nat Neurosci. 2013;16:1896–905.

23. Chiu IM, Morimoto ET, Goodarzi H, Liao JT, O'Keeffe S, Phatnani HP, et al. A neurodegeneration-specific gene-expression signature of acutely isolated microglia from an amyotrophic lateral sclerosis mouse model. Cell Rep. 2013;4:385–401.

24. Beers DR, Zhao W, Liao B, Kano O, Wang J, Huang A, et al. Neuroinflammation modulates distinct regional and temporal clinical responses in ALS mice. Brain Behav Immun. 2011;25:1025–35.

25. Liu B, Li D, Guan YF. BRCA1 regulates insulin-like growth factor 1 receptor levels in ovarian cancer. Oncol Lett. 2014;7:1733–7.

26. Werner H, Bruchim I. IGF-1 and BRCA1 signalling pathways in familial cancer. Lancet Oncol. 2012;13:e537–44.

27. Henkel JS, Beers DR, Zhao W, Appel SH. Microglia in ALS: the good, the bad, and the resting. J Neuroimmune Pharmacol. 2009;4:389–98.

28. David S, Kroner A. Repertoire of microglial and macrophage responses after spinal cord injury. Nat Rev Neurosci. 2011;12:388–99.

29. Mantha AK, Sarkar B, Tell G. A short review on the implications of base excision repair pathway for neurons: relevance to neurodegenerative diseases. Mitochondrion. 2014;16:38–49.

30. Pulvers JN, Huttner WB. Brca1 is required for embryonic development of the mouse cerebral cortex to normal size by preventing apoptosis of early neural progenitors. Development. 2009;136:1859–68.

31. Pao GM, Zhu Q, Perez-Garcia CG, Chou SJ, Suh H, Gage FH, et al. Role of BRCA1 in brain development. Proc Natl Acad Sci U S A. 2014;111:E1240–8.

32. Gowen LC, Johnson BL, Latour AM, Sulik KK, Koller BH. Brca1 deficiency results in early embryonic lethality characterized by neuroepithelial abnormalities. Nat Genet. 1996;12:191–4.

33. King TM, Au KS, Kirkpatrick TJ, Davidson C, Fletcher JM, Townsend I, et al. The impact of BRCA1 on spina bifida meningomyelocele lesions. Ann Hum Genet. 2007;71:719–28.

34. Evans TA, Raina AK, Delacourte A, Aprelikova O, Lee HG, Zhu X, et al. BRCA1 may modulate neuronal cell cycle re-entry in Alzheimer disease. Int J Med Sci. 2007;4:140–5.

35. Nakanishi A, Minami A, Kitagishi Y, Ogura Y, Matsuda S. BRCA1 and p53 tumor suppressor molecules in Alzheimer's disease. Int J Mol Sci. 2015;16:2879–92.

36. Jeon GS, Kim KY, Hwang YJ, Jung MK, An S, Ouchi M, et al. Deregulation of BRCA1 leads to impaired spatiotemporal dynamics of gamma-H2AX and DNA damage responses in Huntington's disease. Mol Neurobiol. 2012;45:550–63.

37. Brain L, Croft PB, Wilkinson M. Motor neurone disease as a manifestation of neoplasm (with a note on the course of classical motor neurone disease). Brain. 1965;88:479–500.

38. Chio A, Brignolio F, Meineri P, Rosso MG, Tribolo A, Schiffer D. Motor neuron disease and malignancies: results of a population-based study. J Neurol. 1988;235:374–5.

39. Forsyth PA, Dalmau J, Graus F, Cwik V, Rosenblum MK, Posner JB. Motor neuron syndromes in cancer patients. Ann Neurol. 1997;41:722–30.

40. Rojas-Marcos I, Rousseau A, Keime-Guibert F, Rene R, Cartalat-Carel S, Delattre JY, et al. Spectrum of paraneoplastic neurologic disorders in women with breast and gynecologic cancer. Medicine. 2003;82:216–23.

41. Sadot E, Carluer L, Corcia P, Delozier Y, Levy C, Viader F. Breast cancer and motor neuron disease: clinical study of seven cases. Amyotroph Lateral Scler. 2007;8:288–91.

42. Berghs S, Ferracci F, Maksimova E, Gleason S, Leszczynski N, Butler M, et al. Autoimmunity to beta IV spectrin in paraneoplastic lower motor neuron syndrome. Proc Natl Acad Sci U S A. 2001;98:6945–50.

43. Evans BK, Fagan C, Arnold T, Dropcho EJ, Oh SJ. Paraneoplastic motor neuron disease and renal cell carcinoma: improvement after nephrectomy. Neurology. 1990;40:960–2.

44. Forman D, Rae-Grant AD, Matchett SC, Cowen JS. A reversible cause of hypercapnic respiratory failure: lower motor neuronopathy associated with renal cell carcinoma. Chest. 1999;115:899–901.

45. Kiewe P, Gueller S, Komor M, Stroux A, Thiel E, Hofmann WK. Prediction of qualitative outcome of oligonucleotide microarray hybridization by measurement of RNA integrity using the 2100 Bioanalyzer capillary electrophoresis system. Ann Hematol. 2009;88:1177–83.

46. Hubbell E, Liu WM, Mei R. Robust estimators for expression analysis. Bioinformatics. 2002;18:1585–92.

47. Liu WM, Mei R, Di X, Ryder TB, Hubbell E, Dee S, et al. Analysis of high density expression microarrays with signed-rank call algorithms. Bioinformatics. 2002;18:1593–9.

48. Noristani HN, Olabarria M, Verkhratsky A, Rodriguez JJ. Serotonin fibre sprouting and increase in serotonin transporter immunoreactivity in the CA1 area of hippocampus in a triple transgenic mouse model of Alzheimer's disease. Eur J Neurosci. 2010;32:71–9.

13

Calcium-responsive transactivator (CREST) protein shares a set of structural and functional traits with other proteins associated with amyotrophic lateral sclerosis

Michail S Kukharsky[1,2†], Annamaria Quintiero[1†], Taisei Matsumoto[3], Koji Matsukawa[3], Haiyan An[1], Tadafumi Hashimoto[3], Takeshi Iwatsubo[3], Vladimir L Buchman[1*] and Tatyana A Shelkovnikova[1,2*]

Abstract

Background: Mutations in calcium-responsive transactivator (CREST) encoding gene have been recently linked to ALS. Similar to several proteins implicated in ALS, CREST contains a prion-like domain and was reported to be a component of paraspeckles.

Results: We demonstrate that CREST is prone to aggregation and co-aggregates with FUS but not with other two ALS-linked proteins, TDP-43 and TAF15, in cultured cells. Aggregation of CREST affects paraspeckle integrity, probably by trapping other paraspeckle proteins within aggregates. Like several other ALS-associated proteins, CREST is recruited to induced stress granules. Neither of the CREST mutations described in ALS alters its subcellular localization, stress granule recruitment or detergent solubility; however Q388stop mutation results in elevated steady-state levels and more frequent nuclear aggregation of the protein. Both wild-type protein and its mutants negatively affect neurite network complexity of unstimulated cultured neurons when overexpressed, with Q388stop mutation being the most deleterious. When overexpressed in the fly eye, wild-type CREST or its mutants lead to severe retinal degeneration without obvious differences between the variants.

Conclusions: Our data indicate that CREST and certain other ALS-linked proteins share several features implicated in ALS pathogenesis, namely the ability to aggregate, be recruited to stress granules and alter paraspeckle integrity. A change in CREST levels in neurons which might occur under pathological conditions would have a profound negative effect on neuronal homeostasis.

Keywords: Amyotrophic lateral sclerosis (ALS), Calcium-responsive transactivator (CREST), SS18L1, Fused in sarcoma (FUS), TAR DNA-binding protein 43 (TDP-43), Protein aggregation, Stress granule, Neurodegeneration, Paraspeckle, Nuclear enriched abundant transcript 1 (NEAT1), Transgenic fly

Background

Amyotrophic lateral sclerosis (ALS) is a fatal adult-onset neurodegenerative condition characterized by aetiologically diverse pathomechanisms, which ultimately results in loss of upper and lower motor neurons, paralysis and death. In a rapidly growing group of genes mutated in ALS the most represented are the genes encoding proteins directly or indirectly involved in RNA metabolism [1-3]. Structural and functional studies of ALS-associated proteins and their disease-linked variants have significantly contributed to our current understanding of the mechanisms of disease development and progression. Characterization of pathological signatures for each ALS-associated protein is crucial in delineating common pathways in the disease pathogenesis and eventually understanding how altered metabolism of proteins with diverse functions results in the same clinical phenotype.

* Correspondence: buchmanvl@cardiff.ac.uk; shelkovnikovat@cardiff.ac.uk
†Equal contributors
[1]School of Biosciences, Cardiff University, Museum Avenue, CF10 3AX Cardiff, UK
Full list of author information is available at the end of the article

Recently, using exome sequencing in sporadic ALS trios Chesi and co-workers [4] have identified two mutations in the SS18L1 gene which encodes calcium-responsive transactivator (CREST) protein. Subsequently two additional mutations in CREST, this time in patients with familial form of ALS, were reported [5]. CREST is a nuclear protein discovered in 2003 in a screen for calcium-responsive genes involved in transcriptional activation [6]. The same year the gene encoding CREST was independently described as translocated in some cases of synovial sarcoma [7]. CREST is important for normal development of the nervous system, and CREST-deficient mice display defective dendritic branching, motor disturbances and early lethality [6]. Importantly CREST interacts with CREB-binding protein (CBP), a histone acetylase known for its neuroprotective properties [8]. In the original study CREST was also shown to bind chromatin remodeling proteins BAF250 and BRG-1 [6]. Subsequently it was demonstrated that CREST and a highly homologous protein, SS18, are dedicated subunits of chromatin remodeling complex Brg/Brm-associated factor (BAF), which is an important modulator of transcription of specific gene sets at various stages of neural development [9]. Mutations in components of the BAF complex have been identified in autism, schizophrenia and other neurodevelopmental disorders, arguing that its function is crucial for normal development of the nervous system [10,11].

Structurally, CREST consists of a C-terminal transactivation domain, which is characterized by low sequence complexity and satisfies the criteria for a prion-like domain [4,6]; an N-terminal autoregulatory domain, which suppresses transactivation at basal state [6]; a central methionine-rich domain, and so called multifunctional domain (MFD) implicated in the protein dimerisation, regulation of transactivation and subcellular localization of the protein [12]. In the nucleus, CREST was shown to be recruited to nuclear bodies of unknown origin [13]. More recently, CREST was identified in a screen for paraspeckle proteins [14].

The majority of ALS-associated proteins are characterized by high aggregation propensity, which is attributable to the presence of a prion-like domain in their structure [15]. The ability to aggregate reversibly is indispensable for their normal function in RNA-protein macromolecular complexes, such as RNA transport granules, stress granules, paraspeckles and Gems; at the same time, pathological aggregation of these proteins is also governed by prion-like domains [16,17]. Despite the confirmed presence of a prion-like domain in CREST structure, the aggregation propensity of wild type CREST and its ALS-associated variants has not been addressed. Furthermore, dysfunction of paraspeckles/paraspeckle proteins has recently emerged as possible pathogenic factor in ALS [18,19]. The role of CREST in the paraspeckle is not clear, nor is it known if the protein

can be recruited to other RNP complexes. Thus far, it has been shown that an ALS-associated CREST mutation leading to the deletion of the 9 C-terminal amino acids, Q388stop [4], abolishes its binding to CBP, suggesting that the missing amino acids act as an interface for interaction between the two proteins [6]. Both Q388stop and a mutation in autoregulatory domain, I123M, reduce depolarization-induced branching in cultured neurons [4]. In vivo effects of the other two mutations involving MFD and methionine-rich domain [5] have not been examined.

Therefore, in current study we aimed to characterize the aspects of CREST structure and interactions relevant to ALS pathogenesis in vitro and in vivo, primarily its aggregation propensity and possible involvement in the formation of nuclear and cytoplasmic RNA granules.

Results

CREST protein is prone to form aggregates in the cell nucleus

Previous studies have demonstrated that in transfected cells exogenous CREST localizes to nuclear dot-like structures designated as nuclear bodies [12]; however their identity has not been determined. We generated constructs to express either untagged CREST or CREST tagged with GFP or Flag peptide. All three proteins displayed predominantly nuclear distribution in neuroblastoma SH-SY5Y and COS7 cells (Figure 1A, Additional file 1: Figure S1). In agreement with the results of the above study, we also observed formation of nuclear dot-like structures upon expression of tagged or untagged CREST (Figure 1A, Additional file 1: Figure S1). In cells with profound accumulation of CREST in the nucleus, the presence of the expressed protein in the cytoplasm and its cytoplasmic aggregation were also evident, particularly for CREST-GFP (Figure 1A, large + cyt panel, Additional file 1: Figure S1). To establish if nuclear dot-like structures formed by CREST were related to known nuclear bodies, transfected cells were co-stained for various nuclear body markers. In SH-SY5Y cells with a diffuse/fine-granular nucleoplasmic distribution of CREST-GFP the protein was excluded from nucleolar region identified by ethidium bromide staining, was not enriched in SMN-positive Gems, coilin p80-positive Cajal bodies or PML bodies but we detected its enrichment around MALAT1-positive nuclear speckles (Figure 1B). CREST was reported to be a paraspeckle component [14]; we also observed CREST-GFP enrichment in paraspeckles visualized by NEAT1 FISH, but only in cells with low levels and diffuse distribution of the protein (Figure 1B, bottom panel). Large dot-like nuclear structures formed by CREST did not overlap with any of the above nuclear bodies, including paraspeckles, though they often surrounded speckles (Figure 1C). Hereafter, these nuclear structures as well as cytoplasmic CREST accumulations of any appearance will be referred as "aggregates".

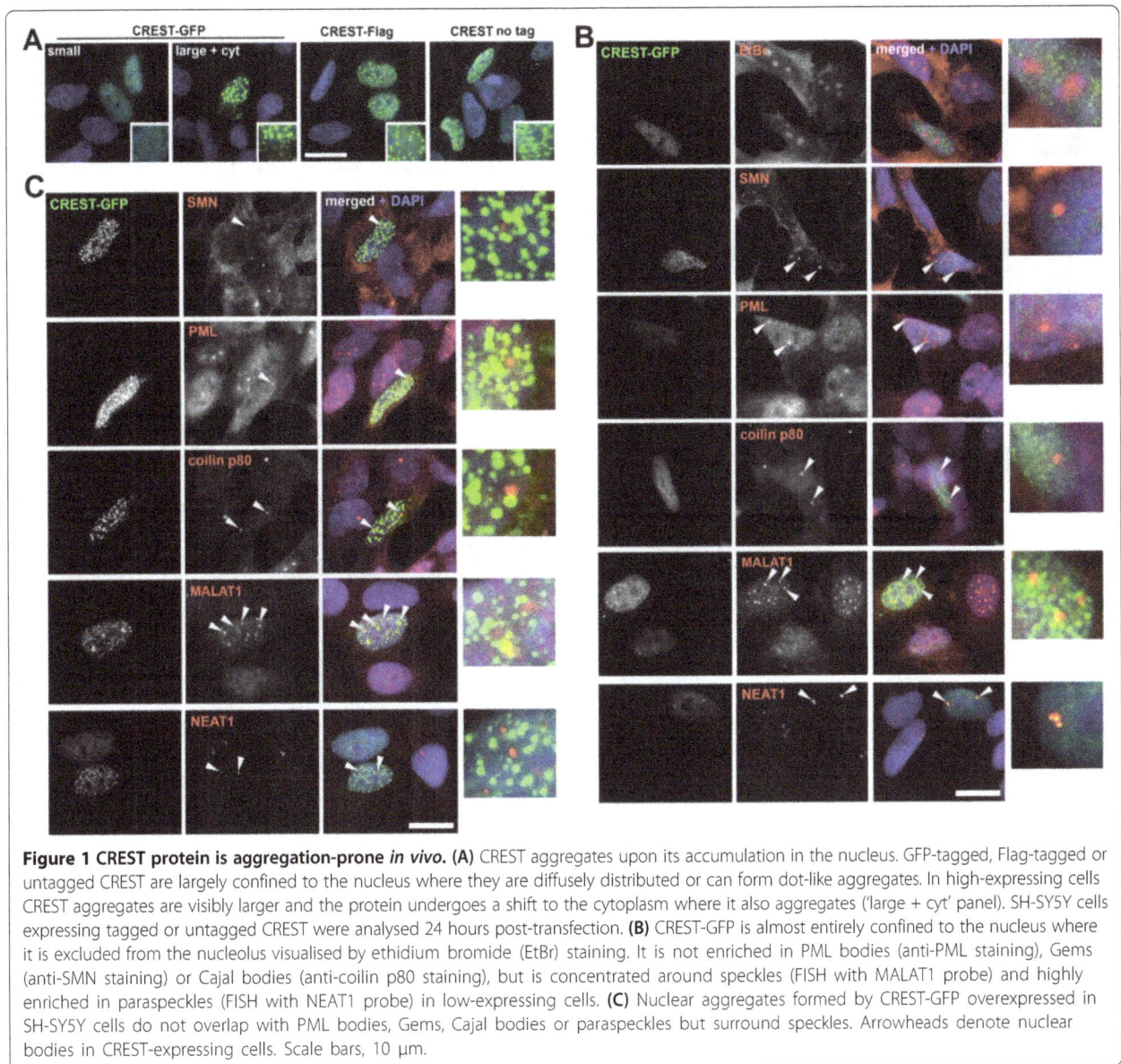

Figure 1 CREST protein is aggregation-prone *in vivo*. (A) CREST aggregates upon its accumulation in the nucleus. GFP-tagged, Flag-tagged or untagged CREST are largely confined to the nucleus where they are diffusely distributed or can form dot-like aggregates. In high-expressing cells CREST aggregates are visibly larger and the protein undergoes a shift to the cytoplasm where it also aggregates ('large + cyt' panel). SH-SY5Y cells expressing tagged or untagged CREST were analysed 24 hours post-transfection. **(B)** CREST-GFP is almost entirely confined to the nucleus where it is excluded from the nucleolus visualised by ethidium bromide (EtBr) staining. It is not enriched in PML bodies (anti-PML staining), Gems (anti-SMN staining) or Cajal bodies (anti-coilin p80 staining), but is concentrated around speckles (FISH with MALAT1 probe) and highly enriched in paraspeckles (FISH with NEAT1 probe) in low-expressing cells. **(C)** Nuclear aggregates formed by CREST-GFP overexpressed in SH-SY5Y cells do not overlap with PML bodies, Gems, Cajal bodies or paraspeckles but surround speckles. Arrowheads denote nuclear bodies in CREST-expressing cells. Scale bars, 10 μm.

Consistent with the previous observation for Venus-tagged CREST [14], GFP-tagged, Flag-tagged and un-tagged CREST also redistributed to nucleolar caps in actinomycin D-treated cells expressing low levels of CREST (Figure 2A and data not shown). We argued that if dot-like CREST structures are stable, irreversibly aggregated entities they will not be affected by transcriptional arrest. Indeed, preformed nuclear aggregates of CREST remained intact following actinomycin D treatment (Figure 2B), although formation of weakly CREST-positive nuclear caps could be observed, probably due to protein redistribution from the pool of not yet aggregated protein (Figure 2B, arrowheads). Using live cell imaging, we also demonstrated that nuclear CREST aggregates are characterized by time- and concentration-dependent fusion and growth (Additional file 2: Video S1).

To explore CREST aggregation biochemically, we expressed untagged protein with subsequent sequential extraction in detergent-containing buffers (see Methods section for details). As shown in Figure 2C, approximately 10% of CREST remained in the TritonX-100/RIPA-insoluble fraction which could only be solubilised by boiling in the presence of 4% SDS. However, similar to some other ALS-associated proteins that form non-amyloid aggregates, neither tagged nor untagged CREST formed SDS-resistant amyloidogenic species, as was evident from detection of only monomeric forms of the protein in semidenaturing detergent agarose gel (SDD-AGE) assay (Figure 2D).

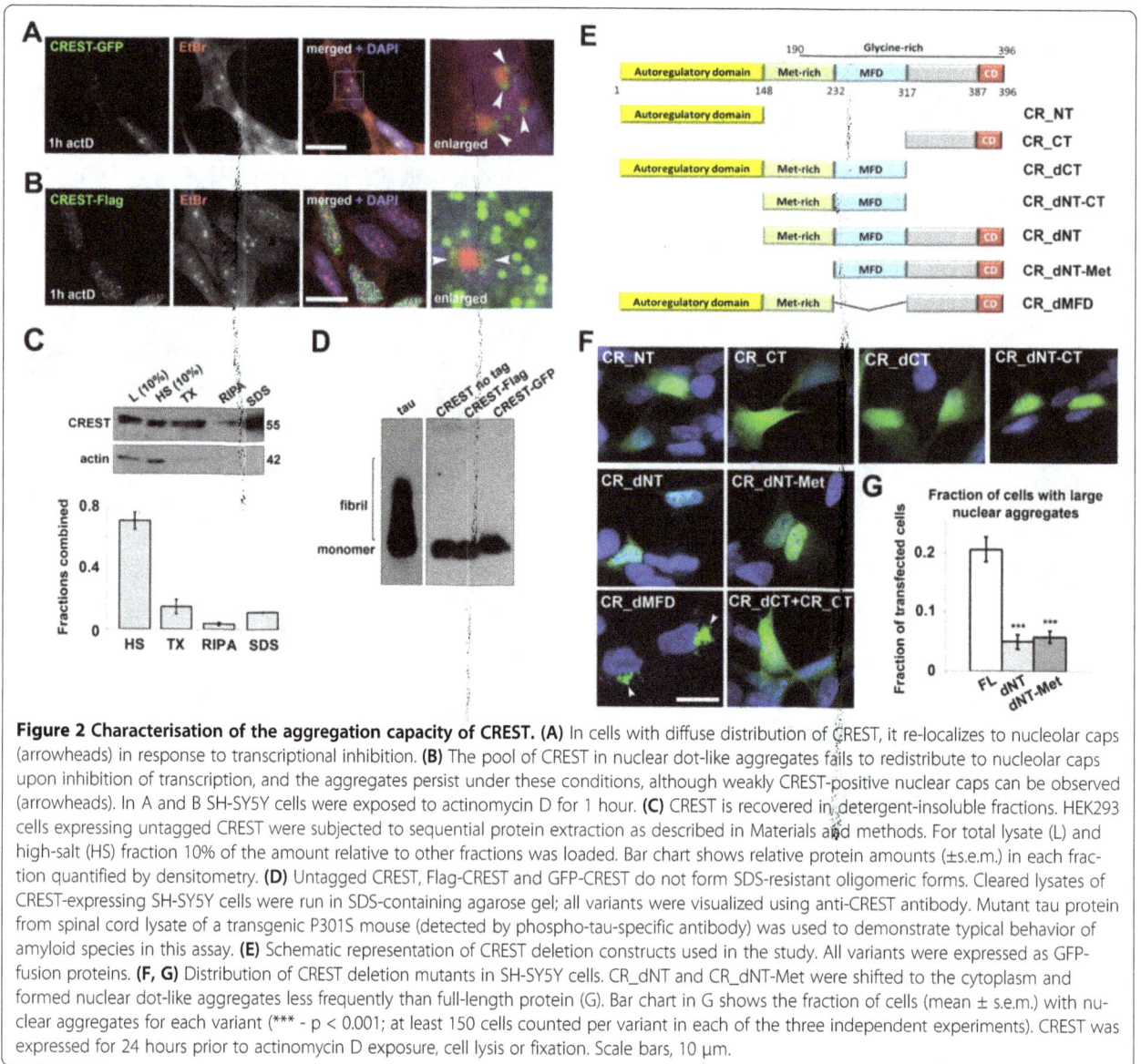

Figure 2 Characterisation of the aggregation capacity of CREST. (A) In cells with diffuse distribution of CREST, it re-localizes to nucleolar caps (arrowheads) in response to transcriptional inhibition. **(B)** The pool of CREST in nuclear dot-like aggregates fails to redistribute to nucleolar caps upon inhibition of transcription, and the aggregates persist under these conditions, although weakly CREST-positive nuclear caps can be observed (arrowheads). In A and B SH-SY5Y cells were exposed to actinomycin D for 1 hour. **(C)** CREST is recovered in detergent-insoluble fractions. HEK293 cells expressing untagged CREST were subjected to sequential protein extraction as described in Materials and methods. For total lysate (L) and high-salt (HS) fraction 10% of the amount relative to other fractions was loaded. Bar chart shows relative protein amounts (±s.e.m.) in each fraction quantified by densitometry. **(D)** Untagged CREST, Flag-CREST and GFP-CREST do not form SDS-resistant oligomeric forms. Cleared lysates of CREST-expressing SH-SY5Y cells were run in SDS-containing agarose gel; all variants were visualized using anti-CREST antibody. Mutant tau protein from spinal cord lysate of a transgenic P301S mouse (detected by phospho-tau-specific antibody) was used to demonstrate typical behavior of amyloid species in this assay. **(E)** Schematic representation of CREST deletion constructs used in the study. All variants were expressed as GFP-fusion proteins. **(F, G)** Distribution of CREST deletion mutants in SH-SY5Y cells. CR_dNT and CR_dNT-Met were shifted to the cytoplasm and formed nuclear dot-like aggregates less frequently than full-length protein (G). Bar chart in G shows the fraction of cells (mean ± s.e.m.) with nuclear aggregates for each variant (*** - p < 0.001; at least 150 cells counted per variant in each of the three independent experiments). CREST was expressed for 24 hours prior to actinomycin D exposure, cell lysis or fixation. Scale bars, 10 μm.

To assess the contribution of different CREST domains to its aggregation propensity, we produced a set of deletion constructs tagged with GFP at their N-terminus (Figure 2E) and expressed them in SH-SY5Y cells (Figure 2F). N-terminal autoregulatory domain (CR_NT) or C-terminal part of CREST (CR_CT) in isolation did not aggregate and were present both in the nucleus and in the cytoplasm. Deletion of C-terminal part completely abolished the protein's ability to aggregate. In contrast, CREST lacking the autoregulatory domain only (CR_dNT) or in combination with Met-rich domain (CR_dNT-Met) was distributed and aggregated in a very similar manner to the full-length protein, i.e. these variants were detected mainly in the nucleus where they formed multiple puncta (Figure 2F). However, for these two variants, cytoplasmic delocalisation was more pronounced and aggregation capacity was diminished compared to full-length CREST (Figure 2F,G). The middle region of CREST comprising Met-rich and MFD domains (CR_dNT-CT) was efficiently targeted to the nucleus where it accumulated inside the nucleolus. Deletion of MFD domain rendered the protein highly aggregation-prone, and this variant was found almost exclusively in the form of aggresome-like cytoplasmic aggregates (Figure 2F). Co-expression of two complementary variants both displaying diffuse cellular distribution, CR_dCT and CR_CT, was not sufficient to trigger aggregation (Figure 2F), suggesting that this process requires the presence of the domains in cis. Therefore, both N-terminal and C-terminal parts of CREST are required for efficient aggregation, while central MFD might limit it.

CREST is recruited to stress-induced stress granules

A growing number of ALS-associated proteins have been shown to be the components of stress granules (SGs), cytoplasmic RNP foci assembled by cells in response to adverse conditions and facilitating translational shutdown under severe stress [20]. We examined CREST behaviour under various stresses and showed that CREST is also a resident of SGs. SH-SY5Y cells expressing full-length CREST-GFP or CREST-Flag were exposed to sodium arsenite, thapsigargin or a prostaglandin 15d-PGJ2 to trigger SG formation by inducing oxidative stress, ER stress or inhibiting translation elongation factor eIF4E [21], respectively. In cells with small aggregates or diffuse staining in the nucleus all three stimuli led to weak but reproducible CREST recruitment to SGs visualised with SG markers TIAR, G3BP1 or FMRP (Figure 3A), which was facilitated by the emergence of typically nuclear CREST in the cytoplasm of stressed cells (Figure 3B). Only two CREST deletion mutants – those lacking N-terminal domains, namely CR_dNT and CR_dNT-Met, – were recruited in SGs, moreover, they were detected at higher levels within SGs compared to the full-length protein (Figure 3C,D and data not shown). This was likely due to their cytoplasmic redistribution rather than enhanced propensity for SG recruitment since fluorescence intensity ratio SG/cytoplasm was similar for CR_dNT and full-length protein (Figure 3D). It was not possible to establish if CR_dMFD was recruited to SGs due to its high aggregation propensity. These results indicate that CREST recruitment to SGs is restricted by its limited occurrence in the cytoplasm and that the presence of C-terminal domain (CT, aa. 317-396) and MFD is necessary and sufficient for SG targeting of CREST.

Cytoplasmic aggregates of full-length CREST-GFP observed in a fraction of cells that also display large nuclear aggregates (similar to illustrated in Figure 1A) were negative for SG or P-body markers under basal conditions or after stress, although in stressed cells these aggregates were found in the vicinity of SGs (Figure 3E,F). Large cytoplasmic aggregates formed by CR_dMFD protein also did not contain core SG proteins even in stressed cells (Figure 3G).

CREST aggregation affects paraspeckles

Dysfunction of the paraspeckle has been recently implicated in pathogenesis of ALS [18,19]. Although the role of CREST in this nuclear body is not clear, it is unlikely to be essential for paraspeckle assembly because the majority of stable cell lines display normal paraspeckles despite very low levels of CREST expression. To further examine the involvement of CREST in these nuclear bodies, we used COS7 cells, which possess prominent paraspeckles. In the majority of cells displaying nuclear dot-like aggregates of CREST-Flag, these structures were

clearly distinct from paraspeckles visualized by staining for a core paraspeckle protein NONO/p54nrb (Figure 4A, top panel). However, careful examination revealed that a fraction of CREST aggregates was adjacent to paraspeckles (Figure 4A, bottom panel). Consistently, similar to paraspeckles, these aggregates are often seen on the border of speckles (Figure 1C). Therefore, sites of paraspeckle assembly might serve as sites of nucleation of CREST aggregates that radiate from paraspeckles and subsequently become scattered in the nucleoplasm. CREST behaves as a typical paraspeckle protein upon transcriptional repression, i.e. becomes recruited to nucleolar caps (Figure 2A) and Ref. [14]). These nucleolar caps match those formed by other paraspeckle proteins such as FUS, and are distinct from nucleolar caps formed by coilin p80 (Figure 4B). Furthermore, CREST deletion variants lacking an autoregulatory domain, CR_dNT and CR_dNT-Met, unlike other deletion mutants, are highly enriched in paraspeckles regardless expression levels and can be readily recruited to actinomycin D-induced nucleolar caps (Figure 4C and data not shown).

We next asked if CREST is able to recruit other paraspeckle proteins into its nuclear aggregates. Indeed, a core paraspeckle component, FUS, was efficiently sequestered into virtually all nuclear aggregates formed by CREST-Flag or CREST-GFP regardless their size and abundance (Figure 4E, Additional file 3: Figure S2B). However, FUS is not essential for CREST aggregation, since siRNA-mediated FUS knockdown did not affect nuclear aggregate formation by CREST-Flag (Figure 4D). Other major paraspeckle proteins, NONO/p54nrb and PSPC1, were not detected in small CREST aggregates (Figure 4F,G, top panels) but co-aggregated with CREST in those nuclei where most of CREST pool was present in the form of larger aggregates (Figure 4F,G, bottom panels). These observations suggest that FUS recruitment to CREST aggregates is highly specific while NONO/p54nrb and PSPC1 can be non-specifically trapped in these aggregates upon their growth. Since FUS is essential for paraspeckle integrity and contributes to the maintenance of NEAT1 levels [14,19], its entrapment in aggregates can negatively affect paraspeckles, including via NEAT1 downregulation. Indeed, COS7 cells expressing CREST-Flag and developing nuclear aggregates, contained paraspeckles (visualised with anti-NONO/p54nrb staining) less frequently than cells with diffuse protein only (Figure 4I). Similarly, among CREST-GFP expressing COS7 cells significantly fewer aggregate-containing cells possessed NEAT1-positive paraspeckles compared to non-transfected cells or cells with diffuse CREST distribution (Figure 4H,I). Furthermore, when we measured NEAT1 levels in neuroblastoma cells expressing untagged CREST or GFP vector, we observed a significant decrease in the transcript abundance in CREST-expressing cells (Figure 4J).

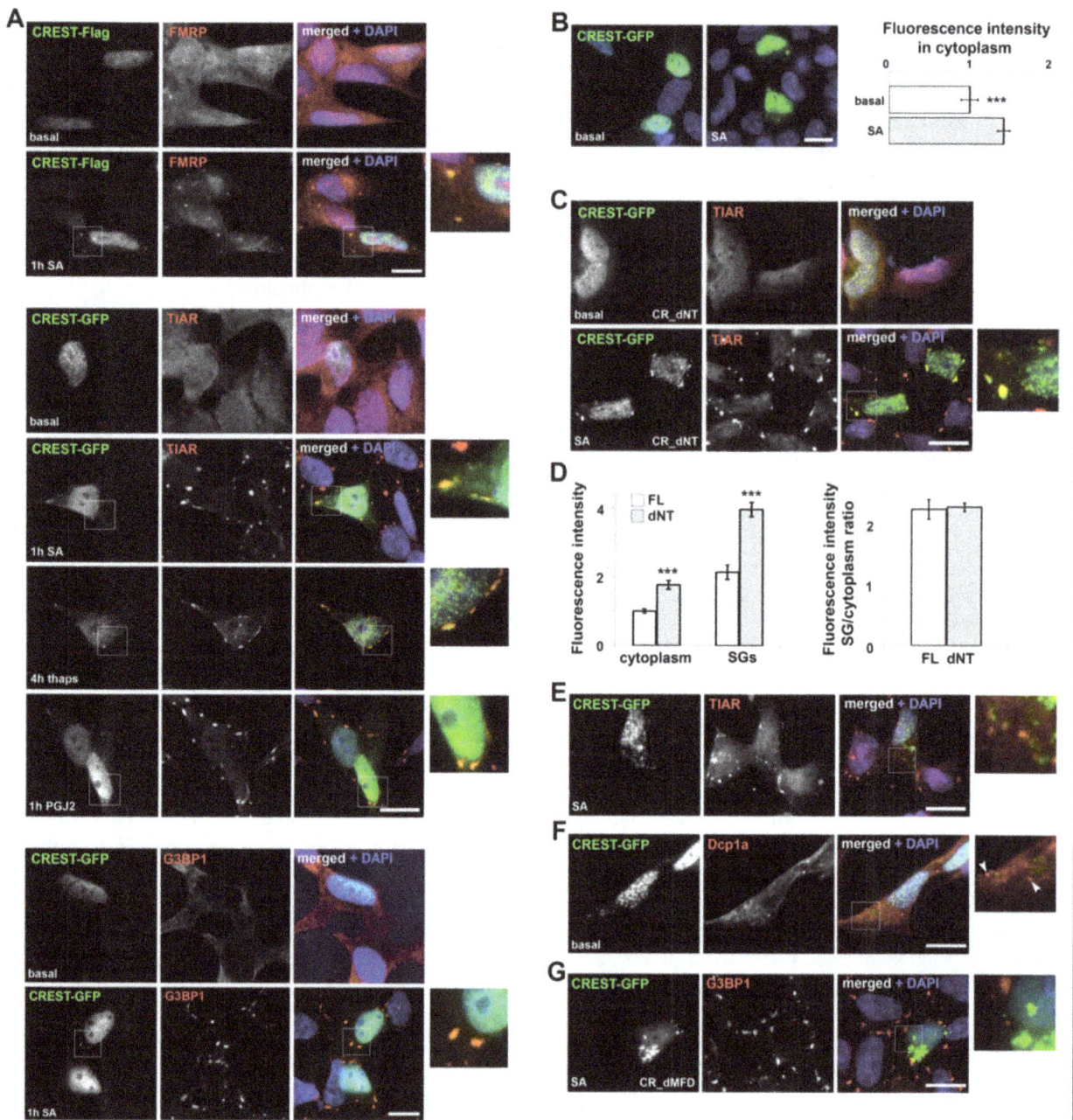

Figure 3 CREST is targeted to stress granules by various stresses. (A) CREST-Flag (top panel) and CREST-GFP (three bottom panels) are detected in stress granules induced by oxidative stress (sodium arsenite, SA), ER stress (thapsigargin, thaps) or inhibition of eIF4E (15d-PGJ2) and visualized with stress granule markers TIAR, FMRP and G3BP1. SA and 15d-PGJ2 were applied to SH-SY5Y cells for 1 hour and thapsigargin – for 4 hours. **(B)** In SH-SY5Y cells subjected to oxidative stress (SA for 1 hour) CREST-GFP undergoes significant shift to the cytoplasm. **(C, D)** CREST deletion mutant lacking autoregulatory domain (CR_dNT) is readily recruited to stress granules **(C)** and shows higher enrichment in these structures compared to full-length protein **(D**, left graph). This phenomenon is related to higher cytoplasmic levels of CR_dNT since the fluorescence intensity ratio stress granules/cytoplasm is similar for full-length and truncated protein **(D)**. **(E)** Cytoplasmic aggregates of CREST-GFP do not overlap with SA-induced stress granules but are found in their immediate vicinity. **(F)** Cytoplasmic aggregates of CREST-GFP do not overlap with P-bodies (visualized by anti-Dcp1a staining, arrowheads in the enlarged panel). **(G)** Aggresomes formed by GFP-tagged CREST lacking MFD domain are negative for a SG marker G3BP1. In **B** and **D**, fluorescence was measured in stress granules and/or cytoplasm of GFP-positive cells as described in Materials and methods, and cytoplasmic intensity for non-stressed cells **(B)** or full-length CREST-GFP **(D)** (mean ± s.e.m.) was taken as equal 1 (***p < 0.001). Scale bars, 10 μm.

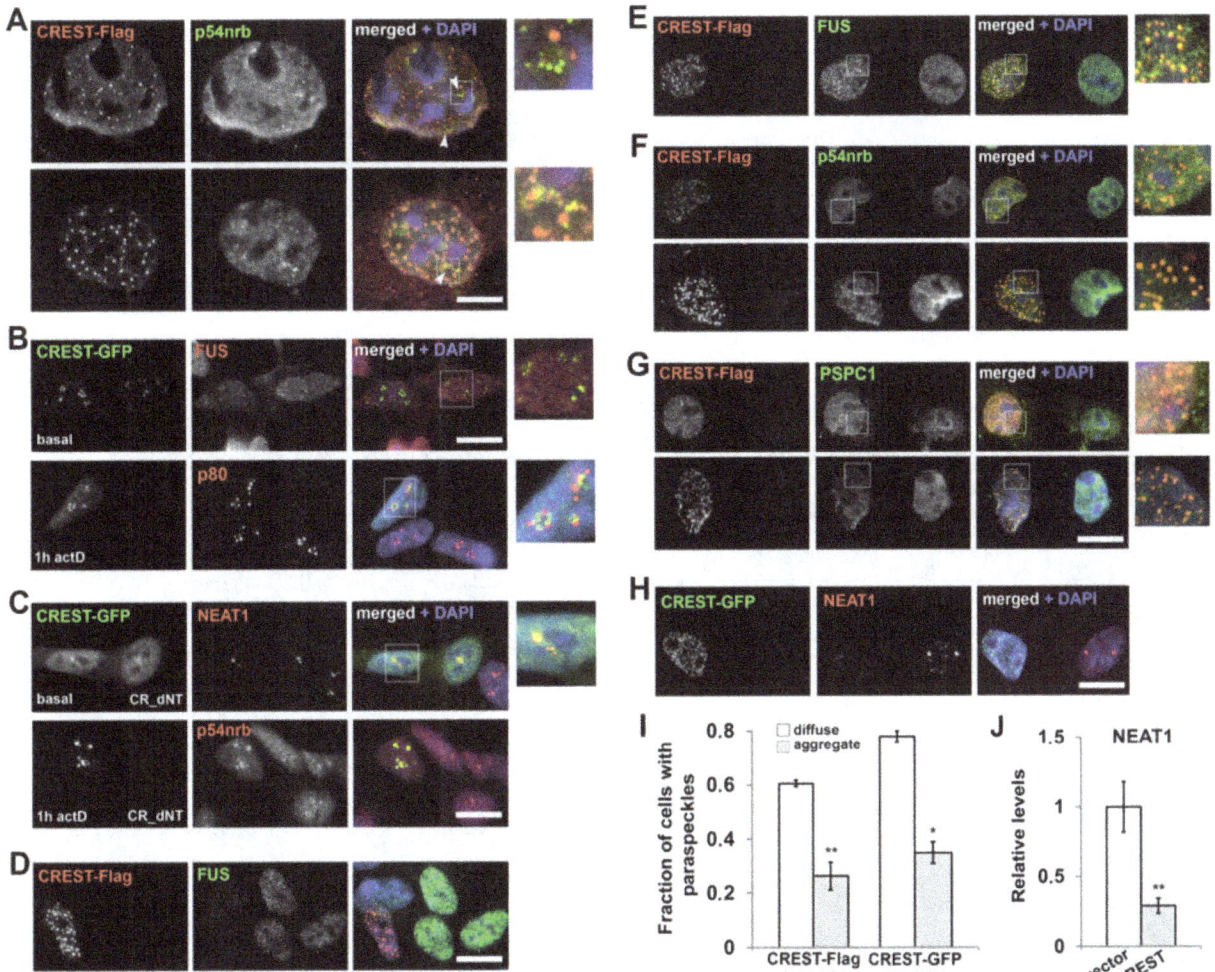

Figure 4 CREST aggregation disrupts paraspeckles. (A) CREST aggregates might originate from the sites of paraspeckle formation. Paraspeckles (anti-NONO/p54nrb staining, arrowheads) and CREST nuclear aggregates exist as distinct structures in COS7 cells (top panel). In a fraction of cells CREST aggregates are found in close apposition to/partially overlapping with paraspeckles (bottom panel). **(B)** In response to transcriptional inhibition CREST redistributes to the same nucleolar caps as a typical paraspeckle protein FUS but not to the caps formed by coilin p80. **(C)** CREST lacking autoregulatory domain is efficiently recruited in paraspeckles (top panel) and redistributes to nucleolar caps (bottom panel). **(D)** Endogenous FUS is not essential for nuclear aggregation of CREST. Cells were co-transfected with FUS siRNA and a plasmid to express CREST-Flag and were analysed 48 hours post-transfection. **(E-G)** CREST efficiently sequesters endogenous FUS into dot-like nuclear aggregates in COS7 cells. In contrast, two other paraspeckle components, p54nrb and PSPC1, are not recruited to small and medium-sized CREST aggregates (F and G, top panels), and are detected in aggregates only in nuclei with extensive CREST aggregation (F and G, bottom panels). **(H, I)** Presence of CREST aggregates in the nucleus negatively affects paraspeckles. The fraction of cells with paraspeckles among COS7 cells expressing CREST-Flag (anti-p54nrb staining) or CREST-GFP (FISH with NEAT1 probe) was quantified separately for cells with diffuse CREST distribution and with nuclear CREST aggregates (mean ± s.e.m, *p < 0.05, **p < 0.01; 150-250 cells counted from each of the four or three independent experiments). **(J)** NEAT1 levels are decreased in CREST-expressing cells. Untagged CREST or GFP (vector) were expressed in SH-SY5Y cells for 24 hours; NEAT1 levels were measured by qPCR (**p < 0.01; results from four independent experiments run in duplicates). Scale bars, A – 5 μm; B-G – 10 μm.

CREST co-aggregates with FUS but not ALS-associated proteins TDP-43 or TAF15

Previously reported results of co-immunoprecipitation experiments demonstrated that two ALS-associated proteins, CREST and FUS, interact in vivo [4]. However, we identified a significant cross-reactivity of the anti-CREST antibody used in the above study with FUS protein (Additional file 4: Figure S3). Nevertheless, we also found that endogenous FUS is efficiently recruited into nuclear

CREST aggregates (Figure 4E). To confirm CREST-FUS interaction in vivo, we transfected cells with a construct to express CREST-GFP and performed immunoprecipitation using GFP-Trap beads. Endogenous FUS was co-immunoprecipitated with CREST in this cellular system indicating that the proteins indeed interact in vivo (Figure 5A).

We went on to study FUS-CREST co-aggregation in more detail and establish if it is specific for FUS. Co-

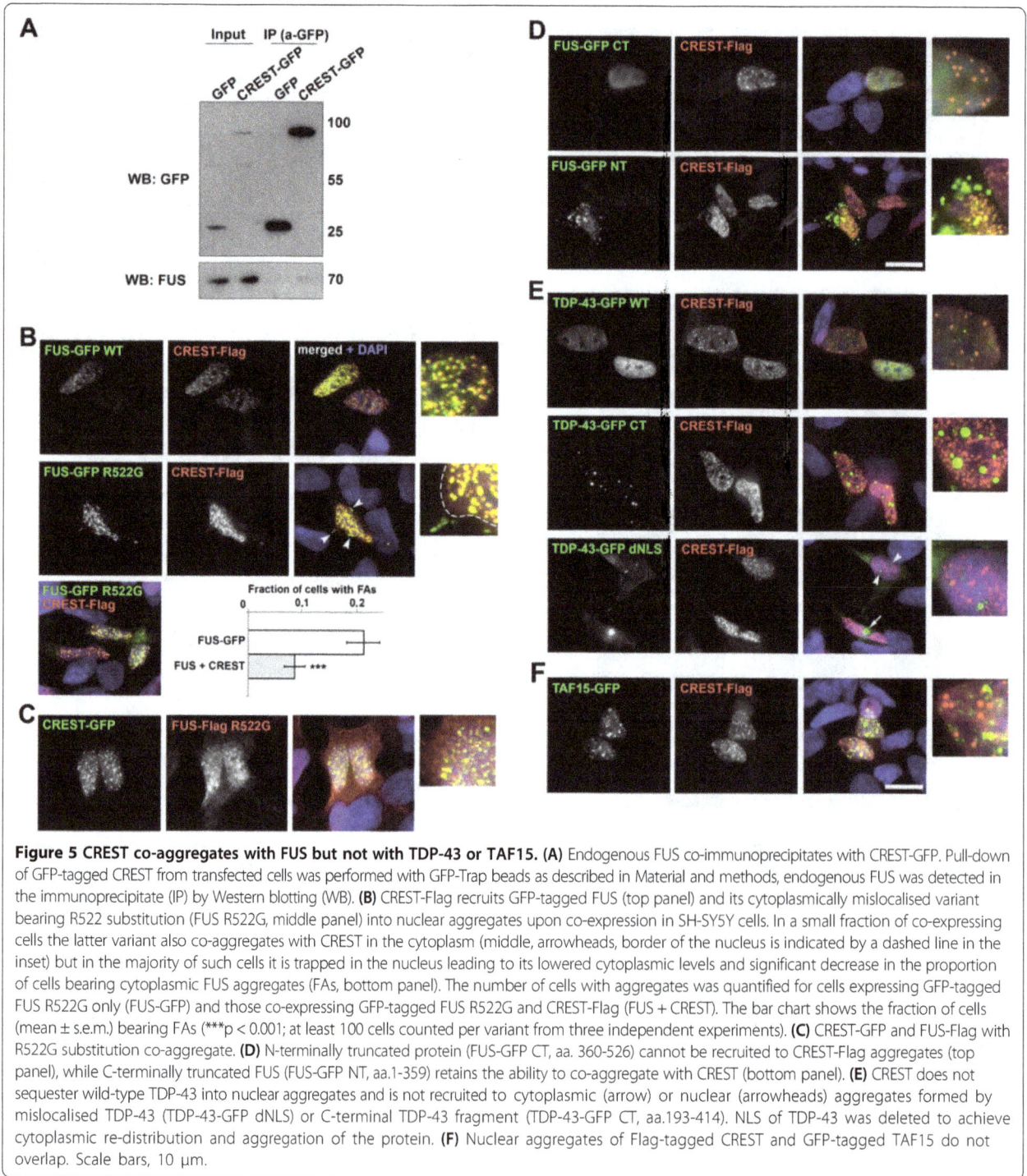

Figure 5 CREST co-aggregates with FUS but not with TDP-43 or TAF15. (A) Endogenous FUS co-immunoprecipitates with CREST-GFP. Pull-down of GFP-tagged CREST from transfected cells was performed with GFP-Trap beads as described in Material and methods, endogenous FUS was detected in the immunoprecipitate (IP) by Western blotting (WB). **(B)** CREST-Flag recruits GFP-tagged FUS (top panel) and its cytoplasmically mislocalised variant bearing R522 substitution (FUS R522G, middle panel) into nuclear aggregates upon co-expression in SH-SY5Y cells. In a small fraction of co-expressing cells the latter variant also co-aggregates with CREST in the cytoplasm (middle, arrowheads, border of the nucleus is indicated by a dashed line in the inset) but in the majority of such cells it is trapped in the nucleus leading to its lowered cytoplasmic levels and significant decrease in the proportion of cells bearing cytoplasmic FUS aggregates (FAs, bottom panel). The number of cells with aggregates was quantified for cells expressing GFP-tagged FUS R522G only (FUS-GFP) and those co-expressing GFP-tagged FUS R522G and CREST-Flag (FUS + CREST). The bar chart shows the fraction of cells (mean ± s.e.m.) bearing FAs (***p < 0.001; at least 100 cells counted per variant from three independent experiments). **(C)** CREST-GFP and FUS-Flag with R522G substitution co-aggregate. **(D)** N-terminally truncated protein (FUS-GFP CT, aa. 360-526) cannot be recruited to CREST-Flag aggregates (top panel), while C-terminally truncated FUS (FUS-GFP NT, aa.1-359) retains the ability to co-aggregate with CREST (bottom panel). **(E)** CREST does not sequester wild-type TDP-43 into nuclear aggregates and is not recruited to cytoplasmic (arrow) or nuclear (arrowheads) aggregates formed by mislocalised TDP-43 (TDP-43-GFP dNLS) or C-terminal TDP-43 fragment (TDP-43-GFP CT, aa.193-414). NLS of TDP-43 was deleted to achieve cytoplasmic re-distribution and aggregation of the protein. **(F)** Nuclear aggregates of Flag-tagged CREST and GFP-tagged TAF15 do not overlap. Scale bars, 10 μm.

expression of CREST-Flag and FUS-GFP led to their robust co-aggregation in the nucleus (Figure 5B, top panel), seemingly, via sequestration of FUS into dot-like CREST aggregates. This was also true for cytoplasmically mislocalised FUS mutant bearing a substitution in its nuclear localisation signal, FUS R522G (Figure 5B, middle panel). Although R522G mutation leads to dramatic shift to the cytoplasm and subsequent cytoplasmic aggregation

of FUS [22,23], when co-expressed with CREST-Flag, FUS-GFP R522G was present in the cytoplasm at low levels and the percent of cells bearing cytoplasmic FUS aggregates was significantly decreased (Figure 5B, bottom panel). We concluded that aggregating CREST-Flag is able to recruit and retain FUS in the nucleus leading to its lowered cytoplasmic levels and interfering with its cytoplasmic aggregation. Interestingly, cells that formed cytoplasmic FUS R522G aggregates also contained overexpressed CREST within those aggregates (Figure 5, middle panel, arrowheads). Similarly, CREST-GFP co-aggregated with FUS-Flag R522G (Figure 5C). The region responsible for co-aggregation of FUS with CREST lies in the N-terminal part of the FUS molecule, since a variant lacking all domains downstream of the RRM (NT-RRM, aa. 1-359) was still able to co-aggregate with CREST, but no recruitment into CREST aggregates was observed for the C-terminal FUS fragment (CT, aa.360-526) (Figure 5D). In contrast, neither normal TDP-43, nor TDP-43 rendered cytoplasmic by deletion of its NLS, nor C-terminal TDP-43 fragment (aa.193-414), showed co-aggregation with CREST (Figure 5E). Furthermore, aggregates formed in the nucleus by another ALS-associated protein structurally highly similar to FUS, TAF15, were clearly distinct from nuclear CREST aggregates (Figure 5F).

Q388stop mutation alters steady-state levels and aggregation propensity of CREST protein

Recently four mutations were identified in CREST in ALS patients [4,5]. However, the basis of their pathogenicity is still not clear. The mutations do not cluster but are spread along the molecule, each found in a different domain (Figure 6A). We created constructs for the expression of these four variants as untagged proteins. The proteins displayed predominantly nuclear distribution indistinguishable from the wild-type protein (Figure 6B). All variants occasionally formed nuclear dot-like aggregates similar to those shown in Figure 1A for untagged wild-type CREST; the frequency of cells bearing such aggregates was comparable between the variants except Q388stop, a mutant lacking eight amino acids at its C-terminus. The latter aggregated in the nucleus significantly more often than wild-type protein or any other studied mutant (p = 0.0169; Figure 6C). All CREST variants were expressed in cell lines studied at similar levels, however, densitometric analysis revealed that steady-state levels of Q388stop variant were elevated (p = 0.0483) compared to other variants despite insignificant differences at mRNA level (Figure 6D). To assess if CREST mutations alter protein stability, we estimated the proteins' half-lives using a pulse chase with cycloheximide. Overexpressed CREST was stable, with half-life of approximately 36 hours, without significant differences between the variants but again with the exception of Q388stop, which displayed increased stability (Figure 6E). The propensity of CREST mutants to aggregate was estimated using the sequential extraction protocol described above. All variants behaved very similarly to the non-mutated CREST without marked changes in the abundance in different fractions (Figure 6F). We did not observe any differences between the mutants in their ability to be recruited to SGs or paraspeckles, or

co-aggregate with FUS protein (Figure 6G, Additional file 3: Figure S2).

CREST overexpression negatively affects dendritic complexity in cultured hippocampal neurons and causes retina degeneration in transgenic Drosophila

In a previous study an inhibitory effect of mutant CREST variants Q388stop and I123M on KCl-induced neurite outgrowth in cultured mouse cortical neurons has been reported [4]. Because CREST is prone to aggregation and sequesters some important proteins into aggregates, it is feasible that its overexpression per se might be deleterious to neurons. We therefore examined the effect of normal CREST and its mutants on the complexity of dendritic tree in unstimulated primary mouse hippocampal neurons. In these cells both GFP-tagged and untagged CREST displayed similar distribution with mainly nuclear localization, and frequent aggregation in the nucleus and occasionally in the processes (Figure 7A); aggregation increased in a concentration-dependent manner. Untagged CREST was used for further analysis due to its more physiological nature. Hippocampal neurons isolated from mice on postnatal day 3 and cultured for 5 days were co-transfected with a vector for GFP expression to visualise neuronal morphology, and each of the CREST variants. The cells were allowed to express the proteins for 48 hours (see Methods for details). Total dendritic length was significantly decreased in CREST-expressing neurons compared to neurons transfected with vector only and was comparable between the variants (Figure 7B). However, this parameter was lower (p = 0.049983) for Q388stop variant compared to wild-type CREST (Figure 7B). Similarly, CREST-expressing cells exhibited fewer dendritic trees, and for Q388stop and to a lesser extent A264T, this effect was even more pronounced than for wild-type protein (Figure 7B). Sholl analysis of CREST expressing neurons also revealed a significant difference only for the Q388stop mutant: the number of shell intersections for neurons expressing this protein was significantly lower compared to that for wild-type protein (Figure 7C).

To address possible effects of elevated CREST levels in vivo, we generated Drosophila melanogaster lines overexpressing untagged normal or mutant human protein using GAL4-UAS system (Additional file 5: Figure S4, Figure 8A). UAS-CREST wild-type, I123M and Q388stop transgenic lines were crossed with gmr-GAL4 line to drive the expression of proteins in the retinal photoreceptor neurons. External morphology of the heads of 5-day-old flies overexpressing these variants was characterized by rough and de-pigmented eyes compared to those overexpressing lacZ as a control protein, without obvious differences between the lines (Figure 8B). Histological analysis revealed marked disruption of the regularly ordered arrays of photoreceptor neurons with thinned retina (Figure 8C).

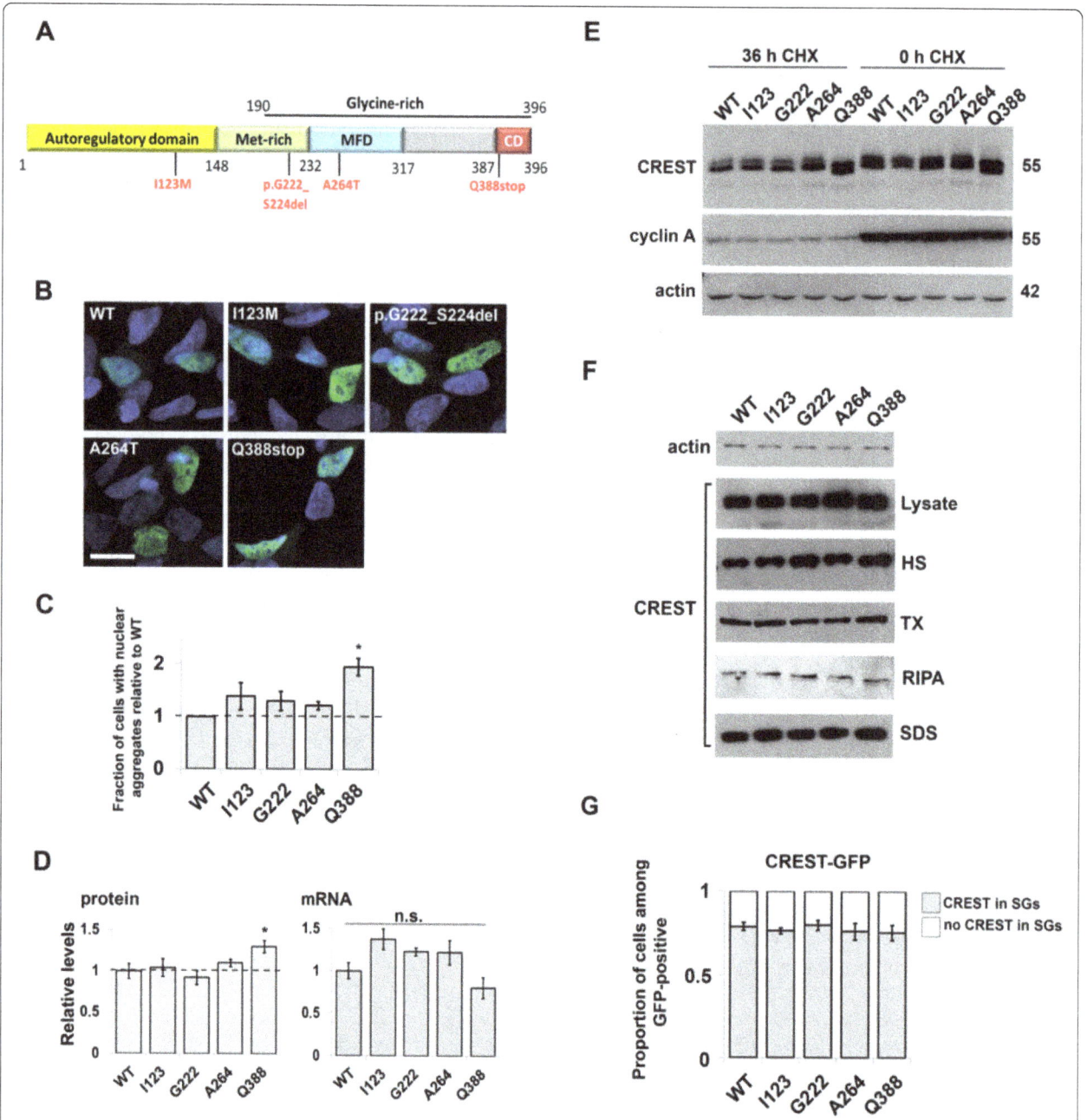

Figure 6 ALS-associated CREST mutation Q388stop increases steady-state levels of the protein and its ability to aggregate. (A) A map of CREST with the positions of single amino acid substitutions or a deletion found in ALS indicated. (B) All CREST variants are localized predominantly to the nucleus in SH-SY5Y cells. (C) Q388stop mutant aggregates in the nucleus more often compared to the normal protein and other mutants. Among cells expressing each of the untagged CREST variants those with aggregates in the nucleus were quantified on the entire coverslip 24 hours post-transfection and obtained values were normalized against the value for wild-type CREST. The bar chart shows means ± s.e.m. of these normalized values from four independent experiments (*p < 0.05). (D) Steady-state protein levels for Q388stop mutant variant are increased compared to the wild-type protein without significant difference at the transcript level. The bar charts show means ± s.e.m. of seven independent experiments (*p < 0.05, Mann-Whitney U-test). (E) All CREST variants are stable proteins with half-lives of approximately 36 hours. Cycloheximide was used to block protein synthesis; levels of a short-lived protein, cyclin A, were measured to confirm successful block of translation. (F) Solubility of mutant CREST variants upon sequential protein extraction was comparable to that of wild-type protein. Fractionation was performed as described in Materials and methods. (G) CREST mutants do not affect the ability of the protein to be recruited to stress granules. The fraction of cells with CREST-positive stress granules after sodium arsenite exposure was quantified in the population of CREST-GFP expressing cells for each variant (at least 100 cells counted per variant in each of the two independent experiments). Scale bar, 10 μm.

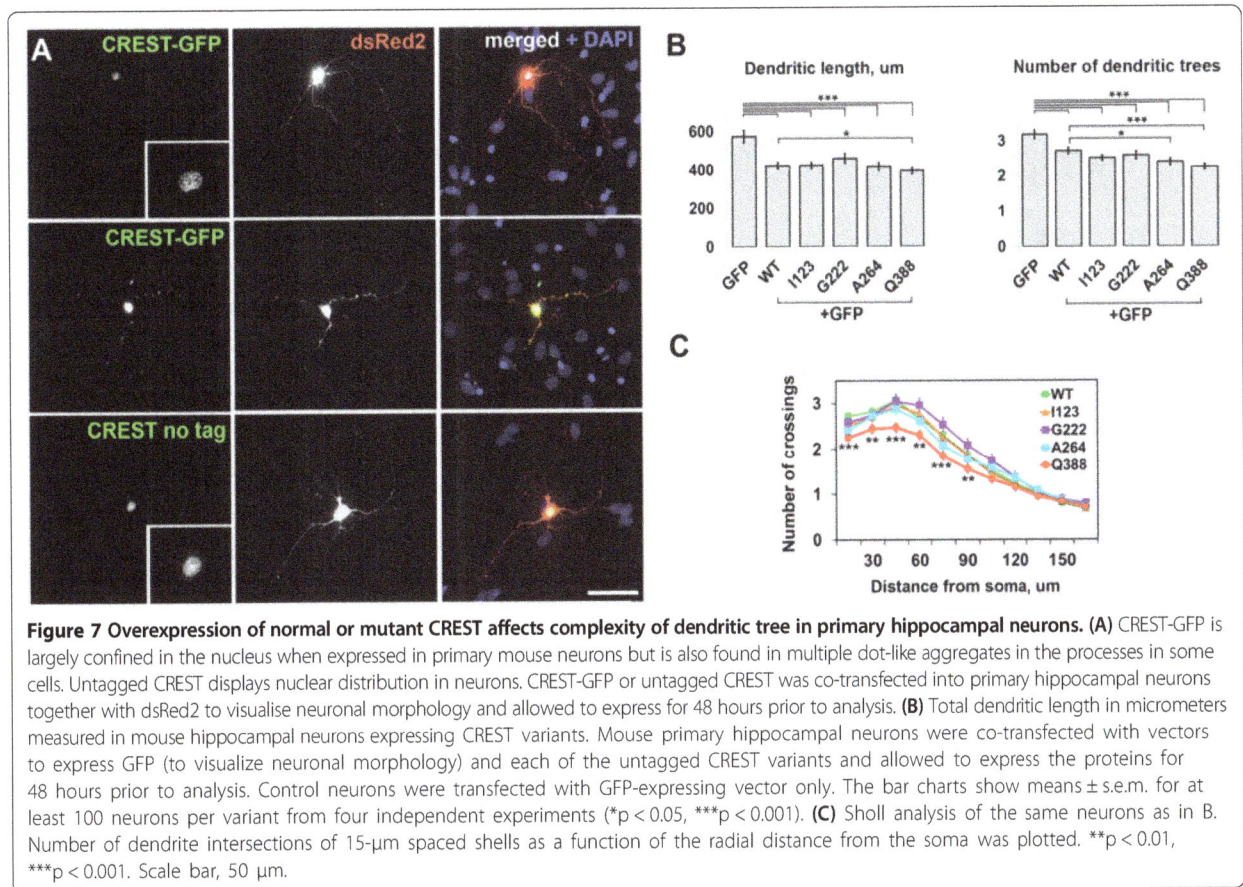

Figure 7 Overexpression of normal or mutant CREST affects complexity of dendritic tree in primary hippocampal neurons. (A) CREST-GFP is largely confined in the nucleus when expressed in primary mouse neurons but is also found in multiple dot-like aggregates in the processes in some cells. Untagged CREST displays nuclear distribution in neurons. CREST-GFP or untagged CREST was co-transfected into primary hippocampal neurons together with dsRed2 to visualise neuronal morphology and allowed to express for 48 hours prior to analysis. **(B)** Total dendritic length in micrometers measured in mouse hippocampal neurons expressing CREST variants. Mouse primary hippocampal neurons were co-transfected with vectors to express GFP (to visualize neuronal morphology) and each of the untagged CREST variants and allowed to express the proteins for 48 hours prior to analysis. Control neurons were transfected with GFP-expressing vector only. The bar charts show means ± s.e.m. for at least 100 neurons per variant from four independent experiments (*p < 0.05, ***p < 0.001). **(C)** Sholl analysis of the same neurons as in B. Number of dendrite intersections of 15-μm spaced shells as a function of the radial distance from the soma was plotted. **p < 0.01, ***p < 0.001. Scale bar, 50 μm.

Thus, overexpression of either normal or mutant CREST in photoreceptor neurons of a fly is sufficient to induce severe degeneration.

Discussion

Our study presents evidence that CREST possesses three properties common to several proteins associated with ALS: i) high propensity to aggregate in cells; ii) recruitment into stress granules; and iii) ability to modulate paraspeckle integrity. There is a growing body of evidence that protein aggregation and altered function of SGs (and likely, paraspeckles) are important factors in ALS pathogenesis, and our observations also point to these processes as potential culprits for the development of pathological changes in ALS cases with CREST mutations.

In the previous studies devoted to cellular localization and functions of CREST it has been proposed that nuclear structures formed by CREST represent a type of nuclear body that recruits CBP protein and thereby regulates its functions [13]. Here we show that CREST structures appearing upon protein accumulation in the nucleus correspond to irreversibly aggregated entities formed due to the high aggregation propensity of CREST, since they grow in time- and concentration-dependent manner and do not dissipate in response to transcriptional repression like genuine nuclear bodies, paraspeckles and Cajal bodies [24,25]. In line with this, CREST accumulates in detergent-insoluble fractions when overexpressed in cultured cells. It cannot be ruled out that at early stages of their formation, nuclear CREST aggregates represent physiologically relevant and functional foci recruiting factors such as CBP to certain genome locations. However, in certain conditions CREST in these foci may start aggregating uncontrollably thereby transforming them into pathological aggregates. This can be caused by abnormally high accumulation of CREST in the nucleus and, consequently, in the foci, or by lower concentration threshold of uncontrollable aggregation for mutated CREST. A similar scenario has been suggested for transformation of cytoplasmic RNA granules enriched in proteins with prion-like domains into proteinaceous inclusions in proteinopathies [22,23]. CREST also has a prion-like domain in its structure, and the latter was proposed to play a role both in physiological and pathological aggregation [15-17]. Since at present the nature of these CREST structures is unclear, in this study they are collectively referred as "aggregates" regardless their physiological significance. It should be kept in mind that accumulation of very high levels of the protein observed in some cells upon its

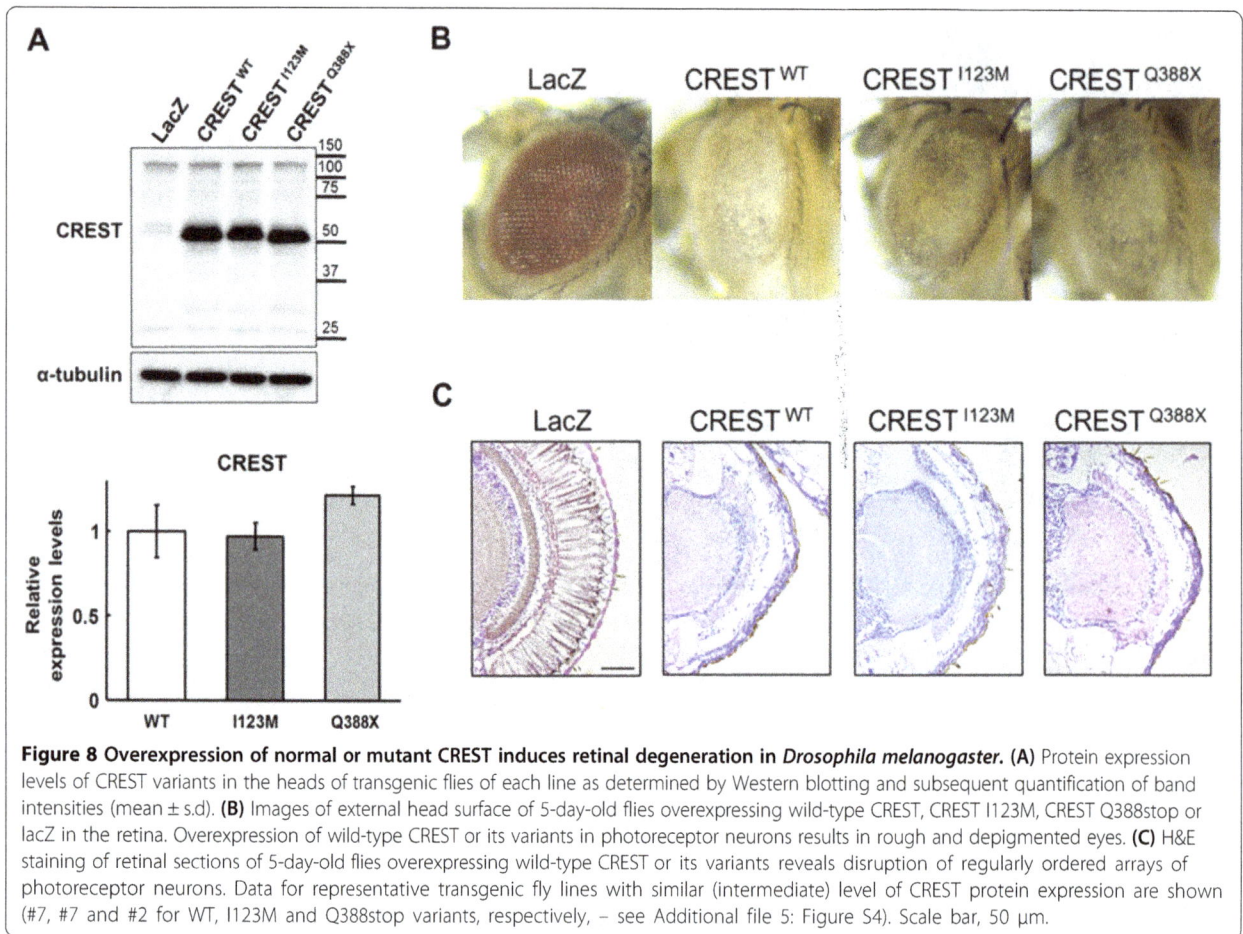

Figure 8 Overexpression of normal or mutant CREST induces retinal degeneration in *Drosophila melanogaster*. (A) Protein expression levels of CREST variants in the heads of transgenic flies of each line as determined by Western blotting and subsequent quantification of band intensities (mean ± s.d). **(B)** Images of external head surface of 5-day-old flies overexpressing wild-type CREST, CREST I123M, CREST Q388stop or lacZ in the retina. Overexpression of wild-type CREST or its variants in photoreceptor neurons results in rough and depigmented eyes. **(C)** H&E staining of retinal sections of 5-day-old flies overexpressing wild-type CREST or its variants reveals disruption of regularly ordered arrays of photoreceptor neurons. Data for representative transgenic fly lines with similar (intermediate) level of CREST protein expression are shown (#7, #7 and #2 for WT, I123M and Q388stop variants, respectively, – see Additional file 5: Figure S4). Scale bar, 50 μm.

overexpression is unlikely to be achieved for the endogenous protein. However, in our study nuclear CREST aggregates started appearing already in cells with low levels of exogenous protein indicating a low threshold for its multimerization. Further studies using more physiological models, such as neurons differentiated from iPS cells of patients with CREST mutations or cells with modified CREST gene, are required to establish the molecular nature of CREST aggregates at different stages of their formation as well as functional relevance of CREST multimerization.

It has been shown previously that the N-terminal autoregulatory domain of CREST is largely dispensable for its localization to nuclear aggregates [13] however we also noted that the CR_dNT mutant lacking this domain has diminished aggregation propensity. Interestingly, unlike similar domains of FUS and TDP-43 [26-28], the C-terminal transactivation domain of CREST cannot aggregate in isolation despite its prion-like properties. Thus, the aggregation propensity of CREST is defined by cooperative action of its C-terminal and N-terminal domains, while MFD may limit it. Importantly, in our study only CREST deletion variants with preserved ability to

aggregate were capable of SG and paraspeckle recruitment. This correlation provides further support for the notion that the ability of proteins bearing a prion-like domain to aggregate reversibly (i.e. "physiological" aggregation) is prerequisite for their entry into RNA granules such as SGs and paraspeckles [15-17]. Seemingly, such proteins have to be tightly regulated, and modulation of CREST aggregation propensity by autoregulatory domain and MFD is an example of such regulation. Even subtle changes in the structure of such domains may lead to uncontrollable aggregation and downstream events deleterious for neurons. We also demonstrated that both autoregulatory domain and MFD of CREST contribute to nuclear localization of the protein. Impairment of these domains' function may therefore result in cytoplasmic redistribution of the protein, similar to redistribution of FUS bearing ALS-linked mutations in its nuclear localization signal [22,23].

We also showed that nuclear aggregates of CREST are able to trap certain proteins such as FUS, which could lead to loss of their function. Therefore, changes in CREST levels (e.g. due to increased stability) or its solubility, triggered by any external or internal factor including mutation, could initiate aggregation of the protein in the nervous system, which in turn would affect CREST binding partners important for neuronal homeostasis. There are several reports of increased stability [29-31] and/or higher aggregation propensity [28,32,33] of ALS-associated TDP-43 mutants compared to non-mutated protein. Similarly, we have demonstrated that at least one of the ALS-linked mutations in CREST, Q388stop, affects protein stability and renders it more aggregate-prone. An opposite situation, where CREST would be sequestered into aggregates formed by other proteins, particularly FUS, is also possible. Our attempts to establish if CREST pathology is present in FUSopathies were precluded by cross-reactivity of the anti-CREST antibody, suitable for histological staining, with FUS. When a truly specific antibody becomes available it would be interesting to determine the extent of CREST involvement in histopathology typical of FUSopathies.

Altered metabolism of SGs is now widely acknowledged to be contributory to ALS pathogenesis [3,34-38], and recently dysfunction of another RNA granule, the paraspeckle, has emerged as a possible factor in ALS pathology. Paraspeckles are built on a long non-coding RNA NEAT1 and recruit a subset of proteins, including FUS and to a lesser extent TDP-43 [14]. Functionally, this RNA granule is involved in the nuclear retention of specific RNAs [39], regulation of gene expression and possibly the cellular stress response [40,41]. Results of several studies suggest a role for paraspeckle proteins and NEAT1 in ALS/FTLD disease pathogenesis [42-49]. Furthermore, it has been specifically demonstrated that paraspeckle assembly triggered by upregulated NEAT1 synthesis occurs in motor neurons at the early stage of ALS development, suggesting a protective role against various insults, which might be particularly important for motor neuron welfare [18]. We have also established links between loss and gain of function of FUS protein and disrupted paraspeckle assembly in ALS-FUS [19]. This allowed us to propose a model whereby aggregation of FUS in the cytoplasm leads to its nuclear loss accompanied by depletion of other paraspeckle proteins, which in turn may disable protective paraspeckle assembly and contribute to neurodegeneration in FUSopathies. A similar scenario may occur in ALS cases caused by CREST mutations, where aggregating protein can sequester FUS (and perhaps other paraspeckle proteins) into aggregates and attenuate protective paraspeckle formation.

We observed no overt phenotypes specific to identified ALS-associated CREST mutations except for Q388stop. Instead, we showed that excess of CREST affects neuron morphology independently of the presence of mutations. Moreover, in transgenic fly models, all studied protein variants, including non-mutated protein, were highly toxic and induced severe retinal degeneration. Therefore,

alterations of CREST stability and consequently, intracellular protein level, which might occur as a result of mutation or triggered by external factors, would be deleterious for neurons, the only type of cells expressing high levels of CREST. Q388stop mutation was predicted to be highly damaging since it affects the prion-like domain and removes a CBP-interaction motif of CREST [4]. We showed that this mutation also increases steady-state protein levels, promotes CREST aggregation and perhaps as a result, negatively affects branching and outgrowth of neuritis in cultured neurons. No gross differences in subcellular localization, aggregation capacity, stability, SG/paraspeckle recruitment or in vivo toxicity of other mutants compared to wild-type protein were registered indicating the need for fine structural and functional assays to further probe their pathogenicity. The fact that alterations in the structure and properties of CREST are not immediately recognizable is not surprising as a similar trend was revealed in the studies of mutant variants of other ALS-associated proteins. For example, only some ALS-causative FUS variants with mutations in NLS are redistributed to the cytoplasm in cultured cells, whereas others do not visibly affect nuclear import [50,51]. Similarly, prion-like and glycine-rich domains of TDP-43 are the hot-spots of mutations, but functional consequences of different mutations in these domains are highly variable [51,52]. Studies on post-mortem tissue of patients bearing mutations in CREST would be highly informative for establishing if CREST is indeed another protein whose aggregation leads to neurodegeneration. CREST is essential for the nervous system homeostasis as evidenced by the severe neurological phenotype of CREST deficient mice [6] as well as its high expression levels specifically in postmitotic neurons [9]. Therefore, it is highly likely that mutations identified in ALS only slightly compromise the protein structure allowing normal development of the nervous system, but nevertheless are sufficient to trigger a severe neurodegenerative disorder in the adulthood. Our studies in vitro and in vivo suggested that altered protein stability and hence its increased levels may be behind this effect. Interestingly, one ALS patient with CREST mutation also carried an amino acid substitution in OPTN gene [5]. It is plausible that in this case the presence of both mutations was necessary for manifestation of the clinical phenotype, providing another example in support of the emerging concept of ALS as an oligogenic disease [53].

In summary, our study provides experimental evidence that CREST can be considered another member of the growing group of ALS-linked aggregation-prone proteins capable of recruitment to SGs and other RNA granules. Until very recently, members of this group were exclusively RNA-binding proteins. However, together with the report on profilin1 recruitment to SGs [54], our study links ALS aetiology with dysfunction of RNA granule components other than RNA-binding proteins.

Methods

Expression plasmids, stable cell lines, transfection and treatments

DNA fragments encoding full-length CREST, FUS, TDP-43 and TAF15 and their deletion and mutant variants were produced by RT-PCR amplification with SuperScript III and AccuPrime polymerases (Invitrogen, Life Technologies) from human (SH-SY5Y cells or fetal brain) total RNA using respective primers and cloned into pCR-BluntII-TOPO vector (Invitrogen, Life Technologies). After sequence validation the fragments were subcloned into the pEGFP-C1 vector (Clontech) downstream and in-frame with GFP to produce proteins bearing N-terminal GFP tag; into the pEGFP-N1 vector (Clontech) upstream and separated by a stop codon from GFP to obtain non-tagged proteins; and into the pCMV4-Flag vector (Sigma) for the expression of Flag-tagged wild-type CREST. SH-SY5Y, HEK293 and COS7 cells were maintained in Dulbecco modified Eagle medium supplemented with 10% foetal bovine serum (Invitrogen, Life Technologies). For immunofluorescence cells were grown on poly-L-lysine coated coverslips. Cells were transfected with expression plasmids or mixture of a plasmid and FUS siRNAs using Lipofectamine2000 (Invitrogen, Life Technologies) according to the manufacturer's instructions. For plasmid co-transfections equal amounts of plasmid DNA were taken into the reaction. For FUS knockdown FUS-specific SiGENOME SMART pool (M-009497-02, Thermo Scientific) was used. For nucleolus staining living cells were exposed to 10 µg/ml of ethidium bromide for 1 hour prior to fixation. To block transcription, cells were treated with 5 µg/ml actinomycin D (Calbiochem, Merck Millipore) for 1 hour. To induce formation of stress granules, cells were subjected to 5 mM sodium arsenite (Sigma) for 1 hour, 2 µM thapsigargin (Sigma) for 4 hours or 50 µM 15-deoxy-delta 12,14-prostaglandin J2 (15d-PGJ2, Cayman Chemical) for 1 hour.

Immunofluorescence on coverslips

Cells were fixed with 4% paraformaldehyde on ice for 15 min, followed by washes with PBS and 5 min permeabealization in cold methanol. After three washes with PBS and blocking in 5% goat serum/PBS/0.1% Triton-X100 for 1 h at room temperature coverslips were incubated with primary antibodies diluted in blocking solution for 1 h at room temperature or at 4°C overnight. Alexa Fluorconjugated anti-mouse or anti-rabbit immunoglobulins (Molecular Probes, Life Technologies) were used as secondary antibodies (1:1000 in PBS/0.1% Triton-X100) and cell nuclei were visualized with DAPI. For RNA-FISH, a commercially available NEAT1 and MALAT1 probes

(Stellaris® FISH Probes against human NEAT1 5′ segment and human MALAT1, Biosearch Technologies) was used according to the protocol provided by the manufacturer. Fluorescent images were taken using BX61 microscope (Olympus) and processed using CellF software (Olympus). For assessing cytoplasmic redistribution of CREST under stress, fluorescence intensity was measured 24 hours after transfection in naïve and sodium-arsenite treated cells in three 2.5 × 2.5 µm squares randomly chosen in the cytoplasm of a transfected cell using free-access ImageJ software. To estimate the enrichment of full-length CREST and CR_dNT in SGs, fluorescence intensity was measured in three 0.5 × 0.5 µm squares in the cytoplasm free from SGs and in three 0.5 × 0.5 µm squares within SGs of a transfected cell. Mean intensities per cell were calculated and used to calculate standard deviation and standard error of the mean (s.e.m.), as well as ratio SG/cytoplasm.

Live cell imaging

Time-lapse images were obtained using Leica TCS SP2 MP confocal microscope, equipped with an on-scope incubator with temperature control. SH-SY5Y cells were plated on glass-bottomed dishes (Mattek) and transfected with a plasmid to express CREST-GFP. Before imaging, regular culture media was replaced with HEPES-buffered media (10 mM HEPES-KOH, pH7.5). Cells were visualized under Fluotar L 63 × 1.4 oil objective. A sequence of images was further transformed into a video clip using Leica Application Suite AF software.

Primary mouse hippocampal cultures

All reagents used for preparation of hippocampal cultures were purchased from Invitrogen, Life Technologies unless stated otherwise. Hippocampi were dissected from mice at postnatal day 3, digested for 40 minutes in 0.1% trypsin in HBSS supplemented with 10 mM Hepes and 1 mM pyruvate. After mechanical dissociation in Neurobasal A medium containing 50 U/ml penicillin/streptomycin, 0.2% β-mercaptoethanol, 500 µM L-Glutamine and 10% horse serum, hippocampi were centrifuged for 5 minutes at 1,500 rpm. Pellets were resuspended in fresh medium and plated on poly-L-lysine coated coverslips. One day after plating the medium was changed to serum-free medium containing B27. Mixed neuronal-glial cultures were transfected on DIV5 using Lipofectamine2000 according to the standard procedure, except Lipofectamin-DNA complexes which were left for 1 hour and subsequently replaced with normal culture medium. Cells were fixed and stained 48 hours after transfection. Estimation of dendritic length, number of dendritic trees and Sholl analysis were performed using Matlab5 software. At least 100 neurons from four independent experiments were analysed per variant.

Primary antibodies

Commercially available primary antibodies against the following antigens were used: CREST (rabbit polyclonal, 12439-1-AP, Proteintech); FUS (mouse monoclonal against C-terminus, Santa Cruz, sc-47711; rabbit polyclonal, ab84078, Abcam); p54nrb (rabbit polyclonal C-terminal, Sigma); TIAR (mouse monoclonal, BD Biosciences); G3BP1 (mouse monoclonal, BD Biosciences); Dcp1a (rabbit polyclonal C-terminal, Sigma); anti-Flag M2 (mouse monoclonal, Sigma); PSPC1 (rabbit polyclonal C-terminal, Sigma); GFP (Living Colours® rabbit polyclonal, Clontech, #632593); SMN (mouse monoclonal, BD Biosciences); cyclin A (rabbit polyclonal, Santa Cruz, sc-751); p80 coilin (mouse monoclonal, BD Biosciences); PML (chicken polyclonal, a kind gift from Prof. Ronald Hay, Dundee); phosphorylated tau (mouse monoclonal, clone AT8, Thermo Scientific); beta-actin (mouse monoclonal, clone AC15, Sigma); alpha-tubulin (mouse monoclonal, clone DM1A, Sigma). Primary antibodies were used at 1:1,000 dilution for all applications.

Protein stability

SH-SY5Y cells were transfected with corresponding constructs and allowed to express the protein for 24 hours. To block translation, cycloheximide (Sigma) was added to a final concentration of 20 µg/ml; cells were harvested after 8, 12, 24, 36 and 48 hours of exposure.

Sequential protein extraction

HEK293 cells were transfected with corresponding constructs and harvested 24 hours post-transfection. Cells were disrupted mechanically in high-salt buffer containing protease inhibitors and centrifuged at 13,000 rpm to remove cell debris; a small amount was kept as total lysate. Samples were subjected to ultracentrifugation at 48,000 rpm for 20 min and supernatant was recovered as high-salt soluble fraction (HS). Resulting pellets were resuspended in high-salt buffer supplemented with 1% Triton-X100 and centrifuged again under the same conditions. Supernatant was labelled as Triton-X100 soluble fraction (TX). The same steps were repeated with RIPA buffer to obtain RIPA-soluble fraction (RIPA). Final pellets were lysed directly in SDS-PAGE loading buffer to yield SDS-soluble fraction (SDS). Protein amounts in different fractions were normalized against the protein amount in the high-salt fraction. For total lysate (L) and high-salt (HS) fraction 10% of the amount relative to other fractions was loaded.

RT-PCR and qPCR

Total RNA was isolated using RNeasy mini kit (Qiagen) and possible DNA contamination removed using RNase free DNase kit (Qiagen). First-strand cDNA synthesis was carried out on 500 ng of RNA using SuperScript III reverse transcriptase (Invitrogen, Life Technologies) and random hexamers (Promega) according to manufacturer's instructions. Quantitative real-time PCR was run in triplicate on an ABI StepOne™ real-time PCR instrument and data were analyzed using StepOne™ Software v2.0 (Applied Biosystems, Life Technologies). cDNA amount for each gene was normalized to that of GAPDH. Primer sequences used were as follows: CREST - forward: 5'-ggttacgcagcaaaccatcc-3', reverse: 5'-ggatctgctggtactg cgtg -3'; NEAT1 - forward: 5'-cttcctccctttaacttatccattcac-3', reverse: 5'-ctcttcctccaccattaccaacaatac-3'; GAPDH - forward: 5'-tcgccagccgagcca-3'; reverse: 5'-gagttaaaagcag ccctggtg-3'.

Immunoprecipitation

Cells were washed with PBS, lysed in ice cold IP buffer (PBS/1% Triton-X100) on ice with periodic vortexing for 10 min. Unbroken cells and cell debris were pelleted at 13000 rpm for 15 min, input sample was taken at this point. Cell lysates were incubated with GFP-Trap® agarose beads (ChromoTek) for 2 hours at 4°C. Beads were washed four times with ice cold high-salt buffer (20 mM Tris, 300 mM NaCl, 1% Triton-X100) and bound complexes were eluted from beads by boiling for 5 min at 100°C in SDS-PAGE loading buffer. To remove beads, samples were centrifuged at $13000 \times g$ for 5 min. Samples were then analyzed by Western blotting. For input 10% of final IP sample was loaded.

Western blotting

For SDS-PAGE loading buffer was used to lyse cells on dishes, followed by denaturation at 100°C for 5 min. After SDS-PAGE, proteins were transferred to PVDF membrane by semi-dry blotting followed by blocking, incubation with primary and HRP-conjugated secondary (GE Healthcare) antibodies and ECL detection as described previously [55]. Equal loading was confirmed by re-probing membranes with antibodies against beta-actin or alpha-tubulin.

Semi-Denaturating Detergent Agarose Gel Electrophoresis (SDD-AGE)

A protocol described previously [56] was used with modifications indicated below. Briefly, SH-SY5Y cells were harvested 24 hours post transfection in PBS-1% Triton-X100, left on ice for 20 min with periodic vortexing and centrifuged at $17,000 \times g$. To obtain a positive control for the presence of amyloid aggregates the spinal cord of a 6-month old transgenic TauP301S mouse was processed in parallel with cell lysates. Supernatants were mixed with equal amounts of 2X SDD-AGE loading buffer (1XTAE, 5% glycerol and 1% SDS) and run in 1.5% agarose containing 0.1% SDS. Proteins from the gel were transferred to nitrocellulose membrane using capillary transfer and the membrane was subjected to Western blotting using anti-CREST and anti-phosphorylated tau antibodies as described above.

Generation and characterization of transgenic flies

Constructs encoding human wild-type or mutant CREST, or lacZ in pUAST vector, were injected into w1118 embryos to produce transgenic flies as described previously [57,58]. At least three independent transformant lines were analyzed per construct. gmr-GAL4 and UAS-lacZ lines were obtained from the Bloomington Drosophila stock center. For immunoblot analysis, heads of 5-day-old flies were dissected and lysed in Laemmli sample buffer for SDS-PAGE containing 2% SDS. For external surface observation, 5-day-old flies were anesthetized with CO_2 and observed with zoom stereo microscopy (Olympus SZ-PT). For histochemical analyses, heads of 5-day-old adult transgenic flies were dissected, collected, briefly washed in phosphate buffered saline (PBS), and fixed with 4% paraformaldehyde containing 0.1% Triton X-100 at room temperature for 2 hours. After brief wash in PBS, tissues were dehydrated by graded ethanol, cleared in butanol and embedded in paraffin. Four-micrometer thick coronal sections were stained with hematoxylin and eosin (H&E) [58].

Statistics

Statistical analysis was performed with Mann-Whitney *U*-test using STATISTICA 6.0 software.

Additional files

Additional file 1: Figure S1. Overexpressed CREST aggregates in a dose-dependent manner in COS7 cells. Flag- or GFP-tagged CREST protein displays diffuse and fine-granular distribution in the nucleus of low-expressing COS7 cells and forms dot-like aggregates as it accumulates. In cells with high levels of the protein, large nuclear aggregates together with cytoplasmic accumulation/aggregation are observed. Cells were analysed 24 hours post-transfection. Scale bar, 10 μm.

Additional file 2: Video S1. Time- and concentration-dependent aggregation of CREST in the nucleus. SH-SY5Y cells were transfected with the expression plasmid encoding CREST fused to GFP and imaged 8 hours post-transfection. Note the fusion of dot-like CREST aggregates to each other and aggregate growth with time. QuickTime Player file (.mov).

Additional file 3: Figure S2. ALS-linked CREST mutations do not alter the protein's ability for stress granule or paraspeckle recruitment. (A) All CREST variants are recruited to sodium arsenite induced stress granules. (B) All CREST mutants sequester endogenous FUS protein into nuclear aggregates. (C) Mutations in CREST do not affect its enrichment in paraspeckles in low-expressing SH-SY5Y cells. Scale bars, A, B - 10 μm, C - 5 μm.

Additional file 4: Figure S3. Polyclonal anti-CREST antibody is cross-reactive to human FUS protein. (A) Aggregates formed by FUS-GFP R522G or FUS deletion mutant NT-RRM lacking C-terminal domains displayed high immunoreactivity with CREST antibody. Aggregates of GFP-tagged TDP-43 with deleted NLS were not recognised by this antibody ruling out possible cross-reactivity with GFP tag or non-specific recognition of aggregated protein species. (B) Full-length FUS and its deletion mutants are recognized by CREST antibody on Western

blots. Specific bands corresponding to GFP-tagged FUS and its deletion mutants dRRM (lacking RRM), dR-R (lacking RRM and RGG3) and NT-RRM (lacking entire C-terminus, amino acids 360-526) are indicated with asterisks. Open arrow points to endogenous CREST protein and black arrows point to non-specific bands. Scale bar, 10 μm.

Additional file 5: Figure S4. CREST overexpression in *Drosophila melanogaster* retinal neurons results in retinal degeneration. (A) Transgenic fly lines expressing normal human CREST or its mutants I123M and Q388stop in retinal photoreceptor neurons with different levels of protein expression were generated. Protein levels were measured in the heads of transgenic flies by Western blotting using anti-CREST antibody and band intensities were quantified (bar chart shows mean ± s.d., CREST WT line #2 = 1.0). (B,C) Expression of wild-type or mutant CREST leads to severe retinal degeneration as evidenced by eye depigmentation (B) and its abnormal histology (C, H&E staining). The chromosome with transgene insertion (Ch) for each line is indicated.

Abbreviations

15d-PGJ2: 15-deoxy-delta 12, 14-prostaglandin J2; ALS: Amyotrophic lateral sclerosis; FTLD: Frontotemporal lobar degeneration; MFD: Multifunctional domain; NEAT1: Nuclear enriched abundant transcript 1; RNP: Ribonucleoprotein; RRM: RNA recognition motif; SA: Sodium arsenite; SDD-AGE: Semidenaturating detergent agarose gel electrophoresis; SG: Stress granule.

Competing interests

The authors declare that they have no competing interests.

Authors' contributions

TAS, MSK, AQ, TM, KM and HA performed experiments; TAS, MSK, AQ, TH, TI and VLB designed experiments and analyzed data; TAS, TH and VLB wrote manuscript. All authors read and approved the final version of the manuscript.

Acknowledgements

We are grateful to Johnathan Cooper-Knock for critical reading of the manuscript. This work was supported by Research Grants from Motor Neuron Disease Association (Buchman/Apr13/6096); Russian Scientific Fund (No. 14-14-01138); Russian Foundation for Basic Research (No.14-04-00796 and No.14-04-01243). AQ was supported by Erasmus studentship.

Author details

[1]School of Biosciences, Cardiff University, Museum Avenue, CF10 3AX Cardiff, UK. [2]Institute of Physiologically Active Compounds Russian Academy of Sciences, 1 Severniy proezd, Chernogolovka, 142432 Moscow Region, Russian Federation. [3]Department of Neuropathology, The University of Tokyo, Tokyo, Japan.

References

1. Robberecht W, Philips T. The changing scene of amyotrophic lateral sclerosis. Nat Rev Neurosci. 2013;14:248–64.
2. Droppelmann CA, Campos-Melo D, Ishtiaq M, Volkening K, Strong MJ. RNA metabolism in ALS: when normal processes become pathological. Amyotroph Lateral Scler Frontotemporal Degener. 2014;15:321–36.
3. Ramaswami M, Taylor JP, Parker R. Altered ribostasis: RNA-protein granules in degenerative disorders. Cell. 2013;154:727–36.
4. Chesi A, Staahl BT, Jovicic A, Couthouis J, Fasolino M, Raphael AR, et al. Exome sequencing to identify de novo mutations in sporadic ALS trios. Nat Neurosci. 2013;16:851–5.
5. Teyssou E, Vandenberghe N, Moigneu C, Boillee S, Couratier P, Meininger V, et al. Genetic analysis of SS18L1 in French amyotrophic lateral sclerosis. Neurobiol Aging. 2014;35(1213):e1219–1212.
6. Aizawa H, Hu SC, Bobb K, Balakrishnan K, Ince G, Gurevich I, et al. Dendrite development regulated by CREST, a calcium-regulated transcriptional activator. Science. 2004;303:197–202.
7. Storlazzi CT, Mertens F, Mandahl N, Gisselsson D, Isaksson M, Gustafson P, et al. A novel fusion gene, SS18L1/SSX1, in synovial sarcoma. Genes Chromosomes Cancer. 2003;37:195–200.

8. Walton MR, Dragunow I. Is CREB a key to neuronal survival? Trends Neurosci. 2000;23:48–53.

9. Staahl BT, Tang J, Wu W, Sun A, Gitler AD, Yoo AS, et al. Kinetic analysis of npBAF to nBAF switching reveals exchange of SS18 with CREST and integration with neural developmental pathways. J Neurosci. 2013;33:10348–61.

10. Neale BM, Kou Y, Liu L, Ma'ayan A, Samocha KE, Sabo, et al. Patterns and rates of exonic de novo mutations in autism spectrum disorders. Nature. 2012;485:242–5.

11. O'Roak BJ, Vives L, Girirajan S, Karakoc E, Krumm N, Coe BP, et al. Sporadic autism exomes reveal a highly interconnected protein network of de novo mutations. Nature. 2012;485:246–50.

12. Pradhan A, Liu Y. A multifunctional domain of the calcium-responsive transactivator (CREST) that inhibits dendritic growth in cultured neurons. J Biol Chem. 2005;280:24738–43.

13. Pradhan A, Liu Y. The calcium-responsive transactivator recruits CREB binding protein to nuclear bodies. Neurosci Lett. 2004;370:191–5.

14. Naganuma T, Nakagawa S, Tanigawa A, Sasaki YF, Goshima N, Hirose T. Alternative 3′-end processing of long noncoding RNA initiates construction of nuclear paraspeckles. EMBO J. 2012;31:4020–34.

15. King OD, Gitler AD, Shorter J. The tip of the iceberg: RNA-binding proteins with prion-like domains in neurodegenerative disease. Brain Res. 2012;1462:61–80.

16. Han TW, Kato M, Xie S, Wu LC, Mirzaei H, Pei J, et al. Cell-free formation of RNA granules: bound RNAs identify features and components of cellular assemblies. Cell. 2012;149:768–79.

17. Kato M, Han TW, Xie S, Shi K, Du X, Wu LC, et al. Cell-free formation of RNA granules: low complexity sequence domains form dynamic fibers within hydrogels. Cell. 2012;149:753–67.

18. Nishimoto Y, Nakagawa S, Hirose T, Okano HJ, Takao M, Shibata S, et al. The long non-coding RNA nuclear-enriched abundant transcript 1_2 induces paraspeckle formation in the motor neuron during the early phase of amyotrophic lateral sclerosis. Mol Brain. 2013;6:31.

19. Shelkovnikova TA, Robinson HK, Troakes C, Ninkina N, Buchman VL. Compromised paraspeckle formation as a pathogenic factor in FUSopathies. Hum Mol Genet. 2014;23:2298–312.

20. Kedersha N, Stoecklin G, Ayodele M, Yacono P, Lykke-Andersen J, Fritzler MJ, et al. Stress granules and processing bodies are dynamically linked sites of mRNP remodeling. J Cell Biol. 2005;169:871–84.

21. Kim WJ, Kim JH, Jang SK. Anti-inflammatory lipid mediator 15d-PGJ2 inhibits translation through inactivation of eIF4A. EMBO J. 2007;26:5020–32.

22. Dormann D, Rodde R, Edbauer D, Bentmann E, Fischer I, Hruscha A, et al. ALS-associated fused in sarcoma (FUS) mutations disrupt Transportin-mediated nuclear import. EMBO J. 2010;29:2841–57.

23. Shelkovnikova TA, Robinson HK, Southcombe JA, Ninkina N, Buchman VL. Multistep process of FUS aggregation in the cell cytoplasm involves RNA-dependent and RNA-independent mechanisms. Hum Mol Genet. 2014;23:5211–26.

24. Bond CS, Fox AH. Paraspeckles: nuclear bodies built on long noncoding RNA. J Cell Biol. 2009;186:637–44.

25. Tapia O, Bengoechea R, Berciano MT, Lafarga M. Nucleolar targeting of coilin is regulated by its hypomethylation state. Chromosoma. 2010;119:527–40.

26. Shelkovnikova TA, Robinson HK, Connor-Robson N, Buchman VL. Recruitment into stress granules prevents irreversible aggregation of FUS protein mislocalized to the cytoplasm. Cell Cycle. 2013;12:3194–202.

27. Ju S, Tardiff DF, Han H, Divya K, Zhong Q, Maquat LE, et al. A yeast model of FUS/TLS-dependent cytotoxicity. PLoS Biol. 2011;9:e1001052.

28. Nonaka T, Kametani F, Arai T, Akiyama H, Hasegawa M. Truncation and pathogenic mutations facilitate the formation of intracellular aggregates of TDP-43. Hum Mol Genet. 2009;18:3353–64.

29. Austin JA, Wright GS, Watanabe S, Grossmann JG, Antonyuk SV, Yamanaka K, et al. Disease causing mutants of TDP-43 nucleic acid binding domains are resistant to aggregation and have increased stability and half-life. Proc Natl Acad Sci U S A. 2014;111:4309–14.

30. Ling SC, Albuquerque CP, Han JS, Lagier-Tourenne C, Tokunaga S, Zhou H, et al. ALS-associated mutations in TDP-43 increase its stability and promote TDP-43 complexes with FUS/TLS. Proc Natl Acad Sci U S A. 2010;107:13318–23.

31. Watanabe S, Kaneko K, Yamanaka K. Accelerated disease onset with stabilized familial amyotrophic lateral sclerosis (ALS)-linked mutant TDP-43 proteins. J Biol Chem. 2013;288:3641–54.

32. Johnson BS, Snead D, Lee JJ, McCaffery JM, Shorter J, Gitler AD. TDP-43 is intrinsically aggregation-prone, and amyotrophic lateral sclerosis-linked mutations accelerate aggregation and increase toxicity. J Biol Chem. 2009;284:20329–39.

33. Guo W, Chen Y, Zhou X, Kar A, Ray P, Chen X, et al. An ALS-associated mutation affecting TDP-43 enhances protein aggregation, fibril formation and neurotoxicity. Nat Struct Mol Biol. 2011;18:822–30.

34. Falsone A, Falsone SF. Legal but lethal: functional protein aggregation at the verge of toxicity. Front Cell Neurosci. 2015. doi: 10.3389/fncel.2015.00045.

35. Shelkovnikova TA. Modelling FUSopathies: focus on protein aggregation. Biochem Soc Trans. 2013;41:1613–7.

36. Li YR, King OD, Shorter J, Gitler AD. Stress granules as crucibles of ALS pathogenesis. J Cell Biol. 2013;201:361–72.

37. Wolozin B. Regulated protein aggregation: stress granules and neurodegeneration. Mol Neurodegener. 2012;7:56.

38. Vanderweyde T, Youmans K, Liu-Yesucevitz L, Wolozin B. Role of stress granules and RNA-binding proteins in neurodegeneration: a mini-review. Gerontology. 2013;9:524–33.

39. Zhang Z, Carmichael GG. The fate of dsRNA in the nucleus: a p54(nrb)-containing complex mediates the nuclear retention of promiscuously A-to-I edited RNAs. Cell. 2001;106:465–75.

40. Hirose T, Virnicchi G, Tanigawa A, Naganuma T, Li R, Kimura H, et al. NEAT1 long noncoding RNA regulates transcription via protein sequestration within subnuclear bodies. Mol Biol Cell. 2014;25:169–83.

41. Imamura K, Imamachi N, Akizuki G, Kumakura M, Kawaguchi A, Nagata K, et al. Long noncoding RNA NEAT1-dependent SFPQ relocation from promoter region to paraspeckle mediates IL8 expression upon immune stimuli. Mol Cell. 2014;53:393–406.

42. Kim HJ, Kim NC, Wang YD, Scarborough EA, Moore J, Diaz Z, et al. Mutations in prion-like domains in hnRNPA2B1 and hnRNPA1 cause multisystem proteinopathy and ALS. Nature. 2013;495:467–73.

43. Tollervey JR, Curk T, Rogelj B, Briese M, Cereda M, Kayikci M, et al. Characterizing the RNA targets and position-dependent splicing regulation by TDP-43. Nat Neurosci. 2011;14:452–8.

44. Seyfried NT, Gozal YM, Donovan LE, Herskowitz JH, Dammer EB, Xia Q, et al. Quantitative analysis of the detergent-insoluble brain proteome in frontotemporal lobar degeneration using SILAC internal standards. J Proteome Res. 2012;11:2721–38.

45. Dammer EB, Fallini C, Gozal YM, Duong DM, Rossoll W, Xu P, et al. Coaggregation of RNA-binding proteins in a model of TDP-43 proteinopathy with selective RGG motif methylation and a role for RRM1 ubiquitination. PLoS One. 2012;7:e38658.

46. Johnson JO, Pioro EP, Boehringer A, Chia R, Feit H, Renton AE, et al. Mutations in the Matrin 3 gene cause familial amyotrophic lateral sclerosis. Nat Neurosci. 2014;17:664–6.

47. Couthouis J, Hart MP, Erion R, King OD, Diaz Z, Nakaya T, et al. Evaluating the role of the FUS/TLS-related gene EWSR1 in amyotrophic lateral sclerosis. Hum Mol Genet. 2012;21:2899–911.

48. Couthouis J, Hart MP, Shorter J, DeJesus-Hernandez M, Erion R, Oristano R, et al. A yeast functional screen predicts new candidate ALS disease genes. Proc Natl Acad Sci U S A. 2011;108:20881–90.

49. Page T, Gitcho MA, Mosaheb S, Carter D, Chakraverty S, Perry RH, et al. FUS immunogold labeling TEM analysis of the neuronal cytoplasmic inclusions of neuronal intermediate filament inclusion disease: a frontotemporal lobar degeneration with FUS proteinopathy. J Mol Neurosci. 2011;45:409–21.

50. Bosco DA, Lemay N, Ko HK, Zhou H, Burke C, Kwiatkowski Jr TJ, et al. Mutant FUS proteins that cause amyotrophic lateral sclerosis incorporate into stress granules. Hum Mol Genet. 2010;19:4160–75.

51. Pesiridis GS, Lee VM, Trojanowski JQ. Mutations in TDP-43 link glycine-rich domain functions to amyotrophic lateral sclerosis. Hum Mol Genet. 2009;18:R156–62.

52. Gendron TF, Rademakers R, Petrucelli L. TARDBP mutation analysis in TDP-43 proteinopathies and deciphering the toxicity of mutant TDP-43. J Alzheimers Dis. 2013;33 Suppl 1:S35–45.

53. van Blitterswijk M, van Es MA, Hennekam EA, Dooijes D, van Rheenen W, Medic J, et al. Evidence for an oligogenic basis of amyotrophic lateral sclerosis. Hum Mol Genet. 2012;21:3776–84.

54. Figley MD, Bieri G, Kolaitis RM, Taylor JP, Gitler AD. Profilin 1 Associates with Stress Granules and ALS-Linked Mutations Alter Stress Granule Dynamics. J Neurosci. 2014;34:8083–97.

55. Al-Wandi A, Ninkina N, Millership S, Williamson SJ, Jones PA, Buchman VL. Absence of alpha-synuclein affects dopamine metabolism and synaptic markers in the striatum of aging mice. Neurobiol Aging. 2010;31:796–804.

56. Halfmann R, Lindquist S. Screening for amyloid aggregation by Semi-Denaturing Detergent-Agarose Gel Electrophoresis. J Vis Exp. 2008;17:838.

57. Kanda H, Igaki T, Kanuka H, Yagi T, Miura M. Wengen, a member of the Drosophila tumor necrosis factor receptor superfamilym is required for Eiger signaling. J Biol Chem. 2002;277:28372–5.

58. Ihara R, Matsukawa K, Nagata Y, Kunugi H, Tsuji S, Chihara T, et al. RNA binding mediates neurotoxicity in the transgenic Drosophila model of TDP-43 proteinopathy. Hum Mol Genet. 2013;22:4474–84.

Permissions

All chapters in this book were first published in MN, by BioMed Central; hereby published with permission under the Creative Commons Attribution License or equivalent. Every chapter published in this book has been scrutinized by our experts. Their significance has been extensively debated. The topics covered herein carry significant findings which will fuel the growth of the discipline. They may even be implemented as practical applications or may be referred to as a beginning point for another development.

The contributors of this book come from diverse backgrounds, making this book a truly international effort. This book will bring forth new frontiers with its revolutionizing research information and detailed analysis of the nascent developments around the world.

We would like to thank all the contributing authors for lending their expertise to make the book truly unique. They have played a crucial role in the development of this book. Without their invaluable contributions this book wouldn't have been possible. They have made vital efforts to compile up to date information on the varied aspects of this subject to make this book a valuable addition to the collection of many professionals and students.

This book was conceptualized with the vision of imparting up-to-date information and advanced data in this field. To ensure the same, a matchless editorial board was set up. Every individual on the board went through rigorous rounds of assessment to prove their worth. After which they invested a large part of their time researching and compiling the most relevant data for our readers.

The editorial board has been involved in producing this book since its inception. They have spent rigorous hours researching and exploring the diverse topics which have resulted in the successful publishing of this book. They have passed on their knowledge of decades through this book. To expedite this challenging task, the publisher supported the team at every step. A small team of assistant editors was also appointed to further simplify the editing procedure and attain best results for the readers.

Apart from the editorial board, the designing team has also invested a significant amount of their time in understanding the subject and creating the most relevant covers. They scrutinized every image to scout for the most suitable representation of the subject and create an appropriate cover for the book.

The publishing team has been an ardent support to the editorial, designing and production team. Their endless efforts to recruit the best for this project, has resulted in the accomplishment of this book. They are a veteran in the field of academics and their pool of knowledge is as vast as their experience in printing. Their expertise and guidance has proved useful at every step. Their uncompromising quality standards have made this book an exceptional effort. Their encouragement from time to time has been an inspiration for everyone.

The publisher and the editorial board hope that this book will prove to be a valuable piece of knowledge for researchers, students, practitioners and scholars across the globe.

List of Contributors

Su Min Lim
Department of Translational Medicine, Graduate School of Biomedical Science and Engineering, Hanyang University, Seoul 133-792, Republic of Korea
Cell Therapy Center, Hanyang University Hospital, Seoul 133-792, Republic of Korea

Seung Hyun Kim
Department of Translational Medicine, Graduate School of Biomedical Science and Engineering, Hanyang University, Seoul 133-792, Republic of Korea
Cell Therapy Center, Hanyang University Hospital, Seoul 133-792, Republic of Korea
Department of Neurology, College of Medicine, Hanyang University, Seoul 133-792, Republic of Korea

Ji Young Choi, Sung Hoon Kim, Minyeop Nahm and Min-Young Noh
Cell Therapy Center, Hanyang University Hospital, Seoul 133-792, Republic of Korea

Won Jun Choi
Department of Neurology, Sheikh Khalifa Specialty Hospital, Ras Al Khaimah, United Arab Emirates

Ki-Wook Oh
Cell Therapy Center, Hanyang University Hospital, Seoul 133-792, Republic of Korea
Department of Neurology, College of Medicine, Hanyang University, Seoul 133-792, Republic of Korea

Yuanchao Xue
Key Laboratory of RNA Biology, Institute of Biophysics, Chinese Academy of Sciences, Beijing 100101, China

Young-Eun Kim and Chang-Seok Ki
Department of Laboratory Medicine and Genetics, Samsung Medical Center, Sungkyunkwan University School of Medicine, Seoul 135-710, Republic of Korea

Jinhyuk Lee
Korean Bioinformation Center, Korea Research Institute of Bioscience and Biotechnology, Daejeon 305-806, Republic of Korea

Department of Bioinformatics, University of Sciences and Technology, Daejeon 305-806, Republic of Korea

Seungbok Lee
Department of Brain and Cognitive Sciences, College of Natural Sciences, Seoul National University, Seoul 110-744, Republic of Korea

Sejin Hwang
Department of Anatomy and Cell Biology, College of Medicine, Hanyang University, Seoul 133-792, Republic of Korea

Xiang-Dong Fu
Department of Cellular Molecular Medicine, University of California, La Jolla, San Diego, CA 92093, USA

Sighild Lemarchant, Yuriy Pomeshchik, Iurii Kidin, Virve Kärkkäinen, Piia Valonen, Sarka Lehtonen, Gundars Goldsteins, Tarja Malm, Katja Kanninen and Jari Koistinaho
Department of Neurobiology, A. I. Virtanen Institute for Molecular Sciences, Biocenter Kuopio, University of Eastern Finland, 70211 Kuopio, Finland

Sarah Bellouze, Gilbert Baillat, Dorothée Buttigieg and Georg Haase
Institut de Neurosciences de la Timone, UMR 7289, Centre National de la Recherche Scientifique (CNRS) and Aix-Marseille Université, 27 bd Jean Moulin, 13005 Marseille, France

Pierre de la Grange
GenoSplice technology, iPEPS - ICM, Hôpital Pitié Salpêtrière, 47/83, bd de l'Hôpital, 75013 Paris, France

Catherine Rabouille
Department of Cell Biology, Hubrecht Institute of the KNAW & UMC Utrecht, Uppsalalaan 8, 3584 CT Utrecht, Netherlands

Alexander McGown, Dame Pamela J. Shaw and Tennore Ramesh
Sheffield Institute for Translational Neuroscience (SITraN), University of Sheffield, 385A Glossop Road, Sheffield, UK

Eiichi Tokuda, Itsuki Anzai, Takao Nomura, Keisuke Toichi and Yoshiaki Furukawa
Laboratory for Mechanistic Chemistry of Biomolecules, Department of Chemistry, Keio University, 3-14-1 Hiyoshi, Kohoku, Yokohama, Kanagawa 223-8522, Japan

Masahiko Watanabe
Department of Anatomy, Hokkaido University Graduate School of Medicine, Sapporo 060 8638, Japan

Shinji Ohara
Department of Neurology, Matsumoto Medical Center, Matsumoto 399-0021, Japan

Seiji Watanabe and Koji Yamanaka
Department of Neuroscience and Pathobiology, Research Institute of Environmental Medicine, Nagoya University, Nagoya 464-8601, Japan

Yuta Morisaki and Hidemi Misawa
Division of Pharmacology, Faculty of Pharmacy, Keio University, Tokyo 105-8512, Japan

Peter E. A. Ash, Ali Al Abdulatif, Heather I. Ballance, Samantha Boudeau and Amanda Jeh
Department of Pharmacology, Boston University School of Medicine, 72 East Concord St., R614, Boston, MA 02118-2526, USA

Elizabeth A. Stanford, Alejandra Ramirez-Cardenas and David H. Sherr
Department of Environmental Health, Boston University School of Public Health, Boston, MA 02118, USA

James M. Murithi and George J. Murphy
Center for Regenerative Medicine, Boston University, Boston, MA 02118, USA

Yorghos Tripodis
Department of Biostatistics, Boston University School of Public Health, Boston, MA 02118, USA

Benjamin Wolozin
Department of Pharmacology, Boston University School of Medicine, 72 East Concord St., R614, Boston, MA 02118-2526, USA
Department of Neurology, Boston University School of Medicine, 72 East Concord St., R614, Boston, MA 02118-2526, USA

Qian-Qian Wei, Yongping Chen, Bei Cao, Ru Wei Ou, Lingyu Zhang, Yanbing Hou and Huifang Shang
Department of Neurology, West China Hospital, Sichuan University, 37 Guoxue Xiang, Chengdu, Sichuan 610041, China

Xiang Gao
Department of Nutritional Science, The Pennsylvania State University, 109 Chandlee Lab, University Park, PA 16802, USA

Csaba Konrad, Hibiki Kawamata, Kirsten G. Bredvik, Andrea J. Arreguin, Steven A. Cajamarca and Giovanni Manfredi
Feil Family Brain and Mind Research Institute, Weill Cornell Medicine, 407 East 61st Street, RR507, New York, NY 10065, USA

Jonathan C. Hupf and Hiroshi Mitsumoto
Department of Neurology, Columbia University, New York, NY, USA

John M. Ravits
Department of Neuroscience, University of California San Diego, La Jolla, CA, USA

Timothy M. Miller
Department of Neurology, Washington University School of Medicine, St. Louis, MO, USA

Nicholas J. Maragakis
Department of Neurology, Johns Hopkins University School of Medicine, Baltimore, MD, USA

Chadwick M. Hales and Jonathan D. Glass
Department of Neurology, Emory School of Medicine, Atlanta, GA, USA

Steven Gross
Department of Pharmacology, Weill Cornell Medicine, New York, NY, USA

Pamela J. Shaw and Richard J. Mead
Sheffield Institute for Translational Neuroscience (SITraN), Department of Neuroscience, Faculty of Medicine, Dentistry and Health, University of Sheffield, 385a Glossop Rd S10 2HQ, Sheffield, UK

Yuri Ciervo and Ke Ning
Sheffield Institute for Translational Neuroscience (SITraN), Department of Neuroscience, Faculty of Medicine, Dentistry and Health, University of Sheffield, 385a Glossop Rd S10 2HQ, Sheffield, UK
Tongji University School of Medicine, 1239 Siping Rd, Yangpu Qu, Shanghai, China

Xu Jun
Tongji University School of Medicine, 1239 Siping Rd, Yangpu Qu, Shanghai, China

Rafaa Zeineddine, Jay F. Pundavela, Lisa Corcoran, Dzung Do-Ha, Monique Bax, Kara L. Vine, Heath Ecroyd, Lezanne Ooi, Mark R. Wilson and Justin J. Yerbury
Illawarra Health and Medical Research Institute, Wollongong, Australia 2522
School of Biological Sciences, Faculty of Science, Medicine and Health, University of Wollongong, Wollongong, Australia 2522

Elise M. Stewart
Intelligent Polymer Research Institute, University of Wollongong, Wollongong, Australia2522

Gilles Guillemin
Australian School for Advanced Medicine, Macquarie University, Sydney, Australia2109

Danny M. Hatters
Department of Biochemistry and Molecular Biology and Bio21 Molecular Science and Biotechnology Institute, University of Melbourne, Parkville, Australia3010

Christopher M. Dobson
Department of Chemistry, University of Cambridge, Cambridge CB2 1EW, UK

Bradley J. Turner
Florey Institute of Neuroscience and Mental Health, University of Melbourne, Parkville, Australia3010

Neil R. Cashman
Department of Medicine (Neurology), University of British Columbia and Vancouver Coastal Health Research Institute, Brain Research Centre, University of British Columbia, Vancouver, CanadaV6T 2B5

Carolina Ceballos-Diaz, Awilda M. Rosario, Paramita Chakrabarty, Amanda Sacino, Pedro E. Cruz, Zoe Siemienski, Nicolas Lara, Corey Moran and Todd E. Golde
Center for Translational Research in Neurodegenerative Disease, Department of Neuroscience, University of Florida, 1275 Center Dr, Gainesville, FL 32610, USA

Hyo-Jin Park, Natalia Ravelo and Nikolaus R. McFarland
Center for Translational Research in Neurodegenerative Disease, Department of Neuroscience, University of Florida, 1275 Center Dr, Gainesville, FL 32610, USA
Department of Neurology, College of Medicine, University of Florida, 1149 S Newell Dr, L3-100, Gainesville, FL 32610, USA

Harun Najib Noristani and Marisa Teigell
Institute for Neurosciences of Montpellier (INM), INSERM U1051, 80, rue Augustin Fliche, 34091 Montpellier, Cedex 5, France

Yannick Nicolas Gerber
Institute for Neurosciences of Montpellier (INM), INSERM U1051, 80, rue Augustin Fliche, 34091 Montpellier, Cedex 5, France
"Integrative Biology of Neurodegeneration", IKERBASQUE Basque Foundation for Science and Neuroscience Department, University of the Basque Country, Bilbao, Spain

Jean Charles Sabourin
"Integrative Biology of Neurodegeneration", IKERBASQUE Basque Foundation for Science and Neuroscience Department, University of the Basque Country, Bilbao, Spain

Andreas Sommacal and Markus Weber
Kantonspital St. Gallen. FachMuskelzentrum/ALS clinic, St. Gallen, Switzerland

Maria dM Vivanco
CIC bioGUNE, Cell Biology & Stem Cells Unit, Technological Park of Bizkaia, Derio, Spain

Florence Evelyne Perrin
Institute for Neurosciences of Montpellier (INM), INSERM U1051, 80, rue Augustin Fliche, 34091 Montpellier, Cedex 5, France
"Integrative Biology of Neurodegeneration", IKERBASQUE Basque Foundation for Science and Neuroscience Department, University of the Basque Country, Bilbao, Spain
Department "Biologie-Mécanismes du Vivant" Faculty of Science, University of Montpellier, Montpellier, France

Nicola J. Rutherford, Amanda N. Sacino, Mieu Brooks, Carolina Ceballos-Diaz, Thomas B. Ladd, Jasie K. Howard, Todd E. Golde and Benoit I. Giasson
Center for Translational Research in Neurodegenerative Disease, Department of Neuroscience, University of Florida, 1275 Center Drive, Room BMS J-483, Gainesville, FL 32610, USA

Annamaria Quintiero, Haiyan An and Vladimir L Buchman
School of Biosciences, Cardiff University, Museum Avenue, CF10 3AX Cardiff, UK

Michail S Kukharsky and Tatyana A Shelkovnikova
School of Biosciences, Cardiff University, Museum Avenue, CF10 3AX Cardiff, UK
Institute of Physiologically Active Compounds Russian Academy of Sciences, 1 Severniy proezd, Chernogolovka, 142432 Moscow Region, Russian Federation

Taisei Matsumoto, Koji Matsukawa, Tadafumi Hashimoto and Takeshi Iwatsubo
Department of Neuropathology, The University of Tokyo, Tokyo, Japan

Index

www.ingramcontent.com/pod-product-compliance
Lightning Source LLC
Chambersburg PA
CBHW082027190326
41458CB00010B/3299